INTRODUCTORY MANAGEMENT AND LEADERSHIP FOR NURSES

AN INTERACTIVE TEXT

THE JONES AND BARTLETT SERIES IN NURSING

SECOND EDITION

INTRODUCTORY MANAGEMENT AND LEADERSHIP FOR NURSES

AN INTERACTIVE TEXT

Russell C. Swansburg, RN, PhD
Consultant in Nursing and Hospital Administration
San Antonio, Texas

Richard J. Swansburg, RN, BSN, MSCIS
Management Systems Specialist II
University of South Alabama
Mobile, Alabama

JONES AND BARTLETT PUBLISHERS
Sudbury, Massachusetts
BOSTON   TORONTO   LONDON   SINGAPORE

World Headquarters

Jones and Bartlett Publishers
40 Tall Pine Drive
Sudbury, MA 01776
978-443-5000
800-832-0034
info@jbpub.com
www.jbpub.com

Jones and Bartlett Publishers Canada
P.O. Box 19020
Toronto, ON M5S 1X1
CANADA

Jones and Bartlett Publishers International
Barb House, Barb Mews
London W6 7PA
UK

ACQUISITIONS EDITOR: *Greg Vis*
SENIOR PRODUCTION EDITOR: *Lianne Ames*
MANUFACTURING BUYER: *Therese Bräuer*
DESIGN: *The Clarinda Company*
ILLUSTRATIONS: *The Clarinda Company*
TYPESETTING: *The Clarinda Company*
COVER DESIGN: *Dick Hannus*
PRINTING AND BINDING: *Courier/Westford*

Library of Congress Cataloging-in-Publication Data

Swansburg, Russell C.
    Introductory management and leadership for clinical nurses : an
interactive text / Russell C. Swansburg. — 2nd edition.
        p.   cm.
    Includes bibliographical references and index.
    ISBN 0-7637-0640-X
    1. Nursing services—Administration.   I. Title.
    [DNLM: 1. Nursing, Supervisory.   2. Nurse Administrators.
3. Administrative Personnel.   4. Nursing, Supervisory.   5. Nurse
Administrators.   6. Administrative Personnel.   WY 105 S972i 1998]
    RT89.S885   1998
    362.1′73′068—dc21
    DNLM/DLC
    for Library of Congress   98-21155
                                                                              CIP

Printed in the United States of America
02   01   00   99   98   10   9   8   7   6   5   4   3   2   1

This book is dedicated to the memory of our beloved grandson and nephew, James Russell Swansburg.

CONTENTS

5

THE PLANNING PROCESS   71

6

FOUNDATIONS FOR PLANNING—MISSION, PHILOSOPHY, OBJECTIVES, AND MANAGEMENT PLANS   93

7

STAFFING AND SCHEDULING   113

11

MANAGING A CLINICAL PRACTICE DISCIPLINE   271

12

DECISION MAKING AND PROBLEM SOLVING   305

13

IMPLEMENTING PLANNED CHANGE   321

14

THE ORGANIZING PROCESS   355

15

COMMITTEES AND OTHER GROUPS   398

16

DECENTRALIZATION AND PARTICIPATORY MANAGEMENT   420

17

THE DIRECTING (LEADING) PROCESS   445

22

23

24

25

FOREWORD

Chaos—dynamic, complex, and unpredictable—rules the health care scene! And nursing is in the swirling middle!

In his first edition, Russell Swansburg alerted us to the handing over of typical management functions to staff nurses, as typical managerial positions disappear. The first edition not only asked questions about how nursing would continue to exist in a de-jobbed chaos, but detailed what tasks/functions staff nurses or mini-managers would need to undertake along with their other responsibilities. He prepared us for these new responsibilities.

That information continues in the second edition. But now we are in the middle of the dynamic scene he predicted, the chaos swirling about us. Now the emphasis is on "clinical nursing management," the patient at the center.

Necessary managerial functions are still the organizational framework of the second edition—planning, organizing, directing or leading, and controlling or evaluating. Overlaid on these basic functions of management are the steps of the nursing process which the ANA (1995) so beautifully integrated into the managerial scene in *Scope and Standards for Nurse Administrators* (Washington: American Nurses Publishing, 1995). Truly, nursing management is "clinical nursing management," and the complexity and chaos begins to lift as we finally address management concepts in the nursing process format.

The health care chaos is not to be feared, but rather utilized by nurses to assure quality in health care. Shaping the environment for success is more possible in dynamic chaos than in stasis.

This second edition of *Introductory Management and Leadership for Nurses* has been updated and expanded to meet the demands put upon staff nurses in the chaotic environment of health care.

Barbara Fuzard, PhD, RN, FAAN
Professor Emeritus
Medical College of Georgia
Augusta, GA

PREFACE

This book is organized around the four major management functions of planning, organizing, leading, and evaluating. It is specifically designed to expose beginning students to a professional approach to management. It can be used in all nursing programs as a first course in nursing management as well as in staff development programs in health care agencies.

Among the goals are to provide theoretical and practical knowledge that will aid each clinical nurse manager in meeting the demands of constantly changing patient care services. Clinical nurses oversee many tasks involving many people with specialized knowledge and skills. This book is intended as a reference for improving communication, enhancing assignment planning and priority setting, and developing training and education programs that lead to staff satisfaction. Through the evaluation process, clinical nurse managers determine whether they are satisfied with the results, from both their own viewpoints and those of their constituents. Financial considerations have dominated the health care industry in recent years, making the job of managing in an environment of decreased human and material resources even more important. As health care has moved out of hospitals, nurse management positions have increased in skilled nursing facilities, ambulatory care centers, hospices, home health agencies, and staffing agencies. In addition, new nurse management positions are evolving.

This book focuses on management competencies needed by clinical nurse managers, including fostering clinical competencies in nursing assessment, diagnosis, interventions, and evaluation. Among the essential theoretical and practical knowledge covered is learning about leadership skills and employee motivation, and learning to make sound decisions that contribute to progress.

This second edition of *Introductory Management and Leadership for Nurses* has been updated and expanded. Because of its importance, Critical Thinking, Chapter 1, has been made the introductory chapter of the text. Chapter 2 Introduction to Managed Care, Chapter 4 Introduction to Theory of Human Resource Development, Chapter 9 Introduction to Collective Bargaining, Chapter 22 Staff Development, Chapter 25 Theory of Quality Management, and Chapter 28 Pay for Performance, are entirely new chapters. In addition, Chapter 22 Staff Development introduces an entirely new application of the theory of critical thinking to nursing education.

Other concepts introduced in this edition include autonomy and empowerment, andragogy, human capital, vision and values statements, temporary workers, collective bargaining, self-managed work teams, total quality management, multiculturalism, and pay for performance, among others. Chapters have been rewritten to provide a new format with learning objectives, key concepts, web exercises that enable students to seek out current management information on the internet, a major manager behavior box, and a major leader behavior box.

WEB ENHANCED EDITION

Introductory Management and Leadership for Nurses, Second Edition, connects students and faculty to the Internet!

New to this edition is a companion web site, www.jbpub.com/swansburg, that connects users of *Introductory Management and Leadership for Nurses*, Second Edition, to an extensive site developed by Jones and Bartlett Publishers and the author. The site offers a variety of activities designed to make your students' independent studying more satisfying. Students will soon discover how the Internet can enhance the learning process.

Features of the companion web site include:

- End of chapter Web Activities to help make the connection between chapter topics and the resources available on the Internet. See example below.
- Suggested links for each chapter's activities are provided along with descriptions of the links.
- Additional practice questions for students.
- Additional instructor support including lesson plans, additional questions and transparency masters.

Unparalled quality and reliability make teaching easier: The site is maintained and updated by Jones and Bartlett and the author so that you don't have to! New sites and additional features are added as they become available. Broken links are quickly repaired or replaced. Bookmark this site for a rich new teaching and learning experience.

Russell Swansburg

Richard Swansburg

WEB ACTIVITIES

- Visit www.jbpub.com/swansburg, this text's companion website on the Internet, for further information on Human Resource Management.
- What types of recruiting strategies can you find on the web that differ from those outlined in the book?
- Are there resources available to help you create your own career development plan?

CRITICAL THINKING

OBJECTIVES

- Compose an illustration of a definition of critical thinking.
- Use a decision-making process to make a personal decision confronting you.
- Evaluate a situation in which public officials are involved in debate and argumentation (critical thinking).

KEY CONCEPTS:

critical thinking
concept analysis

Manager behavior: Promote critical thinking.

Leader behavior: Coach staff to become critical thinkers and to use critical thinking to promote positive patient outcomes and effective interpersonal relationships.

Nurses use critical thinking for several reasons including pursuing higher education and applying professional and technical knowledge and skills in caring for clients. Critical thinking is the best guarantee that nurses will have successful outcomes in either instance. In the eighth edition of his book *Argumentation and Debate,* Freeley indicates that critical thinking is necessary for developing one's ability to analyze, criticize, and advocate ideas. Freeley also indicates that the ability to perform deductive and inductive reasoning and the ability to reach successful conclusions based on facts and judgments are outcomes of critical thinking.[1] These behaviors are essential to a nurse's role as clinician, manager, researcher, or teacher.

Freeley identifies seven methods of critical thinking:

1. Debate. Debate involves inquiry, advocacy, and reasoned judgment on a proposition. A person or a group may debate or argue the pros and cons of a proposition in coming to a reasoned judgment. Usually a debate entails opposing positions as well as specific rules.
2. Individual decisions. An individual may debate a proposition in his or her own mind using problem-solving or decision-making processes. When consent or cooperation of others is needed, the individual may secure it through group discussion, persuasion, propaganda, or coercion or through a combination of these methods.
3. Group discussion. Five conditions for reaching decisions through group discussion are that the group members "(1) agree that a problem exists,

(2) have comparable standards of value, (3) have compatible purposes, (4) are willing to accept the consensus of the group, and (5) are relatively few in number."[2]

4. Persuasion. Persuasion is communication to influence the acts, beliefs, attitudes, and values of others by reasoning, urging, or inducement. Debate and advertising are two forms of communication whose intent is to persuade.

5. Propaganda. Multiple media communication designed to persuade or influence a mass audience, propaganda can be good or bad. Propagandists may debate and argue. Their tactics need to be subjected to critical analysis.

6. Coercion. Threat or use of force is the communication of coercion. An extreme example is brainwashing, in which subjects are completely controlled physically for an indefinite period of time.

7. Combination of methods. Some situations require a combination of the foregoing communication techniques to reach a decision.[3]

A general consensus is emerging that critical thinking should augment or even replace the nursing process within nursing education programs. Critical thinking is generally regarded by academicians as essential to the educated mind, to be superordinate to problem solving and the nursing process.[4] The nursing process should involve critical thinking in problem solving and decision making. Exhibit 1–1 lists several definitions and characteristics of critical thinking from which one can see the relationship of the concept of critical thinking to decision making, problem solving, and standards.

Exhibit 1–1   Critical Thinking

Definitions

The word *critical* is derived from the Greek and means to question, to discuss, to choose, to evaluate, to make judgment.

Greek *kritein*—to choose, to decide

Greek *krites*—judge

English *criterion*—a standard, rule, or method

- Critical thinking is reflecting on a situation, a plan, an event under the rule of standards and antecedent to making a decision. (McKenzie)
- "Critical thinking is both a philosophical orientation toward thinking and a cognitive process characterized by reasoned judgment and reflective thinking." (Jones and Brown)
- "[Critical thinking] is an investigation whose purpose is to explore a situation, phenomenon, question, or problem to arrive at a hypothesis or conclusion about it that integrates all available information and that can be convincingly justified." (Kurfiss)

- "[Critical thinking] is (1) an attitude of being disposed to consider in a thoughtful way, the problems and subjects that come within the range of one's experiences, (2) knowledge of the methods of logical inquiry and reasoning, and (3) some skill in applying those methods." (Glaser)
- "Critical-thinking abilities include defining a problem, selecting pertinent information for the solution, recognizing stated and unstated assumptions, formulating and selecting relevant and promising hypotheses, drawing conclusions, and judging the validity of the inferences." (Hickman; Watson and Glaser)
- "[Critical thinking] is the intellectually disciplined process of actively and skillfully conceptualizing, applying, analyzing, synthesizing, and evaluating information gathered from or generated by observation, experience, reflection, reasoning, and communication, as a guide to belief and action. (National Council for Excellence in Critical Thinking Instruction)

Exhibit 1–1 *Critical Thinking (Continued)*

Characteristics

- Critical thinking is a multidimensional cognitive process. It requires a skillful application of knowledge and experience for the sophisticated judgment and evaluation needed in complex situations. It is interactive—individual with interpretations made of the world.
- It is process oriented.
- It uses structure as a means rather than an end.
- It is a framework within which to interpret knowledge, challenge assumptions, generate contradictory hypotheses, and develop modifications. (Jones and Brown)
- It is affective learning, including moral reasoning and development of values guiding decisions and activities.
- It is awareness of self as the basis of building relationships with a client; conscious awareness of feelings, beliefs, values, and attitudes.
- It is empathy and empowerment. (Woods; Reilly and Oermann).
- It includes social learning theory.
- It is an important outcome of professional socialization.
- It involves cognitive skills of comprehension, application, analysis, synthesis, and evaluation. (Saarmann et al.)
- It is an attitude of critical inquiry that enhances professionalism. (Brooks and Shepherd)
- It is fallible.
- It may lead to bad decisions and errors in judgment.

- It will consistently lead to superior decisions but is sometimes imperfect.
- It includes feelings, images, and intuitional prompts.
- It employs psychological as well as logical or linear patterns. (McKenzie)

Sources: L. McKenzie, "Critical Thinking in Health Care Supervision," *Health Care Supervisor,* June 1992, 1–11; S. A. Jones and L. N. Brown, "Alternative Views on Defining Critical Thinking Through the Nursing Process," *Holistic Nurse Practitioner,* April 1993, 71–76; J. G. Kurfiss, *Critical Thinking: Theory and Practice* (Washington, D.C.: Association for the Study of Higher Education, 1988), 2; E. M. Glaser, *An Experiment in the Development of Critical Thinking* (New York: Teacher's College, 1941), 5–6; J. S. Hickman, "A Critical Assessment of Critical Thinking in Nursing Education," *Holistic Nurse Practitioner,* April 1993, 36–47; G. Watson and E. M. Glaser, *Watson-Glaser Critical Thinking Appraisal Manual* (New York: Harcourt, Brace & World, 1964); *Critical Thinking: Shaping the Mind of the 21st Century* (Rohnert Park, Calif.: Sonoma State University Center for Critical Thinking and Moral Critique, 1992), 7; J. H. Woods, "Affective Learning: One Door to Critical Thinking," *Holistic Nurse Practitioner,* April 1993, 64–70; D. E. Reilly and M. H. Oermann, "Affective Learning in the Clinical Setting," in *Clinical Teaching in Nursing Education,* ed. D. E. Reilly and M. H. Oermann (New York: National League for Nursing, 1992, Pub. 15-2471); L. Saarmann, L. Freitas, J. Rapps, and B. Riegel, "The Relationship of Education to Critical Thinking Ability and Values Among Nurses: Socialization into Professional Nursing," *Journal of Professional Nursing,* January–February 1992, 26–34; K. L. Brooks and J. M. Shepherd, "Professionalism Versus General Critical Thinking Abilities of Senior Nursing Students in Four Types of Nursing Curricula," *Journal of Professional Nursing,* March–April 1992, 87–95.

Exercise 1–1   In your own words, write a definition of critical thinking. Relate your definition to your use of the nursing process in caring for clients.

RESEARCH

A number of research studies have been done relative to critical thinking and nursing education. Using the *Health Care Professional Attitude Inventory* to measure professionalism and the *Watson-Glaser Critical Thinking Appraisal* (CTA) to measure general critical-thinking abilities, Brooks and Shepherd sampled 200 associate-degree, diploma, generic-baccalaureate, and upper-division baccalaureate nursing students and found the following:

1. Upper-division and generic-program seniors exhibited significantly higher critical-thinking abilities than did associate-degree and diploma seniors.
2. Positive correlation between critical-thinking abilities and professionalism was almost as strong among generic and associate-degree seniors as it was for the upper-division seniors.
3. The diploma seniors exhibited the lowest levels of professionalism and critical thinking.
4. Upper-division seniors achieved higher professionalism scores than seniors from the four-year generic programs and showed almost identical levels of critical-thinking abilities.[5]

Saarmann, Freitas, Rapps, and Riegel used the Watson and Glaser CTA scale on a sample of thirty-two subjects in each of the following groups: nursing faculty, BSN-prepared registered nurses, ADN-prepared registered nurses, and entering sophomore nursing students in Southern California. They found that "the critical thinking ability of faculty was not significantly higher than that of sophomore nursing students when the influence of age was controlled statistically. The values of all three groups of nurses were strikingly similar, although faculty valued achievement most highly (P = 0.0001), while sophomore students valued goal orientation most highly (P = 0.001). All subjects valued support highly, but only sophomore students valued benevolence highly."[6]

Hickman analyzed eighteen studies of critical thinking in nursing education and reached the conclusion that "there is not a strong research base supporting a relationship between nursing curricula and critical thinking."[7] However, nursing schools strive to meet the mandates of the National League for Nursing Council of Baccalaureate and Higher Degree Programs that require program outcomes of critical thinking, communication, and therapeutic nursing interventions. Meanwhile, nurse administrators and managers will need to do their own teaching of critical-thinking skills and research of the effects of experience on the level of critical thinking.

More descriptive research studies are needed in nursing management. This will require that more nurse managers be trained in nursing research and suggests that the members of the nursing community ought to unify to implement a theory of nursing management encompassing critical theory. Nurse managers employing a critical-thinking approach would determine how their subordinates interpret organizational phenomena. They would discuss possible falsities of interpretations with their subordinates, bringing out illusions and delusions.[8]

Exercise 1–2 All of us make personal decisions every day. These decisions may relate to work, home, family, community, or other aspects of our lives. State a personal problem you face. What outcome do you want? What means are available to achieve this outcome? List pros and cons of each means and decide which means you will use. Then do it!

APPLICATIONS OF CRITICAL THINKING

Concept analysis is advocated as a strategy for promoting critical thinking.[9] The prepared nurse manager at any level should know the rudiments of critical thinking: recalling facts, principles, theories, and abstractions to make deductions, interpretations, and evaluations in solving problems, making decisions, and implementing changes. Concept analysis uses critical thinking to advance the knowledge base of nursing management as well as nursing practice.

A class of nursing students developed a method of concept analysis using critical thinking. The students did literature searches prior to each class in preparation for concept analysis. In their first session, they developed the following format for concept analysis:

1. Identification and clarification of the concept, including philosophy and content analysis.
2. Characteristics and attributes of the concept—concrete, abstract, quality/quantity.
3. Perceptions—what people think, interpretations, selling, marketing, customers (determine whom the concept affects and what is perceived as needed).
4. Use or application—policy, procedure, practice (skills), knowledge.
5. Researchable and synergistic, evaluation—promote change, create energy, validate theory.

This format was used to study and analyze such concepts as organizational climate, legal and ethical nursing practices, nursing care delivery systems, theory of nursing management, standards of nursing practice, evaluation of patient care, and research in nursing administration.[10]

Application of critical thinking theory to nursing management requires the nurse manager to first have knowledge of the theory. Nursing staff development faculty also must have knowledge of the theory as well as the teaching skills that will stimulate critical thinking and test it at the highest cognitive, affective, and psychomotor domains, not only in process but also in outcomes.

Exercise 1–3   Refer to your local daily newspaper and identify an issue being discussed related to local (city or county) government. What are the arguments involved? Which ones do you support? What can you do about the issue?

You could have a debate on the issue. Form a group of your peers and do the following:

1. Determine the pros and cons of the issue.
2. Elect a team captain to represent each side of the issue.
3. Identify members for each team.
4. Set the rules for the debate, including choosing the monitor; determining the speaking sequence and length of time for each team member to speak; and deciding whether there will be summaries by the team captains, who will judge the debate, and when and where the debate will take place.
5. Make an evaluation.

Lectures are the least effective teaching method for critical thinking. Teaching methods to develop and test the higher level of the cognitive domain and competencies of the affective and psychomotor domains should be a part of the staff development process.[11] Critical-thinking skills can be developed through the study of logic, problem-solving observation, analytic reading of books and articles about nursing and management, and group discussion.[12]

WEB ACTIVITIES

- Visit www.jbpub.com/swansburg, this text's companion website on the Internet, for further information on Critical Thinking.
- What resources are available through the Internet for developing critical thinking skills?
- Are there separate sites on the Internet for each of Freeley's seven methods of critical thinking?

SUMMARY

While critical thinking has been advocated in education for many decades, it is lately receiving attention in defining nursing curricula. Critical thinking is consistent with the nursing process and should be evident in higher-level learning objectives in the cognitive, affective, and psychomotor domains.

NOTES

1. A. J. Freeley, *Argumentation and Debate*, 8th ed. (Belmont, Calif.: Wadsworth, 1993), 1–3.
2. Ibid., 8.
3. Ibid., 9–13.
4. S. A. Jones and L. N. Brown, "Alternative Views on Defining Critical Thinking Through the Nursing Process," *Holistic Nurse Practitioner*, April 1993, 71–76.
5. K. L. Brooks and J. M. Shepherd, "Professionalism Versus Critical Thinking Abilities of Senior Nursing Students in Four Types of Nursing Curricula," *Journal of Professional Nursing*, March–April 1992, 87–95.
6. L. Saarmann, L. Freitas, J. Rapps, and B. Riegel, "The Relationship of Education to Critical Thinking Ability and Values Among Nurses: Socialization into Professional Nursing," *Journal of Professional Nursing*, January–February 1992, 26–34.
7. J. S. Hickman, "A Critical Assessment of Critical Thinking in Nursing Education," *Holistic Nurse Practitioner*, April 1993, 36–47.
8. B. D. Steffy and A. J. Grimes, "A Critical Theory of Organizational Science," *Academy of Management Review*, April 1986, 332–336.
9. V. H. Kemp, "Concept Analysis as a Strategy for Promoting Critical Thinking," *Journal of Nursing Education*, November 1985, 382–384.
10. Graduate students in the master's program in nursing management at Louisiana State University School of Nursing, New Orleans, La., fall 1993.
11. J. H. Woods, "Affective Learning: One Door to Critical Thinking," *Holistic Nurse Practitioner*, April 1993, 64–70.
12. L. McKenzie, "Critical Thinking in Health Care Supervision," *Health Care Supervisor*, June 1992, 2.

INTRODUCTION TO MANAGED CARE

"The HMO revolution has already forced some 53 million people from Marcus Welby-style medicine into the Wal-Mart model of health care."

Source: E. Spragins, "Does Your HMO Stack Up?" *Newsweek*, June 24, 1996, pp. 56–63.

OBJECTIVES

- Locate sources and discuss the comparative costs of various health-care services.
- Show how the development of health insurance influences health-care delivery in today's world.
- Describe the changes occurring in the U.S. health-care system.
- Describe the elements of managed care and their impact upon patients.
- Explain the effects of managed care relative to managers, nurses, physicians, health-care organizations, and other providers.

KEY CONCEPTS

managed care; fee-for-service reimbursement; indemnity insurance plans; point-of-service option; health maintenance organization (HMO); capitation

Manager Behavior: Solve problems resulting from managed care and promote interests of patients and personnel.

Leader Behavior: Empower professional nurses to produce quality outcomes for patients, personnel, and insurers within an environment influenced by managed care.

INTRODUCTION

Headlines and topics related to the high cost of health care have emerged as a major impetus for the evolution of the health-care system into one of managed care. A nurse manager need only examine a few days' mail to note the importance of this occupational phenomenon. New publications abound exhibiting such titles as *Inside Medicaid Managed Care* and *Managed Care Quarterly*.

All major health-care publications carry articles on managed care that posit such questions as "Will the Cost Cutting in Health Care Kill You?"[1] Major newspapers and news weeklies include articles entitled "HMOs Tell Courts They Aren't Liable" and "Does Your HMO Stack Up?"[2] Writers have reported that quality health care is busting the budgets of consumers, companies, and the government. As a result, managed care has become the dominant health-care delivery system in the United States.

THE COSTS OF HEALTH CARE

National health expenditures have risen from $12.7 billion, or 4.4 percent of the gross domestic product (GDP), in 1950 to $988.5 billion, or approximately 13.7 percent of the GDP, in 1995 (see Exhibit 2–1). Health-care costs topped one trillion dollars in 1997.

In 1996, approximately 90.5 percent of federal spending went to national defense, payments to individuals, Social Security, Medicare, Medicaid, and interest on the national debt. Medicare is financed almost exclusively by payroll taxes, with expenditures growing at a faster rate than the wage-base tax. The primary contribution to this disparity once again is rising medical costs. Solutions to the problem include reduced health-care cost increases, higher cost sharing by beneficiaries, reduced provider reimbursement, and increased payroll taxes.

Expenditure of Health-Care Dollars

During the years 1950–1995, the amount of private health expenditures went from $8.9 billion to $532.1 billion, an increase of approximately 5,980 percent. Public expenditures rose from $2.8 billion to $456.4 billion, an increase of 16,300 percent. The ratio of public to private expenditures actually decreased (see Exhibit 2–1).

The ultimate solution to controlling costs is fast becoming managed care.

While direct patient (out-of-pocket) payments rose from $7.1 billion in 1950 to $182.5 billion in 1995, they actually decreased from 80.3 percent to 34.3 percent of the total private health expenditures. Insurance premiums rose from $1.3 billion to $310.6 billion during the same period. (See Exhibits 2–1 and 2–2.)

In the public domain, the health-care dollar is spent for Medicare, Medicaid, Veterans Administration, public health services, and other public assistance programs. Medicare increased from $7.7 billion in 1970 to an estimated $187 billion in 1995. Public assistance, including Medicaid, rose from $6.3 billion to an estimated $146.4 billion between 1970 and 1995 (see Exhibit 2–1.)

Exhibit 2–2 shows the average annual per capita expenditures for physicians' services, hospital care, and total medical care services for the years 1970 to 1995.

Exercise 2–1   Pick several managed-care products. Identify the costs to the patient enrolled in a managed-care plan and compare them to the costs to a patient in an indemnity health insurance plan.

Exhibit 2–1 National Health Expenditures: 1950 to 1995

Year	Total (Billions) $	Per Capita (Dollars) $	Percent of GDP %	Private Total (Billions) $	Out-of-Pocket Payments Total (Billions) $	Insurance Premium (Billions) $	Public Total (Billions) $	Medicare (Billions) $	Public Assistance (Billions) $	Medicaid (Billions) $
50	12.7	0	4.4	8.9	7.1	1.3	2.8	—	0.1	—
55	17.7	0	4.4	12.9	9.1	3.2	4.0	—	0.2	—
60	26.9	141	5.1	19.5	13.1	5.9	5.7	—	0.5	—
65	41.1	202	5.7	29.4	18.5	10.0	8.3	—	1.7	—
70	73.2	341	7.1	43.0	24.9	16.3	24.9	7.7	6.3	5.1
75	130.7	582	8.0	72.3	38.1	31.3	50.1	16.4	14.5	12.3
80	247.2	1,002	8.9	142.5	60.3	69.7	104.8	37.5	28.0	23.3
85	428.2	1,666	10.2	253.9	100.6	132.3	174.3	72.2	44.4	37.5
90	697.5	2,588	12.1	413.1	148.4	232.4	284.3	112.1	80.4	64.8
95	988.5	3,509	13.7	532.1	182.6	310.6	456.4	187.0	146.4	120.1

Source: U.S. Bureau of the Census, *Statistical Abstract of the United States 1997*, 117th ed., Washington, D.C., 1997.

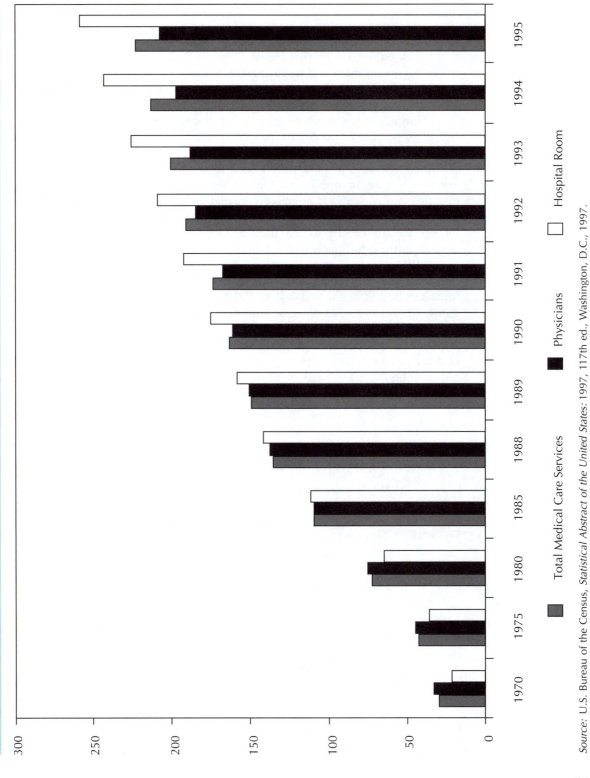

Exhibit 2–2 Indexes of Medical Care Per Capita Expenditures 1980–1996.

Source: U.S. Bureau of the Census, *Statistical Abstract of the United States: 1997,* 117th ed., Washington, D.C., 1997.

11

HEALTH-CARE SYSTEM USA

Is the health-care system of the United States really a system? One could argue that it is a nonsystem. Rising health-care costs have spawned health-care policy issues to control them and to encourage wellness or fitness care as a viable alternative to illness care. In addition, ambulatory care continues to expand as an alternative to inpatient care.

During the twentieth century, heart disease and cancer, which account for nearly 60 percent of all deaths, have surpassed infectious and parasitic diseases, which once accounted for over 40 percent of all deaths, as the major causes of death. Antibiotic drugs are widely used to treat and prevent infections and parasites, urban water supplies are filtered and chlorinated, milk is pasteurized, and infectious individuals are effectively treated using isolation procedures. Although we have many safe, efficient, and cost-effective vaccines, these vaccines, such as the vaccine for rubella for children between ages 1 and 4 years, are not being utilized to their full potential.[3]

Life expectancy at birth increased from 54.1 years in 1920 to 75.8 in 1995. Life expectancy is predicted to increase to 76.7 years in 2000 and 77.9 years (74.1 for males and 80.6 for females) in 2010.[4] Increased life expectancy changes the nature of health care as older persons develop more degenerative diseases.

Maintenance of community health is affected by social, economic, and political factors. Suicides, homicides, and accidents are among the leading causes of death among persons ages 1 through 39 years. Suicide and homicide rates doubled among the 10–24 age group from 1961 to 1994.[5] Solutions to these problems must take the behavioral component into account.

Historical Development of Health Insurance

1929	Blue Cross
1935	Social Security Act
1946	Hospital Survey and Construction Act (Hill-Burton)
1964	Hill-Harris Hospital and Medical Facilities Amendments
1965	P.L. 89-97 Medicare and Medicaid
1982	TEFRA
1983	P.L. 98-21 Social Security Amendments Prospective Payment System (PPS)
1985	Consolidated Omnibus Budget Reconciliation Act (COBRA)
1986	Gramm-Rudman Deficit Reduction Amendment and Omnibus Budget Reconciliation Act
1987, 1988	Omnibus Budget Reconciliation Acts (OBRA)
1989	Physician Payment Review Commission
1994	Medicare Choice Act
1996	Health Insurance and Accountability Act
1997	Balanced Budget Act

Blue Cross

Prepaid health-care plans began in 1929 with Blue Cross. By the 1940s, one fifth of the U.S. population was covered; by 1966, one third. By 1984, approximately 57 percent of the U.S. population was covered by employer- or employer-union-provided group plans. By 1994, 179.6 million persons, or 70.3 percent of the population, were covered by government or private insurance for the entire period; 54.7 million, or 22.1 percent, were covered for part of the period; and 11.9 million, or 4.8 percent, were not insured. At any one time, approximately 40 million, or 15.2 percent of the U.S. population, were not insured.[6]

To update these and previous data on the internet (http://census.gov/).

Social Security

The Social Security Act of 1935 provided funds for maternal and child health-care services, education and training of public health workers, research in nutrition and industrial hygiene, and aid to children with disabilities.[7]

Exercise 2–2   Set up an appointment with your local Social Security office personnel. Determine what services have been added since 1935.

Hospital Survey and Construction Act

Hospital construction in areas of severe shortage was stimulated by the Hospital Survey and Construction Act of 1946 (Hill-Burton). This act equalized the relative availability of hospital facilities between urban and rural areas and among the states.[8]

Hill-Harris Hospital and Medical Facilities Amendments

The Hill-Harris Hospital and Medical Facilities Amendments, enacted in 1964, dealt with modernization grants, area-wide planning, and long-term care facilities.[9]

Social Security Amendments of 1965

Medicare and Medicaid were created in 1965 by Public Law 89-97. With this law, the federal government assumed a major role in health-care financing. As a result, approximately one tenth of the U.S. population was aided in 1965. This represented about one third of hospital patient days, bringing the proportion covered by third-party players to two thirds at the time the law went into effect. By 1996, approximately 37.5 million persons were covered by Medicare and over 36.3 million by Medicaid. This represented over 27.8 percent of the U.S. population.[10]

TEFRA

Public Law 97-248, the Tax Equity and Fiscal Responsibility Act (TEFRA), was passed by Congress in 1982 and went into effect in 1983. It ushered into effect the prospective payment system (PPS), as it made reimbursement for Medicare patients prospective, creating a system of cost-per-case limits. This was the prelude to the diagnosis-related groups (DRGs) reimbursement system.

Social Security Amendments of 1983

Public Law 98-21, the Social Security Amendments of 1983, was signed in April 1983 by President Reagan. It was enacted to head off potential deficits in the Hospital Insurance Trust Fund of the Social Security program. This law established a prospective payment system (PPS) for hospital care based on diagnosis-related groups (DRGs). Prospective payment means the expected payment for a particular diagnosis-related group (DRG).

Exercise 2–3 How many DRGs currently exist? Interview the financial officer of a hospital to find out how DRGs are currently impacting the agency's budget.

COBRA

The Consolidated Omnibus Budget Reconciliation Act (COBRA) of 1985 was followed by the Omnibus Budget Reconciliation Act in 1986. This act modifies the reimbursement provisions of the prospective payment system.

Physician Payment Review Commission

In 1989, the Physician Payment Review Commission was created. This system introduced a new payment system for Medicare limiting amounts physicians could charge above a resource-based fee schedule within a neutral budgetary environment.

Medicare Choice Act of 1994

This law allows seniors to opt out of Medicare and into integrated health plans. It allows for choice of Medicare fee-for-service, employer-sponsored, or other managed-care health plans during open enrollment periods.

Health Insurance and Accountability Act

Signed into law on August 21, 1996, the Health Insurance and Accountability Act established favorable federal tax treatment for the benefits and premiums of qualified long-term care services. Benefits received from a qualified long-term care insurance policy are not taxable. Also, premiums for qualified long-term care insurance policies (up to a specified limit based on age) and expenses not reimbursed for qualified long-term care services will be tax-deductible, similar to medical expenses. The act also protects the portability of health insurance for employees changing jobs and establishes law for medical savings accounts.

Balanced Budget Act of 1997

President Clinton signed into law the Balanced Budget Act of 1997 on August 5, 1997. The act offers a new level of health-care options called Medicare + Choice. Among these choices are preferred provider organizations (PPOs) and provider-sponsored organizations (PSOs). Other changes include redistributed payments between rural and urban areas and restricted movements among plans.[11]

The result of these third-party payer programs have been a mixed blessing. Many people have good health and good health care because they are insured by such programs. Out-of-pocket costs to them have been dramatically reduced, but third-party payer programs have been weak incentives to consumers, who have seldom questioned the need for many services or sought out less costly providers or styles of care.

COMPONENTS OF THE U.S. HEALTH-CARE SYSTEM

Components of the U.S. health-care system include patients, insurers, and providers such as hospitals, ambulatory care services, home health services, long-term care facilities, physicians, nurses, allied health personnel, pharmacies, providers of durable medical equipment, and federal, state, and local public health services. As costs have increased, physicians who have been fee-for-service reimbursed are increasingly being reimbursed by capitation through contracts with managed-care insurers or have become employees of the managed-care insurers. Employees have switched from indemnity insurance plans to managed-care plans.

The heart of the managed care revolution is money not medicine.

George Anders[13]

Indemnity insurance plans cover bills from most providers and pay most health-care bills by charges or costs with some deductibles or copayments. Indemnity plans are fast disappearing as employers and governments switch to managed care. As health-care costs have soared, employers have increased employees' share of indemnity insurance premiums. Indemnity insurance plans do not keep costs down. Indemnity insurers are changing to become organizers and administrators of managed-care networks and subsequently deliverers of health care. This transformation is reducing the number of insurers.[12]

In the new managed-care environment, many providers are integrated into the insurance plan services through individual contracts and subcontracts.

Clients accept the providers of these contract services, thus limiting their choice of most health-care provider services. Clients receive a total package of health care dictated by the contracts between employers and insurers.

MANAGED CARE

Managed care is a patient care system that includes insurance companies, providers, and clients. Most enrollees of managed care are employees of businesses that contract for health insurance as a benefit. Many plans accept individual enrollees, particularly those plans that enroll Medicare beneficiaries. Managed care is the process by which health-care benefits are monitored for cost-management purposes, resulting in limitation of benefit coverage and access to health-care benefits. Managed-care organizations manage the distribution of health-care dollars, utilization of services, and access to benefits.

Managed-Care Organizations (Alternative Delivery Systems)

Patients are beginning to accept health-care plans that limit their freedom of choice. The following sections discuss some of these plans.

Health Maintenance Organizations (HMOs).   Financing of HMOs is done by capitation, in which there is a predetermined payment per patient or per service. Managed care is designed to cut costs.

The HMO is defined under the HMO Act as an organized system for providing health care in a geographic area, for which the HMO is responsible for providing or otherwise assessing its delivery. It operates under an agreed-upon set of basic and supplemental health maintenance and treatment services (defined products). The HMO is a voluntarily enrolled group of people and has a community rating.[14] HMOs have the following characteristics:

- Utilization risks are shifted from payer to provider.
- Competition draws consumers to less costly services when they have a choice of plans.
- Use of preventive care and ambulatory facilities decreases hospital admission rates, lowering insurance costs by 10 percent to 40 percent.
- Use of primary care physicians at fixed salaries decreases use of expensive surgeons and specialists.
- HMOs eliminate unneeded facilities such as hospitals, operating rooms, or radiation therapy units.
- Paperwork and overhead are reduced.
- HMOs provide organized, cooperative care for individuals and families.
- Enrollees make appointments with gatekeeper physicians or nurses, mostly family practice, internal medicine, and pediatrics.
- Gatekeepers control all referrals to specialists.
- Enrollees pay a small fee per visit and for medications.
- Gatekeepers control unneeded procedures, both diagnostic and therapeutic.

- HMO plans contract with providers such as hospitals, laboratories, radiology, physician specialists, and druggists for discounted prices.
- HMO plans emphasize complete patient care, management of chronic illness, education, disease prevention, and wellness. Oxford Health Plans recently hired twenty nurse practitioners because they are trained to do disease prevention and health promotion. These RNs will be reimbursed at the same rate as MDs. They do more preventive care.
- HMOs make physicians business-oriented practitioners.
- HMO plans do mass customization to give each of a mass of customers what the customer desires.
- HMOs offer capitated payments, one price per enrollee.
- HMOs reduce the risk of unneeded procedures, such as caesarian sections and hysterectomies.
- Fifty percent of HMO physicians are paid flat fees that are incentives to reduced care.

Pilot programs of Medicare HMOs indicate that hospitalization of Medicare clients could be decreased 30 percent. HMO membership increased from 9.1 million in 1980 to 46.2 million in 1995.

Hospitals that do not succeed in the growing competition will be faced with empty beds, unused ancillaries, decreasing reimbursement revenues, closings, and layoffs. Hospital administrators will learn not to respond to physicians at all costs. Many will employ physicians, give up beds and services, seek out special markets and relationships, adopt aggressive marketing strategies and techniques, and look outward. Hospitals will save management fees by managing their own HMOs.

Wolfe indicates that HMOs do not decrease costs, because they increase profits. Forty-five percent are owned by eight insurance companies. Their average profit from first quarter 1992 to first quarter 1993 was 40 percent.[15]

As HMOs expand, health costs increase. In California, with 80 percent of employees covered by managed care, costs are 19 percent above the national average and rising more rapidly.[16]

Although HMOs are the most common type of managed-care organization, many more millions of people belong to other types, discussed in the following paragraphs.

Preferred Provider Organizations (PPOs). In a PPO, a group of providers act as health-care brokers providing services to a group of patients at reduced fees. PPOs have the following characteristics:

- PPOs contract with consumers through employers and insurers and with providers, including physicians, hospitals, and allied services.
- Services are discounted, and patients have no out-of-pocket expenses.
- Patients are limited to using the listed providers.
- PPOs are intermediaries between payer and subscriber groups, furnishing marketing and administrative services.

- PPOs set their own size, number of staff specialists, geographic availability, time limits for claims and payments, and other features.
- PPOs place hospitals but not physicians at risk.

Arguments that the traditional physician-patient relationship will be destroyed are relatively inconsequential. These relationships will soon disappear anyway. Working people want efficiency and do not want to sit in a physician's office waiting hours past their appointed time. Given adequate information, they will make choices about their care, and they should. The old concept of withholding information is outmoded and dangerous. The objective of all competitive health-care plans is to provide good-quality care more cheaply.

Health Care Cost Coalitions (HCCCs).   HCCCs are organizations of employers, and sometimes unions, for effectively bargaining for better rates and parity with Medicare, Medicaid, and other insurers. They work to develop PPOs and utilization review programs.

Prudent Buyer Systems.   Prudent buyer systems are characterized by joint purchasing arrangements, purchasing consortia composed of multiple providers, and competitive bidding for exclusive contracts.

Health Promotion and Wellness Programs.   Increased education and awareness enable such programs to emphasize illness prevention.

Hospital Physician Organizations (HPOs).   HPOs are a relatively new entity. Their objective is to combine and reduce overhead, which can be done by sharing such services as billing.

Managed care is a fact of life. It will not go away, and most Americans will eventually belong to a managed-care plan.

Provider-Sponsored Organizations (PSOs).   PSOs are networks of hospitals and physicians who are their owners. There are approximately eighty-four in the United States. Supporters of PSOs say they are health providers engaged in treating patients, while HMOs are insurance companies that invest in stocks, bonds, and other liquid assets. PSOs offer less risk to providers than do HMOs, as providers get only part of their income from the PSO.[17]

Exercise 2–4   Attend a marketing session given by a managed-care company. Analyze the presentation. What do you see as advantages to the patient? Disadvantages?

Managed Care Plan Enrollments.   Over 60 million people are enrolled in managed care plans, the bulk of them in HMOs, with 103.2 million enrollment predicted by the year 2000. This includes 5 million to 5.5 million of Medicare's 38 million beneficiaries. Medicare's HMO patients are 12 percent healthier than the average Medicare patient. More than three fourths of active employees are enrolled in managed care plans. Average annual premiums went from $3,741 in 1994 to $3,915 in 1996.[18]

Advantages and Strengths, Problems and Solutions of Managed Care

Advantages of Managed Care.   Managed care has a number of advantages, including the following:

- Managed care has reined in skyrocketing medical costs. Medical care inflation is the lowest since 1973, although it rose in 1997 to pay for two years of rollbacks and sagging profits.
- Managed care puts patients first by making clinical decisions before economic ones.
- Managed care limits patients' time to get appointments.
- Managed care offers fast-track treatment for life-threatening conditions.
- Department of Health and Human Services is responsible for ensuring due process of Medicare HMO enrollees. It can require a written notice describing the reason for denial of service and giving clear information on how to appeal an HMO decision, and it can require expedited consideration in time-sensitive medical situations.
- Managed care puts interests of third party at bay.
- Medicare rules limit financial penalties against managed-care plan physicians for referrals or expensive procedures.
- By law, new mothers in managed-care plans cannot be forced out of hospitals in less than 48 hours.
- Gag rules can be limited by law.
- Most HMO enrollees get the care they need.[19]
- Some plans pay for prescription drugs.
- Federal law changes would allow HMOs to be sued for malpractice and held accountable for mistakes.
- Profit motive may be checked.
- Managed-care plans receive better-quality report cards.
- Managed care plans can keep out physicians who have malpractice judgments.

Strengths of Managed Care.   If improvements are made, managed care will lead to better-informed consumers. Treatment guidelines of managed-care plans will be developed that people can trust. Conservative treatment may cost less and have better outcomes. For example, $1,000 worth of physical therapy may be better for herniated disks than a 15-thousand-dollar operation. In a study of Californians under 65 who had appendicitis, 25.8 percent of HMO members had ruptured appendixes, versus 29.3 percent of fee-for-service patients. Patients in managed-care plans have a place to complain. Ninety-five percent of female HMO members at Scripps Clinic, LaJolla, California, get mammograms, while the national average is around 75 percent. Mammograms can detect breast cancer and result in earlier treatment.[20]

Problems with Managed Care.   The following are among the problems with managed care:

- Medicare enrollees in HMOs may not regain Medigap insurance if they return to fee-for-service choice.
- Gag clauses in contracts between plan and physician forbid disclosures that advise patients of medically necessary but expensive treatment options. Gag clauses limit care, undermine trust, and are negative to clinical independence. Executive orders prohibit gag rules for Medicare patients (5 million, or 13 percent of beneficiaries) and 13.3 million Medicaid recipients. The managed-care industry has promised not to restrict patient-doctor communications.
- Managed care limits choices by denial of referral to specialists.
- Managed care does less research.
- Patients receive a decline in compassion, communication, and quality of care.
- Plans have conflicting formularies and incompatible information systems.
- Physicians must chase approvals and correct inappropriate denials. They are rewarded for providing less care.
- Money goes to corporate salaries and profits (20 percent).
- High-risk patients are screened out. Service to sick and disabled is limited. Patients are dumped into public facilities. The poor, the sick, and the elderly have lower access, satisfaction, and outcomes.
- Medical service accounts (MSAs) are opposed by managed-care insurers because unused money in the savings account goes to the employee, not the insurance company.
- Women have a harder time getting needed medical care from HMOs.
- Since more people are getting into the managed-care system, they are having a harder time accessing needed care and so visit doctors more frequently because they become sicker.
- Appropriate treatment of members with rare medical conditions is sometimes a problem. This can be solved with a point-of-service option that permits the client to go to any physician by paying an additional fee.
- Patients are being moved through the system by decisions of clerks rather than nurses. Example: Patient was observed in recovery room for 45 minutes and then was moved to floor against the nurse's better judgment. Patient went bad and had to be moved to ICU.
- Plans have a tendency to look only at statistical averages while failing to understand the individuality of patients. As a result, plans fail to recognize that complex medical problems cannot always be standardized into predetermined treatment paths.
- HMO enrollees with mental-health problems often receive poorer detection and treatment.

Exercise 2–5   From information in this chapter, prepare a short questionnaire (10–15 questions) pertaining to the services provided for managed-care enrollees. Identify and interview two persons, a managed-care plan enrollee and an indemnity insurance plan enrollee. Compare problems and advantages of the two plans.

Solutions to Managed-Care Problems. Some of these problems do have solutions. Four hundred bills representing backlash legislation were introduced in state legislatures in 1996. Among the goals of such bills are the following:

- Managed-care programs would be forced to pay the physician or the hospital the client uses.
- Clients would see specialists without preapproval.
- Emergency-room care would be paid for even if the emergency was imagined.
- HMOs would be banned from paying physicians for withholding treatments.
- Gag clauses would be outlawed.
- HMOs could not fire physicians who speak out against policies they feel endanger patients.[21]

In 1997, the Texas state legislature passed, and the governor signed into law, a bill making managed care plans responsible when they withhold medical treatment. Texas is the first state to pass legislation allowing managed-care groups to be sued for withholding treatment resulting in harm to the client. About 4.3 million Texans are enrolled in managed-care plans.[22]

Economic Implications

Managed care has as its ultimate goal the making of a profit. This is true whether the organization is a not-for-profit or a for-profit one. The not-for-profit organization needs to make a profit to stay in business. By law, any profits must be reinvested in the business or used to reduce premiums.

For-profit organizations want to make profits for their shareholders. Business is about providing employment, providing value for customers, developing skills of employees, and developing capabilities of suppliers as well as earning money for shareholders.

Managed-care whether by for-profit or by nonprofit organizations, has a number of economic implications. Profits of mental-health managed-care plans are enormous. Administrative and profit-loading costs are seldom below 40 percent.[23] Unnecessary mastectomies, heart bypasses, and prostate surgeries are reduced under managed-care plans. Health-care premiums for these plans rose only 2 percent in 1995. Some companies encourage workers to choose the best HMOs by discounting monthly premiums.[24]

Overuse of medical services and administrative inefficiencies result in $200 million in unnecessary costs.[25]

Having reached maximum savings through managed care, health-care costs were expected to rise as much as 5 percent in 1997 and 10 percent in 1998. This will be partly due to higher technology and prescription costs, which have risen three times faster than other components of health care. Also, legislators and employers tell the insurers they must cover a certain minimum level of service as well as a minimum number of persons with preexisting or serious conditions. Physicians are thus demanding higher compensation.[26]

Managed-care organizations are making tremendous profits. Oxford Health Plans, an HMO, has over $2 billion in annual sales. It grows 125 percent

Managed care is creating an economic upheaval.

annually, and its earnings compound at over 75 percent. In four years, its stock went from $4 a share to over $47 a share. The big earners are medical device companies and national health-care providers. Healthsouth does $6 billion worth of rehabilitation and outpatient surgery a year at 1,000 locations. Its specialty is sports medicine. Heart valves cost less than $1,000 to manufacture, yet they sell for $3,000. St. Jude Medical has the patents and FDA approval and few competitors. Phycor, which buys and runs physician practices, imposes management practices that cut costs.[27]

Exercise 2–6   John Kay, director designate of Oxford University's new School of Management Studies, asks the question: What is a company's purpose if it is not to maximize shareholder value? With a group of your peers, discuss how the values evident in a world of managed care can be used to integrate the goals of this statement with the goals of quality health care for people.

Source: J. Kay, "Shareholders Aren't Everything," *Fortune*, 17 February 1997, 133–134.

Ethical Implications

Successful managed-care organizations will recognize all players as stakeholders in a community. These organizations will conduct business in an ethical manner. They will make long-term commitments to employees, customers, suppliers, and other stakeholders. This will give these organizations a competitive advantage.

Whether myth or fear, the following are some of the ethical questions implied by managed care: Will pressure of legalization for physician-assisted suicides and cost management by managed-care organizations affect patient outcomes? Will the poor, the elderly, and the uninsured be forced to accept fewer costly procedures and face early death? Will patients' rights force physicians to inform patients of the right to physician-assisted suicide? Should people, including those in need, receive uncompensated care?

Exercise 2–7   Locate and read five recent articles on managed care published in nursing journals. Summarize the implications for the nursing profession, including economic, ethical, consumer, practice, education, research, quality, and management.

Consumer Implications

Most consumers are not in managed-care plans voluntarily; their employers put them there. Consumers need to be informed and vigilant so they will use the services effectively and efficiently. Many physicians belong to several plans, and several plans have many physicians to choose from. Thus, physician choice for consumers is broadened.

The following are some examples of managed-care problems for the consumer:

1. A 61-year-old woman waited four hours in an HMO hospital emergency room while a blood clot starved her body of oxygen. She had no call button and was not monitored. Her daughter blamed her death on the HMO-owned hospital.[28]

2. A woman claimed that an HMO stopped an orthopedist from mending her broken, infected leg because it would cost too much. Approval for treatment took much persuasion by the doctor. The HMO wanted to amputate the woman's leg; the orthopedist saved it.[29]

3. Patients get sicker while waiting six to ten weeks to see a colon cancer specialist or get CAT scans.[30]

4. A six-month-old baby is sick, feverish, moaning, and panting. Parents call hotline nurse, who refers them to HMO contract hospital 42 miles away. Parents drive through torrential rain, past a nearby non-HMO hospital. A potentially fatal infection resulted in amputation of both of the child's hands and feet.[31]

5. "In Massachusetts, 22 percent of HMO patients are afraid that their doctors would not provide needed care, and only two-thirds have confidence in their physicians."[32]

6. "Twenty percent of Medicare HMO enrollees dropped out within 12 months of joining."[33]

7. "Your policy may say you'll get quality treatments and hospitalization, but in the brave new world of managed care your actual treatments will probably be determined by someone who never saw you."[34]

Wellness Example

A 91-year-old patient in a nursing home existed in a terrified state, requiring oxygen and medication to sustain her breathing. She refused to leave her room. Then, the Eden Alternative was introduced to change the environment of nursing homes. This alternative brings pets—cats, birds, and fish—into the resident's environment. In this new environment, the patient-become-resident cares for a cat and a parakeet. She lunches with friends and participates in activities with other residents. She no longer needs an oxygen tank, and her medications have been reduced.

Other modifications of this environment include interior decoration, large, luxurious inside plants, raised outside flowerbeds, birdfeeders, and validation therapy. All aspects of the environment are designed to include the residents. The nursing home is managed by autonomous, self-directed teams of nurses, housekeepers, aides, and therapists. Families participate. Employee turnover is reduced. A playground is provided where residents can watch the children of employees and of residents' relatives play. Schoolchildren visit with residents. The environment is one in which wellness prevails over illness. Spirits are nurtured and soar over apathy. This is holistic care that raises the quality of the residents' lives.

Clients need to be convinced to modify risk-taking behavior: smoking, skipping medications, abusing alcohol, driving without fastened seat belts, poor nutrition, inadequate exercise, unprotected sex, and other lifestyle practices negative to good health.[35]

Practice Implications

Nurse midwife numbers are increasing. Nurse midwives are being hired by physicians and hospitals. Because nurse midwives are less expensive than physicians and they score high in patient satisfaction, managed-care organizations are interested in hiring them. Nurse midwives provide quality time, personal attention, and expert state-of-the-art skills to patients.

In other areas, registered nurses are being replaced by less-skilled employees. Shifts are understaffed. Inferior supplies include surgical gloves that break easily, smaller alcohol sponges, and chest suction with valves that do not indicate whether they are on or off.

HMOs are determining practitioners' credentials and setting practice guidelines.

Education Implications

Education is unprofitable in the managed-care environment. Future generations of caregivers may push distance learning technology, which has inconveniences: compressed videos, logistical or mechanical problems, lack of laughter and spontaneous reactions, and distracted students. Research indicates, however, that students learn as well or better and there is a wider audience with distance education. Distance education still has a long way to go.[36]

Research Implications

Research is unprofitable in the managed-care environment. Since research expands the frontiers of medical knowledge, less-funded research has serious implications for health care.

Quality Implications

A system for rating HMO quality allows "consumers to differentiate between an HMO that's great at answering the phone from one that's doing a great job of detecting breast cancer."[37]

Criteria for rating HMOs may include the following:

1. Meets industry standards of NCQA accreditation. The Health Plan Employer Data and Information Set (HEDIS) measures such aspects of plans as physicians' credentials checked, affiliation with (Joint Commission on Accreditation of Health Care Organizations) accredited hospitals, and board certification of physicians.
2. Measures satisfaction of physicians and members.

3. Tracks members' health, measuring and addressing risk-taking behavior.
4. Uses hard-nosed outcomes measures, including morbidity and mortality.
5. Develops prevention and screening tools to keep people healthy through early detection.
6. Encourages perinatal care during first trimester of pregnancy, resulting in low caesarian rate and high normal delivery rate.
7. Employers do independent surveys of contract plans using outcomes measures.[38]

Quality isn't examined very closely when most employers choose group health-insurance plans. In a recent study of the chronically ill, the elderly and the sickest poor fared much worse in three urban HMOs than their counterparts did in traditional plans.

Jane Bryant Quinn[39]

The following are major contenders in the health-care-quality movement:

1. National Committee for Quality Assurance (NCQA). The commission's findings do not say much: The NCQA has accredited 18 percent of HMOs fully and 17 percent temporarily, and 4 percent of HMOs that have applied have flunked. Fifty percent of HMOs have not even applied.
2. John Ward's *Medical Outcomes Survey*. The survey evaluates people's general health. It may be effective over time.
3. Foundation for Accountability (FACCT). FACCT develops standards for judging how well HMOs handle specific illnesses.

Quality measurements are difficult to standardize and for different people to agree on. Insurers and providers often select the cheapest outcome rather than base their decisions on morbidity and mortality. Consumers need knowledge if they are to access quality. This knowledge consists of ways providers deliver care without raising costs to consumers. It includes knowledge of how consumers can be assertive about getting needed services. It also includes data linked to expected outcomes of care and treatment. Knowledge consists of benchmarked best practices, including critical paths for specific diagnoses and procedures. It includes data about morbidity and mortality related to all health-care providers.

HMOs with thick rosters of physicians may be laggards in providing quality care. Their MDs practice medicine the way the HMO wants them to. Best

---

How You, the Consumer, Can Find Quality Care

1. Learn the best medical technique for the procedure or treatment facing you.
2. Check public information about providers caring for you.
3. Check member satisfaction surveys before choosing an HMO.
4. Assert yourself in dealing with your HMO and file a grievance if dissatisfied.
5. Switch health plans if dissatisfied. If unable to, nag your boss.

HMOs may have fewer physicians and a central office. Aetna, U.S. Healthcare, and PruCare go for large numbers of MDs and offer money as motivation for them to keep costs down. In 1996, the average MD worked for thirteen HMOs with thirteen sets of criteria. HMO-salaried MDs use treatments that work best and so maintain quality. This is a provable fact, as Kaiser Permanente HMO scores higher on quality measures than Aetna or U.S. Healthcare.[40]

Hospitals are beginning to use a GM-developed program for measuring quality, called PICOS (Purchased Input Concept Optimization with Suppliers). PICOS purports to eliminate waste, streamline operations, and improve customer satisfaction. The hospital using PICOS guides a small team of eight to ten key employees to examine a process, identify the waste, and redesign the process to reduce or eliminate the waste. Health-care providers look at waiting times, billing procedures, and duplication of work.[41]

Patients may be satisfied with physicians and access to them, although physicians may not know the latest treatment for a patient's condition. It is easy to find satisfied customers who are healthy.

Self-surveys may inflate customer satisfaction. Independent surveys are best, although they may comply with the wishes of those who pay for them. Among good independent surveyors are the Sachs Group, Evanston, Illinois; Care Data; Center for the Study of Services Annual Guide, which rates 400 HMOs; and National Committee for Quality Assurance, HEDIS 3.0 report.

Management Implications

As managed-care plans and enrollments increase, managers of all health-care provider organizations face the necessity for maintaining financial stability. To do this, they become experts in negotiating contracts, planning new ventures, and reorganizing their organizations to make maximum use of human resources. Successful managers provide leadership that empowers employees to provide maximum quality outcomes for their patients. As managers pursue these functions, they oversee evaluation techniques that are simple to administer and lead to quality improvement.

WEB ACTIVITIES

- Visit www.jbpub.com/swansburg, this text's companion website on the Internet, for further information on Managed Care.
- Managed care has created volumes of debate within society and on the Internet. Search for sites that are for or against managed care and note the arguments on both sides.
- The American Association of Managed Care Nurses is an organization offering information on managed care. Locate their site and review.

SUMMARY

Managed care is fast replacing fee-for-service and indemnity insurance plans. The object of this transformation is reduced costs and increased profits. While managed care has many problems, such problems are gradually being solved, some with federal and state legislation. The most prominent form of managed care is the health maintenance organization (HMO). Managed care has important implications for practice, research, education, and management.

NOTES

1. E. Faltermayer, "Will the Cost Cutting in Health Care Kill You?" *Fortune,* 31 October 1994, 221–222, 224, 226, 228, 230, 232.
2. "HMOs Tell Courts They Aren't Liable," *San Antonio Express-News,* 17 November 1996, 28A; E. Spragins, "Does Your HMO Stack Up?" *Newsweek,* 24 June 1996, 56–61, 63.
3. U.S. Bureau of the Census. *Statistical Abstract of the United States:* 1997, 117th ed., Washington, D.C., 1997, 188.
4. Ibid, 96, 102, 103.
5. Ibid, 120–121; T. C. Tillock, "Cost Containment in the Health Care Industry," *Aging & Leisure Service,* February 1981, 5–15.
6. Ibid.
7. Ibid.
8. Ibid.
9. Ibid.
10. Ibid.
11. J. Rother, "Managed Care and Medicare Part 1," *Modern Maturity,* November–December 1997, 34–43, 75–76, 80.
12. C. J. Loomis, "The Real Action in Health Care," *Fortune,* 11 July 1994, 149–153, 155–157.
13. "Book Review: How HMOs Are Destroying Medical Trust," G. Anders, *Health Against Wealth: HMOs and the Breakdown of Medical Trust* (Boston, MA: Houghton Mifflin, 1996), in *Public Citizen Health Research Group Health Letter,* January 1997, 1–4.
14. U.S. Bureau of the Census, op. cit., 121.
15. S. M. Wolfe, ed., "$1.06 Trillion for Health in 1994, $1.2 Trillion by 1995, $2 Trillion by 2000," *Public Citizen Health Research Group Health Letter,* February 1994, 1–2.
16. J. Canham-Clyne, S. Woolhandler, and D. Himmelstein, *The Rational Option for a National Health Care Program* (Stony Creek, Conn.: Pamphleteer's Press, 1995), 400.
17. "Health Care Battle Pits Doctors Against Insurance Firms," *San Antonio Express-News* 30 March 1997, 13A; B. B. Gray, "The Big Squeeze: Managed Care Will Have to Change," *Healthweek,* 5 January 1998, 1, 6.
18. "Health Premiums Will Go Up This Year and Next, Study Says," *Healthweek,* 10 February 1997, 24; B. B. Gray. "Managed Care Enrollment: Big and Getting Bigger," *Healthweek,* 16 December 1996, 1.
19. "Study Says Health Care Costs, Access Troubling to Many," *San Antonio Express-News,* 23 October 1996, 6A.
20. E. Faltermayer, op. cit.
21. "HMO Backlash Spurs Wave of Restrictive Legislation," *San Antonio Express-News,* 15 March 1996, 10B.

22. L. Tolley, "Bush Clears Bill to OK HMO Suits," *San Antonio Express-News*, 23 May 1997, 1E, 3E.

23. C. Olian, "HMO: Managed or Mangled?" *Public Citizen Health Research Group Health Letter*, March 1997, 3–5.

24. "HMO Backlash," op. cit.

25. C. J. Loomis, op. cit.

26. P. Lamiell, "With Savings Peaked, Health-Care Costs May Rise," *Austin American-Statesman*, 12 April 1997, D2.

27. A. E. Serwer, "Health Care Stocks: The Hidden Growth Stars," *Fortune*, 14 October 1996, 74, 79–80, 82.

28. "HMO Backlash," op. cit.

29. Ibid.

30. Ibid.

31. "Book Review," op. cit.

32. S. Woolhandler and D. H. Himmelstein, "Annotation: Patients on the Auction Block," *Public Citizen Health Research Group Health Letter*, March 1997, 1–2.

33. Ibid.

34. C. Olian, op. cit.

35. A. McDonald, "Nursing Homes Teach Elders to Live Again," *San Antonio Express-News*, 14 April 1997, 10, 100.

36. S. Gandy, "Distance Learning May Take You Where You Want to Go, But It's Still a Bumpy Ride," *Healthweek Houston/San Antonio*, 21 April 1997, 1, 10.

37. E. E. Spragins, "Does Your HMO," op. cit.

38. Ibid.

39. J. B. Quinn, "Is Your HMO OK—Or Not?" *Newsweek*, 10 February 1997, 52.

40. E. E. Spragins, "Take My Freedom, Please!" *Newsweek*, 7 April 1997, 81.

41. K. Driscoll, "Hospitals Take Lesson in Quality Improvements from GM," *San Antonio Express-News*, 13 April 1997, 3H.

INTRODUCTION TO THEORY OF NURSING MANAGEMENT

OBJECTIVES

- Define such terms as *manager, managing, management,* and *nursing management.*
- Differentiate among concepts, principles, and theories.
- Discuss *systems theory.*
- Illustrate selected principles of nursing management.
- Describe roles for nurse managers.
- Distinguish between two cognitive styles: intuitive thinking and rational thinking.

KEY CONCEPTS

theory
concept
principle
management theory
general systems theory
nursing management theory
management development
management roles
cognitive styles (intuitive versus rational)
nursing management levels

Manager behavior: Applies a personal theory or style of nursing management.

Leader behavior: Develops the management knowledge and skills of nursing personnel, working with them to formulate and test a theory of nursing management that will succeed in the work environment.

WHAT IS MANAGEMENT?

Modern management theory evolved from the work of Henri Fayol, who identified the administrator's activities or functions as planning, organizing, coordinating, and controlling.[1] Fayol defined management in these words:

> To manage is to forecast and plan, to organize, to command, to coordinate, and to control. To foresee and provide means examining the future and drawing up the plan of action. To organize means building up the dual structure, material and human, of the undertaking. To command means binding together, unifying and harmonizing all activity and effort. To control means seeing that everything occurs in conformity with established rule and expressed demand.[2]

While some believed that these were technical functions to be learned only on the job, Fayol believed that they could be taught in an educational setting if a theory of administration could be formulated.[3] He also stated that the need for managerial ability increased in relative importance as an individual advanced in the chain of command.[4]

Fayol listed the principles of management as follows:[5]

I. Division of work
II. Authority
III. Discipline
IV. Unity of command
V. Unity of direction
VI. Subordination of individual interests to the general interests
VII. Remuneration
VIII. Centralization
IX. Scalar chain (line of authority)
X. Order
XI. Equity
XII. Stability or tenure of personnel
XIII. Initiative
XIV. Esprit de corps

Another theorist in the development of the science and art of management was L. Urwick, who indicated that administrative skill is a practical art that improves with practice and requires hard study and thinking. The administrator has to master intellectual principles, the process being reinforced by general reflection about actual problems. From his work, Urwick concluded that there are three principles of administration. He described the first principle as that of *investigation* and stated that all scientific procedure is based on investigation of the facts. Investigation takes effect in *planning*. The second principle is *appropriateness*, which underlines *forecasting*, entering into process with *organization* and taking effect in *coordination*. Exercising the third principle, the administrator looks ahead and organizes *resources* to meet future needs. Planning enters into process with *command* and is effected in *control*.[6]

Throughout management literature, the original functions of planning, organizing, directing (command and coordination), and controlling as defined by Fayol, Urwick, and others have been accepted as the principal functions of managers. Managing means accomplishing the goals of the group through effective and efficient use of resources. The *manager* creates and maintains an internal environment in an enterprise in which individuals work together as a group. *Managing* is the art of doing, while *management* is the body of organized knowledge underlying the art. In modern management, staffing is frequently separated from the planning function, directing has been labeled "leading," and "controlling" is used interchangeably with "evaluating."

Theory, Concepts, and Principles

The knowledge base of management science includes theory, which in turn includes concepts, methods, and principles. The principles are related and can be observed and verified to some degree when they are translated into the art or practice of management. *Concepts* are thoughts, ideas, and general notions about a class of objects that form a basis for action or discussion. They tend to be true, but not always. *Principles* are fundamental truths, laws, or doctrine on which other notions are based. Principles provide guidance to concepts and to thought or action in a situation.[7] In nursing management, research—Urwick's "investigation of facts"—becomes part of the theory of the field.

If nursing is going to base its theory on laws, nurses will need to validate principles through research. This is a difficult task, as theorists in the social sciences have discovered. It is difficult to reduce human behavior to laws. Nurses deal with human behavior in all roles, but particularly so in nursing management.

White explores a viewpoint on nursing theories in which she addresses prescriptive theories. She notes that their use as practice guidelines "must be broad enough to encourage a wide range of practice situations but not so broad as to be meaningless." A theory of decision making might be more beneficial than a theory of nursing in the practice arena. Nurses believe that for nursing to be a real profession, it should have a scientific and theoretical base. Nursing is thus a practice profession based on the physical and social sciences.[8]

Nurse managers learn to merge the disciplines of human relations, labor relations, personnel management, and industrial engineering into a unifying force for effective management. Many nurse managers would add the theory of nursing to this list. A successful synthesis of these disciplines would promote employee commitment, increased productivity, good labor relations, and competitiveness in health care. If these goals are not achieved, the workforce is poorly managed.

Contradictions exist in management theory because of lack of agreement about sets of ideas and concepts among and within disciplines.[9] General systems theory is one such contradiction.

General Systems Theory

General systems theory is an organismic approach to the study of the general relationships of the empirical universe of an organization and human thought. It grew out of biology as an analogy between an organism and a social organization. Boulding describes nine levels of a general systems theory:[10]

1. A static structure or level of frameworks.
2. A moving level of predetermined necessary motions or clockworks.
3. A control mechanism level—the thermostat.
4. The level of the open-system or self-maintaining structure—the cell.
5. The genetic-societal level.
6. The "animal" level.
7. The "human" level.
8. The level of social organization.
9. Transcendental systems.

Another version of the key concepts of general systems theory is summarized in Exhibit 3–1; the author's model of an open system is Exhibit 3–2.

Exhibit 3–1   Key Concepts of General Systems Theory

Subsystems or Components
A system, by definition, is composed of interrelated parts or elements. This is true for all systems—mechanical, biological, and social. Every system has at least two elements, and these elements are interconnected.

Holism, Synergism, Organicism, and Gestalt
The whole is not just the sum of the parts; the system itself can be explained only as a totality. Holism is the opposite of elementarism, which views the total as the sum of its individual parts.

Open-Systems View
Systems can function in one of two ways: closed or open. Open systems exchange information, energy, or material with their environments. Biological and social systems are inherently open systems; mechanical systems may be open or closed. The concepts of open and closed systems are difficult to defend in the absolute. We prefer to think of open–closed as a continuum; that is, systems are relatively open or relatively closed.

Input-Transformation-Output Model
The open system can be viewed as a transformation model. In a dynamic relationship with its environment, it receives various inputs, transforms these inputs in some way, and exports outputs.

System Boundaries
It follows that systems have boundaries that separate them from their environments. The concept of boundaries helps us understand the distinction between open and closed systems. The relatively closed system has rigid, impenetrable boundaries, whereas the open system has permeable boundaries between itself and a broader suprasystem. Boundaries are relatively easily defined in physical and biological systems but are harder to delineate in social systems such as organizations.

Negative Entropy
Closed physical systems are subject to the force of entropy, which increases until eventually the entire system fails. The tendency toward maximum entropy is a movement to disorder, complete lack of resource transformation, and death. In a closed system, the change in entropy must always be positive; however, in open biological or social systems, entropy can be arrested and may even be transformed into negative entropy—a process of more complete organization and ability to

transform resources—because the system imports resources from its environment.

Steady State, Dynamic Equilibrium, and Homeostasis
The concept of a steady state is closely related to that of negative entropy. A closed system eventually must attain an equilibrium state with maximum entropy—death or disorganization. However, an open system may attain a state in which the system remains in dynamic equilibrium through the continuous inflow of materials, energy, and information.

Feedback
The concept of feedback is important for understanding how a system maintains a steady state. Information concerning the outputs or the process of the system is fed back as an input into the system, perhaps leading to changes in the transformation process or in future outputs. Feedback can be positive or negative, although the field of cybernetics is based on negative feedback. Negative feedback is informational input that indicates that the system is deviating from a prescribed course and should readjust to a new steady state.

Hierarchy
A basic concept in systems thinking is that of hierarchical relationships among systems. A system is composed of subsystems of a lower order and is also part of a suprasystem. Thus, there is a hierarchy of the components of the system.

Internal Elaboration
Closed systems move toward entropy and disorganization. In contrast, open systems appear to move in the direction of greater differentiation, elaboration, and a higher level of organization.

Multiple Goal Seeking
Biological and social systems appear to have multiple goals or purposes. Social organizations seek multiple goals, if for no other reason than that they are composed of subunits and individuals with different values and objectives.

Equifinality of Open Systems
In mechanistic systems, there is a direct cause-and-effect relationship between the initial condition and the final state. Biological and social systems operate differently. Equifinality suggests that certain results may be achieved with different initial conditions and in dif-

Exhibit 3–1   Key Concepts of General Systems Theory *(Continued)*

ferent ways. This view suggests that social organizations can accomplish their objectives with diverse inputs and with varying internal activities (conversion processes).

Source: F. E. Kast and J. E. Rosenzweig, "General Systems Theory: Applications for Organization and Management," *Academy of Management Journal* (December 1972): 447–464. Reprinted with permission.

Exhibit 3–2   An Open System

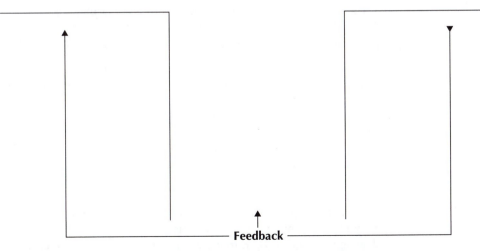

External Environment

Transformation process

INPUT   **OUTPUT**

INPUT	Transformation	OUTPUT
Nursing personnel	Planning	Organizing, leading, controlling
Supplies	Management of nursing care of clients by nursing personnel	Resolution of nursing problems of clients
Equipment	Critical thinking	Outcomes: client improvement; client health-care goals met; peaceful death
Physical plant	Application of nursing theory in management and clinical care	
Clients		
Knowledge, values, ethics, skills, and beliefs		

Feedback

Exercise 3–1   Read the original article by Boulding listed in Note 10. With a group of peers, formulate a systems theory of nursing management that illustrates these nine levels.

With the emerging changes in health-care systems, nurse leaders will need to accelerate changes in nursing organizations. The goal may be nursing modules centered around closely related operations, such as differentiated practice delivery models matched with intensity of care, specialized services, or both. Standardization and flexibility can be melded with systems developed based on a requirement for a theory of nursing practice as a foundation for all modules, but with different theories being used in different modules by choice of professional clinical nurses.[11]

Full realization of systems theory is as far away in nursing as it is in manufacturing. Nursing management and practice are the integrators that tie the parts of the health-care system together. Transformational nurse leaders will be fully knowledgeable of the work being done by their constituents, since they will be the coaches and facilitators. To integrate people, materials, machines, and time, followers of the systems concept must do as well as think.[12]

Nursing Theory-Based Conceptual Models of Nursing Administration

Self-Care Nursing.   Dr. Sarah E. Allison established Orem's theory as the basis for nursing practice at the Mississippi Methodist Rehabilitation Hospital and Center over twenty years ago. Allison, McLaughlin, and Walker state that a theory-based nursing systems design for a population of patients does the following:[13]

- Describes the nursing characteristics of the patient population to be served.
- Uses these characteristics to predict the types of client problems for which nursing is needed.
- Identifies appropriate nursing technologies.
- Determines the types and number of nursing personnel needed.
- Organizes nursing personnel for effective performance.
- Defines outcomes or results based on nursing theory.

Examination of a theory-based nursing system will reveal the following:[14]

- Mission, philosophy, and objectives statements.
- Documentation tools or forms, the data from which provide a nursing database.
- Standards of care and practice.
- Staff education.
- Quality assurance outcomes audits.
- Patient classification systems.
- Job descriptions.
- Policies and procedures.
- Career development programs that attract and retain the best nurses as they motivate by clarifying the role of the nurse.
- The support given by nursing administration's commitment.

Iowa Model.   A conceptual model for nursing administrative practice will assist in solving problems of change. It will serve as a visual image to guide thinking in planning, decision making, and communicating. The Iowa Model of Nursing Administration "provides for the critical interdependence of both clinical activities and management activities or outcomes." The Iowa model may be used to guide decision making and evaluating change.[15] This model is depicted in Exhibit 3–3, with definitions applied to the Iowa Model of Nursing Administration in Exhibit 3–4.

Exhibit 3–3   The Iowa Model of Nursing Administration

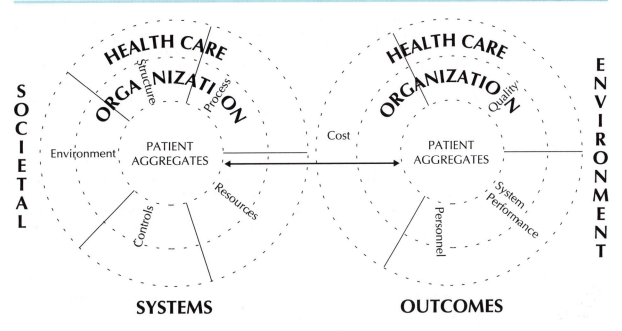

Source: Copyright 1990 by the NSA Program, University of Iowa College of Nursing. Reprinted with permission.

Exhibit 3–4   Definitions Applied to the Iowa Model of Nursing Administration

Patient aggregates	A grouping of patients who have similar basic care characteristics (e.g., medical diagnosis) within a nursing unit
Organization	A group of employees acting together to achieve the goals of the employing institution (e.g., quality patient care)
Health-care system	All financial, political, legal, and professional groups in the United States involved in the delivery of health-care services to the public
Systems	A set of interrelated and interdependent parts that form a complex whole or work together to deliver health care to the public
Outcomes	Desired results; the degree to which goals and objectives are met in the delivery of health care to the public

Source: Copyright 1990 by the NSA Program, University of Iowa College of Nursing. Reprinted with permission.

NURSING MANAGEMENT

In nursing, management relates to performing the functions of planning, organizing, staffing, leading [directing], and controlling [evaluating] the activities of a nursing enterprise and departmental subunits. A nurse manager performs these management functions to deliver health care to patients. Nurse managers or administrators work at all levels to put into practice the concepts, principles, and theories of nursing management. They manage the organizational environment to provide a climate optimal for the provision of nursing care by clinical nurses.

Management knowledge is universal, as is nursing management knowledge. The latter uses a systematic body of knowledge that includes concepts, principles, and theories applicable to all nursing management situations. A nurse manager who has applied this knowledge successfully in one situation can be expected to do so in new situations. Nursing management occurs at unit and executive levels. At the executive level, it is frequently termed "administration." The theories, principles, and concepts remain the same. They can all be classified under the major functions of nursing management or nursing administration.

With decentralization and participatory management, the supervisory or middle-management level is fast being eliminated. Nurse managers of clinical units are being educated in management theory and skills at a master's level. Clinical nurses are being educated in management skills, empowering them to take action in managing groups of employees as well as patients and families. Clinical nurse managers are doing more in the coordinating duties among units, departments, and services.

Exercise 3–2   In your own words, define nursing management as it relates to your job. If you are a student, observe the work of a nurse manager and define management in terms of your observations.

Who Needs Nursing Management?

All types of health-care organizations, including nursing homes, hospitals, home-health-care agencies, ambulatory care centers, and student infirmaries, need nursing management. The nurse working with one client and family needs management knowledge and skills to help people work together to accomplish a common goal. Primary nurses working with several clients prioritize their care to assist their clients in achieving improved health or, sometimes, in accepting peaceful death.[16]

General Principles of Nursing Management

The following are some major principles of nursing management that are discussed in more detail in succeeding chapters.

1. Planning is a major function of nursing management that is primary to all other activities or functions of management.

2. Effective utilization of time is essential to effective nursing management that performs in the present while planning for future performance, growth, and change.

3. Decision making is a primary element of nursing management at every level.

4. Nurse managers manage a clinical practice discipline in which professional nurses are primarily knowledge workers, applying their knowledge to the gathering of data, the making of nursing diagnoses and nursing prescriptions, the supervision of the implementation of the nursing care plan by skilled workers, and the evaluation and adjustment of the plan.

5. Social goals are formulated by nurse managers and achieved by clinical nurses.

6. Organizing is a second major function of nursing management.

7. Change is a major element in nursing management, with exponentially increasing change being the only constant in today's world.

8. Organizational cultures should be managed to reflect values and beliefs, with managers in nursing having a common purpose of making productive the values, aspirations, and traditions of employees, who are individuals as well as members of communities and of society.

9. Directing or leading is a third major function of nursing management, empowering employees, improving quality, and leading to excellence of production.

10. Motivation is a basic element of the directing function of nursing management, resulting in satisfactory performance, which results from job satisfaction, a condition requiring that nurse managers stimulate motivation of nurse employees.

11. Effective communication is a primary element of nursing management, resulting in fewer misunderstandings and giving employees a common vision, common understanding, and unity of direction and effort.

12. Staff development is a primary element of the directing function of nursing management that maintains the competency of all practicing nurses.

13. Controlling or evaluating is the fourth major function of nursing management and includes the processes of evaluating the carrying out of the adopted plan, the given orders, and the established principles through establishing standards, comparing performance with standards, and correcting deficiencies.

14. All of these major functions of nursing management operate independently and interdependently.

Exercise 3–3   Describe a belief you have about nursing management in the organization in which you work or are doing clinical practice as a student. Discuss your belief with your clinical group of practicing peers or students and nurse manager or instructor.

(continued)

Exercise 3–3
(continued)

Summarize the conclusions. Is your belief valid? Totally? Partly? Not at all? Validity can be established by comparing your conclusions with viewpoints found in publications or by obtaining agreement from practicing nurse managers. You will be codifying selected theory of nursing management.

Management Development

Management development is big business: 500,000 managers take management education programs at least once every year, 7,800 minicourses for executives are conducted at the University of Pennsylvania Wharton School in one year, and 14,000 managers are enrolled annually in management seminars at AT&T. In the new health-care environment, home-health-care agencies, ambulatory care centers, and similar health-care agencies are increasing. They are no less complex than hospitals and, like hospitals, need cost controls and increased productivity to thrive. Unless nurses are educated to manage in these new environments, they will lose out to other professions or will manage poorly and be unhappy and unsuccessful.[17]

Nurses require preparation for their management jobs, including synthesis of nursing and management knowledge. The nurse manager is prepared to manage other nurses, who will provide the clinical care. Education of nurses will provide human resource management skills, including preceptor and mentor assignments. A model of progression from nursing expertise to management expertise is illustrated in Exhibit 3–5.

A system for developing nurse administrators has been published by Fralic and O'Connor, who make frequent reference to the work of Katz and of Charns and Schaefer. Katz classifies management skills into three categories:

1. Conceptual skills, which are an innate ability, or thinking skills.
2. Technical skills, which include methods, processes, procedures, or techniques.
3. Human skills, which relate to leadership ability and intergroup relations.

In nursing, technical skills are divided into nursing management technology and nursing practice technology. Fralic and O'Connor relate the conceptual, human, and technical skills to three management levels, with the chief nurse executive needing the highest level of conceptual competence and the nurse manager needing the highest level of nursing practice technology. The needed staff development is evident in the role requirements.[19]

Spicer indicates that scientific management knowledge is the basis of the nurse manager's role, including knowledge of a model role and the ability to conceptualize it. Preparation for management and support during the transition are needed for the change from clinical nurse to manager nurse. The role model would demonstrate the relationships between politics and strategy, between power and influence.[20]

Preparation of nurse managers includes knowledge of legal labor practices and institutional policy in managing employees. It includes preparation for in-

Exhibit 3–5 Management Progression for Nursing

Skill requirements and training focus

Senior Management Executive	Management expertise	Conceptual ability 75% Management of human resources 20% Technical expertise 5% In-service focuses on planning, forecasting, and marketing
Assistant Director		Conceptual ability 50% Management of human resources 40% Technical expertise 10% This position can be line or staff; therefore, in-service focus depends on the circumstances of the particular agency
Middle-Management Supervisor	Leadership ability Leadership ability	Conceptual ability 20% Management of human resources 70% Technical expertise 10% In-service focuses on management/leadership principles and upgrading of technical skills to the same degree as the staff nurse
Entry-Level Management Assistant Supervisor	Gray area	Conceptual ability 20% Management of human resources 35% Technical expertise 45% In-service focuses on management/leadership principles along with upgrading of technical skills
Level III	THRESHOLD	Conceptual ability 15% Management of human resources 15% Technical expertise 70% In-service begins to include exposure to management/leadership principles along with upgrading of technical skills
Level II	Nursing expertise	Conceptual ability 10% Management of human resources 5% Technical expertise 85% In-service focuses on upgrading of technical skills
Level I		Conceptual ability 5% Management of human resources 5% Technical expertise 90% In-service training focuses on upgrading of technical skills

Source: S. Gleason, O. W. Nestor, and A. J. Riddell, "Helping Nurses Through the Management Threshold," *Nursing Administration Quarterly* (Winter 1983): 14. Reprinted with permission of Aspen Publishers, Inc., 1983.

service training, including understanding principles of adult education, performing a needs survey, and preparing, presenting, and evaluating programs. Money matters concern all levels of nurse managers and include budgeting, managing cost and revenue centers, and increasing productivity. Nurse managers use performance appraisal as a continuum directed toward results. Preparation of nurse managers assists them in becoming self-directed.[21]

In the new management culture, nurses will survive and prosper by updating their skills. Entrepreneurial managers invest in their employees with pay, fiscal quality in the workplace, and training.[22]

Leadership is a huge industry. Content of leadership training includes feedback, personnel growth, skill building, and conceptual awareness. Training is for values-based leadership; values are those shared by leaders and constituents. Investing in training and technology will improve efficiencies.[23]

Exercise 3–4   Translate the management of time as nursing management theory into an example, such as "A nurse who practices good management will know how to use time effectively." The example may be one that applies to you as manager or to observed behavior of another nurse manager. To do this, keep a log for a day. Make entries at 15-minute intervals on separate paper, using the following format:

Time	*Activity*	*Delays, Bottlenecks*

Analyze your log. How much of your day was productive? How much was unproductive? What can be done to increase productive time? Using the following format, make a management plan to use your time better.

Management Plan

Goal:

Actions	*Target Dates*	*Assigned To*	*Accomplishments*

Based on your observations from this exercise, write a theory statement that describes management as the effective use of time.

NURSING MANAGEMENT AND ROLES

Role Development

The nurse manager draws from the best and most applicable theories of management to create an individual management style and performance. This requires knowledge and the skill to use it. The nurse manager continues to acquire management knowledge and to use it to solve managerial problems. This requires a contingency approach, as no single approach works for all situations. The nurse manager acts with the assumption that clinical nurses and other personnel want to be competent and that with managerial support they will be motivated to achieve competence. As each competence goal is achieved, a higher goal is set. Clinical nurses will seek out the organization that fits their needs.[24]

McClure vividly points out that nurse managers are managing a clinical discipline performed by professional nurses. Nurses are predominantly female and often experience conflict between being a nurse and being a homemaker. The nurse manager devises strategies to deal with such conflict. Blue-collar nurses often lack knowledge of nursing research and do not read to keep up-to-date. They want nurse managers to do everything. White-collar nurses, who want to be treated differently, look for job enrichment with primary nursing and professional autonomy. They want to be organized like the medical staff, with staff appointments and peer review. The nurse manager manages these two groups differently.[25]

Exercise 3–5   The following functions originate from a theory of the institution or organization and the division of nursing: Plans for accomplishing objectives are made, strategies for accomplishing them are formulated, activities are organized by priority, work is assigned, managerial jobs are designed, and an organizational structure evolves. Describe how each of these activities is evident in your place of practice as a student or in your workplace as a practicing professional nurse.

Cognitive Styles: Intuitive Thinking Versus Rational Thinking

Nugent states that management science is based on the assumption that reason or rational thinking is the only form of thought. Rational modes of thought are based on a cognitive style of learning, deciding, and solving problems that is systematic, analytic, reflective, and field-independent.

An intuitive mode of thought also exists. Intuitive modes of thought are based on a different cognitive style of learning, deciding, and problem solving that is intuitive, global-relational, active, and field-dependent.[26] Differences between rational and intuitive modes of thought are summarized in Exhibit 3–6.[27]

Rational and intuitive modes alternate in real life. Intuitive thinkers are frequently blocked when confronted by rational thinkers. They have to think in causal terms rather than in terms of meaning and significance, and this stifles and frustrates them, making them inarticulate. Rational thinkers, in turn, can become frustrated and uncomfortable when confronted with intuitive thinkers. Many people do not know that these different cognitive domains exist.[28]

Nurse managers and clinical nurses can benefit from having both intuitive and rational thinkers who set and evaluate goals. Intuitive thinkers will formu-

Exhibit 3–6 Characteristics of the Rational and Intuitive Modes of Thought

Aspect	Rational Mode	Intuitive Mode
Ordering of the mode	Linearity, sequence	Iteration, cycles
	Discrete steps	Simultaneity, interaction, association
Elements and their relationships	Discrete entities	Gestalts, integrated wholes
	Logically interrelated categories	Many experience forms (difficult to categorize)
		Integration through meaning and significance
Reliance on context	Little reliance on context	Strong reliance on context
	Assumption of boundaries	Unbounded or difficult to bound
	Explicitness	Large amount of implicitness
Movement and control of the process	Completion of one step before passing to another	Emergence and evolution of gestalts
	Relative inflexibility	Relative flexibility
	Great control over process	Little control over the process

Source: P. S. Nugent, "Management and Modes of Thought," *Journal of Nursing Administration* (February 1982): 19–25. Reprinted with permission of Lippincott. © February 1982.

late goals that are flexible, generating ideas and images of hopes, desires, and expectations. They will describe the future. The resulting gestalt can then be translated by rational thinkers into structure, with specificity of goals, objectives, means, and actions. The processes can alternate, with new ideas and goals emerging. Knowledge of intuitive and rational thinking should be applied to the job of managing nurses.[29]

Whole-brain thinking, the combining of logical and intuitive thinking, may improve managerial ability and skills. Techniques that assess whole-brain thinking are listed in Exhibit 3–7.[30]

Management Levels

Nurse managers perform at several levels in the health-care organization, including first-line patient-care management at the unit level, middle management at the department level, and top management at the executive level. In some organizations, decentralization displaces the middle-management level and redistributes department-level functions to staff functions under a matrix or other organizational structure. The roles of managers are developmental, building upon knowledge and skills as the scope of the nurse manager's role increases in breadth and depth. Middle nurse manager roles are fast being eliminated as clinical nurses are being empowered and given management education.

Operational Nurse Managers.   The following are some of the knowledge and skills needed by nurses in operational management roles:[31]

Exhibit 3–7 Accessing the Left and Right Hemispheres

Left	Right
Writing: Words foster clear and effective left brain thinking.	Brainstorming: allows thinking to flow, free of critique.
Sorting thoughts: Outlining ideas in a logical sequence after classifying like thoughts into groups.	Relaxation techniques: Relaxation produces alpha brain waves which access the right brain.
Computer use: Input requires exact, sequential ordered data which stimulates the left hemisphere.	Music: Slow rhythmic musical pattern produces alpha brain waves, creating an internal cerebral atmosphere that allows for easy entry to "lateral thinking."
Stimulate left brain by note taking, analyzing body language, tone of voice, organizing, prioritizing, writing, outlining, controlling the environment.	Functions that activate right brain: Visualizing; daydreaming; *responding* to body language; tone of voice; hugging; smiling; laughing; allowing events to happen; drawing; doodling; printing.

Source: D. C. Veehoff. "Whole Brain Thinking and the Nurse Manager," *Nursing Management* (August 1993): 34. Reprinted with permission of Springhouse.

1. Financial management—knowledge and skills to prepare and defend a budget for expenses of unit personnel, supplies, capital equipment, and revenues to meet expenses. Ability to manage scarce and expensive resources for performance.
2. Ability to match moral choices related to human needs, moral principles for behavior, and individual feelings in making decisions.
3. Recognition of and advocacy for patients' rights.
4. Active and assertive effort to share power within the organization, including shared power for nursing's practitioners. This includes nursing autonomy, which is threatened by authoritarian management. In turn, practicing nurses are involved in solving managerial problems.
5. Ability to communicate and to promote effective communication among nursing staff and others; presentation skills.
6. Knowledge of internal factors related to purpose, tasks, people, technology, and structure.
7. Knowledge of external factors related to economy, political pressures, legal aspects, sociocultural characteristics, and technology.
8. Ability to study situations and use management concepts and techniques, analyze them, make correct diagnoses of problems, and tie the process together as decisions.
9. Ability to provide for staff development.
10. Ability to provide a climate in which nurses clearly perceive that they are pursuing meaningful and worthwhile goals through their individual efforts.
11. Ability to effect change through an orderly process.
12. Knowledge of how to empower clinical nurses through committee assignments, quality circles, primary nursing, and even titles.

13. Commitment to maintain self-development through reading and attending workshops and other educational programs.

To these could be added staffing and scheduling, management reports, hiring, performance appraisal, job productivity and satisfaction, constructive discipline dealing with stress and conflict, personnel management, computers, and values, norms, and ways of doing things (organizational culture).[32] While these may be done as staff development, master's-level management preparation is essential.

While this list is in no way complete, it is a solid beginning that will be built upon in succeeding chapters.

Executive Nurse Managers.   Executive nurse managers increase their knowledge and skills by building on what they learned as lower-level managers. Nurse managers at this level should be able to do the following:

1. Apply financial management principles to costing and pricing nursing care and convey this knowledge to the nurses providing care.
2. Coordinate the division budget.
3. Empower lower-level nurse managers.
4. Undertake corporate self-analysis of what nursing can do (skills, capabilities, weaknesses); make assumptions about nursing, its environment, and its beliefs. Convey results to employees.
5. Specify, weigh, interrelate, and accomplish multiple goals simultaneously.
6. Abandon obsolete principles of standardization, centralization, specialization, and concentration.
7. Share authority and power through decentralization with participatory management, employee involvement, and quality-of-worklife programs.
8. Establish and use a matrix organization with task forces and project teams with project leaders.
9. Set the stage for clinical nursing practice. (This does not necessarily require that the nurse executive be clinically competent.)
10. Promote application of a theory of nursing within a nursing care delivery system.
11. Advise nursing educators on content of nursing administration programs.
12. Set depth and breadth of nursing research programs.
13. Anticipate future of health care and of nursing.
14. Manage strategic planning.
15. Serve as mentors, role models, and preceptors to lower-level managers, graduate students, and others.
16. Recognize and use authority and power potential.

Research data indicate that executive nurses prepared at the Ph.D. level need courses in ethical and accountable decision making, including missions and goals, policies, human resources, financial and material resources, databases, and communication management. These courses would be organized under organizational structure and governance, resources, and information management.[33] See Exhibit 3–8.

Exhibit 3–8 Summary of Findings: Decision Making

Organizational Structure and Governance		Resources		Information Management	
*Missions and Goals**	*Policies and Politics*	*Human†*	*Financial and Material*	*Databases*	*Communication*
History	Environment	Organizational	Acquire	Delimit	Processing
Philosophy	Administrative	behavior	Allocate	Establish	Managing
Purpose	process	Leadership	Budget	Utilize	Diplomacy
Objectives	Procedures/	Market	Monitor	Maintain	Interpersonal skills
Systems analysis	guidelines	Recruit	Manage	Evaluate	Team-building
Strategic planning/	Legalities	Appoint/admit/hire	Cost analysis	Revise	Problem-solving
forecasting	Regulations	Assign work			Conflict resolution
Change agentry	Obstacles	Develop			Writing
	Bureaucratic/	Educate			
	professional	Counsel/consult/			
	conflict	mentor			
	Power	Evaluate			
		Promote/progress			
		Retire/release/			
		graduate			
		Collective			
		bargaining			

* Refers to the missions and goals either of the nursing school and the broader academic institution in which the school is a part or of the nursing department and the broader health-care services institution in which the department is a part.
† Refers to faculty, students, staff.

Source: J. C. Princeton, "Education for Executive Nurse Administrators: A Databased Curricular Model for Doctoral (PhD) Programs," *Journal of Nursing Education* (February 1993): 62. Reprinted with permission.

Exercise 3–6 Write a short theory of nursing management based on information presented in this chapter. Remember that a theory of nursing management is an accumulation of concepts, methods, and principles that can be or have been observed and verified to some degree when translated into the art or practice of nursing management.

Exercise 3–7 Examine the following periodicals for the past 12-month period:
The Journal of Nursing Administration
Nursing Research
Nursing Management
Nursing Administration Quarterly
Note the following:

1. The number of articles on nursing theory versus nursing management theory.

(continued)

Exercise 3–7
(continued)

2. The theory of nursing that can be incorporated into a theory of nursing management. Did the research indicate that the theory fulfilled its claim? Explain.
3. The theory of nursing management that is being used (applied) in the organization in which you participate for clinical experience as a student or in which you are employed.
4. The theory of nursing management that could be used (applied) in the organization in which you are gaining clinical experience as a student or in which you are employed. Consider the value the research has for meeting the goals of the organization, the division of nursing, and the nursing unit.
5. Make a management plan for putting the research results into practice.

WEB ACTIVITIES

- Visit www.jbpub.com/swansburg, this text's companion website on the Internet, for further information on The Theory of Management.
- What journals or organizations could you search for information on management?
- Try searching under the names of some of the leading theorists and theories discussed in this chapter. What do you find?

SUMMARY

A main thrust of nursing management is that the focus is on human behavior. Nurse managers educated in the knowledge and skills of human behavior manage both professional nurses and nonprofessional nursing workers to achieve the highest level of productivity in patient care services. To do this, they must acquire the management competencies of leadership to stimulate motivation through communication with the workforce.

Among the general principles of effective nursing management are those related to planning, effective utilization of time, decision making, managing a clinical practice discipline, social goals formulation, change, organizing, organizational cultures, directing or leading, motivation, communication, staff development, and controlling or evaluating.

All of the major functions of planning, organizing, directing or leading, and controlling or evaluating operate dependently and interdependently.

The primary role of the nurse manager is to manage a clinical practice discipline. To accomplish this requires numerous competencies that are supported by a theory of nursing management.

NOTES

1. H. Fayol, trans., *General and Industrial Management,* by C. Storrs (London: Pitman & Sons, 1949), 3.
2. Ibid., 5–6.
3. R. M. Hodgetts, *Management: Theory, Process, and Practice,* 5th ed. (Orlando, Fla.: Harcourt Brace, 1990), 38.
4. Fayol, op. cit., 8–9.
5. Ibid., 19–20.
6. L. Urwick, *The Elements of Administration* (New York: Harper & Row, 1944), 14–15.
7. L. C. Megginson, D. C. Mosley, and P. H. Pietri, Jr., *Management: Leadership in Action,* 5th ed. (New York: Harper & Row, 1996), 15–20.
8. V. White, "Nursing Theory: A Viewpoint," *Journal of Nursing Administration,* July–August 1984, 6, 15.
9. W. Skinner, "Big Hat, No Cattle: Managing Human Resources, Part I," *Journal of Nursing Administration,* July–August 1982, 27–29.
10. K. E. Boulding, "General Systems Theory—The Skeleton of Science," *Management Science,* April 1956, 197–208.
11. P. F. Drucker, "The Emerging Theory of Manufacturing," *Harvard Business Review,* May–June 1990, 94–100.
12. Ibid.
13. S. E. Allison, K. McLaughlin, and D. Walker, "Nursing Theory: A Tool to Put Nursing Back into Nursing Administration," *Nursing Administration Quarterly,* spring 1991, 72–78.
14. Ibid.
15. D. L. Gardner, K. Kelly, M. Johnson, J. C. McClosky, and M. Maas, "Nursing Administration Model for Administrative Practice," *Journal of Nursing Administration,* March 1991, 37–41.
16. V. Henderson, *The Nature of Nursing* (New York: Macmillan, 1966), 15.
17. S. Gleeson, D. W. Nestor, and A. J. Riddell, "Helping Nurses Through the Management Threshold, *"Nursing Administration Quarterly,* winter 1983, 11–16.
18. Ibid.
19. M. F. Fralic and A. O'Connor, "A Management System for Nurse Administrators, Part 1," *Journal of Nursing Administration,* April 1983, 9–13; M. F. Fralic and A. O'Connor, "A Management Progression System for Nurse Administrators, Part 2," *Journal of Nursing Administration,* May 1983, 32–33; M. F. Fralic and A. O'Connor, "A Management Progression System for Nurse Administrators, Part 3," *Journal of Nursing Administration,* June 1983, 7–12.
20. J. G. Spicer, "Dispelling Illusions with Management Development," *Nursing Administration Quarterly,* winter 1983, 46–49.
21. Ibid.
22. D. Osborne and T. Gaebler. 1992. *Reinventing Government.* New York: Plume.
23. J. Huey, "The Leadership Industry," *Fortune,* 21 February 1994, 54–56; N. J. Perry, "How to Mine Human Resources," *Fortune,* 21 February 1994, 96.
24. M. L. McClure, "Managing the Professional Nurse: Part I, The Organizational Theories," *Journal of Nursing Administration,* February 1984, 15–21; M. L. McClure, "Managing the Professional Nurse: Part II, Applying Management Theory to the Challenges," *Journal of Nursing Administration,* March 1984, 11–17.
25. Ibid.
26. P. S. Nugent, "Management and Modes of Thought," *Journal of Nursing Administration,* February 1982, 19–25.

27. Ibid.
28. Ibid.
29. Ibid.
30. D. C. Veehoff, "Whole Brain Thinking and the Nurse Manager," *Nursing Management,* August 1993, 33–34.
31. J. O'Leary, "Do Nurse Administrators' Values Conflict with the Economic Trend?" *Nursing Administration Quarterly,* summer 1984, 1–9; M. L. McClure. "Managing the Professional Nurse: Part I. The Organizational Theories," *Journal of Nursing Administration,* February 1984, 15–21; M. A. Maidique, "Point of View: The New Management Thinkers," *California Management Review,* Fall 1983, 151–160; M. A. Poulin, "Future Directions for Nursing Administration," *Journal of Nursing Administration,* March 1984, 37–41; M. A. Fralic and A. O'Connor, "A Management Progression System for Nurse Administrators, Part I," *Journal of Nursing Administration,* April 1983, 9–13; G. Gentleman, "Power at the Unit Level," *Nursing Administration Quarterly,* winter 1983, 27–31; M. A. Poulin, "The Nurse Executive Role: A Structural and Functional Analysis," *Journal of Nursing Administration,* February 1984, 9–14.
32. J. J. Mathews, "Designing a First Line Manager Development Program Using Organization-Appropriate Strategies," *Journal of Continuing Education in the Health Professions,* vol. 8, no. 3 (summer) 1988, 181–188.
33. J. C. Princeton, "Education for Executive Nurse Administrators: A Databased Curricular Model for Doctoral (Ph.D.) Programs," *Journal of Nursing Education,* February 1993, 59–63.

INTRODUCTION TO THEORY OF HUMAN RESOURCE DEVELOPMENT

The most exciting breakthroughs of the 21st century will occur not because of technology but because of an expanding concept of what it means to be human.[1]

John Naisbitt and Patricia Aburdene

OBJECTIVES

- Define and give examples of the concept of human resource development (HRD).
- Define and give examples of the concepts of autonomy and empowerment.
- Illustrate the notion of self-help by applying it to nursing management.
- Give examples of the elements of HRD.
- Define andragogy and discuss its relevance in HRD.
- Apply a typology of adult education to goals for an HRD program.
- Define the concept of human capital and describe its relevance to HRD in nursing management.
- Project future changes in nursing HRD.

KEY CONCEPTS

human resource development (HRD)
science of behavioral technology
autonomy
empowerment
self-help
human resource planning
role theory
andragogy
typologies and taxonomies of adult education and HRD
human capital

Manager Behavior: Plans, organizes, directs, and controls all aspects of a human resource development program.

Leader Behavior: Establishes direction, aligns people, stimulates motivation, and inspires people to cause drastic and useful change in performing their nursing roles.

INTRODUCTION

Much of the voluminous theory of human resource development (HRD) comes from the generic fields of business and management. HRD is grounded in the theory of personnel or human resource management and the science of behavioral technology. One process through which HRD is applied is nursing management.

Because the success pattern of the industrial age is a liability to the information age of the 1990s, corporations will have to reshape their policies and structures to recruit employees. By the year 2000, we may have coined a new name for the 1990s, such as "The Age of the Individual" or "The Age of the Human Being." We are already well into the information age, and during the next several decades, the following changes will continue to occur within the United States:[2]

1. Agriculture will be reduced in manpower and productivity.
2. Only 10 percent of the population will be employed in manufacturing.
3. Sixty-five percent to 70 percent of the workforce will be employed in service industries.
4. The information/electronic industry will continue to create jobs. It is currently creating 4 million to 4.5 million jobs a year.
5. Education will be a dominant industry because services are education-intensive.
6. Training budgets will increase to $10 trillion per year.
7. There will be approximately 350 million people in the United States.
8. Income will average $40,000 per capita at a 2 percent per year compound model of growth in the gross national product (GNP).
9. A new accounting system will evolve to depreciate people as human capital with education becoming the capital to replace losses.
10. There will be more organizations, with fewer employees per organization.

Nursing as a service industry will continue to grow, be education-intensive to develop new roles, and require increased capital for staff development and maintenance.

DEFINITION

Human resource development is the process by which corporate management stimulates the motivation of employees to perform productively. HRD provides the stimuli that motivate nursing personnel to provide nursing-care services to clients at quality and quantity standards that keep the health-care entity reputable and financially solvent, the nurses satisfied with their professional accomplishments and quality of work life, and the clients treated successfully.[3]

HRD practices the concepts of democracy. In HRD, people grow and prosper from learning to use the skills of problem solving, application of logic, inquiry, critical thinking, and decision making. HRD is a lifelong process, hence its relationship to adult education and lifelong learning. It is also a process of helping and sharing that leads to competence and satisfaction with both the process and the outcomes. The HRD process facilitates self-direction, self-discipline, focus on immediate problems, and satisfaction related to employee participation in problem solving and decision making.[4]

Obviously, nurse administrators and managers of today's workforce must be well-schooled in human resource development. HRD theory includes the theory of change, problem solving and decision making, leadership, motivation, communication, participatory management, decentralization, and adult education. In nursing, HRD should be a proactive program as well as a part of strategic planning.

Health-care organization administrators and nurse managers at all levels are learning that efficiency and effectiveness result from advanced HRD programs. These advanced programs facilitate human relationships, reliability, initiative, autonomy, and talents. They do so through policies, procedures, and leadership that are fair, promote trust, reduce stress, communicate through feedback, and increase productivity without undue emphasis on costs. Keeping employees satisfied with the work environment decreases turnover, an expensive aspect of human resource management. Good HRD programs are therefore cost-effective.

THE SCIENCE OF BEHAVIORAL TECHNOLOGY

The science of behavioral technology has as its basis the premise that consequences will influence behavior. It can be used to improve employee performance. People will work more willingly if supervisors or managers exercise concern for their feelings and needs. A basic question here is, What will the employee work for? Three applications of the science of behavioral technology are analyzing problems, influencing job behavior, and designing learning systems.

Exercise 4–1   Identify an HR problem from the area in which you work. How is this problem being resolved? How could it be resolved using the science of behavioral technology? You may form a quality circle or a focus group to solve this problem. Make a management plan for solving the problem using the following format. Consider these aspects: the degree to which the problem and the solution influence job behavior and the degree to which staff development can be used as a learning system in implementing the solution.

Objective:

Activities	Date to Be Completed	Persons Responsible	Accomplishments

Staff development aligned with HRD needs to decide which education and training strategies to follow to satisfy the needs of employees with broad educational backgrounds, employees with high-level or specialized educational preparation, and all other categories of employees. This should be supported by consensus building, collaboration, partnership, and mutually agreed-upon objectives. See Exhibit 4–1 for differences between ACE (adult continuing education) and HRD.

Other applications of the science of behavioral technology will be found in the chapters on decentralization and participatory management, leadership, motivation, and communication.

AUTONOMY AND EMPOWERMENT

As part of HRD, health-care corporations should increasingly develop programs to enlarge the authority of professional nurses, increase their voice in management of their clinical practice discipline, and improve their career development possibilities. Both the organization's administration and the employees want control over HRD events. As stakeholders in the health-care system, clinical nurses and managers both have an obligation to keep the enterprise healthy. As economic stakeholders, nurses need security of income through wages and benefits, while management's stake is on profits and, in some cases, dividends for shareholders. Nurses have a psychological stake in their need for dignity. Both nurses and managers have potential stakes related to rights and obligations, efficiency and controls, and the trend toward greater employee influence in decisions and subsequent outcomes. These stakes should be spelled out in policies. The leader who balances motivation with control will manage effectively as "human beings strive to be involved and to gain influence over their lives to the extent that they are psychologically ready to do so and to the extent that economic organizational conditions allow them to do so."[5]

People want to work hard, perform well, learn new skills, and be involved in decisions about their work. Employees want to have input into placement and promotion. Managers who support the professional autonomy of nurses support empowerment of this group. Professional nurses thus gain control of their lives through feeling and using their own strength and power. Empowerment is therapeutic and spiritual; it is healthy for both employees and organizations. It stems from and gives support to useful experiential feelings or ideologies.[6]

Nurses are empowered when administrators and managers share authority with them. Nurses seek community with other nurses as a form of empowerment. Their power is extended by new technologies and the ability to use them. They are empowered by computers with modems, cellular phones, FAX machines, and access to e-mail systems. Nurses are empowered when society rewards their initiative as individuals.[7]

Empowerment motivates. Self-managed teams are empowered teams. They are used by one in five U.S. employers, with resulting drops in labor cost, increases in morale, and signs of eased alienation. In 1986, the United Auto Workers (UAW) and Chrysler created self-managed teams at the rundown New Castle, Indiana, plant. Workers were renamed "technicians," and line supervisors

Exhibit 4–1 The Differences Between Adult Continuing Education and Human Resource Development

ACE	HRD
Purpose and Mission	
Primary focus is on individual development and personal growth.	Primary focus is on organizational development and the role of employees in that development.
Education is the primary means for changing people, e.g., classes, courses, workshops, and individualized instruction.	Education is one dimension of organizational change. Others include job rotation/enrichment, organizational restructuring, and incentive plans.
Programming	
Programming is primarily marketed for the general public.	Programs are for employees only. Some may be marketed, but on a space-available basis.
Program identification is communitywide, with needs analysis tapping a wide variety of groups and organizations.	Program identification is within the organization, with intensive needs analysis of management, employees, customers, competitors, and environment.
Participants (Learners)	
The learners usually select the program to meet personal needs and goals.	The learner's performance is evaluated and training and development needs identified.
The learner is the primary client. The learner's employer is secondary to the learner's meeting his/her own goals.	The needs of the organization are primary. The employee's needs are met within the needs of the employer.
Instructional Resources	
Resources are primarily from education, as use of faculty is desired, if not required.	Resources are from any source (expertise in or out of the organization) that meets the organization's needs and can be afforded (bought).
Certification is often required and ranges from a teaching certificate to approval by a faculty department.	The test of acceptance is, Can the person/program meet the present needs of the organization? Accountability is driven by the bottom line.
Finances (Payment of Fees)	
Payment for the program is by the participant. Payment by participant's employer is usually through tuition reimbursement.	Payment is by the employer and usually includes salary while in training. Employee-selected courses must be approved by the employer.
Major Players (Roles)	
Directors/deans of ACE under a chief executive for instruction/academic affairs, coordinators, instructors (full/part-time)	Chief executive for human resources, director of HRD, instructional and content specialists, trainers, and consultants.
Prefer experience in ACE, with coursework in adult education desired. Increasingly, people with content expertise are being hired and trained in adult education. Terminal degree (master's/doctorate) preferred to relate with others in the school/college.	Prefer people from the organization or HRD experience in base industry (banking, manufacturing, retailing, etc.). Coursework in adult education is not considered necessary, but coursework will be paid if desired. Performance is required; terminal degree is optional but increasingly becoming a plus.

Source: D. H. Smith, "Adult and Continuing Education and Human Resource Development—Present Competitors, Potential Partners," *Lifelong Learning: An Omnibus of Practice and Research* 12, no. 7 (1989). Used by permission of the author.

became "team advisers." Seventy-seven teams were created that assign tools, confront sluggish performers, order repairs, talk to customers, hire new employees, and even alter work hours after consulting a labor-management steering committee. Team members are paid for extra training. As a result, absenteeism went from 7 percent to 2.9 percent, union grievances from more than 1,000 a year to 33, and defects per million parts made from 300 a year to 20; production costs keep shrinking.[8]

Autonomy and empowerment are achieved through collaboration and mutual planning, leading to commitment, satisfaction, and productivity. Malcolm Knowles states that as adults mature, they move toward autonomy, activity, objectivity, enlightenment, large abilities, responsibilities, and altruism, focusing on principles, deep concerns, originality, and tolerance for ambiguity.[9] For more information, see Chapter 16, Decentralization and Participatory Management.

Exercise 4–2   Discuss the meaning of autonomy and empowerment. List work conditions that keep professional nurses from autonomy and empowerment in the organization in which you work. Make management plans for resolving each condition using the format of exercise #1.

SELF-HELP

One goal of HRD is the development of a self-reliant learner who remains a knowledgeable and skilled worker on into the future. Another goal is the development of a worker who learns and uses the skills of self-help and of diagnosing his or her learning needs, being able to explore options in learning, thinking divergently, making decisions, and evaluating his or her own role in cooperation at work and in the world.[10] The HRD program uses leadership, staff development, and the theory of adult education to accomplish these goals.

Self-help is a unique form of self-directed learning that spans one's life cycle. A person does not necessarily help himself or herself independent of others. Self-help is also a process that occurs within small, voluntary, peer-run support groups, offering participants the opportunity to work together to overcome or cope with a common concern or problem.

According to Hammerman, the self-help movement began with Alcoholics Anonymous (AA). Participants tend to be white-collar, middle-class, with employment capability and the strong support of concerned spouses. Self-help groups provide, among other things, a network of information, support, and help from peers. Authenticity being a strength of self-help, HRD programs can use the self-help process to validate the authenticity of the learning. Sometimes issues of peer versus management leadership and agency sponsorship arise. These can be prevented or resolved through a warm, supporting, accepting environment that lowers defenses and allows for open, trusting, authentic dialogue. Members learn things not available elsewhere. Professionals put interests of group members first, and the group agrees on each professional person's tools for self-help.[11] As workers, professional nurses benefit from the self-help groups.

Role theory supports the notion of self-help. Changing environments—between external forces and the organization and between the organization and its members—lead to role ambiguity, which increases with redesigned and new relationships. This can lead to role conflict as a result of competing role behaviors, particularly among members of multidisciplinary teams. This role conflict increases with increased interaction on new turf. Role overload occurs as added work crowds time allotments, particularly if new programs are added and old ones retained. HRD and staff development programs provide the organizational support needed to cope with role changes and deal with role overload. They include the skills of priority setting and assertiveness.[12]

HUMAN RESOURCE PLANNING

Human resource planning is undertaken as part of the strategic planning process. This is essential to retain outstanding professional talent. It is not enough to address only the business activities of nursing, such as management processes and functions, budgets, objectives, and staffing. Nurse managers serve in dual roles, as managers of human resources and as managers of nursing operations. Nurse managers need to enlist the support of the human resources department. They also need to develop an understanding between other operational departments and nursing.[13]

Other elements of strategic human resource planning include the following:[14]

1. Projection for future growth, changes in the employment market, external demographics, and balancing human resources against finances.
2. Development of a strategic human resource planning approach that describes actions, roles, authorities, and responsibilities of the human resource department, line management, and individual employees.
3. Inventory of human resource planning skills that include future issues, a system for translating business plans into human resource requirements and programs, career development, two-way communication, attitude surveys, employee sensings, group feedback sessions, and exit interviews.
4. Analysis of current and future macro issues of major world influences that will affect the strategic business plan (SBP) and the human resources plan (HRP). These influences include such factors as the age of the population, productivity in U.S. industry, inflation, politics, unions, technology, and expectations of nurses.
5. Analysis of current and future micro issues of major organizational influences, including geographic location, availability of skills, potential in-house promotions, living costs, and unions.
6. Development of programs to support the SBP and the HRP.
7. Provision for periodic and timely audits.
8. Support and commitment of all management levels.

As part of strategic planning, nurse managers will develop goals and objectives that

1. Address increased automation of nursing information systems.
2. Project changes that will occur in nursing products and services.
3. Project the organization and types of employees that will be needed for changed products and services.
4. Trace trends in the corporate culture: values, cultural rituals, social processes, and learning patterns of clients and employees.
5. Address the retraining of employees in outmoded jobs.
6. Explore future leads through content analysis, trends extrapolation forecasting, simulation forecasting, modeling, scenario projection, and trend impact analysis. These complex techniques can improve forecasting.
7. Assess new management techniques that include open work systems, quality of work life programs, quality circles, and participatory management techniques.
8. Promote job security and career development, including management of nurses who are "fast burners," or stars, the top 5 percent to 10 percent of the nursing force.
9. Lower barriers to women, minorities, older workers, new workers, and immigrants.
10. Keep employees updated in knowledge and skills and provide more resources to learning and development.
11. Develop policies to deal with dual careers of employees, changing careers and life values, changes in the work ethic related to personal and leisure activities, downgrading and demoting employees.[15] The implication for those responsible for the staff development are varied, comprehensive, and demanding.
12. Are futuristic. What services can nurses provide as product lines? Some examples are services to customers desiring help with filing claims and appealing decisions of third-party payers and a clinical nursing consultation service.

HRD planning should create a climate for the personal growth of learners, who should be included in the planning. The organizational structure should be planned to encourage member participation, goal understanding and acceptance, the seeking and sharing of information, the handling of disagreement and conflict, participation in decision making, an atmosphere that encourages expression of feelings, and leadership.[16]

Planning should provide for time to do the job because time is a precious human resource that must be protected.[17] In nursing, the HRD program should encourage nurse managers to understand and decide which programs will support the business strategy of the organization. Strategic plans will provide for the development of employees to maintain and upgrade competence, leading to increased productivity. Exhibit 4–2 provides an example. Phases and stages in the process of strategic planning are summarized in Exhibit 5–3 in chapter 5.

Exhibit 4–2 Scenario

HRD. To develop long-range (strategic) plans for the long-term care facility, the administrator involved representatives of all levels and all departments at a series of meetings at which long-range goals were defined. Physicians were included. These goals were catego-

rized by top managers, and the organized list was integrated into a master plan that included budgetary projections and key personnel responsibilities. After ratification by the board of trustees, the plan was publicized and implementation begun.

Operational Human Resource Planning

Planning encompasses the writing of personnel policies that will assist in recruiting and maintaining a qualified staff. Data to help develop these policies will need to be collected and analyzed in cooperation with the human resource division and representatives of the entire nursing staff. Nursing management has an ethical responsibility to inform nurses about needed information compiled on them and to ensure that only needed information is retained. This information should be used to develop jobs and to recruit, select, assign, retain, and promote nursing personnel based on individual qualifications and capabilities and without regard to race, sex, creed, or color. The information will be used to develop personnel policies to classify personnel according to competence and to establish salary scales commensurate with qualifications and positions of comparable responsibility within the community and agency. Written copies of personnel policies, job descriptions, and job standards will be made available to all nursing personnel.

Model of HRM

Strategic human resource management (SHRM) is the process of building a human organization that makes a business successful. SHRM integrates HRM with the strategic needs of the firm. SHRM includes the components of policies, culture, values, and practices that are linked or integrated across levels of the organization. The 5-P Model of SHRM of Schuler includes philosophy, policies, programs, practices, and processes systematically linked to the strategic needs of the organization (see Exhibit 4–3).

HRM is linked to the organization's strategic plan for survival, growth, adaptability, and profitability. To apply Schuler's 5-P Model of SHRM to nursing, one should do the following:

1. Take on the HR philosophy—look at statements of business values of nursing. Also, look at the culture of the organization regarding empowerment, training and education, teamwork, careers, and values. This culture includes all activities affecting the behavior of workers in their efforts to formulate and implement the strategic needs important to the success of the business, the participatory processes needed to link HR practices and strategy, a systematic and analytical mindset, and opportunity for HR departments to impact through strategic initiatives.

ORGANIZATIONAL STRATEGY

Initiates the process of identifying strategic business needs and provides specific qualities to them

| INTERNAL CHARACTERISTICS | EXTERNAL CHARACTERISTICS |

STRATEGIC BUSINESS NEEDS

Expressed in mission statements or vision statements and translated into strategic business objectives

STRATEGIC HUMAN RESOURCES MANAGEMENT ACTIVITIES

Human Resources Philosophy
Expressed in statements defining business values and culture

} **Expresses** how to treat and value people

Human Resources Policies
Expressed as shared values (guidelines)

} **Establishes** guidelines for action on people-related business issues and HR programs

Human Resources Programs
Articulated as human resources strategies

} **Coordinates** efforts to facilitate change to address major people-related business issues

Human Resources Practices
For leadership, managerial, and operational roles

} **Motivates** needed role behaviors

Human Resources Processes
For the formulation and implementation of other activities

} **Defines** how these activities are carried out

Source: R. S. Schuler, "Strategic Human Resources Management: Linking the People with the Strategic Needs of the Business," *Organizational Dynamics* (1992): 20. © 1992 American Management Association, New York. All rights reserved.

2. Adopt HR policies—link the HR philosophy with particular people-related business needs.
3. Follow HR programs—make changes needed to effect strategic business needs. HR programs may be HR strategies.
4. Use HR practices—provide leadership, managerial, and operational practices. Cue and reinforce role performance. Leadership involves establishing direction, aligning people, motivating and inspiring individuals, and causing dramatic and useful change. Management involves planning, directing, delegating, organizing, and coordinating. Operational involves delivering services and making products.
5. Use HR processes—combine interaction of strategic education with line management. Promote empowerment, ownership, and participation.[18]

An SHRM system has two general responsibilities:

1. Competence management—use the skills needed to execute given organizational strategy: competence acquisition, utilization, retention, and displacement.
2. Behavior management—control activities to control employee behavior leading to organization goals and coordinate individuals to support organizational strategy.

"A good theory enables one to both predict what will happen given a set of values for certain variables, and to [sic] understand why this predicted value should result."[19] Traditionally, HRM has been viewed as the aggregate of practices of managing people in organizations: selection, training, appraisal, and rewards. Strategic human resource management (SHRM) is "the pattern of planned human resource deployments and activities intended to enable an organization to achieve its goals." SHRM links HRM practices, the strategic management process, and coordination or congruence among the various HRM practices. Theory of HRM models is a recent movement of the past ten to fifteen years. It is subject to consistent, rigorous empirical tests. SHRM theory is grounded in the theory of organizations.[20]

ANDRAGOGY

In HRD and staff development, learners are adults, and educational programs are based on theories of adult education. Andragogy is a concept and theory of adult education based upon assumptions about adults as learners. According to Knowles, the concept is a behavioral one and incorporates the following beliefs:[21]

1. The adult learner needs to be self-directing and treated with respect.
2. An environment needs to be established that allows adults to participate in making decisions affecting their lives.
3. Since adults have experiences to share with others, experiential techniques should be a part of adult education. Because adults are more closed to new concepts, they need to be "unfrozen."

4. Adults should be able to immediately apply what they learn. Learning should relate to doing something or learning a skill.
5. Social role development determines the adult's readiness to learn.
6. Adults go through a sequence of learning.

Knowles recommends the construction of a six-point process design for adult learners to produce a content design as follows:[22]

1. Self-directed mutual planning by the adult learners.
2. Creation of a social climate that is an adult learning environment: informal, comfortable, friendly, caring; each student is treated as a unique individual and is listened to.
3. Diagnosis of needs: students' needs plus teacher's needs plus negotiation leads to successful learning.
4. Sequential learning experiences: follow the problem-solving process with sequence, continuity, and unity.
5. Construction of a training plan of self-directing activities that meet objectives. The teacher acts as facilitator.
6. Evaluation to redirect learning: identify competencies → assess level of competence → identify gaps in competence as needs that motivate learners → raise level of competency to reduce gaps.

Adult education reflects lifelong learning and is well-established in our society and in nursing. Since staff development in nursing relates to adults, it should follow the precepts of adult learning.

Exercise 4–3   Describe those learning activities in your life that are self-directed. Decide where you want to expand your self-directed learning, and make a plan for doing so. List knowledge and skills you wish to acquire as a citizen, an employee, and an individual.

Teaching Adult Patients

Writing on the topic of teaching adult patients, Goodwin-Johansson notes the increasing number of adult patients. She states that education is an integral part of the health care of adult patients, the goal being the achievement, maintenance, and protection of health. She describes patient education as "planned combinations of learning activities designed to help people who had experience with illness make changes in their behavior conducive to good health."[23] The conduct of hospitals affects application of the principles of andragogy.

Providers expect patients to be compliant rather than choose their own goals and learning experiences. The patient has decreased energy and will for risk taking, as opposed to being involved in solving problems, making immediate application of treatments, and participating voluntarily. The patient is surrounded by experts, with staff controlling the patient's time schedule. The patient faces such social barriers as involuntary attendance, rules that limit freedom, decreased geographic boundaries, decreased privacy, and decreased personal identity. These conditions prevent the exercise of such adult education principles as taking into account life experiences, having a teacher who functions as a facilitator rather than as an authority, and individualization.[24]

Facilitators of adult education should be technically proficient, effective leaders who engender images of interpersonal skills of caring, trust, and encouragement. Also, they need instructional planning skills that include needs assessment, context analysis, setting educational objectives, organizing learning activities, and evaluation. They also need teaching and learning skills that produce a favorable educational climate and offer teaching and learning interactions that provide challenge, closure, practice, feedback, and reinforcement. They should make learners think critically and reflectively.[25]

Adult educators respect learners. They mediate between information and individuals, organize opportunities, and stimulate learners. Adult educators exercise patience in coaching learners to take control of learning tasks. They may have to assist learners to "unlearn." As they relinquish control, they praise and communicate, motivate with deeds rather than words, control intimidation of students, and are always concerned with what is right.[26]

Adult education enriches one's life, as more education leads to better employment. To pursue higher education is a personal decision that can be advanced by management. Completion of the bachelor of science in nursing (BSN) by associate degree in nursing (ADN) or diploma graduates is an example. Research has validated the fact that increased productivity comes from investing in people and their education.

TYPOLOGIES AND TAXONOMIES OF ADULT EDUCATION

Various typologies and taxonomies exist in education. The most commonly known taxonomies, or classifications, are the taxonomies of educational objectives addressed to cognitive, affective, and psychomotor domains. Taxonomies and typologies help to connect the parts of an educational system, clarify the field, serve as a basis for allocating resources, design curricula, and eliminate duplication. Several taxonomies and typologies of adult education exist, including that of Rachal, who has proposed his typology of adult education based on six major types and their subtypes (see Exhibit 4–4):[27]

1. Liberal: individual or group structured study of humanities, arts, and sciences where there is free inquiry, curiosity, and intellectual growth. Such studies include university lecture series, Great Decisions programs, Great Books programs, reading circles, and writing clubs.
2. Occupational: technological changes.
3. Self-help: knowledge, information, skills, or recreational learning related to adjusting to the environment.
4. Compensatory: knowledge to meet new standards and to combat illiteracy, including adult basic education (ABE) and adult secondary education (ASE).
5. Scholastic: graduate study and research.

Exhibit 4–4 Typology of Adult Education

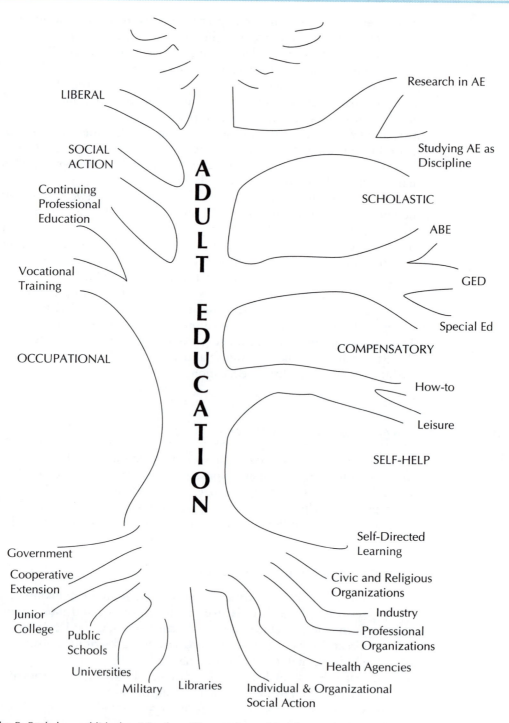

LIBERAL

SOCIAL
ACTION

Continuing
Professional
Education

Vocational
Training

OCCUPATIONAL

A
D
U
L
T

E
D
U
C
A
T
I
O
N

Research in AE

Studying AE as
Discipline

SCHOLASTIC

ABE

GED

Special Ed

COMPENSATORY

How-to

Leisure

SELF-HELP

Self-Directed
Learning

Government

Cooperative
Extension

Junior
College

Public
Schools

Universities

Military   Libraries

Civic and Religious
Organizations

Industry

Professional
Organizations

Health Agencies

Individual & Organizational
Social Action

Source: John R. Rachal, unpublished revision from "Taxonomies and Typologies of Adult Education," *Lifelong Learning* 12, no.
2 (1988): 20–23. Reprinted with permission of John R. Rachal.

6. Social action: peace education, environmental education, drug education, and the fostering of understanding of major public issues. Since social action is, by definition, political, the adult educator would describe rather than prescribe and would focus on the educative rather than the political orientation of the social action agents.

Exercise 4–4   Application of brainstorming technique (also see chapter on committees). As a group technique, brainstorming seeks to develop creativity by free association of ideas. The object is to generate as many ideas as possible. All members of the group should respond positively. A member must never criticize the suggestions of another member, because this stifles free expression of ideas.

1. Have the following materials available:
   poster pad (or chalkboard)
   marker pen (or chalk)
   masking tape
2. Select any current topic of interest to the group that presents problems for which the group can create solutions. If the group has no topic, it could discuss one of the following ideas:
   Principles of adult learning (andragogy) as they are being practiced in the group workplace.
   Middle management needs to be eliminated in health-care organizations.
   There is no such thing as a lifetime job anymore.
3. Plan a one-hour session. Elect a facilitator and a recorder for the group. The facilitator (a) explains the process and the topic to the group, (b) tells members to say whatever comes into their mind as quickly as possible, (3) manages criticism by one member of another, and (4) encourages free expression of ideas throughout the process. Everyone is encouraged to participate; the wilder the ideas, the better.
4. The recorder writes the ideas on the poster pad. The goal is to get as many ideas as possible. If ideas fit together, the recorder combines them. When a page is filled, the recorder tears it off and tapes it to the wall or some other visible place.
5. After 45 minutes have elapsed, the facilitator uses the remaining time to evaluate the ideas. All ideas are evaluated positively, and the group decides how to proceed with the outcomes.

HUMAN CAPITAL

An emerging theory for HRD is that employees are human capital who can be treated as assets because they have high economic value. In a technological world, human beings' assets are their knowledge and skills, which depreciate as new technology emerges. Employers invest in their human capital by providing

HRD programs in the form of staff development and continuing education. "Human capital economics is a system of inputs, processes, outputs, and adjustments which individuals, firms, government agencies, institutions, and societies make toward the increases of potential and performance which the individual human or humans as groups may contribute to society, the economy, specific employers, or themselves."[28]

In nursing, the inputs are newly employed nurses who come to organizations with a continuum of assets, such as specialty certification, graduate education, certification in life support systems, and skills in management, teaching, and research.

Processes provided by management include orientation, internships, preceptorships, staff development, certification, and continuing education. Self-directed continuing education, including courses and reading, add to the RN's assets. All of these processes lead to adaptation and growth, maintaining and increasing the value of the RN's assets.

Outputs of this system of management of human capital are competence, specialists, profits or return on equity, and value added to the human assets. Adjustments include retraining as new jobs emerge and rehabilitation after lapses in employment. Human capital—professional nurses—are kept valuable through HRD programs that promote motivation or job satisfaction.

Odiorne indicates that community colleges are a proven investment in human capital because their products increase the personal disposable income of people who complete college courses. Education promotes upward mobility. Educated citizens are informed citizens who make better citizenship decisions. Investment in education by minorities leads to increased social status. Investment in human capital increases capital promotion through increased earnings.[29]

A Typology for HRD of Personnel

Odiorne suggests a four-category typology for HRD of personnel: stars, workhorses, problems, and deadwood. He suggests training each group separately as follows:[30]

Stars.   These are a small group of personnel with high potential whose performance lives up to that potential. Managers should educate stars to increase performance and develop their potential once they have been identified by assessment center method, review board method, or staff analysis method.

Top managers still pick successors like themselves with perceived star qualities, such as adaptability to change, company and career orientation, ability to manage self-expression, lateral and upward mobility, dedication, loyalty, adaptivity, quiet differentiation, early achievement, ability to work in a web of tensions, gamesmanship, flexibility, and ability to generalize.

The star of the future will be surrounded by technology, be comfortable with high-level decision making and problem analysis, do less traveling, have more span of control over work, and be a collaborative group leader. Future stars will also be innovative. On their way to stardom, they will acquire a master's degree in business administration (MBA), use skills, be creative, create new jobs, and be entrepreneurs in technology, engineers, and scientists. They will appreciate the liberal arts as the accumulated knowledge of civilization. Future stars will have skills of rational thought, decision making, problem solving, ethical evaluation, communication, knowledge of government, and special education and experiences. Future stars will be trained by stars as mentors who are goal oriented, are superior performers, behave to be imitated, support and help, delegate responsibility, give feedback, exhibit positive attitudes, mentor women and minorities, are sponsors, and provide support groups. Some nurses are stars inculcated with the success ethic. Nursing leaders can develop HRD programs that will provide the ingredients.

Workhorses.   These persons can be trained to improve their performance. They can be motivated using theories of Maslow, McGregor, and Herzberg, among others. They should be well paid for their work, participate in decision making by merging personal and organizational goals, and be provided with job enrichment. Organizational development will motivate workhorses through job design, working conditions, increased variety of tools, development of higher skills, assignment of increased responsibility, job rotation, content change, and team competition. Workhorses thrive on HRD programs that provide for personal growth, self-fulfillment, and use of abilities to perform meaningful work in a pleasant workplace.

Problems.   Problem employees exhibit undesirable behavior that can be corrected by remedial training. They may exhibit emotional outbursts or immaturity, ignore important things, be overcome by trivia, be slow to respond to change, retain obsolete ideas and procedures, treat people unfairly, enforce rules too rigidly, retain authority, fail to communicate, be too lax, and lack sense of timing and the ability to anticipate. To avoid or remedy their poor performance, training should be preceded by specifying performance standards, removing obstacles to success, providing the needed training, providing favorable consequences for doing right, providing feedback, encouraging self-control, and helping them with their personal problems.

Deadwood.   These are workers who do not respond to training or developmental discipline. They should be fired, using appropriate human resource procedures. Not only are they nonproductive, but also they negatively influence personnel who are workhorses and problems.

Nurse managers may want to turn workhorses into stars. This will require need and drive on the part of the workhorse. It has been tried at Bell Laboratories and Dupont Company with considerable success. Stars say the most important skills include technical competence and taking initiative to go beyond basic job duties.[31]

THE FUTURE

Strategic HRD will envision future change so that the quality of work life and standard of living for nursing personnel will continue to improve into the next century. This will include proactive involvement of nurses in the formulation of health-care policy. Nursing leaders need to communicate the needs of the future, including skills and job requirements.[32]

Electronic technology is intrusive, and as it becomes more intensive, it will increase time-based stress. This will be an area for further research, including reaction to demands on time and the social influences of electronic technology intrusion.[33]

The positive approach to the twenty-first century is echoed by Naisbitt and Aburdene, who view the future as providing more upward mobility for women and minorities as they gain credentials and tenure. An abundance of good jobs will be available for which people will be educated and trained. Two million new jobs—managerial, administrative, and technical—will be created annually. The entire workforce must be upgraded constantly. More people will start their own businesses, or they will become highly skilled professionals who will not be managed authoritatively. "The dominant principle of organization has shifted, from management in order to control an enterprise to leadership in order to bring out the best in people and to respond quickly to change."[34]

The primary challenge of leadership in the 1990s is to encourage the new, better-educated worker to be more entrepreneurial, self-managing, and oriented toward lifelong learning. Leaders will coach, inspire, and gain people's commitment. They will set personal examples of excellence. Leaders will manage to bring out the best in people and respond quickly to change. They will encourage self-management, autonomous teams, and entrepreneurial units. Leaders will move people in a direction without carrying them. They will inspire loyalty by giving it. Leaders will create vision and sell it to their constituents. They will be ethical, open, empowering, and inspiring as teachers, counselors, and facilitators who will keep people excited by managing accelerated change.

In their book *Megatrends 2000,* Naisbitt and Aburdene propose the following *millenial* trends:[35]

1. The Booming Global Economy of the 1990's
2. A Renaissance in the Arts
3. The Emergence of Free-Market Socialism
4. Global Lifestyles and Cultural Nationalism
5. The Privatization of the Welfare State
6. The Rise of the Pacific Rim
7. The Decade of Women in Leadership
8. The Age of Biology
9. The Religious Revival of the New Millennium
10. The Triumph of the Individual

Exercise 4–5   Application of nominal group technique (also see chapter on committees). The nominal group process is a method for structuring a group meeting to obtain a large number of ideas from the group and to order and set priorities for those ideas.

1. Supplies needed:
   pencils or pens and paper or 5×8 file cards
   poster pad or chalkboard
   marker pen or chalk
   masking tape
2. Choose a topic of interest to the group or discuss the following idea: Professional nurses have limited autonomy and empowerment.
3. Time required: one and one-half to two hours
4. Elect a leader or facilitator to define the process and assign the topic to the group.
5. Give each member a pencil or pen and a sheet of paper or a 5×8 file card. Ask everyone to write down all possible ideas about the assigned topic. Allow five to ten minutes.
6. Have each group member present an idea, one at a time, to the group until all lists are exhausted. Do not allow discussion at this point. If an idea occurs to a group member as another is speaking, that person can add the idea to the bottom of his or her list to be shared later.
7. The leader or facilitator writes all ideas on the poster pad or chalkboard as they are shared, according to the following rules:
   a. No discussion or evaluation of ideas during the round-robin sharing and listing on the poster pad.
   b. No debate about equivalency of ideas. All are written on the chart even if they appear to be the same or closely related to another on the chart.
   c. No rewording of an idea while it is being listed on the chart.
   d. No talking out of turn. If the process suggests a new idea to an individual, that person can give the idea at his or her next turn.
8. As pad pages fill up, they are torn off and taped to the wall or other surface so they can be seen by group members.
9. Once all ideas are listed, each recorded idea is discussed for clarification, elaboration, defense, and evaluation. New items can be added or categories suggested for ideas.
10. After all ideas are discussed, the group votes on and gives priority to each idea.
11. The results are averaged, and the final group decision is taken from the pool and prescribed to the appropriate entity for implementation.

WEB ACTIVITIES

- Visit www.jbpub.com/swansburg, this text's companion website on the Internet, for further information on Introduction to Theory of Human Resource Development.
- Search for Human Resources as a topic, what can you find?
- What resources are listed on the Internet for andragogy?

SUMMARY

As the clinical practice discipline of nursing evolves, so does the concept of wholeness. Staff development thus becomes a component of the larger domain of human resource development. Business and industry leaders have found that productivity is positively influenced by a focus on development of personnel to their fullest potential. As a consequence, the assembly lines in factories have given way to self-directed work teams. Given responsibility for making decisions and accomplishing the organization's mission, employees rise to fulfill expectations.

The new management practice eliminates middle management and places trust in the worker. With this trust, workers are energized and are empowered by the autonomy, the control they have over the productive work of the enterprise.

Workers learn to work in teams and to rotate within the group roles, including being able to perform several jobs. They learn to support each other and to respect the varied talents of individual team members.

Adult education, or andragogy, is the process by which employees are kept updated to achieve both the goals of the organization and their own personal goals. It is also the process by which they develop their roles as citizens and benefit themselves, society, and the organization for which they work.

People are viewed and valued as human capital. As technology advances, they depreciate in knowledge capacity and ability to perform their jobs. Adult education as staff development is an investment that keeps human value from depreciating. This entire process represents the science of behavioral technology. Satisfied employees achieve organizational and personal objectives, satisfy customers, and make an organization successful. Included in the science of behavioral technology are such theories as decision making, decentralization and participatory management, leadership, motivation, and the growing need for adult education that maintains the human capital and keeps the organization productive. The theory of HRD will be developed further in succeeding chapters.

NOTES

1. J. Naisbitt and P. Aburdene, *Megatrends 2000* (New York: William Morrow & Company, 1990), 16.
2. P. A. Strassman and S. Zuboff, "Conversation with Paul A. Strassman," *Organizational Dynamics,* fall 1985, 19–34; A. J. Rutigliano, "Naisbitt & Aburdene on 'Re-Inventing' the Workplace," *Management Review,* October 1985, 33–35.
3. M. Beer, B. Spector, P. R. Lawrence, D. Q. Mills, and R. E. Walton, *Managing Human Assets* (New York: The Free Press, 1984).
4. P. D. Carter, "Revitalizing Society: Practicing Human Resource Development Through the Life Span," *Lifelong Learning: An Omnibus of Practice and Research* vol. 11, no. 6 (1988): 27–31.
5. M. Beer et al., op. cit., 43.
6. M. L. Hammerman, "Adult Learning in Self-Help Mutual/Aid Support Groups," *Lifelong Learning: An Omnibus of Practice and Research* vol. 12, no. 1 (1988): 25–27, 30.

7. J. Naisbitt and P. Aburdene, op. cit.

8. J. S. Lublin, "Trying to Increase Worker Productivity, More Employers Alter Management Style," *The Wall Street Journal,* 14 February 1992, B1, B7.

9. P. D. Carter, op. cit.; M. S. Knowles, *The Modern Practice of Adult Education* (New York: Associated Press, 1980).

10. D. Cassivi, "The Education of Adults: Maintaining a Legacy," *Lifelong Learning: An Omnibus of Practice and Research* vol. 12, no. 5 (1989): 8–10.

11. M. L. Hammerman, op. cit.

12. B. L. Wells and S. C. Padgitt, "Timebinds: Mediating Organizational and Professional Role Expectations of the Adult Educator," *Lifelong Learning: An Omnibus of Practice and Research* vol. 12, no. 7 (1989): 22–25.

13. E. J. Metz, "The Missing 'H' in Strategic Planning," *Managerial Planning,* May/June 1984, 19–23, 29.

14. E. C. Smith, "How to Tie Human Resource Planning to Strategic Business Planning," *Managerial Planning,* September–October 1983, 29–34.

15. E. J. Metz, op. cit.

16. D. Cassivi, op. cit.

17. B. L. Wells and S. C. Padgitt, op. cit.

18. R. S. Schuler, "Strategic Human Resources Management: Linking the People with the Strategic Needs of the Business," *Organizational Dynamics,* summer 1992, 18–22.

19. P. M. Wright and G. C. McMahan, "Theoretical Perspectives for Strategic Human Resource Management," *Journal of Management* 18, no. 2 (1992): 295–320.

20. Ibid.

21. M. S. Knowles, "Gearing Adult Education for the Seventies," *Journal of Continuing Education in Nursing,* May 1970, 11–17.

22. Ibid.

23. C. Goodwin-Johansson, "Educating the Adult Patient," *Lifelong Learning: An Omnibus of Practice and Research.* vol. 11, no. 7, 1988, 10–13.

24. Ibid.

25. M. W. Galbraith, "Essential Skills for the Facilitator of Adult Learning," *Lifelong Learning: An Omnibus of Practice and Research* 12, no. 6 (1989): 10–13.

26. D. Cassivi, op. cit.

27. J. Rachal, "Taxonomies and Typologies of Adult Education," *Lifelong Learning: An Omnibus of Adult Education* vol. 12, no. 2, 1988, 20–23.

28. G. S. Odiorne, *Strategic Management of Human Resources* (San Francisco: Jossey-Bass, 1984), 5.

29. Ibid.

30. Ibid.

31. J. E. Rigdon, "Using New Kinds of Corporate Alchemy, Some Firms Turn Lesser Lights into Stars," *The Wall Street Journal,* 3 May 1993, B1, B13.

32. M. Beer et al. op. cit.

33. M. L. Wells and S. C. Padgitt, op. cit.

34. J. Naisbitt and P. Aburdene, op. cit., 218.

THE PLANNING PROCESS

OBJECTIVES

- Define planning.
- Discuss and differentiate among examples of the purposes of planning.
- Discuss and differentiate among examples of the characteristics of planning.
- Discuss and differentiate among examples of the elements of planning.
- Describe the strategic planning process.
- Describe operational planning.
- Differentiate between examples of strategic and tactical planning.
- Write a business plan.

KEY CONCEPTS

planning
strategic planning
functional planning
operational planning
business plan

Manager Behavior: Develops operational and strategic plans for the agency and makes them available for personnel.

Leader Behavior: Solicits input from personnel in making and using operational and strategic plans for the agency.

WHAT IS PLANNING?

Planning, a basic function of management, is a principal duty of all managers. It is a systematic process and requires knowledgeable activity based on sound managerial theory. The first element of management defined by Fayol was planning, which he defined as making a plan of action to provide for the foreseeable future. This plan of action must have unity, continuity, flexibility, and precision. Fayol outlined the contents of a plan of action for his business, a large mining and metallurgical firm. The plan included annual and ten-year forecasts, taking advantage of input from others. Planning improves with experience, gives sequence in activity, and protects a business against undesirable changes. Fayol's concept was that planning facilitates wise use of resources and selection of the best approaches to achieving objectives. Planning facilitates the art of handling people. It requires moral courage, since it can fail. Effective planning requires continuity of tenure. Good planning is a sign of competence.[1]

Urwick wrote that research in administration provides needed information for forecasting. According to Urwick, investigations should be carried out and their results expressed in terms of the concrete. Planning should be based on objectives that should be framed in terms of making a product or providing a service for the community. Simplification and standardization are basic to sound planning procedures. The product or service should be of the right pattern. Planning provides information to coordinate work effectively and accurately. A good plan should be based on an objective, be simple, have standards, be flexible, be balanced, and use available resources first.[2]

Planning is a continuous process, beginning with the setting of goals and objectives and then laying out a plan of action for accomplishing them, putting them into play, reviewing the process and the outcomes, providing feedback to personnel, and modifying plans as needed. As planning is put into action, the management functions of organizing, leading, and evaluating are implemented, making all management functions interdependent.

Planning is a thinking or mental process of decision making and forecasting. It is future oriented and ensures desirable probable outcomes. Planning involves determining objectives and strategies, programs, procedures, and rules to accomplish the objectives.[3] In nursing, planning helps to ensure that clients or patients will receive the nursing services they want and need and that these services are delivered by satisfied nursing workers.

Purposes of Planning

The following are some reasons for planning:[4]

1. Planning increases the chances of success by focusing on results, not on activities.
2. It forces analytic thinking and evaluation of alternatives, therefore improving decisions.
3. It establishes a framework for decision making that is consistent with top management objectives.
4. It orients people to action instead of reaction.
5. It includes day-to-day and future-focused managing.
6. It helps to avoid crisis management and provides decision-making flexibility.
7. It provides a basis for managing organizational and individual performance.
8. It increases employee involvement and improves communication.
9. It is cost-effective.

Among the activities of planning that Douglass addresses are assessment by collection, classification, analysis, interpretation, and translation of data; strategic planning; development of standards; identification of needs and priority setting; management by objectives; and formulation of policies, rules, regulations, methods, and procedures.[5]

Donovan wrote that planning has several benefits, among which are satisfactory outcomes of decisions; improved functions in emergencies; assurance of economy of time, space, and materials; and the highest use of personnel. She included decision making, philosophies, and objectives as key elements in planning.[6]

Characteristics of Planning

What is the nature of planning? What is so distinctive about it that requires a nurse to have the knowledge and skills requisite to engage in planning? In an environment of changing technology, mounting costs, and multiple activities, a need exists for professional nurses to plan. The forecasting of events and the laying out of a system of activities or actions for accomplishing the work of nursing and of the organization are prerequisites to success. Koontz and Weihrich define planning as "selecting missions and objectives and the actions to achieve them; [planning] requires decision making, that is, choosing future courses of action from among alternatives."[7] They viewed planning as an elementary function of management. In planning, the nurse would avoid leaving events to chance; she or he would apply an intellectual process to consciously determining the course of action to take in accomplishing work. Donovan stated that the planning process must be deliberate and analytic to produce carefully detailed programs of action that will achieve objectives.[8]

The nurse manager plans effectively to create an environment in which nursing personnel will provide the nursing care desired and needed by clients. In such an environment, clinical nurses will make decisions about the form or modality of practice, and nurse managers will work with nursing personnel to establish and meet their personal objectives while meeting the objectives of the organization.

According to Hodgetts, planning forces a firm to forecast the environment, gives direction in the form of objectives, provides the basis for teamwork, and helps management to learn to live with ambiguity.[9] It should be comprehensive, with professional nurses carefully determining objectives and making detailed plans to accomplish them. All managers and representative clinical nurses should provide input into strategic planning, and every unit should have a strategic plan.

Planning involves the collection, analysis, and organization of many kinds of data (the how) that will be used to determine both the nursing care needs of patients and the management plans that will provide the resources and processes to meet those needs.

The following are some of the kinds of data that will need to be collected and analyzed for planning purposes:

1. Daily average patient census.
2. Bed capacity and percentage of occupancy.
3. Average length of stay.
4. Number of births.
5. Number of operations.
6. Trends in patient populations.
   a. Diagnoses.
   b. Age groups.

  c. Acuity of illness.
  d. Physical dependency.
 7. Trends in technology.
  a. Diagnostic procedures.
  b. Therapeutic procedures.
 8. Environmental analysis.
  a. Forces impacting upon nursing from within: availability of nurses, turnover, other departments, delivery systems including nursing modalities, theory-based practice, and physicians.
  b. Forces impacting upon nursing from without: government, education, accreditation bodies, third-party payers, and others.
  c. Trends in health care and in nursing, including changes in characteristics.
  d. Threats to the nursing profession.
  e. Opportunities for the nursing profession.

Exhibit 5–1 gives examples of data that might be collected and analyzed for planning purposes by nursing managers.

Data on diagnostic and therapeutic procedures will be used to plan for new procedures, to revise old procedures, and to make new procedures known to nursing personnel. The preceding is certainly not an exhaustive list of sources of data that will be used for planning purposes, and other sources are listed in this chapter.

Exercise 5–1   With case management and disease management becoming common roles for professional nurses,[10] identify and list the kinds of data used in planning for such management. Use the internet to obtain a database for management of clinical outcomes.

Exhibit 5–1   Planning Data for Nurse Managers

- Live births have decreased 30 percent in the three years since the institution of a family planning program.
- Sixty-three percent of live births are discharged within a 24-hour period.
- The number of deliveries with complications has increased from 210 to 257 in one year.
- A new cardiac catheterization laboratory has been completed.
- The hospital planning board has decided to coordinate with other hospitals in the area to consolidate specialty services for newborn care, cardiovascular surgery, and neuroscience services.

- Enrollment of students for clinical nursing affiliation has increased from 450 to 792 in one year.
- Enrollment of students in the nursing cooperative education program has increased from 102 to 187 students.
- Medicare reimbursement pays $__ per patient for days of home care.
- Early discharge has decreased average daily census from 381 to 304.
- Patient acuity has increased by 0.6 percent points overall.

Planning a dynamic, organizational process, has the characteristics of an open system. It leads to success rather than failure. It prevents crisis and panic, which are costly, unrealistic, chaotic, distorting of achievement, and dominated by a single person. Planning thus improves nursing division performance. It identifies future opportunities and expectations based on conditions through forecasting techniques that range from simple to complex. Simple forecasting techniques follow the process of gathering data and analyzing them to determine alternative decisions and the effects each decision will produce. Strengths, weaknesses, opportunities, and threats are part of this analysis, which leads to decision, choice, and implementation. In complex forecasting, computer-based mathematical models are available that are becoming less expensive, require a lot of time and specialized skills, and extend from three to fifteen years. New simulation models are constantly improving and are essential to modern planning.

Planning is viewed as resting on logical, reflective thinking that is neither cast in concrete nor all-encompassing. If needed, leadership or top management will effect change to undertake effective planning. It will obtain input from all levels to ensure success through format, procedures, time frames, maintenance, and input review.

Planning is the key element of nursing that gives the profession direction, cohesion, and thrust. It causes all nursing personnel to focus on goals and objectives and stimulates their motivation. Through the planning process, nurse managers select and retain the elements of past and present plans that work. They focus on the future, and they implement and evaluate. Thus, they successfully manage nursing personnel and material resources to achieve the objectives of the nursing enterprise.

Elements of Planning

While planning is characterized as being a conceptual or thinking process, it produces readily identifiable specific elements or constituents, including written statements of mission or purpose, philosophy, objectives, and detailed management or operational plans—the blueprints by which the purpose, philosophy, and objectives are put into measurable actions. Management or operational plans include decision-making and problem-solving processes. They include strategies, policies, and procedures.

Planning includes assessment of the nursing agency's strengths and weaknesses, covering factors that affect performance and facilitate or inhibit the achievement of objectives. This assessment process will have objectives of its own, both long-range and short-range. As an example, if the clinical promotion ladder is a strength in nurse retention but is weakly applied by selective nurse managers, the problem can be addressed by written objectives.

Planning entails writing specific, useful, realistic objectives (the why) that will reflect both strategic and operational goals for the agency and its personnel. Objectives become the reasons for an operational nursing management plan (the what) that will detail the activities to be performed, the target dates or time frames for their accomplishment (the when), the persons responsible for accomplishing them (the who), and strategies for dealing with technical, economic, social, and political aspects. These operational plans will have control systems for monitoring performance and providing feedback. They will address the budget. Objectives and operational plans are discussed in detail in chapter 6.

Good management, according to Meier,[11]

> starts with a coordinated purposeful organization of people who collectively on a functional responsibility basis are responsible for:
>
> 1. Setting objectives
> 2. Planning strategy
> 3. Setting goals—short-term objectives
> 4. Developing company philosophy
> 5. Setting policies—the plan
> 6. Planning the organization
> 7. Providing personnel
> 8. Establishing procedures
> 9. Providing facilities
> 10. Providing capital
> 11. Setting performance standards
> 12. Development of management information systems
> 13. Activating people.

Good management keeps the nursing agency successful, ensuring its growth, success, and direction and a return on investment in the future.

Exercise 5–2	Write a summary of a nursing or health-care agency that describes its work, the volume of products and services, marketing activities, trends, financial summary, and impact upon employees.

STRATEGIC PLANNING

Nursing administrators can increase effectiveness through strategic panning, which can promote professional nursing practice and the long-range goals of the organization and the division of nursing. Drucker defines strategic planning as "a continuous, systematic process of making risk-taking decisions today with the greatest possible knowledge of their effects on the future; organizing efforts necessary to carry out these decisions and evaluating results of these decisions against expected outcome through reliable feedback mechanisms."[12]

Strategic planning in nursing is concerned with what nursing should be doing. Its purpose is to improve allocation of scarce resources, including time and money, and to manage the agency for performance. Strategic planning provides strategic forecasting from one year up to more than twenty years. It should involve top nurse managers and representatives of all levels of nursing management and practice. It will include analysis of such factors as projected technological advances, the internal and external environments, the nursing and health-care market and industry, the economics of nursing and health care, availability of human and material resources, and judgments of top management.[13]

In today's world, the strategic planning process is used to acquire and develop new health-care services and product lines, including new nursing services and products. Strategic planning is also used to divest outdated services and products. Both activities present moral and ethical dilemmas for the managers and practitioners of nursing. Strategic planning can foster better goals, better corporate values, and better communication about corporate direction. It can lead to changes in operating management and organization. Strategic planning can produce better management strategy and analysis and can forecast and mute external threats.

Odiorne recommends the following process for crafting a strategic plan:[14]

1. Identify the major problems of your organization, determining where you are headed and where you want to be. This is "gap analysis," a technique to examine markets, products, customers, employees, finances, technology, and community relations. Cabinets or task forces from each area may be helpful in doing gap analysis and identifying major problems.
2. Examine outside influences that relate to the key problems of your organization. Focus on the few major issues.
3. List the critical issues—those that affect the entire organization, have long-term impact, and are based on irrefutable evidence rather than media hype.
4. Rank the critical issues according to their importance to your organization and plan accordingly: "must do" and "to do" and "important but not urgent." Then divide them into "success producers" and "failure preventers."
5. Decide the critical issues to all organization managers.
6. Include time in the budget.

Exercise 5–3   Apply this process to personal career planning for yourself. Where and what do you want to be with regard to career in five years? ten years? What obstacles to your goals exist externally and internally? These obstacles might be family, finances, health, employer. List them as critical issues and make a plan to overcome them.

Strategic plans should be developed from the bottom up, the front line where business occurs. The written plan should be shared with everyone, should not be slavishly followed, as it will be constantly affected by change, and should be modified every year.[15]

Exhibit 5–2 lists ways in which strategic planning can be used to improve management. The process of strategic planning has several phases, as summarized in Exhibit 5–3.

Exercise 5–4   Interview a chief executive officer and a chief nurse executive officer of an organization. Determine each one's orientation to strategic planning. Compare the results. Exhibit 5–4 lists some possible interview questions.

Exhibit 5–2 How Strategic Planning Can Be Used to Improve Nursing Management

- To provide accountability and monitoring of performance; to tie merit to performance.
- To set up more formal planning programs and require divisional and unit planning.
- To integrate strategic plans with operational and financial plans.
- To think and concentrate more on strategic issues.
- To improve knowledge of and training in strategic planning.
- To increase top management involvement and commitment.
- To improve focus on competition, market segments, and external factors.
- To improve communication from top administration and nursing management.

- To allow better execution of plans.
- To be more realistic, and less rationalizing and vacillating.
- To improve the development of nursing management strategies.
- To improve the development and communication of nursing management goals.
- To put less emphasis on raw numbers.
- To anticipate the future and plan for it.
- To develop the annual budget.
- To focus on quality outputs that will improve nurse performance and productivity, decrease losses, and increase return on equity.

Exhibit 5–3 Summary of Phases of Strategic Planning Process

PHASE 1 The Mission and the Creed
Develop statements that define the work, the aims, and the character of the division of nursing. These include idea statements of shared values and beliefs. They are called mission (or purpose) and creed (or philosophy) statements and relate to personnel, patients, community, and all other potential customers.

PHASE 2 Data Collection and Analysis
Collect and analyze data about the health-care industry and nursing. Such data should include internal forces that define the work and affect employees, clients, stockholders, and creditors; technological advances; threats; opportunities to improve growth and productivity; external forces, such as competition, communities, government and political issues, and legal requirements; marketing and public relations or image; trends in the physical and social work environments; and communication. Use simple and complex forecasting techniques, including trend lines, group consensus, nominal group process, and a qualitative decision matrix that uses probabilities based on conditions of certainty, risk, and uncertainty. Refer to Chapter 20 Appendix for definitions.

PHASE 3 Assess Strengths and Weaknesses
Define those factors from the data analysis that influence the management of the division of nursing. List them as strengths or opportunities that will facilitate effectiveness and achievement of goals and objectives or as weaknesses or threats that will impede achieving goals and objectives. Define the current position and strength of the unit.

PHASE 4 Goals and Objectives
Write realistic and general statements of goals. Break the goals down into concrete written statements of objectives the division of nursing intends to accomplish in the next three to five years.

PHASE 5 Strategies
Identify untoward conditions that could develop in achieving each objective. Note administrative actions to avoid or manage them. Use this information to modify goals and objectives, making contingency plans for alternative actions. Define the organization needed for doing and implementing strategic plans. It should be interactive if cross-functional activities are involved—a matrix organization.

Exhibit 5–3   Summary of Phases of Strategic Planning Process *(Continued)*

PHASE 6 Timetable
Develop a timetable for accomplishing each objective. Identify by geographic units as well. This phase will produce or become part of the plans.

PHASE 7 Operational and Functional Plans
Provide guidelines or general instructions that lead the functional and operational nurse managers to develop action plans to implement the goals and objectives. These will include detailed actions, policies, practices, communication and feedback, controlling and evaluation plans, budgets, timetables, and persons to be held accountable.

PHASE 8 Implementation
Put the plans to work.

PHASE 9 Evaluation
Provide for formative evaluation reports before, during, and after the operational plan is implemented. Provide for summative evaluation that is quantified. Report actual versus expected results. Frequently evaluate the strategic mission and plan. Provide continuous feedback that can be used to modify and update the plan. Use people who implement the plan to evaluate it.

Exhibit 5–4   Planning Interview Questions

1. Do you have a strategic plan?
2. What length of time does it cover?
3. Who develops it?
4. Who uses it?
5. What products and services will be affected by it?
6. How will it impact professional nurses and nursing?
7. How will they impact it?
8. Can professional nurses initiate new products and services?
9. How will managers be updated?
10. Will products and services be divested?
11. What moral and ethical dilemmas could evolve?
12. What new nursing skills and roles will be needed?
13. How will they be obtained?
14. How does the strategic plan position nursing technically?
15. How does it position nursing as a profitable enterprise?
16. What have been the results of employee attitude surveys?
17. How are accomplishments celebrated?
18. How are employees made successful, supportive of one another, more communicative, and more trusting?
19. How will managers be updated?

FUNCTIONAL AND OPERATIONAL PLANNING

Operational management is the organization and directing of the delivery of nursing care. It includes such planning as creating a budget, creating an effective organizational structure that encompasses a quality monitoring process, and directing nurse leaders, an administrative staff, and new programs.[16]

Nursing planning performed at a service or departmental level is referred to as functional planning. It generally relates to a specialty service within a nursing division. For example, the staff development director would be included in development of the strategic plan but would develop operational plans for staff development as a whole and for specific services or units. Likewise, the director of a home-health-care agency would assist in developing the strategic plan for the company but would develop agency mission, philosophy, goals, objectives, and operational plans. With decentralization, each nurse manager would develop a strategic plan for her or his unit to be integrated into the organization's strategic plan.

Operational plans are everyday working management plans developed from both long-range objectives and the strategic planning process and short-range or tactical plans. In development of operational objectives, new strategic objectives can emerge or old ones can be modified or discarded. Strategic and tactical plans are made into operational plans and carried out at all levels of nursing management, not just at the patient-care level.

Operational managers develop goals, objectives, strategies, and targets to set the strategic plan in motion. They match each unit goal or objective to a strategic goal or objective. Their objectives can be much more detailed and specific than the strategic objectives. Numerous operational objectives can support one strategic objective.

All aspects of an operational plan are based on goals and their achievement. The individual leadership style determines whether goal setting will be of the top-down or bottom-up variety. Bottom-up goal setting is participatory, using guidelines from the operational manager.[17] Participatory goal setting is believed to increase workers' commitment and achievement. Increased participation leads to greater group cohesiveness, which in turn fosters increased morale, increased motivation, and increased achievement and productivity. Individuals, including professional nurses, can ensure greater relative success in achievement of goals by building in some slack in terms of projected resources and time. Nurses who reject goals of participating staff should explain their reasons for rejection. Participation in goal setting does not alone ensure success. Exhibit 5–5 suggests a timetable for strategic and operational planning. Like the plan itself, such planning should be flexible.

The goal is to plan, assess progress toward goals and objectives at all levels, and provide feedback to all levels of management. Efficiency is also a goal; all levels of management should guard against unnecessary time spent in meetings. As organizing changes are occurring, controlling activities are in operation and activities are being evaluated.

Business Plans

Business plans are detailed descriptions of the process for ensuring the launching of a new product or product line, project, unit, or service. Business plans meet many of the standards for strategic planning, as they are projected over an extended time period of months or years. Their purpose is to provide sources of information for investors and decision makers within and external to the organization, motivation, and measurement of performance.[18] Business plans are the blueprints for business ventures.

The following are key elements of a business plan as described by Johnson[19] and others:

Exhibit 5–5 Timetable for Strategic and Operational Planning

1. Organization
   Mondays 7–9 A.M. Conference room. Breakfast.
   Attendees: Chief executive officer (CEO), assistants (including for division of nursing), and understudies.
   Agenda: CEO, with input from all others, relates each item to strategic plan. CEO updates and develops written operational plans at meeting or immediately following, then reviews them for next agenda for progress and for strategic plan development.
   Minutes: Prepared and distributed to attendees.

2. Division of Nursing
   Monday 3–4 P.M. Nursing conference room.
   Attendees: Chief nurse executive (CNE), associates, department heads, chairs of clinical consultants, nursing management, and staff nurse committees.

   Agenda: Chairs, with input from CNE and all others, relate each item to strategic plan of division of nursing. These goals and objectives have already been coordinated with the organizational strategic plan. CNE and others update operational plans of division and departments during meeting or immediately following, then review them for next agenda for progress and nursing strategic plan development.
   Minutes: Prepared and distributed to attendees, to CEO, and to selected others.

3. Service and Unit
   CNE and/or associates meet with their nurse managers and representative clinical nurses at mutually determined times and places. The groups have agendas, keep minutes, update written operational plans, and provide feedback to top nurse managers and clinical nurse staff.

1. Introduction—nature, goals, objectives, and desired outcomes of the proposed business.
2. Description of the business—goals, nature, and history of the sponsoring institution, nature and history of the product, and industry trends.
3. Market and competition analysis, including target audience, pricing, promotion, placement, and positioning. Uses data from solid market research.
4. Product development—product description, resources, time frames for development, and quality control plan.
5. Operational plan—location, facilities, labor force, and equipment.
6. Marketing plan—mission, marketing research, measurable goals, strategies, and a staffing and financial plan.
7. Organizational plan—organizational chart and job descriptions.
8. Developmental schedule.
9. Financial plan.
10. Executive summary.

Business plans are often categorized as strategic plans. Many of the key elements are the same, although a business plan would be more detailed than a strategic plan. Actually, a business plan would be developed for each new venture emerging from a strategic plan. Exhibit 5–6 illustrates an operational plan for development of an intermediate cardiac rehabilitation program. The plan was made and carried out by a team led by a cardiovascular clinical nurse specialist.

Exhibit 5–6 Division of Nursing—Cardiac Rehabilitation Program

Strategic Objective
The patient is provided with an effective patient and patient-family teaching program, which will include guidance and assistance in the use of medical center resources and community agencies that can contribute support to the patient's total needs.

Operational Objectives	Actions	Target Dates and Persons Responsible	Accomplishments
Determine cardiologist's perception of the program: goals, resources to be used, breadth of services to be provided, etc.	1. Prepare an agenda for meeting with cardiologist.	Do by July 1, 19xx. Swansburg and Perry	The following agenda was developed: • Need for new services. • What will it be? • What will it cost? • What will be charged? • Who will pay? • Where will it be done? • Who will do it? • How many patients? • What equipment and supplies are needed?
	2. Make appointment with cardiologist.	May 3, 19xx, at 11 A.M. in Dr. C's office; S and P	May 3, 19xx. Had a meeting with Dr. C, the cardiologist. The purpose of this program is to rehabilitate patients following open-heart surgery, angioplasty, and post-MI. It is the intermediate phase between acute care and when they enter "bounce back." The following decision evolved from the meeting: 1. We will undertake this program on a limited basis, as there is no other such service available. 2. The service will include physical exercises, monitoring, progress report by patient, counseling as indicated. 3. Only patients with insurance or with ability to pay will be accepted. 4. It will be done in PT on Mon., Wed., and Fri. from 7 to 9 A.M. 5. Equipment and supplies will be in-house. 6. The CV clinical nurse specialist will be the project director.

Exhibit 5–6   Division of Nursing—Cardiac Rehabilitation Program *(Continued)*

Operational Objectives	Actions	Target Dates and Persons Responsible	Accomplishments
Meet with the CV clinical nurse specialist and plan the program.	3. Make appointment with nurse D to plan the program.	May 4, 19xx, at 8 A.M.; S and P with D.	Plan: 1. D will coordinate with PT director. 2. P will figure cost of program by the hour and set charges with accounting office. 3. D will borrow equipment to run the program until the next capital budget. 4. Accomplish this by May 12, 19xx.
Have plan completed by May 31, 19xx.	4. Set up a control chart to identify when each phase of project will be completed.	May 12, 19xx; P.	May 10, 19xx: Done. Posted.
	5. Write policy and procedure for the program. Include admission and discharge procedures and emergency plan.	May 31, 19xx; D.	May 29, 19xx: Draft presented; minor changes needed. May 31 19xx: Done.
	6. Obtain equipment and supplies.	May 31, 19xx; D.	May 17 19xx: Done.
	7. Coordinate with PT director.	May 12, 19xx; D.	May 17 19xx: Done.
	8. Meet with cardiologist when all of this is done.	June 1, 19xx; P, S, and D.	Met with cardiologist June 2, 19xx. Dr. C is happy with plan and will be ready to start on July 1, 19xx.
Provide for third-party reimbursement.	9. Discuss with insurance companies.	June 15, 19xx; P.	June 15, 19xx: Insurance reps will visit the program and make decision. Appointment made.
Develop marketing plan.	10. Prepare detailed marketing plan.		Marketing plan is already in operation with announcements mailed to all area cardiologists.
Develop evaluation plan.	11. Prepare evaluation plan.	June 30, 19xx; P and D.	D has a good evaluation plan.
	12. Implement program.	July 1, 19xx; D.	July 1, 19xx: Had our first patient today. Cardiologist was there as required by insurance companies. All went well.
	13. Evaluate the program weekly until stabilized.	D, beginning July 8, 19xx.	

Exhibit 5–7   Standards for Planning Process

	Yes	No
1. The plan is written.		
2. It defines the nursing business.		
3. It contains objectives (general and specific goals).		
4. It defines strategies.		
5. It supports the mission.		
6. It details forecasted activities for one year.		
7. It details forecasted activities for longer than one year.		
8. It has been developed with input from clinical nurses and line managers.		
9. It addresses resources (personnel and facilities).		
10. Changes are evident.		
11. Financial plans are included.		
12. Needs are identified and supported.		
13. Priorities are listed.		
14. Time tables are listed.		
15. It is based on current data analysis.		
16. It assesses both strengths and weaknesses.		
17. It derives from a good nursing management information plan.		
18. It is used and modified consistently.		

Exercise 5–5   Determine the length of the planning process for the agency in which you work or are a student. Use the checklist from Exhibit 5–7 above. From your survey, summarize the effectiveness of the planning process. How can it be improved? Can you initiate this improvement? If not, who can?

PRACTICAL PLANNING ACTIONS

Practical day-to-day planning actions of value to the professional nurse include the following exercises.

Exercise 5–6   At the beginning of each day, make a list of actions to be accomplished for the day. Cross off the actions as they are accomplished or at the end of the day. At the beginning of the next workday, carry over actions not accomplished; either do them first or decide whether they are actions that really need to be done. Do not hold tasks over from one day to the next indefinitely.

Exercise 5–7   Plan ahead for meetings. If the meeting is a nursing responsibility, prepare and distribute the agenda in advance. Have a secretary call members for their items to be listed on the agenda. Forward nursing items for the agenda of organizational meetings to the appropriate chair in advance. Prepare for the presentation.

Exercise 5–8   Identify developing problems and put them in the appropriate portion of the agency's operational or management plan.

Exercise 5–9   Review the operational or management plan on a scheduled basis. Do this with key personnel so that each knows responsibilities for accomplishment of activities.

Exercise 5–10   Review the appropriate portions of the agency operational or management plan with other nurses when they are being counseled.

Exercise 5–11   Plan for discussion of ideas gleaned from professional publications. This can be part of a job standard, with different managers assigned specific topics or journals. This may help to integrate research results into practice.

Exercise 5–12   Suggest similar practical planning actions to other nurse managers.

Planning will also be necessary to provide programs for orientation and continued learning of nursing personnel so that all will have current knowledge and be current in practice. Improvement of patient care and of other services necessitates initiation and utilization of and participation in studies or research projects in the health-care field.

To Make Planning Successful

Make decisions about the kind of planning to be undertaken. Which level of personnel should perform specific aspects of planning? Involve personnel in planning activities that they are going to carry out. Teach people the elements of planning and mesh the information with other management functions. Ensure that all personnel are involved. Accept outcomes different from those originally planned, since activities may quickly become outdated and require modified plans.

UNIT PLANNING

Planning extends to the operational units of any health-care agency. The processes involved are the same. It is here that the work for which nursing exists takes place. Planning should be done on a daily, weekly, and long-term basis. Daily planning is related to patient care and includes history taking, assessment, and nursing diagnosis and prescription. It involves matching people to jobs, developing policies and procedures specific to the types of clients cared for, identifying training needs, preparing and conducting training programs, coordinating all patient care activities, supervising personnel, and evaluating. It also includes implementing a theory of nursing into the management and practice of nursing, an effective and efficient nursing care delivery system, and a system of statistical process control.

Unit objectives should be clearly defined and a sound management or operational plan made to achieve them. An operating instruction from one nursing agency states, "The division of nursing has a stated philosophy and objectives. Personnel of each unit within the division will have their own philosophy and will set up their own objectives. The objectives will be continuously evaluated, and a written statement as to progress will be sent to the chair's office each August and February."

Exhibit 5–8 is a modified business plan for accomplishing objectives related to management improvement and resource management for an intensive care unit.

RELATIONSHIPS TO ORGANIZATION

Planning within the nursing organization is intended to assist in fulfilling the mission of the health-care facility. It supports the organization's objectives and meshes with the plans of all other departments contributing to provision of total health-care needs, whether direct or indirect (such as planning for the environment). Planning includes delineation of the responsibilities of professional nurses in relation to activities in other departments with which nursing interrelates. The organizational chart will show the relationship of the division of nursing to the board of control, the administrator, and other departments.

Plans will provide for optimum support of the nursing agency by other departments providing services, supplies, and equipment used by the nursing service. There will be plans for regular meetings with the administrator for participation on all agency committees concerned with general administrative policies and activities and the total program of the organization. There will also be plans for periodic reports to the board of control, through administrators, concerning the programs, major plans, and problems of the division of nursing.

Exhibit 5–8   Operational Plan—Intensive Care Unit

Management Improvement: Unit Objectives February 1, 19xx

1. Precipitate imaginative thinking to improve existing procedures, capitalize on time expenditure, and introduce modern concepts and materials that directly enhance unit accomplishment.
2. Promote creativity in improving the existing patient environment.
3. Provide more modern concepts of total patient care by constant review and revision of unit administrative/managerial policies.

Plans for Achievement of Objectives	Actions	Target Dates	Accomplishments
Plan and implement a continuing unit improvement program.	1. Conduct a continuous review and analysis of unit improvement efforts through:	February	Reviewed and found current for following reasons: Turnover in personnel is fast. Not all objectives were adequately met; need to establish a better way of accomplishing them.
	a. Monthly unit conferences to review and update philosophy and objectives. Strive to accomplish more in each objective area.	February–July	
	b. Patient suggestions	Review each month	
	c. Suggestions of superiors	Daily	
	d. Revise unit procedures	April	Done
	e. Brief all personnel. Discuss philosophy, objectives, job descriptions, performance standards, hospital and nursing service policies and procedures, and unit procedures.	February	Done. In addition, all nurses were counseled by the charge nurse. Nursing technicians are presently receiving counseling, and all is being documented. Counseling had not been documented in six years except for remarks such as, "Things went well and we did our job, so no counseling was needed."
	2. Review equipment and supplies for improvement by addition or deletion.		
	a. Submit work order to alter a locker as a drying cabinet for respirator parts, since moisture provides a growth medium for *Pseudomonas* bacteria.		Disapproved. Disposable tubing was approved, ordered, and in use by June.

(continued)

Exhibit 5–8 Operational Plan—Intensive Care Unit *(Continued)*

Plans for Achievement of Objectives	Actions	Target Dates	Accomplishments
	b. Check on status of new floor, piped-in compressed air system, and cardiac monitors.	February–April	New floor to be done by August 1. Compressed air started by March 15. Cardiac monitors arrived April 3. Patient units 1, 3, and 4 were equipped. Unit 4 was designated the maximum monitoring site and is to be used to monitor patients with Swan-Ganz arterial lines and questionable cardiac conditions.
Review standardized policies and procedures for implementation of more current concepts of improved care accomplishments.	3. Evaluate all areas of management for current standardized efficiency. a. Check all areas of infection sources.		
	(1) Air exchange and pressure checked quarterly.	February	This was done, and cleaning procedures were looked at and improved when they appeared poor. HEPA filters were replaced in February. Wall suction valves were replaced. Pipelines were found to be clogged with secretions, and system had to be purged. Shelves were mounted on wall by four units to replace bedside stands. Respirators, nebulizers, and blenders were mounted on wall above each patient unit. Suction bottles were relocated and outlets changed in an effort to isolate them from the oxygen nebulization units. Swan-Ganz catheters were standardized, and requisitioning was transferred from the unit to central supply. Ambu bags were equipped with corrugated tubing to serve as an oxygen reservoir and deliver a maximum concentration of 99% to 100%. The disposable Aqua-pack nebulizer was deleted, resulting in a $40 per case saving.
	(2) HEPA filters changed quarterly.	February	
	(3) Check wall suction, since filters do not appear to be doing the job.	February	
	(4) Eliminate messy bedside stands.	February	
	b. Improve safety.		
	(1) Secure equipment.	April	
	(2) Isolate oxygen nebulization units from suction.	April	
	(3) Send all equipment to central supply for processing.	April	
	(4) Improve efficiency of Ambu resuscitators.	April	
	4. Projected: An anesthesiologist will be assigned to the intensive care unit. All bronchoscopies will be done here. Open heart surgery is still an open and current topic.		

Exhibit 5–8   Operational Plan—Intensive Care Unit *(Continued)*

Resources Management

1. Provide, secure, and maintain the appropriate and economical use of supplies and equipment that will permit unit personnel to devote maximum time and care to patient activities.
2. Provide the unit with adequate tools for safe and effective patient care.
3. Provide the unit with conservative utilization and centralization of unit supplies and equipment, thus promoting peak efficiency in meeting patients' needs.

Plans for Achievement of Objectives	Actions	Target Dates	Accomplishments
Plan, evaluate, and project needed supplies and equipment that will enhance effective and safe nursing care.	Identify projected needs with unit manager through review of 1. Unit inventories of equipment and budgetary estimate. 2. Standards for supplies. 3. Availability of supplies and equipment. 4. Economical use of supplies and equipment.	February	Items ordered (projected replacements for 19xx–19xx): 1 electronic thermometer 1 IV pump 5 transducers 1 ventilator 1 sphygmomanometer 1 Wright respirometer 4 metal storage cabinets 4 Ambu bags 1 blood gas analyzer New cubicle curtains
Plan and execute appropriate utilization of materials.	1. Economical use of expendable supplies and adequate safeguards to prevent misuse and loss. 2. Knowledge of principles of operation of appropriate mechanical equipment and procedures for effecting prompt servicing and repairs.		Items replaced: ECG and defibrillator portable ECG machine spirometers suction regulators Items deleted: 1 electronic thermometer 1 internal/external defibrillator (to dog lab) 2 compressor units Miscellaneous: file card supply system revamped shelving obtained for lower doors Personnel turnover: Projected losses: Ms. Speich, RN, June Ms. Ullman, RN, August Ms. Urbom, RN, May Ms. Malloy, RN, June Mr. Falco, ward clerk, April Projected gains: Ms. Tishoff, RN, May Mr. Robertshaw, RN, May Mr. Angelus, RN, April Mrs. Figuera, unit secretary, April

Myra C. Breck, R.N.
Charge Nurse, ICU

WEB ACTIVITIES

- Visit www.jbpub.com/swansburg, this text's companion website on the Internet, for further information on The Planning Process.
- Are software tools available on the Internet to help with the planning process?
- Explore the Internet to discover various discussion areas and conferences related to planning.

SUMMARY

Planning is a mental process by which professional nurses use valid and reliable data to develop objectives and determine the resources needed and a blueprint for their use in achieving the objectives. The major purpose of planning is to make the best possible use of personnel, supplies, and equipment.

Strategic planning sets objectives for long-term nursing activities of one to five years or longer. While traditionally done by top managers, it is an important skill for all professional nurses to develop. It assures survival. Human resource planning will assure effective use of a scarce commodity, the professional nurse. Strategic planning has a mission, collects and analyzes data, assesses strengths and weaknesses, sets goals and objectives, uses strategies, operates on a timetable, gives operational and functional guidance to professional nurses, and includes evaluation.

Tactical planning is short-term planning. Operational planning is synergistic, putting strategic and tactical planning in motion. It includes goals, objectives, strategies, actions, a timetable, identification of responsible persons, and note of accomplishments. Operational planning is daily, weekly, and monthly planning and can provide data for further strategic and tactical planning.

Exercise 5–13   List the threats to nursing, their severity, and the probability that they will occur. Consider technological, economic, demographic, politico-legal, and sociocultural forecasting.

Exercise 5–14   List the opportunities in nursing, their attractiveness, and the probability that they will occur. Consider technological, economic, demographic, politico-legal, and sociocultural forecasting.

NOTES

1. H. Fayol, trans. by C. Storrs, *General and Industrial Management* (London: Isaac Pitman & Sons, 1949), 43–50.
2. L. Urwick, *The Elements of Administration* (New York: Harper & Row, 1944), 26–34.

3. H. S. Rowland and B. L. Rowland, *Nursing Administration Handbook,* 4th ed. (Gaithersburg, Md.: Aspen, 1997), 13, 32–36.

4. L. Curtin, "Learning for the Future," *Nursing Management* 25, no. 1 (1994): 7–9.

5. L. M. Douglass. *The Effective Nurse: Leader and Manager,* 5th ed. (St. Louis: Mosby, 1996), 125–151.

6. H. M. Donovan, *Nursing Service Administration: Managing the Enterprise* (St. Louis: Mosby, 1975), 50–64.

7. H. Koontz and H. Weihrich, *Management,* 9th ed. (New York: McGraw-Hill, 1988), 16.

8. H. M. Donovan, op. cit., 63–64.

9. R. M. Hodgetts, *Management: Theory, Process, and Practice,* 5th ed. (Orlando, Fla.: Harcourt Brace Jovanovich, 1990), 123–124.

10. M. Hill, "Disease Management: How to Make the Mission Possible," *The New Definition,* spring 1997, 1–2.

11. A. P. Meier, "The Planning Process," *Managerial Planning,* July/August 1974, 1–5, 9.

12. P. F. Drucker, *Management: Tasks, Responsibilities, Practices,* (New York: Harper & Row, 1973), 125.

13. D. H. Fox and R. T. Fox, "Strategic Planning for Nursing," *Journal of Nursing Administration,* May 1983, 11–16; R. N. Paul and J. W. Taylor, "The State of Strategic Planning," *Business,* January–March 1986, 37–43.

14. G. S. Odiorne, "The Art of Crafting Strategic Plans, *Training* (October 1987): 94–96, 98.

15. T. Peters, *Thriving on Chaos* (New York: Harper & Row, 1987), 615–617.

16. L. J. Johnson, "Strategic Management: A New Dimension of the Nurse Executive's Role," *Journal of Nursing Administration,* September 1990, 7–10.

17. R. Cushman, "Norton's Top-Down, Bottom-Up Planning Process," *Planning Review,* November 1979, 3–8, 48.

18. K. W. Vestal, "Writing a Business Plan," *Nursing Economics,* May–June 1988, 121–124.

19. J. E. Johnson, "Developing an Effective Business Plan," *Nursing Economics,* May–June 1990, 152–154; J. E. Johnson, D. G. Sparks, and C. Humphreys, "Writing a Winning Business Plan," *Journal of Nursing Administration,* October 1988, 15–19.

FOUNDATIONS FOR PLANNING—MISSION, PHILOSOPHY, OBJECTIVES, AND MANAGEMENT PLANS

OBJECTIVES

- Define mission or purpose statement as it obtains to nursing services.
- Use a set of standards to evaluate a purpose or mission statement for a nursing agency.
- Write a purpose or mission statement for a nursing agency. Identify the vision and values to be imparted to clients.
- Define philosophy as it obtains to nursing services.
- Use a set of standards to evaluate the philosophy statement of a nursing agency.
- Write a philosophy statement for a nursing agency.
- Define objectives as they obtain to nursing services.
- Use a set of standards to evaluate the objectives statements of a nursing agency.
- Write objectives for a nursing agency.
- Define operational plan (management plan) as it obtains to nursing services.
- Use a set of standards to evaluate an operational plan of a nursing agency.
- Describe strategy as it relates to the planning function of nursing services.

KEY CONCEPTS

nursing mission (purpose)
nursing vision and values
nursing philosophy
nursing objectives
management or operational plan
strategy

Manager Behavior: Develops statements of mission (purpose), vision and values, philosophy, and objectives for the nursing agency. Uses operational (management) plans.

Leader Behavior: Coaches personnel in the development and use of statements of mission (purpose), vision and values, philosophy, and objectives for the nursing agency. Encourages personnel to use operational (management) plans in appropriate instances.

INTRODUCTION

Statements of mission or purpose, vision and values, philosophy or beliefs, and objectives, and an operational or management plan have already been referred to. This chapter discusses these basic tools of management in greater detail. Knowledge of their use is part of the theory of nursing management. The tools are part of the planning function of nursing management, and skill in using them successfully is part of the strategy of nursing management planning.

Written statements of purpose, vision and values, philosophy, and objectives, and written operational plans are the blueprints for effective management of any enterprise, including the health-care institution. They are a component of planning at each management level. Statements at the corporate level serve the top managers of the organization. Those at the division level serve the managers and personnel of major divisions, such as nursing, operations, or finance. These statements evolve from and support those of the institution. Services, departments, and units each have written statements of purpose, vision and values, philosophy, and objectives, and written operational plans that are developed from and support the documents at division and corporate levels (see Exhibit 6–1).[1]

MISSION OR PURPOSE, VISION, AND VALUES

Mission or Purpose

The mission of an organization describes the purpose for which that organization exists. Mission statements provide information and inspiration that clearly and explicitly outline the way ahead for the organization. They provide vision.[2]

The purpose for any organization is to provide individuals with the means to productive and meaningful lives. Therefore, the purpose of the organization and each unit should be defined, a teamwork approach should prevail, constituents should be properly trained, and all individuals should be treated with respect.[3]

Exhibit 6–1   Evolution of Mission, Vision and Values, Philosophy, and Objectives Statements and Operational Plans

Mission (purpose) statements	Corporate
	↓
Vision and value statements	Division
	↓
Philosophy (beliefs) statements	Department
	↓
Objectives statements	Unit
Operational (management) plans	

Organizational purpose moves, guides, and delivers the organization to a perceived goal. Many writers indicate that the purpose or mission statement should be created from a vision statement that tells what the company stands for. The vision statement is created with the customer's needs in mind. To determine these needs, one must ask and listen to the customer. External customers who purchase the products or services may be given a tour of the organization. In nursing, external customers are prospective patients and families, accreditation and licensing officials, faculty and students, and even taxpayers and shareholders. Internal customers are the employees, both departmental and intradepartmental. The mission or purpose statement incorporates the culture of the organization, including strong leadership, rules and regulations, achievement of goals, and the notion that people are more important than work.[4]

Vision

Employees who participate in developing the vision statement believe in their own abilities and are more committed to the organization than employees who do not participate. The vision statement is shared companywide so that employees may live the vision. It is kept updated to keep pace with technology and trends.[5] A vision statement is sometimes considered more strategic than a mission statement. The mental exercise of creating one is more meaningful than the contents of the statement itself. Vision, values, mission, or purpose statements are meaningful only to their creators.[6]

Values

Values are the moral rationale for business. Examples of values are informality, creativity, honesty, quality, courtesy, and caring. Values statements make employees feel proud and managers feel committed. They give meaning to the right way to do things; they give employees enthusiasm and energy. Values bond people and set the behavior standards of the employees.[7]

Nursing Mission or Purpose

Defining a mission or purpose allows nursing to be managed for performance. It describes what it will be and what it should be. It describes the constituencies to be satisfied. It is the professional nurse's commitment to a specific definition of purpose or mission.

One purpose of a nursing entity is to provide nursing care to clients. Such care can include promotion of self-care concepts. Thus, the mission statement should include definitions of nursing and self-care as defined by professional nurses.

Virginia Henderson has defined nursing as follows:

> The unique function of the nurse is to assist the individual, sick or well, in the performance of those activities contributing to health or its recovery (or to peaceful death) that he would perform unaided if he had the necessary strength, will or knowledge. And to do this in such a way as to help him gain independence as rapidly as possible.[8]

King defined nursing as

a process of action, reaction, interaction, and transaction whereby nurses assist individuals of any age group to meet their basic human needs in coping with their health status at some particular point in their life cycle. Nurses perform their functions within social institutions and they interact with individuals and groups. Therefore, three distinct levels of operation exist: (1) the individual; (2) the group; and (3) society.[9]

Orem defined nursing as follows:

Nursing is an art through which the nurse, the practitioner of nursing, gives specialized assistance to persons with disabilities of such character that more than ordinary assistance is necessary to meet daily needs for self-care and to intelligently participate in the medical care they are receiving from the physician. The art of nursing is practiced by "doing for" the person with the disability, by "helping him to do for himself," and/or by "helping him to learn how to do for himself." Nursing is also practiced by helping a capable person from the patient's family or a friend of the patient to learn how "to do for" the patient. Nursing is thus a practical and didactic art.[10]

Emerging from these and other theories of nursing is a commonality of terms central to the definition of nursing: nurse, patient or client, individual, group, society, nursing process, self-care, and health.

A further mission of nursing is to provide a public good, and this should be indicated in the statement of mission or purpose, which tells why the nursing entity exists. The statement is written so that it can be known by all people working within the organizational entity, since it states the reason for their

Exhibit 6–2   Mission Statement of an Organization

Subject: Mission Statement

It is the mission of the University of South Alabama Hospitals & Clinics to:

1. Provide high-quality and continually improving acute and long-term health care services and resources to the people of the community and region without regard to race, creed, color, age, sex, national origin, or handicapping condition, and to provide a high-quality setting conducive to the education and research activities of the University and the community.
2. Provide a dynamic and innovative setting for clinical experiences and post-graduate education of health care professionals.
3. Establish and maintain sound financial practices and procedures while providing cost-effective care, recognizing that patient care and education missions will only be achieved through the protection

and growth of the system's assets. Health care for the medically indigent is the responsibility of society and the community. Our obligation for providing this care is limited to what the community supports.

4. Recognize that our future success is dependent upon developing and utilizing our most important asset—people. Toward that end, we will provide an environment for professional employee growth through career opportunity and continuing education.
5. Work cooperatively with physicians and other health care providers to improve the standards of health care delivery in our community.

Source: Reprinted with permission of the University of South Alabama Medical Center, Mobile, Alabama.

employment. An ultimate strategy is to have nursing personnel participate in developing mission statements and in keeping them updated so that they will know, understand, and support them.

The mission should be known and understood by other health-care practitioners, by clients and their families, and by the community. A statement of purpose must be dynamic, giving action and strength to evolving statements of philosophy, objectives, and management plans. Statements of purpose can be made dynamic by indicating the relationship between the nursing unit and patients, personnel, community, health, illness, and self-care. Exhibits 6–2 (on the previous page), 6–3, and 6–4 are examples of the mission statement of an organization, the division, and the unit, respectively. Exhibit 6–5 lists the standards for evaluation of the mission statements of an organization.

Exhibit 6–3   Mission Statement of a Division

Subject: Statement of Mission and Purpose for the Division of Nursing

The mission and purpose of the Division of Nursing is consistent with the mission and purpose of the University of South Alabama Medical Center. The mission and purpose of the Division of Nursing is fourfold:

1. To provide the patient, at a reasonable cost, a quality of nursing care that can be measured and evaluated.
2. To provide an environment that facilitates nursing research and education and its application to patients under nursing practice.
3. To create a working milieu that encourages professional growth and personal satisfaction for all levels of nursing practice.
4. To foster a positive, professional image of nursing to the public through community involvement and guest relations.

Source: Reprinted with permission of the University of South Alabama Medical Center, Mobile, Alabama.

Exhibit 6–4   Mission Statement of a Unit

Subject: Purpose: Sixth Floor

The purpose of the sixth floor is consistent with the purpose of the Division of Nursing.

1. To assess the physical, emotional, and spiritual needs of patients, their families, and/or significant others so as to provide optimal care.
2. To provide patients with an individualized plan of care, in regard to their needs, in a cost-effective manner to the patient and the hospital.
3. To serve as the patient's, family's, and/or significant other's advocate to assure complete care with regard to the patient's, family's, and/or significant other's needs.
4. To provide and promote continuing education through in-services, research projects, and patient-care conferences to improve the quality of our health care.
5. To incorporate all disciplines related to patient's care in evaluating the needs of the patient, family, and/or significant others.
6. To assess and evaluate our quality of nursing care on an ongoing basis through quality assurance and monthly audits.

Source: Reprinted with permission of the University of South Alabama Medical Center, Mobile, Alabama.

Exhibit 6–5   Standards for the Evaluation of Mission Statements of the Nursing Division and Its Departments, Services, and Units

1. The mission statement tells the reason for the existence of the nursing division, department, service, or unit in relation to the practice of nursing and of self-care as defined by the nursing staff and in relation to the service being provided to the community of clients. Once definitions of nursing and self-care have been developed by the nursing staff and ratified by the nursing administration, they may be quoted in the mission statement.
2. The nursing division mission statement supports the mission of the organization. Unit mission statements are customized by line personnel.
3. The statement indicates that the nursing organization exists to provide a public good.
4. The mission statement is developed by the people who will live by it.
5. It includes a set of core values held by the people who will live by it.
6. It is short, clear, and unambiguous; it has a clear meaning.
7. The mission statement describes the organization's uniqueness.

Exercise 6–1   Use Exhibit 6–5, "Standards for the Evaluation of Mission Statements of the Nursing Division and Its Departments, Services, or Units," to (1) develop a mission statement and (2) evaluate a mission statement.

PHILOSOPHY

A written statement of philosophy sets out values, concepts, and beliefs that pertain to nursing administration and nursing practice within the organization. It verbalizes the visions of both nurse managers and nurse practitioners as to what they believe nursing management and practice are. It states their beliefs as to how the mission or purpose will be achieved, giving direction toward this end. Statements of philosophy are abstract and contain value statements about human beings as clients or patients and as workers, about work that will be performed by nursing workers for clients or patients, about self-care, about nursing as a profession, about education as it pertains to competence of nursing workers, and about the setting or community in which nursing services are provided. The character and tone of service are set by planning that evolves purpose and philosophy statements, one from the other, for the organization and each of its units.

Contents

Among the contents of a philosophy statement are the core values related to a nursing modality, the need for advanced preparation, continuing education, students, research, nursing management, and nursing's role in the organization. Philosophy statements pertain to patients' involvement in their care and to their extended families. Philosophy statements also pertain to nurses' rights, including commitment to staff promotion and a nurse's responsibility to the profession.[11]

As with the mission statement, the philosophy statement is most effective when developed by those who will live by it. Unit statements of philosophy support the organizational philosophy. Philosophy that is communicated zealously and is totally supported by top management is most effective. Unlike mission and objectives statements, the philosophy statement remains constant. As with mission statements, philosophy statements evolve from higher levels of management and practice.

Exhibits 6–6, 6–7, and 6–8 are examples of the philosophy statement of an organization, division, and unit, respectively. Exhibit 6–9 lists the standards for evaluation of philosophy statements of an organization.

Exhibit 6–6   Organizational Philosophy Statement

Subject: Philosophy of the University of South Alabama Medical Center

We believe that:

- The University of South Alabama Medical Center is dedicated to excellence in the fields of patient care, teaching, and research.
- We are dedicated to providing the most effective and efficient patient care.
- We are committed to provide services for patients requiring highly specialized and unique medical treatment.
- We are committed to providing the same level of health care to all patients with the same health problem within the hospital.
- We are committed to providing a safe environment for patients, staff, and guests. We assure the rights of patients to confidentiality, full disclosure of risks involved in care, and involvement in decision making.
- The University of South Alabama Board of Trustees, the Medical Executive Committee, the medical staff at large, and the University of South Alabama Medical Center Administration support both in concept and by resource allocation the implementation and ongoing activities of the Risk Management program designed to reduce risks and losses and promote safety in the hospital setting.
- Continuing education is essential to competence of staff. Professional growth and development is both a personal and organizational responsibility.
- Research should be fostered to the extent possible and should follow acceptable guidelines for protection of human subjects.
- We have an obligation to monitor and continuously improve all activities through quality assessment and improvement as an integral part of Quality Assurance.

- Everyone should be treated with dignity.
- There are fiscal limits to what we can do and every employee must market the hospital to obtain revenues to maintain financial stability.
- Health care for the medically indigent is the responsibility of society and the community from which they come. Our capacity and obligation for providing indigent care is limited to what the community supports.
- We have an obligation to use our finances and limited resources responsibly and to maintain and improve the fiscal integrity of our institution.
- Health care should focus on prevention and wellness in addition to illness. We promote and plan for patients to care for themselves from time of admission.
- We are the leaders in health care in this community. We believe in supporting laws and regulations and in working to make changes that benefit our mission.
- Our staff are our best asset and they will be treated with respect.
- Our staff have a responsibility to serve this Medical Center with total commitment to our philosophy, goals, policies, and procedures to assure a successful organization.
- We have a responsibility to provide learning experience for all students in the health care field, including providing appropriate clinical settings and role models.

Source: Reprinted with permission of the University of South Alabama Medical Center, Mobile, Alabama.

Exhibit 6–7   Philosophy Statement of a Division

Subject: Philosophy of the Division of Nursing

We believe that:

- The philosophy of the Division of Nursing is consistent with the philosophy of the University of South Alabama Medical Center.
- We are dedicated to excellence in patient care, teaching, and research and to providing the most effective and efficient care.
- Everyone should be treated with dignity.
- Health is not merely the absence of disease or infirmity but a state of optimum physical, mental, and social well-being.
- Nursing care promotes self-care concepts, enabling patients to meet their basic human needs in coping with their health status throughout their life cycles. Nursing involves a broad approach of health care aimed at a healthy society through education of the public.
- Professional nursing care at University of South Alabama Medical Center is provided equally to all patients accepted for treatment.
- Patients and their families have a right to be kept informed about all aspects of their health status and to participate in decisions affecting their care to the fullest extent possible.

- The physical, mental, spiritual, and social needs of our patients can be achieved by striving to maintain goal-directed multidisciplinary plans of care.
- The highly specialized care offered at the Medical Center requires qualified staff for all positions. The most important assets of the institution are the staff and they will be treated with respect.
- We have an obligation to manage personnel and finances to achieve maximum productivity.
- Improvement of the quality of nursing is assured by the continuous evaluation of nursing care and positive modifications to nursing techniques and activities.
- Continuing education is essential to the delivery of quality professional nursing and is both a personal and organizational responsibility.
- We have a responsibility to provide appropriate learning experiences and role models for all students in the health care field.
- We accept the responsibility of being involved in nursing research.

Source: Reprinted with permission of the University of South Alabama Medical Center, Mobile, Alabama.

Exhibit 6–8   Philosophy Statement of a Unit

Subject: Philosophy of Sixth Floor

- We believe that all patients should be given equal, individualized care by all nursing staff and that such care should incorporate physical, emotional, and spiritual needs.
- We believe the goal of health care should be to assist the patient to progress toward a level of optimal health.
- We believe that the patient should be encouraged by all nursing staff to progress toward self-care and independence.
- We believe that it is the responsibility of all nursing staff to act as a patient advocate to provide quality care according to the wishes of the patient, family, and/or significant others.

- We believe that continuing education is a necessary component of continuing improvement in health care.
- We believe that nursing is an integral part of health care, and that the nurse is an important member of the health care team.
- We believe that patients, their families, and/or significant others have the right to be well informed about the patient's state of health, prognosis, and care.

Source: Reprinted with permission of the University of South Alabama Medical Center, Mobile, Alabama.

Exhibit 6–9 Standards for Evaluation of Philosophy Statements of the Nursing Division, Department, Service, or Unit

1. A written statement of philosophy should exist for the nursing division and each of its units.
2. A written statement of philosophy should be developed in collaboration with nursing employees, the consumers, and other health care workers.
3. Nursing personnel should share in an annual (or more frequent) review and revision of the written statement of philosophy.
4. The written statement of philosophy should reflect these beliefs or values:
   (1) The meaning of the clinical practice of nursing.
   (2) Recognition of rights of individuals and of the responsibility of nursing personnel to serve as advocates for those rights.
   (3) Selective other statements about humanity, society, health, nursing, nursing process, and self-care relevant to external forces (community, laws, etc.) and internal forces (personnel, clients, material resources, etc.), research, education, and family as are deemed appropriate to accomplishing the mission of the division and each of its units.
5. The nursing philosophy should support the philosophy of the organization as expressed at all levels above the nursing division.
6. The statement of philosophy should give direction to the achievement of the mission.

Exercise 6–2 Use Exhibit 6–9, "Standards for Evaluation of Philosophy Statements of the Nursing Division, Department, Service, or Unit, to (1) develop a philosophy statement and (2) evaluate a philosophy statement.

OBJECTIVES

Objectives are concrete and specific statements of the goals that nurse managers seek to accomplish. They are action commitments through which the key elements of the mission will be achieved and the philosophy or beliefs sustained. They are used to establish priorities. They are stated in terms of results to be achieved and focus on the provision of health-care services to clients. Like the statements of mission and philosophy, they must be meaningful, relevant, and functional. They must be alive. Moore has stated, "If objectives are presented in terms of what can be observed, they can serve as useful tools for evaluation of nursing care and personnel performance, and as a basis for planning educational programs, staffing, requisition of supplies and equipment, and other functions associated with the nursing department."[12]

According to Moore, nursing organizations should have objectives for evaluation of patient care, evaluation of personnel performance, planning of educational programs, staffing, and requisition of supplies and equipment.

Drucker indicates that mission and purpose, as well as the basic definition of a business, have to be translated into objectives if they are to become more than insight, good intentions, and brilliant epigrams never to be achieved. Objectives are concrete statements that become the standards against which performance can be measured. They are the basic tactics of any business, including the business of nursing management. Objectives must be selective rather than global, and they must be multiple rather than single, so as to balance a wide range of needs and goals related to nursing services to clients or patients; productive use of people, money, and material resources; updating through innovation; and the discharge of a social responsibility to the community. Objectives must be used, and one way to use them is to develop them into specific management and operational plans.[13]

Organization and use of all resources—human, financial, and physical—are areas for objectives. Objectives address the need to develop managers, the needs of major groups within the division, including nonmanagerial workers, labor relations, the development of positive employee attitudes, and maintenance and upgrading of employee skills. Objectives provide for attractive job and career opportunities and provide activities to control worker assignment and productivity. They are the means by which productivity in nursing is measured. Objectives are also needed in the areas of social responsibility, innovation, and wellness.

Objectives are the fundamental strategy of nursing, since they specify the end product of all nursing activities. They must be capable of being converted into specific targets and specific assignments so that nurses will know what they have to do to accomplish them. Objectives become the basis and motivation for the nursing work necessary to accomplish them and for measuring nursing achievement. They make possible the concentration of human and material resources and of human efforts. Objectives are needed in all areas on which the survival of nursing and health-care services depends. In nursing, all objectives should be performance objectives that provide for existing nursing services for existing patient groups. They should provide for abandonment of unneeded and outmoded nursing services and health care-products and provide for new nursing services and health-care products for existing patients. They should provide for new groups of patients, for the distributive organization, and for standards of nursing service and performance. Last but not least, there should be objec-

Exhibit 6–10 The Elements of Objectives

- *A performance objective.* The patient receives individualized care in a safe environment to meet total therapeutic nursing needs—physical, emotional, spiritual, environmental, social, economic, and rehabilitative (also illustrates next provision).
- *Existing nursing services for existing patients.* Nurse consultants have been made available from medical nursing, surgical nursing, mental health nursing, and maternal and child health nursing. Their services can be requested by any professional nurse or physician.
- *Abandonment of outmoded nursing services and products.* Universal precautions have been implemented and the old handwashing basins have been discarded.

- *New nursing services for new groups of patients.* Plans are being made to offer consultative nursing services from the general hospital to nursing homes in the area. In the future this will be extended to retirement homes. Both actions are the result of market surveys.
- *Organization for new nursing services.* The nurse manager has evaluated the necessity of restructuring the organization of the division of nursing to provide new nursing services.
- *Standards of nursing service and performance.* The nurse manager has decided to use the Standards of Nursing Practice developed by the ANA Congress for Nursing Practice for all nurses within the division.

tives for research and development of new nursing services and products. Refer to Exhibit 6–10 (p. 102) for a breakdown of the elements of objectives.

Exhibits 6–11, 6–12, and 6–13 are examples of objectives for an organization, a nursing department, and a nursing unit, respectively. Exhibit 6–14 lists the standards for evaluating the objectives of an organization.

Exhibit 6–11   Goals of the University of South Alabama Medical Center

Global Goals

Increase number of paying patients

Increase awareness of resources among public

Short-term plan of what we sell

Long-term plan of what we sell

Increase in services

Educate the staff to sell the formal hospital plan to build hospital on campus

Research provision of differently priced services

Market hospital to university employees

Improve access to hospital

Improve intelligence

Residents to use Medical Center for private practice

Improve management of patients for maximum reimbursement

Create new markets

Improve efficiency

Recognize hospital as a business

Reconcile difference in goals between Foundation and hospital

Definitive Goals

1. Increase number of paying patients
   (1) Plan for incentive for M.D.'s (Steve)
   (2) Who are private M.D.'s using hospital? (Pat)
   (3) Survey private M.D.'s in town (John)
   (4) Market HMO (internal) (Susie and John)
   (5) Input from department heads (Brookley meeting)
   (6) Create new markets and identify opportunities through money arrangements
       (i) Where are they? (Dept. Heads)
       (ii) Maintain ROA
       (iii) Maintain Keesler arrangement
       (iv) Surrounding counties
       (v) HHC

   (vi) Public service (plan for industry) (Pat)
   (vii) Organizations and involvement (clinic and campus)
   (viii) Student organizations on campus
   (7) Market hospital to university employees
2. Increase awareness of resources among public
   (1) PR plan
   (2) Short-term marketing plan of what we sell (identifying what we are selling now)
3. Long-term marketing plan of what we sell
   (1) What new products can we sell (or divert)?
   (2) Formal plan to build hospital on campus
4. Educate the staff to sell the hospital
   (1) Just for the pride of it
   (2) Management people in civic organizations
   (3) Reference 1(4)
   (4) Employees identify with PR and marketing people
   (5) Recognize hospital as a business
5. Research provision of differently priced services
   (1) Innovative ways to bill for services
6. Improve access to hospital
   (1) Parking
   (2) Waiting areas
   (3) Emergency Department
7. Improve intelligence (above board)
   (1) Professional groups
   (2) Reference 4(2)
   (3) Internal network
8. Residents to use Medical Center for private practice
9. Improve efficiency
   (1) Improve management of patients for maximum reimbursement
       (i) Audit bills with charts
10. Improve cooperative relationship between Foundation (C of M) and Medical Center

Source: Reprinted with permission of the University of South Alabama Medical Center, Mobile, Alabama.

Exhibit 6–12   Objectives of the Department of Nursing

Subject: Objectives of the Division of Nursing

The objectives of this Division of Nursing shall be to provide the patient:

1. Individualized care in a safe environment to meet the patient's total needs as assessed by the professional nurse and utilizing the nursing process. This care covers physical, emotional, spiritual, environmental, social, economic, and rehabilitational needs involved in planning total patient care.
2. An effective teaching program which will include guidance and assistance in the use of medical resources and community agencies.
3. Benefits of effective communication, cooperation, and coordination with all professional and administrative services involved in the planning of total patient care.
4. Benefits of a continuous, flexible program of in-service education for all department of nursing personnel adapted to orientation, in-service, continuing education and leadership development.
5. Benefits from Nursing Services' participation in education of students.
6. With cost-effective care by the timely procurement, effective utilization, and proper handling of equipment and supplies.
7. Benefits through a positive work atmosphere in which nurses' job satisfaction is attained.
8. Benefits from a close association between Division of Nursing personnel and community nursing organizations and groups to keep abreast of current trends and advancements in nursing.
9. Maximum nursing care hours by relieving nursing personnel of non-nursing duties.
10. Benefits from the development of a cost-effective balanced budget for the Division of Nursing.
11. Benefits from close supervision by an RN of all personnel who give patient care, and from continuous evaluation of the care given.
12. Benefits from implementation of the results of nursing research.

Source: Reprinted with permission of the University of South Alabama Medical Center, Mobile, Alabama.

Exhibit 6–13   Objectives of a Nursing Unit

Subject: Objectives of Sixth Floor

The objectives of the Sixth Floor shall be to provide the patient, family, and/or significant others:

1. Individualized total patient care based on an assessment by an RN, considering all needs, physical, emotional, and spiritual, of the patient, family, and/or significant others.
2. The nursing process will be the basis of all care given by the professional nurse.
3. To provide quality care in a cost-effective manner to patient and hospital.
4. To coordinate information from all disciplines, to plan for optimum care while hospitalized and after discharge.
5. To involve the patient's family and/or significant others in caring for the patient to meet their needs.
6. To identify problem areas in nursing care through monthly audits to ensure the quality of our nursing care.
7. To increase knowledge and improve nursing care by providing a variety of in-service [training] from all departments involved in the care of the patient.

Source: Reprinted with permission of the University of South Alabama Medical Center, Mobile, Alabama.

Exhibit 6–14   Standards for Evaluation of Statements of Objectives for a Nursing Division, Department, Service, or Unit

1. The objectives for the nursing division, department, service, or unit should be in written form.
2. The objectives should be developed in collaboration with the nursing personnel who will assist in achieving them.
3. Nursing personnel should share in an annual (or more frequent) review and revision of the written statements of objectives.
4. The written statement of objectives should meet these qualitative and quantitative criteria:
   (1) They operationalize the statements of mission and philosophy; they can be translated into actions.
   (2) They can be measured or verified.
   (3) They exist in a hierarchy or sequence that is prioritized.
   (4) They are clearly stated.
   (5) They are realistic in terms of human and physical resources and capabilities.
   (6) They direct the use of resources.
   (7) They are achievable (practical).
   (8) They are specific.
   (9) They indicate results expected from nursing efforts and activities; the ends of management programs.
   (10) They show a network of desired events and results.
   (11) They are flexible and allow for adjustment.
   (12) They are known to the nursing personnel who will use them.
   (13) They are quantified wherever possible.
   (14) They exist for all positions.

Exercise 6–3   Use Exhibit 6–14, "Standards for Evaluation of Statements of Objectives for a Nursing Division, Department, Service, or Unit," to (1) develop objectives and (2) evaluate objectives.

THE OPERATIONAL PLAN

Objectives must be converted into actions: activities, assignments, and deadlines, all with clear accountability. The action level is where nurses eliminate the old and plan for the new. It is where time dimensions are put into perspective and new and different methods can be tried. It is where nurses answer these questions over and over again: What is it? What will it be? What should it be?

An operational plan is the written blueprint for achieving objectives. It specifies the activities and procedures that will be used and sets timetables for the achievement of objectives. It tells who the responsible persons are for each activity and procedure. It describes ways of preparing people for jobs and procedures for evaluating the care of patients. It specifies the records that will be kept and the policies needed. It gives individual managers freedom to accomplish both their own objectives and those of the institution, division, department, or unit. The operational plan is sometimes called a management plan (see Exhibits 6–15 and 6–16).

Exercise 6–4   Use Exhibit 6–16, "Standards for Evaluation of Management Plan of Nursing Division, Department, Service, or Unit," to (1) develop management plans and (2) evaluate management plans.

Exhibit 6–15   Management Plan

Objective

The client receives skilled nursing services to meet his total individual needs as diagnosed by professional nurses. This process is systematic, beginning with the gathering of base data and it is planned, implemented, evaluated, and revised on a continual basis. It covers physical, emotional, spiritual, environmental, social, economical, and rehabilitational needs and includes health teaching involved in the planning of total client care. Its ultimate goal is to assist clients to, or return them to, optimal health status and independence as quickly as possible.

Actions	Target Dates	Accomplishments
Institute primary care nursing	January 1–June 30	Assigned to Ms. Scott. Decision made to attempt to use self-care concepts of Orem: (1) definition, and (2) nursing systems.
1. Assign problem of overall development of a plan	January 31	Assigned to Ms. Longez January 19. In discussion with Ms. Scott and Ms. Longez, a decision was made to
2. Assign development of a self-care concept for application using Orem and Kinlein as references	February 15	investigate application of self-care using the nursing process as described by Kinlein. The nursing staff were particularly interested in the nursing history process described by Kinlein. Ms. Longez has added this dimension to her assignment. She has requested Mr. Jarmann be assigned to assist her and he has agreed.
3. Organize resources	February 28	February 5: Ms. Scott has just updated me on the project. A good portion of her plan has been developed. They are now doing a staffing plan, including job descriptions and job standards. February 27: The plan is completed and has been discussed with me. A few minor adjustments are being made.
4. Coordinate plan	March 31	
(1) Nursing personnel		Done. All want to participate.
(2) Administrator		Done.
(3) Public relations		Announcements made to community through news media.
(4) Physicians		Done and well received.
(5) Other as needed		Presented to board per request of administrator. They want progress reports.
5. Select and train staff	April 30	Assigned to Ms. Finch for training. Will be assisted by Ms. Scott and Ms. Longez. I will select staff with their recommendation.
6. Implement	June 30	Ms. Scott wants to direct implementation and I have concurred.

Exhibit 6–16   Standards for Evaluation of Management Plan of Nursing Division, Department, Service, or Unit

1. The written management plan should operationalize the strategic goals of the organization as well as the objectives of the nursing division, department, service, or unit. It should specify activities or actions, persons responsible for accomplishing them, and target dates or time frames, as well as providing for evaluation of progress. Each activity or action should be listed in problem-solving or decision-making format, as appropriate.
2. The management plan is personal to the incumbent, who should select the standards for developing, maintaining, and evaluating it. The nurse manager should solicit desired input from appropriate nursing persons and others.
3. The actions listed should reflect planning for:
   (1) Nursing care programs to ensure safe and competent nursing services to clients.
       (i) The nursing process, including data gathering, assessment, diagnosis, goal setting and prescription, intervention and application, evaluation, feedback, change, and accountability to the consumer.
       (ii) A process and outcome audit.
       (iii) Promotion of self-care practices.
   (2) Establishment of policies and procedures for employing competent nursing personnel: recruitment, selection, assignment, retention, and promotion based on individual qualifications and capabilities without regard to race, national origin, creed, color, sex, or age.
   (3) Integration of nursing care programs into the total program of the health care organization and community through committee participation in professional and service activities, and credentialing of individuals in organizations, including nursing organizations.
   (4) A budget that is evaluated and revised as necessary.
   (5) Job descriptions that include standards stated as objectives, outcomes, or results, and that are known to the incumbents.
   (6) Specific utilization of personnel. This part of the plan should:
       (i) Conform to a staffing plan that is based on timing nursing activities and rating of patients.
       (ii) Match competencies of people to total job requirements.
       (iii) Place prepared people in practice.
       (iv) Place prepared people in administration.
       (v) Place prepared people in education.
       (vi) Place prepared people in research.
       (vii) Foster identification of non-nursing tasks and their assignment to appropriate other departments or non-nursing personnel.
       (viii) Recognize excellence in all fields: administration, education, research, and practice.
   (7) Provision of needed supplies and equipment for nursing activities.
   (8) Provision of input into remodeling and establishing required physical facilities.
   (9) Orientation and continuing education of all nursing personnel.
   (10) Education of students in the health care field according to a written agreement and collaborative implementation between faculty of the educational institutions and personnel of the service organization.
   (11) Development of nursing research staff, research activities, and application of the research findings of others.
   (12) Evaluation of all objectives—organizational, divisional, departmental, and at the service and unit level, as well as those stated in the individual's job description and standards.
4. The management plans should have mileposts that are reasonable and attainable, with deadlines included.
5. Management plans should be based on complete information.

STRATEGY

Planning is the strategy of an organization and is essential to all businesses, including those providing health care. Planning techniques used in business and industry are being increasingly used in health-care organizations. Strategy is the process by which an organization achieves success in a changing environment. Nursing has only tapped the surface of a business strategy.[14] A myriad of services is available that can be offered to potential clients, such as telephone and e-mail access to information on drug prices, durable-medical-equipment prices, educational services, research briefs, and a host of therapeutic nursing products. A nursing strategy will outline how the organization achieves its strategic goals and objectives in a competitive marketplace.

Cavanaugh relates strategy to power, indicating that organizational power gives nurses the power to do their jobs better. Her suggestions for nurses to strategize are summarized as follows:[15]

1. Use the political system to turn personal power into organizational power.
2. Recognize the self-interests of others in the organization and use them in a win-win manner.
3. Diagnose, plan, and execute an effective political campaign to achieve a well-thought-out, purposeful goal.
4. Define ways to achieve objectives while helping others. Know people and their goals.
5. Disengage from losing issues and from issues in which you have to defend yourself on someone else's turf. A technique for doing this is placing the issue at the end of an agenda or omitting it from the minutes.
6. Defend your territory.
7. Plan and carry out an offense on issues of your own choosing and commitment.
8. Build coalitions.
9. Exploit opportunities, using situations to your advantage. Go after winning issues.
10. Set situations to benefit persons who can benefit you. Then deliver the goods at a cost-effective price.

A political climate exists in any organization, and its democratic nature requires compromise, trade-offs, favors, and negotiation. Nurses must be political to gain their goals and objectives in such a climate. Ehrat identifies four considerations of political strategy:[16]

1. Structure considerations. The first major political concept is to learn the history of the organization, including its past struggles and their outcomes. Budgets reflect one of these political outcomes. What is valued by the organization? The successful professional nurse identifies these valued data and operates within their constraints and boundaries.

2. Economy considerations. What are the costs versus the benefits? Give something in return for gaining something better. All departments expect to gain a fair share of an increased budget. To assure that nursing has equity, nurses develop clientele, confidence, a meaningful network, administrative support, and effective platform skills, and they exploit their opportunities. In gaining and sustaining this influence, they do not go beyond tolerated limits.

3. Process considerations. Timing is important and is learned from leadership experience and maturation. Resolution is needed to prepare for and carry out negotiation and compromise. Impact must be considered from the viewpoint of opposition, support, risks, price, and trade-offs, all of which require strategies.

4. Outcome considerations. The outcome must meet minimum standards of satisfaction and avoid trouble. It must meet some needs of everyone. Consensus means 70 percent to 80 percent approval, agreement, and support.

Resources in the health-care field are scarce, causing political conflicts and power struggles. Nurses should learn the strategy associated with political knowledge and skills.

The nurse moving into a new nursing position plans strategies for success. From day one, this person arrives early, listens, is polite, and does not criticize the predecessor. This nurse makes friends with the boss, assumes authority, gets rid of nonessentials, trains subordinates, and delegates decision making to them. She or he establishes a psychological distance, avoids gripers and treats all employees as adults, maintains an open mind, and follows good communication skills by keeping people informed and accepting their input.

When conflicts occur, the nurse does not take sides. This individual attends to actions that produce quick results, impact the organization, are favorable to employees, and require a small investment. Vision is provided by giving a sense of nursing's mission, its importance, its relevance, and the meaningfulness of nursing work. This is done by listening, sharing, developing mutual ideas, and enlisting support of informal leaders.

Clear, complete plans are developed in seven key results areas:

1. Client satisfaction.
2. Productivity.
3. Innovation.
4. Staff development.
5. Budget goals.
6. Quality.
7. Organizational climate.

These areas will include standards of performance that challenge and inspire. The professional nurse follows the rules. Rewards are given, including praise to relieve anxiety and to recognize accomplishments, and the best pay possible. Back talk, disobedience, insubordination, and malcontents are not tolerated; they are won over or neutralized. Decisions are made on test data and judgment.[17]

RESEARCH

While research could be considered as a key results area under innovation, it is good strategy to separate it into an eighth key results area. Research studies show that 20 percent of small businesses that did *not* do strategic planning failed, while only eight percent of small businesses that did strategic planning failed.[18]

A research study of the relationship between nursing department purpose, philosophy, and objectives and evidence of their implementation examined documents in thirty-five nursing departments. Specific indicators used were patient classification systems and staffing patterns, standards of patient care, and cost-containment activity. Implementation rates of desired nursing activity varied from 9 percent to 25 percent, indicating that a "low rate of implementation negates a causal relationship between references in the documents to desired nursing activity and actual nursing activity." The researchers suggest that purpose statements are sometimes unrealistic and unachievable. The framework for this study should be used to expand the research in this area.[19]

Exercise 6–5   Identify and develop a statement of the planning strategy for a nursing organization or unit.

WEB ACTIVITIES

▪ Visit www.jbpub.com/swansburg, this text's companion website on the Internet, for further information on The Foundations for Planning.

▪ Many organizations post their mission statements or value statements on the Internet. Locate some of these sites that clearly state the organization's objectives.

▪ Can you find sites on the Internet that state nursing visions and values? Do they differ from those you find in the book?

SUMMARY

The basic tools of planning are statements of mission or purpose, vision and values, philosophy or beliefs, and objectives, and an active operational or management plan. All nurses use such documents to accomplish the work of nursing.

The statement of mission or purpose tells the reason an entity, whether an organization, a division, a department, or a unit, exists. The nursing mission statement pertains to the clinical practice of nursing supported by research, education, and management.

The statement of philosophy reflects the values and beliefs of the organizational entity. It is translated into action by nursing personnel.

Objectives are concrete statements describing the major accomplishments nurses desire to achieve. Major categorical areas for objectives include

1. Organization and use of all resources, human, financial, and physical.
2. Social responsibility.
3. Staffing.
4. Requisition of supplies and equipment.
5. Planning of educational programs.
6. Innovation.
7. Marketing.
8. Evaluation of patient care.
9. Evaluation of personnel performance.

Operational or management plans convert objectives into action and include activities, assignments, deadlines, and provision for accountability. A major strategy of an organization is the planning process and the formulation and use of statements of mission, philosophy, and objectives and of organizational plans developed with the broadest possible input.

Statements of mission, philosophy, and objectives support each other at different agency levels, from the unit to the service or department and then to the division and finally to the organization.

NOTES

1. For a classic article on purpose, philosophy, and objectives, refer to M. A. Moore, "Philosophy, Purpose, and Objectives: Why Do We Have Them?" *Journal of Nursing Administration,* May–June 1971, 9–14.
2. D. L. Calfee, "Get Your Mission Statement Working!" *Management Review,* January 1993, 54–57.
3. P. Crosby, *Running Things: The Art of Making Things Happen* (New York: NAL-Dutton, 1989).
4. J. R. Reyes and B. H. Kleiner, "How to Establish an Organizational Purpose," *Management Decision: Quarterly Review of Management Technology* 28, no. 7 (1990): 51–54.
5. Ibid.
6. E. E. Spragins, "Resource—Constructing a Vision Statement," *Inc.,* October 1992, 33.
7. A. Campbell, "The Power of Mission: Aligning Strategy and Culture," *Planning Review,* September/October 1992, 10–12, 63.
8. V. Henderson, *The Nature of Nursing* (New York: Macmillan, 1966), 15.
9. I. M. King, "A Conceptual Frame of Reference in Nursing," *Nursing Research,* January–February 1968, 27–31.
10. D. E. Orem, *Nursing: Concepts of Practice,* 5th ed. (New York: McGraw-Hill, 1995), 7.
11. G. W. Poteet and A. S. Hill, "Identifying the Components of a Nursing Service Philosophy," *Journal of Nursing Administration,* October 1988, 29–33.
12. M. A. Moore, op. cit., 13; D. L. Calfee, op. cit.

13. P. F. Drucker, *Management: Tasks, Responsibilities, Practice* (New York: Harper & Row, 1978), 99–102.

14. D. E. Morris and S. E. Rau, "Strategic Competition: The Application of Business Planning Techniques to the Hospital Marketplace," *Healthcare Strategic Management,* January 1985, 17–20.

15. D. E. Cavanaugh, "Gamesmanship: The Art of Strategizing," *Journal of Nursing Administraiton,* April 1985, 38–41.

16. K. S. Ehrat, "A Model for Politically Astute Planning and Decision Making," *Journal of Nursing Administration,* September 1983, 29–35.

17. V. C. Sherman, "Taking Over: Notes to the New Executive," *Journal of Nursing Administration,* May 1982, 21–23.

18. Ireland, R. D., and M. A. Hitt. 1992. "Mission Statements: Importance, Challenge, and Recommendations for Development." *Business Horizons* (May–June): 34–42.

19. B. J. Trexler, "Nursing Department Purpose, Philosophy, and Objectives: Their Use and Effectiveness," *Journal of Nursing Administration,* March 1987, 8–12.

7

STAFFING AND SCHEDULING

OBJECTIVES

- Describe the components of the staffing process.
- Do a work sampling study covering a specific period of time.
- Determine the responsibility for staffing activities.
- Determine the core staff and the complementary staff for a nursing unit.
- Prepare a staffing plan for a nursing unit.
- Describe the components of a patient classification system (PCS).
- Determine the modified approaches to nurse staffing and scheduling used by a health-care organization.
- Identify methods for improving productivity in a health-care agency.

KEY CONCEPTS

staffing

work sampling

work contracts

core staff

self-scheduling

patient classification system (PCS)

modified work week

productivity

Manager Behavior: Applies principles and techniques for staffing and scheduling to meet agency standards for amount and quality of care needed.

Leader Behavior: Applies principles and techniques for staffing and scheduling to meet personnel needs and agency standards for amount and quality of patient care needed.

STAFFING PHILOSOPHY

Staffing is certainly one of the major problems of any nursing organization, whether it be a hospital, nursing home, home-health-care agency, ambulatory care agency, or another type of facility. Aydelotte has stated, "Nurse staffing methodology should be an orderly, systematic process, based upon sound rationale, applied to determine the number and kind of nursing personnel required to provide nursing care of a predetermined standard to a group of patients in a particular setting. The end result is prediction of the kind and number of staff required to give care to patients."[1]

Components of the staffing process as a control system include a staffing study, a master staffing plan, a scheduling plan, and a nursing management information system (NMIS). The NMIS includes these five elements:[2]

1. Quality of patient care to be delivered and its measurement.
2. Characteristics of the patients and their care requirements.
3. Prediction of the supply of nurse power required for elements 1 and 2.
4. Logistics of the staffing program pattern and its control.
5. Evaluation of the quality of care desired, thereby measuring the success of the staffing itself.

West adds a position control plan and a budgeting plan (see Exhibit 7–1).

Nurse staffing must meet certain regulatory requirements, among which are legal requirements of Medicare. (The Medicare regulations are excerpted in Exhibit 7–2.) This legal standard is further supported by, for example, the standards of the Joint Commission on Accreditation of Healthcare Organizations. Some other standards include the ANA *Scope and Standards for Nurse Administrators,* ANA *Standards of Clinical Nursing Practice,* and state licensing requirements.

From all of these standards and from the expectations of the community, of nurses, and of physicians, the nurse administrator will develop a staffing philosophy as a basis for a staffing methodology. Community expectations will be related to economic status, local value and belief systems, and local standards of culture. Nurses' expectations will be related to the same community standards and, in addition to their perceptions of the practice of nursing and its components, to the results desired and to the workload tolerated. See Appendix 7–1, "Staffing and Assignment Guidelines."

Exhibit 7–1   Components of the Staffing Process

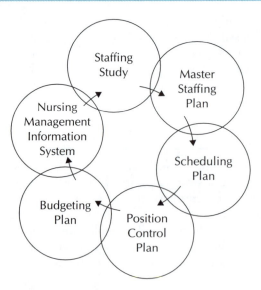

Exhibit 7–2   Medicare and Medicaid Regulations

482.23   Condition of participation: Nursing services.

The hospital must have an organized nursing service that provides 24-hour nursing services. The nursing services must be furnished or supervised by a registered nurse.

(a) *Standard: Organization.* The hospital must have a well-organized service with a plan of administrative authority and delineation of responsibilities for patient care. The director of nursing service must be a licensed registered nurse. He or she is responsible for the operation of the service, including determining the types and numbers of nursing personnel and staff necessary to provide nursing care for all areas of the hospital.

(b) *Standard: Staffing and delivery of care.* The nursing service must have adequate numbers of licensed registered nurses, licensed practical nurses (vocational), and other personnel to provide nursing care to all patients as needed. There must be supervisory and staff personnel for each department or nursing unit to ensure, when needed, the immediate availability of a registered nurse for bedside care of any patient.

  (1) The hospital must provide 24-hour nursing service furnished or supervised by a registered nurse, and have a licensed practical nurse or registered nurse on duty at all times, except for rural hospitals that have in effect a 24-hour nursing waiver granted under §405.1910(c) of this chapter.

  (2) The nursing service must have a procedure to ensure that hospital nursing personnel for whom licensure is required have valid and current licensure.

  (3) A registered nurse must supervise and evaluate the nursing care for each patient.

  (4) The hospital must ensure that the nursing staff develops, and keeps current, a nursing care plan for each patient.

  (5) A registered nurse must assign the nursing care of each patient to other nursing personnel in accordance with the patient's needs and the specialized qualifications and competence of the nursing staff available.

  (6) Non-employee licensed nurses who are working in the hospital must adhere to the policies

and procedures of the hospital. The director of nursing service must provide for adequate supervision and evaluation of the clinical activities of non-employee nursing personnel which occur within the responsibility of the nursing service.

(c) *Standard: Preparation and administration of drugs.* Drugs and biologicals must be prepared and administered in accordance with Federal and State laws, the orders of the practitioner or practitioners responsible for the patient's care as specified under §482.12(c), and accepted standards of practice.

  (1) All drugs and biologicals must be administered by, or under supervision of, nursing or other personnel in accordance with Federal and State laws and regulations, including applicable licensing requirements and in accordance with the approved medical staff policies and procedures.

  (2) All orders for drugs and biologicals must be in writing and signed by the practitioner or practitioners responsible for the care of the patient as specified under §482.12(c). When telephone or oral orders must be used, they must be

    (i) Accepted only by personnel who are authorized to do so by the medical staff policies and procedures, consistent with Federal and State law;

    (ii) Signed or initialed by the prescribing practitioner as soon as possible; and

    (iii) Used infrequently.

  (3) Blood transfusions and intravenous medications must be administered in accordance with State law and approved medical staff policies and procedures. If blood transfusions and intravenous medications are administered by personnel other than doctors of medicine or osteopathy, the personnel must have special training for this duty.

  (4) There must be a hospital procedure for reporting transfusion reactions, adverse drug reactions, and errors in administration of drugs.

Source: Reprinted with permission from CCH's *Medicare and Medicaid Regulations,* copyright 1986, CCH Incorporated, Riverwoods, Ill.

Nurses can discern from the nursing agency's existing statements of purpose, philosophy, and objectives various values related to staffing. A staffing philosophy may encompass beliefs about using a patient classification system for identifying patient care needs. It may cover beliefs about use of skilled personnel as a core staff, with a float pool for supplemental staffing. It may also specify who will be responsible for hiring.[4]

Objectives of nurse staffing are excellent care and high productivity. Professional nurses can develop a statement of purpose that is comprehensive in stating the quality and quantity of performance it is intended to motivate. Purpose statements should be quantified.[5]

Current and future trends indicate extensive structural changes in the health-care system, including downsizing, mergers, closures, and increased ambulatory care services. Managers and clinical nurses will be faced with making staffing decisions to increase productivity. These decisions should be based on lessons learned during the past two decades about management of human resources or human capital.

STAFFING STUDY

A staffing study should gather data about environmental factors within and outside the organization that affect staffing requirements. Aydelotte listed four techniques drawn from engineering to measure the work of nurses. All involved the concept of time required for performance.[6] Aydelotte's techniques are as follows:

1. Time study and task frequency.
   a. Tasks and task elements (procedures).
   b. Point and time started.
   c. Point and time ended.
   d. Sample size.
   e. Average time.
   f. Allowance for fatigue, personal variation, and unavoidable standby.
   g. Standard time = step e + step f.
   h. Frequency of task × standard time = the measurement of nursing activity.
   i. Total of all tasks × standard time = volume of nursing work.
2. Work sampling (variation of task frequency and time). Procedure is as follows:
   a. Identify major and minor categories of nursing activities.
   b. Determine number of observations to be made.
   c. Observe random sample of nursing personnel performing activities.
   d. Analyze observations. Frequency occurring in a specific category = percentage of total time spent in that activity. Most work sampling studies sample direct care and indirect care to determine ratio.
3. Continuous sampling (variation of task frequency and time). Technique is the same as for work sampling except that
   a. Observer follows one individual in the performance of a task.
   b. Observer may observe work performed for one or more patients if they can be observed concurrently.

4. Self-reporting (variation of task frequency and time).
    a. The individual records the work sampling or continuous sampling on himself or herself.
    b. Tasks are logged using time intervals or time tasks start and end.
    c. Logs are analyzed.

Many work sampling studies focus on procedures, ignore standards, and are lacking in objectivity, reliability, and accuracy. The techniques themselves are sound (see Exhibit 7–3).

Exhibit 7–3   Work Sampling Study

RN, LPN, NA (*circle one*)

Task or Procedure	Time Started	Time Ended	Minutes
1. _____			
2. _____			
3. _____			
4. _____			
5. _____			
6. _____			
7. _____			
8. _____			
9. _____			
10. _____			

(A) Total number of tasks and procedures = _____

(B) Total minutes = _____

Average Time

Total minutes	+	Total number of tasks and procedures	=	Average time per procedure or task
(B) _____	+	(A) _____	=	(C) _____

Standard Time

Average time	+	Time allowed for fatigue, personal variation, and unavoidable standby	=	Standard time in minutes
(C) _____	+	(D) _____	=	(E) _____

Measurement of Nursing Activity

Standard time	×	Frequency of an individual task or procedure	=	Measurement of nursing activity
(E) _____	×	(F) _____	=	(G) _____

Volume of Nursing Work

Standard time	×	Total number of tasks and procedures	=	Volume of nursing work
(E) _____	×	(A) _____	=	(H) _____

Source: Adapted from: M. K. Aydelotte, *Nurse Staffing Methodology: A Review and Critique of Selected Literature* (Washington, D.C.: U.S. Government Printing Office, January 1973).

According to West, "There are three cardinal rules for forecasting staffing requirements."[7] The first is to base staffing projections upon past staffing history; Exhibit 7–4 is designed as a data sheet for this purpose. The data can be collected from the patient classification system reports and census reports. Such data are readily available in most hospitals. Some NMISs, such as Medicus, provide numbers of personnel required, including the mix of RNs, LPNs, and NAs (nursing assistants). Other data needed are sick time, overtime, holidays, and vacation time. The attrition rate is also important and is discussed in Chapter 8 as turnover. In some patient classification systems, these data are built into the staffing formula.

The second cardinal rule for staffing is to review current staffing levels. Review of future plans for the institution is the third cardinal rule.[8] Clinical nurses who are involved in staffing plans will have confidence in the plans. These staffing studies can be made with electronic spreadsheets.

Staffing requires much planning on the part of nurses. Data must be collected and analyzed. These data include facts about the product—patient care—as well as diagnostic and therapeutic procedures performed by both physicians and nurses and the knowledge elements of professional nursing translated into

Exhibit 7–4   Staffing History Data Sheet

Year _____   Month _____   Cost Center _____

Day	ADC	Patient Acuity	Personnel				
			Sick Hours	Overtime Hours	Holiday Hours	Vacation Hours	Other
1							
2							
			• • •				
31							
Average							

Source: Adapted with permission from M. E. West, "Implementing Effective Nurse Staffing Systems in the Managed Hospitals," *Topics in Health Care Financing* (Summer 1980). Copyright Aspen Publishers.

professional nursing skills of history taking and assessment, nursing diagnosis and prescription, application of care, evaluation, record keeping, and all other actions related to primary health care of patients.

> Basic to planning for staffing of a division of nursing is the fact that qualified nursing personnel must be provided in sufficient numbers to ensure adequate, safe nursing care for all patients twenty-four hours a day, seven days a week, fifty-two weeks a year.

Each staffing plan must be tailored to the needs of the agency and cannot be arrived at by a simple worker/patient ratio or formula.

Changing, expanding knowledge and technology in the physical and social sciences, the medical field, and economics influence planning for staffing. Healthcare institutions are treating more clients on an outpatient basis. New drugs, improved diagnostic and therapeutic procedures, and reimbursement changes have decreased the lengths of hospitalization. Standards of the Joint Commission on Accreditation of Healthcare Organizations, the American Nurses Association, and other professional and governmental organizations have required upgrading of health care.

Planning for staffing is influenced by the following:[9]

1. Changing concepts of nursing roles for clinical nurse practitioners and specialists.
2. Patient populations that are changing as birthrates decline and longevity increases.
3. Institutional missions and objectives related to research, training, and many specialties.
4. Personnel policies and practices.
5. Policies and practices related to admission and discharge times of patients, assignment of patients to units, and intensive and progressive care practices.
6. The degree to which other departments carry out their supporting services.
7. The number and composition of the medical staff and the medical services offered.
8. Arrangement of the physical plant, which has a large impact on staffing requirements.
9. The organization of the division of nursing.
10. Data to be analyzed that will include numbers of admissions, discharges, and transfers; the amount of supervision needed by assisting personnel; patient teaching; emergency responses; mode of care delivery; and staff mix.

STAFFING ACTIVITIES

Price identified seventeen different staffing activities and suggested that the nurse administrator identify by name the persons responsible for each activity. A modified Price format for gathering data and analyzing responsibility for staffing activities would cover the following: recruitment; interviewing, screening, and hiring of RNs, LPNs, and NAs; assignment to clinical units and shifts; preparing work schedules in advance; maintaining daily schedule; adjusting for staff absences and patients' needs; calculating turnover and hours of care; checking time cards and payroll; policy development; telephone communication; and contract compliance.[10]

Orientation Plan

A main purpose of orientation is to help the nursing worker adjust to a new work situation. This should be a planned program that includes orientation—whether through a buddy system, a special orientation unit, or other method. Those nursing tasks and skills required of each nursing worker who is not proficient in them should be the focus of this program. Productivity is increased, since fewer personnel are needed when workers are fully oriented to the work situation. Exhibit 7–5 is an example of an orientation plan.

Staffing Policies

Written staffing policies should be readily available in at least the following areas:

1. Vacations.
2. Holidays.
3. Sick leave.
4. Weekends off.
5. Consecutive days off.
6. Rotation to different shifts.
7. Overtime.
8. Part-time and temporary personnel.
9. Use of float personnel.
10. Exchangeability of staff.
11. Use of special abilities of individual staff members.
12. Exchanging hours.
13. Requests of personnel.
14. Requests of management.
15. The workweek.

Work Contracts

A work contract should be set up between each employee and the institution. The contract should state the date employment is to commence, the job classification, the hours of work, the rate of pay, whether the job is full-time or part-time, and any other specific points agreed upon between employee and institu-

Exhibit 7–5   Nursing Orientation—Week 1

Monday	Tuesday	Wednesday	Thursday	Friday

8:00–4:30
 	
Personnel Orientation
 	
Benefits
 	
Quality assurance
 	
Employee health
 	
Infection control
 	
Fire & safety
	8:00–10:00
	Introduction
	  Philosophy
	  Dress code
	  Staffing
	  Time/attendance
	  Skills Assessment
	
	10:00–10:15
	Break
	
	10:15–12:15
	Documentation
	
	12:15–1:15
	Lunch
	
	1:15–4:30
	MAR
	Medical Policies
	Medical Exam
		8:00–8:15
		Computer Class
		Assignment
		
		8:15–12:00
		Code 1
		CPR
		
		12:00–1:00
		Lunch
		
		1:00–4:30
		Clinical Skills
		RN/LPN
		  BGM
		  Emergency trach R.
		  TPN dressing C.
		
		NA
		  BGM
		  Vital signs
		  Body mechanics
		  Infection control
		  Legal
			8:00–4:30
			RN IV Therapy
				8:00–8:45
				Alabama Eye Center
				
				8:45–9:30
				Alabama Organ Center
				
				9:30–9:45
				Break
				
				9:45–10:00
				Nutrition Service
				
				10:00–11:00
				Telephone System
				
				11:00–12:00
				Lunch
				
				12:00–4:30
				Team Building

Source: Reprinted courtesy University of South Alabama Medical Center, Mobile, Alabama.

tional representative. Both parties should sign the contract. Work contracts may be superseded by union contracts.

STAFFING THE UNITS

Each patient care unit should have a master staffing plan that includes the basic staff needed to cover the unit each shift. Basic staff is the minimum or lowest number of personnel needed to staff a unit. It includes fully oriented full-time and part-time employees. The number may be based on examination of previous staff records and expert opinion of nurse managers. It includes all categories: registered nurses, licensed practical nurses, and nursing technicians or assistants for each shift. Exhibit 7–6 shows a formula for determining a core staff per shift.

Next the number of *complementary* personnel is determined. Complementary personnel are scheduled as an addition to the basic group, but the total

Exhibit 7–6 Formula for Estimating a Core Staff per Shift

The average daily census for a 25-bed medical-surgical unit over a 6-month period is 19 patients. The basic average daily hours of care to be provided are 5 hours per patient per 24 hours. How many total hours of care will be needed on the average day to meet these standards? $19 \times 5 = 95$ hours. If the workday is 8 hours, this means $95 \div 8 = 11.9$ or 12 full-time-equivalent (FTE) staff are needed to staff the unit for 24 hours. An FTE is one person working full time (40 hours a week) or several persons who together work a total of 40 hours a week. A total of 12 FTE $\times$ 7 days per week = 84 shifts per week, if the staffing is to be the same each day. If each employee works five 8-hour shifts per week, $84 \div 5 = 16.8$ is the number of FTEs needed as basic staff for this unit.

The number of nursing personnel to cover sick leave, vacations, and holidays or other absences can also be determined and added to the basic staff. This information is determined from a study of personnel policies and use. It is frequently included in patient classification system formulas. Such additional staff may be provided from a float pool.

The next determination to be made is the ratio of RNs to other nursing personnel. If the ratio is determined as 1:1, how many of the basic staff of 16.8 should be RNs? One-half of the total, which would be 8.4 RNs and 8.4 others (LPNs, nurse's aides, orderlies, or nursing assistants). A study of staffing patterns in 80 med/surg, pediatrics, and post-partum units in 12 Salt Lake City community hospitals recommends a mix of 58% RNs, 26% LPNs, and 16% aides.[11]

The final determination is how many personnel are needed for each shift. Warstler recommends proportions of: day—47%; evening—35%; and night—17%.[12] This means that for a total staff of 16.8 personnel, 8 would be assigned to days, 6 to evenings, and 2.8 to nights. This is obviously approximate; other patterns could also be chosen by the nurse administrator.

The number of complementary nursing personnel would be added to this basic staff. They could be a group of one RN, one LPN, and one other and assigned accordingly. They are entered into the following table as numbers in parenthesis added to the figure for basic staff.

In today's reimbursement environment, complementary personnel may be budgeted as a pool. They may even exist only as a portion of basic personnel assigned to a pool.

Basic Staffing Plan for 25-Bed Medical-Surgical Unit

Category	Day	Evening	Night	Totals
RNs	4 + (1)	3	1.4	8.4 + (1)
LPNs	2	2 + (1)	1.4	5.4 + (1)
Others	2	1	0 + (1)	3 + (1)
Totals	8 + (1)	6 + (1)	2.8 + (1)	16.8 + (3)

number in both groups will be controlled by financial resources and the availability of personnel. Complementary personnel provide the flexibility needed to meet short-term and unexpected changes. They are not ensured a permanent pattern and are usually scheduled for four-week periods.

Float personnel are employees who are not permanently assigned to a station. They provide flexibility to meet increased patient loads as well as unexpected personnel absences. The number and kinds of float personnel can be accurately determined from general monthly records that show absence rates, personnel turnover, and fluctuations in patient care workloads. Float personnel may be assigned to a pool or by unit.

Some nurse administrators do not hire part-time nursing personnel, who may be an economic or cost-control factor in staffing, since they usually do not receive the same benefits as full-time personnel. Part-time personnel will be better motivated if they receive some benefits, such as a number of paid holidays and vacation days proportionate to days worked and pay increases when they complete the aggregate days worked by full-time personnel. Their total hours worked can be controlled to fill actual shortfalls.

Whatever the staffing policy, it should be arrived at through consultation with clinical nurses. The nursing department personnel budget is also a master staffing plan. The process for developing a master staffing plan is depicted in Exhibits 7–6, 7–7, and 7–8. The basic staff for a unit may be determined by using Exhibit 7–6. It may be translated to a staffing board, using Exhibit 7–7. Exhibit 7–8 may be used for self-scheduling.

Exhibit 7–7 Staffing Board

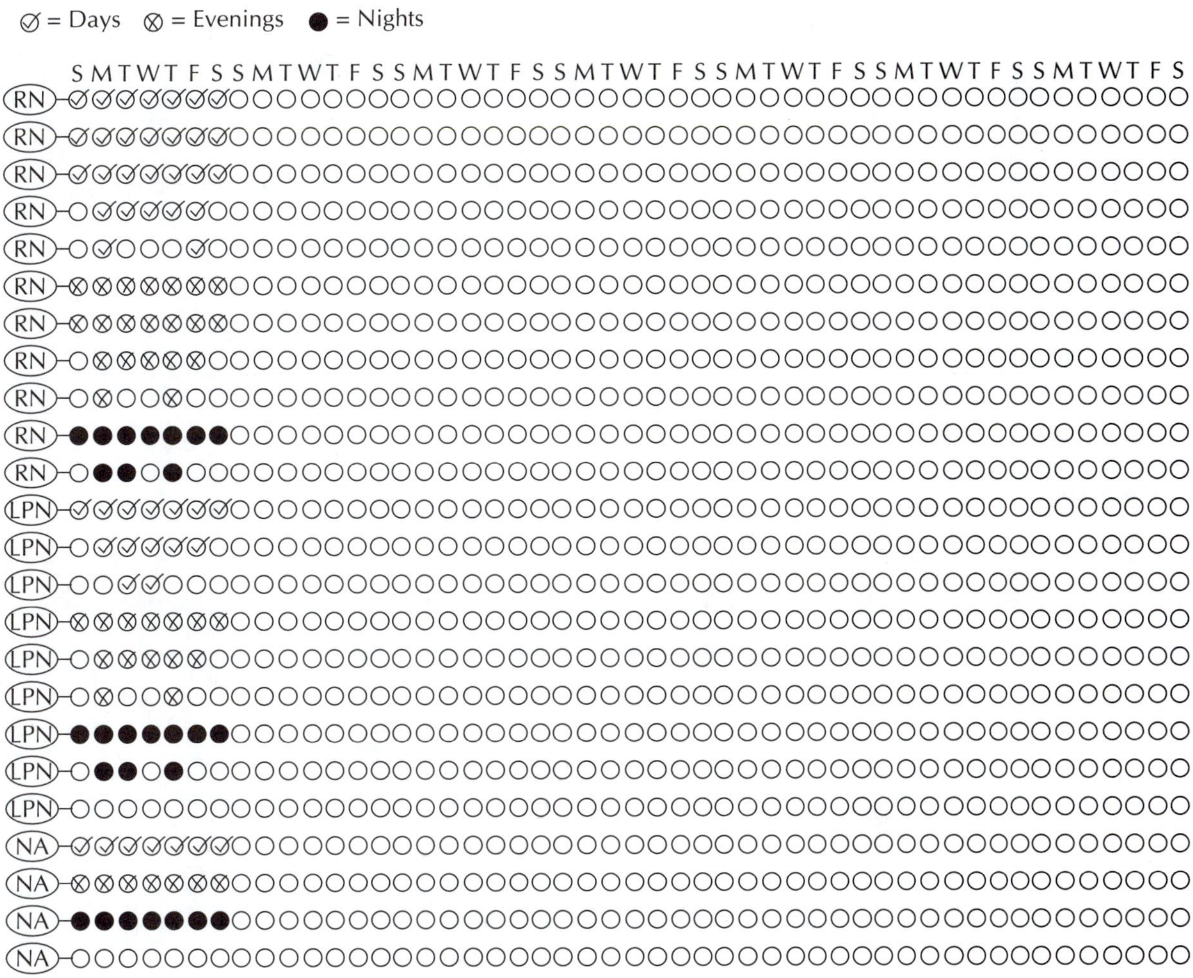

Left row of pegs is coded by category of personnel: RN, LPN, NA (nursing assistant). There are peg holes on the board for 24 persons for seven weeks. Larger boards can be used. Pegs for scheduling would be color-coded for shifts: day, evening, night, weekend, off, etc.

Exhibit 7–8   Self-Scheduling Format

	S	Initials	M	Initials	T	Initials	W	Initials	T	Initials	F	Initials	S	Initials
Week *Jan 15* 11a.m.	3RNs 1LPN 1NA	JH	5RNs 2LPNs 1NA		4RNs 3LPNs 1NA		4RNs 3LPNs 1NA		4RNs 2LPNs 1NA		5RNs 2LPNs 1NA		3RNs 1LPN 1NA	
3p.m..	3RNs 1LPN 1NA	JH	5RNs 2LPNs 1NA		4RNs 3LPNs 1NA		4RNs 3LPNs 1NA		4RNs 2LPNs 1NA		5RNs 2LPNs 1NA		3RNs 1LPN 1NA	
7p.m.	2RNs 1LPN 1NA		4RNs 3LPNs 1NA		3RNs 2LPNs 1NA		3RNs 2LPNs 1NA		4RNs 3LPNs 1NA		3RNs 2LPNs 1NA		2RNs 1LPN 1NA	
11p.m.	2RNs 1LPN 1NA		4RNs 3LPNs 1NA		3RNs 2LPNs 1NA		3RNs 2LPNs 1NA		4RNs 3LPNs 1NA		3RNs 2LPNs 1NA		2RNs 1LPN 1NA	
3a.m.	1RN 1LPN 1NA		2RNs 2LPNs 1NA	JH	2RN 2LPN 1NA	JH	1RN 1LPN 1NA	JH	2RNs 2LPNs 1NA	JH	1RN 1LPN 1NA		1RN 1LPN 1NA	
7a.m.	1RN 1LPN 1NA		2RNs 2LPNs 1NA	JH	2RN 2LPN 1NA	JH	1RN 1LPN 1NA	JH	2RNs 2LPNs 1NA	JH	1RN 1LPN 1NA		1RN 1LPN 1NA	
Week 11a.m.														
3p.m.														
7p.m.														
11p.m.														
3a.m.														
7a.m.														

Each block represents 4 hours of staffing.
Names and Initials:

RN Jane Hatfield JH ____   _____   _____   _____   _____

_____   _____   _____   _____   _____

_____   _____   _____   _____   _____

_____   _____   _____   _____   _____

_____   _____   _____   _____   _____

Exhibit 7–9 Cyclic Schedules

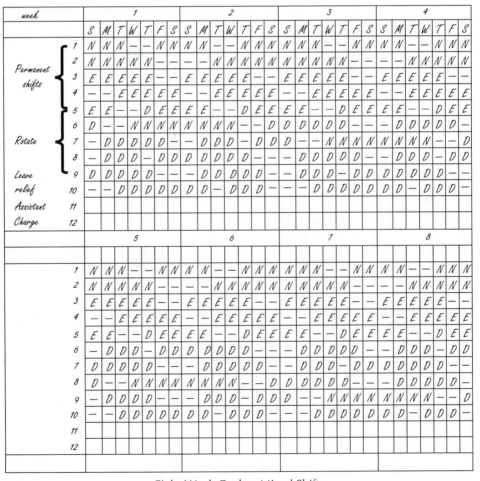

Minimum Basic Schedule

Eight-Week Cycle—Mixed Shifts

Source: Department of the Air Force, *USAF Hospital Nursing Service Manual* (Washington, D.C.: U.S. Government Printing Office, 1971): 4-4–4-14.

The average daily census of a unit is 29 patients, the basic average daily hours of care to be provided are 6 hours per patient per 24 hours, and the workday is 8 hours. Use Exhibit 7–6, "Formula for Estimating a Core Staff per Shift," to determine the following:

1. The total hours of care needed on the average day to meet these standards.
2. The number of full-time equivalents (FTEs) needed to staff the unit for 24 hours.
3. The number of 8-hour shifts needed per week.
4. The number of FTEs needed as basic staff for this unit.
5. Using the Salt Lake City community hospitals' recommendation of staff mix, determine the mix of RNs:LPNs:aides.
6. Using Warsler's proportion for staffing shifts, determine the number of FTEs for days, evenings, and nights.
7. Make a table for basic staffing for this unit. Do not add complementary staff unless there is some rationale for it.

STAFFING MODULES

Cyclic Scheduling

Cyclic scheduling is one of the best ways of staffing to meet the requirements of equitable distribution of hours of work and time off. A basic time pattern for a certain number of weeks is established and then repeated in cycles. Since it is relatively inflexible, cyclic scheduling works only with a staff that rotates by policy and personal choice. It is not generally accepted by personnel who need flexible staffing to meet their personal needs such as those related to family and educational pursuits.

An infinite number of basic cyclic patterns can be developed and tailored to suit the needs of each unit. (Samples are shown in Exhibit 7–9.) Patterns should reflect policy, workload factors, and staff preferences. Nursing personnel may use a staffing board (Exhibit 7–7) to develop a pattern and cycle satisfactory to them. The staffing board is used to show the numbers of nursing personnel required for each day of the week for six weeks. Using the numbers from the basic staffing plan, the nurse manager and staff determined that one fewer RN was needed on weekdays and on Saturday and Sunday and could best be used on Monday and Friday, as these were high- volume workdays as determined by the standards. Also, only two RNs were needed on Saturday and Sunday evenings, while four were needed on Monday and Thursday evenings. One RN was needed on nights, with two on Monday, Tuesday, and Thursday nights.

Similarly, basic staffing for LPNs and others is shown on the staffing board in Exhibit 7–7. These numbers are then transferred to the self-scheduling format shown in Exhibit 7–8.

The numbers of staff are noted by the nurse manager for each four hours of staffing. Nursing personnel insert their initials in each block according to the givens of staffing policies. Additional pages can be used for self-scheduling for four, six, or any other number of weeks. Exhibit 7–9 as illustrated indicates FTEs needed on one week and a blank for one week. Signature and initials indicate that each employee has scheduled themselves for specific dates and hours of work.

It has been stated previously that staffing policies should be established in specific areas. The following are some policies that might be considered:

1. Personnel are scheduled to work their preferred shifts as much as possible.
2. Personnel choices are balanced to meet the needs of the unit and of other employees.
3. An employee is allowed to make her or his own arrangements for special time off or to exchange within specific personnel policies.
4. Policies have been established for making schedule changes.
5. Each employee has a copy of his or her work schedule.
6. Consideration has been given to staffing during hours of clinical experience for students.
7. There is a weekend and holiday schedule policy. It is a common practice in many organizations throughout the United States to plan alternate weekends off for nursing personnel. Weekend coverage can be by "weekends only" employees. Staffing levels needed can be influenced by hospital policies on admissions and discharges and weekend staffing policy.

Self-Scheduling

Self-Scheduling is an activity that could make a staff happier, more cohesive, and more committed. It should be planned carefully on a unit (cost-center) basis. Planning may use either a self-directed work team or a quality circle technique approach. Self-scheduling matches staff to individual preferences. It has been found to shorten scheduling time and reduce conflicts; increase job retention and job satisfaction; and reduce illness time, voluntary absenteeism, and turnover. A nurse manager asked a nurse administrator how she could reduce absentee problems. The nurse manager said she had twelve RNs with absentee problems. A discussion followed about self-scheduling and the procedures to use. Several months later, the nurse manager reported to the nurse administrator that she had implemented self-scheduling and found that only one of the twelve employees still posed an absentee problem. The other eleven absentee problems had disappeared with self-scheduling. The nurse manager then successfully proceeded to implement self-scheduling with all other employees who requested it.

Self-scheduling leads to more responsible employees. It meets such personal goals as family, social life, education, child care, and commuting. It is an example of participatory management with decentralized decision making. The planning must include the givens, or rules, to be followed. These rules should be minimal to meet legal and professional standards.[13]

PATIENT CLASSIFICATION SYSTEMS

A patient classification system (PCS), which quantifies the quality of nursing care, is essential to staffing nursing units of hospitals. In selecting or implementing a PCS, a representative committee of nurse managers and clinical nurses should be used. The committee can include a representative of hospital administration which would decrease skepticism about the PCS.

Purposes

The committee will identify the purposes of the PCS to be purchased or developed. Among these purposes are the following:

1. Staffing. The system will establish a unit of measure for nursing: *time,* which will be used to determine both numbers and kinds of staff needed. Perceived patient needs can be matched with available nursing resources.
2. Program costing and formulation of the nursing budget. A prescribed unit of time will be used to determine the actual cost of nursing service. Profits and losses of nursing can then be determined.
3. Tracking changes in patient care needs. A PCS gives nurse managers the ability to moderate and control delivery of care services, adjusting intensity and cost.
4. Determining values for the productivity equation: output divided by input. Reducing input costs reduces costs of each output (time unit). In the prospective payment system (PPS), this output measure has been the discharged patient. Outputs become the criteria for measuring nursing productivity, regardless of quality. PCSs provide workload indexes as productivity measures.
5. Determining quality. Once a standard time element is established, staffing is adjusted to meet the aggregate times. A nurse manager can elect to staff below the standard time to reduce costs. Thus, the nurse manager makes a decision to reduce quality by reducing time and cost. It is best to do this in collaboration with clinical nurses, who are the personnel who are continually present and can assist with developing and applying more efficient procedures and protocols. This can involve rearrangement of the physical setting and the assembling of equipment and supplies. Involvement by clinical nurses will increase their trust and respect, improve their attendance and work habits, improve workforce stability, and reduce errors. Clinical nurses' input into decision making can be through product evaluation and selection, identification of non-

nursing tasks to be done by lower-priced workers, increased mechanization, and job evaluation.[14]

Nursing Management Information Systems for PCSs

Nursing management information systems (NMISs) are described in more detail in chapter 21. A good system is basic to a sound PCS. It will provide shift reports of personnel needed and assigned, by type; staffing and productivity data, by unit and area; average data on the intensity of care needed, by class of patient; and the cost per time unit of patient care, by class of patient.[15]

Characteristics Desired of PCSs

The following characteristics are desirable of PCSs, which should

1. Differentiate intensity of care among definitive classes.
2. Measure and quantify care to develop a management engineering standard.
3. Match nursing resources to patient care requirements.
4. Relate to time and effort spent on the associated activity.
5. Be economical and convenient to report and use.
6. Be mutually exclusive, counting no item under more than one work unit.
7. Be open to audit.
8. Be understood by those who plan, schedule, and control the work.
9. Be individually standardized as to the procedures needed for accomplishment.
10. Separate requirements for registered nurses from those of other staff.[16]

Components of PCSs

The first component of a PCS is a method for grouping patients or patient categories. Johnson indicates two methods of categorizing patients. Using factor evaluation, each patient is rated on independent elements of care, each element is scored (weighted), scores are summarized, and the patient is placed in a category based on the total numerical value obtained. Using prototype evaluation, each patient is categorized to a broad description of care requirements.[17]

Johnson describes a prototype evaluation with four basic categories and one category for a typical patient requiring one-on-one care. Each category addresses activities of daily living, general health, teaching and emotional support, and treatments and medications. Data are collected on average time spent on direct and indirect care (see Exhibit 7–10).

A second component of a PCS is a set of guidelines describing the way in which patients will be classified, the frequency of classification, and the method of reporting the data (see Exhibit 7–11). The third component of a PCS is the average amount of time required for care of a patient in each category (see Exhibit 7–12).

Exhibit 7–10   Classification Categories—Medical Surgical Units

CATEGORY I—Self-Care

1. Activities of daily living.
   a. Eating—feeds self or needs little assistance.
   b. Grooming—almost entirely self-sufficient.
   c. Excretion—goes to bathroom alone or almost alone. Not incontinent.
   d. Comfort—self-sufficient.
2. General health—good. Admitted for a diagnostic procedure, simple procedure, or surgery that is simple or minor.
3. Teaching and emotional support—routine teaching for simple procedures, follow-up teaching or discharge teaching. No unusual or adverse emotional reactions. Patient may require orientation to time, place, and person once a shift.
4. Treatments and medications—none or simple medications or treatment.

CATEGORY II—Minimal Care

1. Activities of daily living.
   a. Eating—needs help in preparing food, positioning, or encouragement to eat. Can feed self.
   b. Grooming—can do majority of care unassisted or with minimal assistance.
   c. Excretion—needs help getting to bathroom or using urinal. Not incontinent or experiences occasional stress incontinence or dribbling.
   d. Comfort—turns self or turns with minimal encouragement or assistance
2. General health—mild symptoms including more than one mild illness. Requires monitoring of vital signs, diabetic urines, uncomplicated drainage, or infusion.
3. Teaching and emotional support—needs 5–10 minutes per shift for teaching or emotional support. Patient may be mildly confused, belligerent, or agitated but is well-controlled by medications, frequent orientation, or restraints.
4. Treatments and medications—requires 20–30 minutes a shift. Needs evaluation of effectiveness of medication or treatment frequently. May require observation q2h for mental status.

CATEGORY III—Moderate Care

1. Activities of daily living.
   a. Eating—needs to be fed but can chew and swallow.
   b. Grooming—unable to do much for self.
   c. Excretion—needs bedpan or urinal placed or removed. Can only partially turn or lift self. Incontinent two times each shift.

   d. Comfort—completely dependent and needs turning but can be turned by one person.
2. General health—acute symptoms may be impending or subsiding. Requires monitoring and evaluation of physiological or emotional state q2-4h. Has continuous drainage or infusion that requires monitoring q1h.
3. Teaching and emotional support—requires 10–30 minutes a shift. Very apprehensive or mildly resistive to teaching. Patient may be confused, agitated, or belligerent but is fairly well controlled by medications, frequent orientation, or restraints.
4. Treatments and medications—requires 30–60 minutes a shift. Requires frequent observation for side effects or allergic reaction. May require observation q1h for mental status.

CATEGORY IV—Extensive Care

1. Activities of daily living.
   a. Eating—cannot feed self. Difficulty chewing and swallowing. May require tube feeding.
   b. Grooming—complete bath, hair care, oral care. Patient cannot assist at all.
   c. Excretion—incontinent more than two times a shift.
   d. Comfort—cannot turn self or assist with turning. May require two people to turn.
2. General health—seriously ill. Exhibits acute symptoms such as bleeding and/or fluid loss, acute respiratory episodes, or other episodes requiring frequent monitoring and evaluation.
3. Teaching and emotional support—requires more than 30 minutes a shift. Teaching of very resistive patients or care and support of patients with severe emotional reactions. Patient may be confused, belligerent, or agitated and is not controlled by medications, frequent orientation, or restraints.
4. Treatment and medication—requires more than 60 minutes a shift. Elaborate treatments done more than once per shift or requiring two persons. May require observation more frequently than q1h for mental status.

CATEGORY V—Intensive Care

Requires one-to-one observation or continuous monitoring each shift.

Source: K. Johnson, "A Practical Approach to Patient Classification," *Nursing Management,* June 1984, 40. Reproduced by permission.

Exhibit 7–11   Directions for Classifying Patients

1. Patient classification will be reviewed one time each shift by the charge nurse or her designee on the 7–3 and 3–11 shifts.
2. Classification is made by comparing the individual patient with each of the categories. If a charge nurse is unsure as to what category a patient belongs, she should refer to the ADL indicator only and classify by those guidelines.
3. The cue sheet is only a guideline. It is not expected that every patient will be classified in the same category by disease entity alone.
4. After the category is selected, the charge nurse will place a number on the Kardex to denote that patient's classification
   Self-Care   —I
   Minimal Care   —II

Moderate Care   —III
Extensive Care   —IV
Intensive Care   —V

5. The charge nurse (or designee, e.g., secretary) will tally the number of patients in each category. The nursing office will call for the tallies at approximately 1 p.m.–9 p.m.
6. Patients who have private-duty nurses and sitters are classified according to the level of care the staff on the unit must provide to the patients.

Source: K. Johnson, "A Practical Approach to Patient Classification," *Nursing Management,* June 1984. Reprinted with permission.

Exhibit 7–12   Data Collection—Standard Care Hours per Patient Category

Directions: Consider a patient whom you have cared for today in each of the following categories. Indicate, to the best of your ability, the amount of time that was required to care for the patient. If you did not care for a patient in one of the categories this shift, please leave that category blank. Your cooperation in completing these forms is appreciated.

Check one:

RN	_____
LPN	_____
Aide/Attendant	_____

Fill in blank:

_____Shift
_____Unit
_____Date

Please leave this form in the area designated for that purpose on the nursing unit.

Category I	—Self-Care	_____Minutes
Category II	—Minimal Care	_____Minutes
Category III	—Moderate Care	_____Minutes
Category IV	—Extensive Care	_____Minutes

Source: K. Johnson, "A Practical Approach to Patient Classification," *Nursing Management,* June 1984. Reprinted with permission.

A method for calculating required staffing and required nursing care hours is the fourth and final component of a PCS. The formula is "the sum of the standard times for each category multiplied by the number of patients in that category plus the indirect care time equals required hours of patient care. Dividing this value by 7.0 (number of hours staff actually work each shift) results in the number of staff required to work each shift."[18]

The Commission for Administration Services in Hospitals (CASH) system of patient classification appears to be of the prototype evaluation type. CASH is a patient classification design that rates patients by intensity of care and establishes a category relating to nursing hours required based on patients' ability to feed and bathe themselves with supervision; mobility status; special procedures and treatments; and observational, institutional, and emotional needs. This design is quantified by determining the nursing care time associated with the critical indicators. The GRASP® system of patient classification uses a workload measurement design to evaluate the categories of tasks that nurses perform in providing patient care and identifies how much nursing time is required for each task. The time is then totaled.[19] GRASP® is a factor evaluation design, as is Medicus.

There is only general agreement that three to five categories of patient acuity are sufficient for a PCS. Alward argues that four categories are best to reduce variance and statistical probability of error. She also states that the factor evaluation instrument is better than the prototype system, as it prevents ambiguity or overlap among the categories.[20] There are PCSs based on models of nursing, developed in-house, and microcomputer models.

Research.   A research study was conducted at a 1,000-bed acute care, urban, university-affiliated hospital in Canada. The purpose of the research study was to examine whether three methods of patient classification estimate the same hours of care when applied to the same patient population. The three PCSs used were GRASP, PRN (Project Research in Nursing), and Medicus, all factor evaluation designs.

PRN, developed in Canada, includes 154 care activities, organized within a needs approach model, adapted from the Henderson model. GRASP assumes that 15 percent of activities in which nurses are involved take up 85 percent of nurses' time. Classification instruments are developed around these activities and are hospital specific. The Medicus tool has its origins in operations research, with approximately thirty-seven condition indicators rated daily. PRN and Medicus require modification to account for layout and other physical modifications of individual workplaces.

The mean hours of care estimated by each classification system are presented in Exhibit 7–13. It can be seen from Exhibit 7–13 that for the average patient on the average day, PRN predicted more care (9.06 hours) than Medicus

Exhibit 7–13   Means of Total Nursing Care Hours by Different Classification Systems*†

	$\overline{X}$	SD	Min	Max	SEM	CV
Medicus	6.63	6.18	1.75	31.9	0.14	0.93
PRN	9.06	7.04	0	36.0	0.15	0.77
GRASP	6.57	5.21	1.4	22.5	0.12	0.79

* Result of paired *t*-tests:

PRN—Medicus	$t = 35.50$	$p = 0.0001$
Medicus-GRASP	$t = 1.05$	$p = 0.30$
PRN—GRASP	$t = 32.40$	$p = 0.0001$

† $N = 2002$

Source: L. O'Brien-Pallas, P. Leatt, R. Deber, and J. Till, "A Comparison of Workload Estimates Using Three Methods of Patient Classification," *Canadian Journal of Nursing Administration*, September/October 1989, 20. Reprinted with permission.

Exhibit 7–14   Means of Direct Nursing Care Hours by Different Classification Systems*†

	X̄	SD	Min	Max	SEM	CV
Medicus	3.22	3.36	0.79	17.9	0.08	1.04
PRN	4.51	3.77	0	18.29	0.08	0.84
GRASP	3.35	2.66	0	13.81	0.06	0.79

* Result of paired *t*-tests:

PRN—Medicus	$t = 38.16$	$p < 0.0001$
Medicus-GRASP	$t = -4.08$	$p < 0.0001$
PRN—GRASP	$t = 32.14$	$p < 0.0001$

† $N = 2002$

Source: L. O'Brien-Pallas, P. Leatt, R. Deber, and J. Till, "A Comparison of Workload Estimates Using Three Methods of Patient Classification," *Canadian Journal of Nursing Administration,* September/October 1989, 21. Reprinted with permission.

or GRASP (6.63 and 6.57, respectively). No significant difference existed between GRASP and Medicus systems in mean estimates of total care (t = 1.05, p = 0.30).

From Exhibit 7–14 above it can be noted that PRN predicted on the average more direct care time (4.51 hours per patient) than did GRASP or Medicus (3.35 and 3.22, respectively). GRASP estimated an average of 0.13 of an hour of more direct care than did Medicus. All three systems demonstrated significant differences in direct care time estimates (p < 0.0001). PRN fairly consistently estimated more hours of direct care than did the other two systems. Medicus tended to estimate more hours than GRASP in ICU settings but fewer in non-ICU settings.

The following are the results of the study:[21]

- Different PCSs generate different estimates of hours of care and related nursing workload.
- PRN predicts more hours of care than does Medicus or GRASP.
- The GRASP PCS will estimate fewer hours of care than the Medicus or PRN PCSs and so is the least costly of the three.
- The Medicus PCS will estimate fewer hours of care than the PRN and so is less costly than PRN, but it is more costly than GRASP.
- PRN has construct validity.

Problems with PCSs

One of the major problems of PCSs is in maintaining reliability and validity. This can be done through continuing education and quality checks. A calendar can be established to have external personnel from staff development or another nursing department or unit perform a classification following that done by unit personnel (interacter reliability). This can be done monthly or more often, depending upon the results. Patients can be monitored on different days and different shifts, with a stratified random sample of about 15 percent or 20 percent of the patient census. Simple percentage agreement of 90 percent or higher indicates satisfactory reliability. If agreement is below 80 percent, the system should be reviewed and adjusted.

A calendar also can be established to take a unit rotation work sample to determine whether procedures or tasks change with time and technology. This can be an annual spot check. Validating of PCSs varies. A questionnaire can be used to evaluate a nursing staff's satisfaction with hours of care. Validity can also be tested using an expert panel of nurses. Patient category descriptions or critical indicators of nursing intervention and patient requirement lists should be reviewed annually by using standards. The PCSs must be altered if results of quality checks or work samples so indicate.

Orientation and continuing education are the best methods of assuring reliability and validity. The nursing staff must find the PCS credible. If the nurses believe that the classifications are accurate and useful, they will try to rate patients accurately. They need periodic classes to be updated and kept well-informed. Managers must support the use of a valid and reliable PCS, since it indicates the institution's commitment to quality patient care.

Nursing should orient other department heads and physicians to the use of PCSs. Admission and placement of patients are related to PCS outcomes.[22]

Practicing nurses want the PCS to provide more staff. Managing nurses want to use it to validate staffing and scheduling and permit variable staffing. These objectives must be kept in harmony.

Exercise 7–2   Do a literature search for PCSs for long-term care. Summarize your findings.

MODIFIED APPROACHES TO NURSE STAFFING AND SCHEDULING

Many different approaches to nurse staffing and scheduling are being tried in an effort to satisfy the needs of employees and meet workload demands for patient care. They include game theory, modified workweeks (ten- or twelve-hour shifts), team rotation, "premium day" weekend nurse staffing, and "premium vacation" night staffing. Such approaches should support the underlying purpose, mission, philosophy, and objectives of the organization and the division of nursing and should be well-defined in staffing philosophy and policies. Nurses are like other workers in one respect: They would like to live as normal a home life as possible. Shifts have to be staffed and patient care needs met. The successful nurse executive will try to accommodate both by using the best available administrative staffing methodology, which must be considered from the economic or cost/benefit viewpoint.

Staffing and scheduling are reasons for employee turnover and job retention. Understaffing has a negative effect on staff morale, delivery of quality care, and the nursing practice modality. It can close beds. It causes absenteeism from staff fatigue, burnout, and professional dissatisfaction. On the other hand, overstaffing is expensive and has a negative effect on staff morale and productivity since nurse managers want to receive value for their money, they need to know that economic constraints exist that are further stretched by the costs of recruiting, hiring, and orienting new nurses and for overtime and temporary hires when the environment creates turnovers and absenteeism. Staffing and scheduling must balance the personal needs of nurses with the economic and productivity needs of the organization.[23]

Modified Workweeks

Modified workweek schedules using ten- and twelve-hour shifts and other methods are commonplace. A nurse administrator should be sure the work schedules are fulfilling the staffing philosophy and policies, particularly with regard to efficiency. Also, such schedules should not be imposed upon the nursing staff but should show a mutual benefit to employer, employee, and, ultimately, the clients served.

The four-day, ten-hour work schedule for night nurses was studied in a hospital that had difficulty recruiting qualified nurses to the night shift. It had been perceived that ten-hour shifts had stabilized staffing in intensive care, with increased productivity and decreased turnover.

Turnover on the night shift had been 70 percent for an eight-month period. Positions stayed vacant longer than for other shifts, and sick time was higher, which increased recruitment and orientation time. Nurses were involved in planning the four-day, ten-hour night-shift schedule. Night nurses agreed to use overlap hours to assist with day-shift care. The day shift agreed to reduce staff by one FTE. Plans were discussed with and accepted by the union. Making assignments of personnel and meeting schedules were addressed and resolved through participatory management. The results of these changes included reduced sick time on the ten-hour shift, reduced turnover, increased incentive, increased requests for night shift, and decreased labor hours[24] (see Exhibit 7–15).

The Twelve-Hour Shift.
A second scheduling modification is the twelve-hour shift, on which nurses work seven shifts in two weeks: three on, four off; four on, three off. They work a total of eighty-four hours and are paid four hours' overtime. Twelve-hour shifts and flexible staffing have been reported to have improved care and saved money because nurses can manage their home and personal lives better.[25]

A research study was done to measure the effect of fatigue from twelve-hour shifts on critical thinking. Findings: There were "no significant differences between levels of fatigue and critical thinking ability in nurses working eight- and 12 hours."[26]

The Weekend Alternative.
Another variation of flexible scheduling is the weekend alternative. Nurses work two twelve-hour shifts and are paid for forty hours plus benefits. They can use the weekdays to go to school or for other personal needs. The weekend schedule has several variations. Monday-through-Friday nurses have all weekends off.

Exhibit 7–15   A Graph Comparing Casual Absenteeism on One Unit with Different Schedules

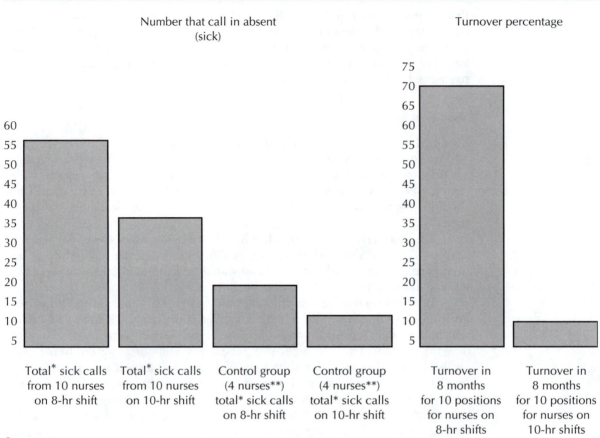

Number that call in absent (sick)

Turnover percentage

Total* sick calls from 10 nurses on 8-hr shift

Total* sick calls from 10 nurses on 10-hr shift

Control group (4 nurses**) total* sick calls on 8-hr shift

Control group (4 nurses**) total* sick calls on 10-hr shift

Turnover in 8 months for 10 positions for nurses on 8-hr shifts

Turnover in 8 months for 10 positions for nurses on 10-hr shifts

* 8-month period
** Same nurses

Source: J. A. Ricci, "10-Hour Night Shift: Cost vs. Savings," *Nursing Management,* January 1984, 38. Reprinted with permission.

Other Modified Approaches

A study by Imig, Powell, and Thorman indicated that while flexible staffing filled vacant positions, it did not increase payroll costs, hours per patient day, or overtime, and it decreased absenteeism by 60 percent. The hospital in this study returned to eight-hour shifts because primary nursing was threatened. In this particular study, there was *no change* in medication errors, patient and staff injuries, quality of care plans, complaints, recruitment, and staff attitudes from before to six months after flexible staffing. Also, use of agency nurses was not reduced.[27]

A Flexible Role: Resource Acuity Nurse.   At West Virginia University Hospital, top nurse executives established a resource acuity nurse position to provide greater flexibility and assure adequate staffing during peak workload periods. The executives envisioned having nurses in positions who would be available to provide immediate relief to units whenever the greatest care needs arose. The resource acuity nurse would stay at the hospital for as long as needed.

The nurse managers developed guidelines for undertaking the following resource acuity nurse responsibilities:

- Assisting with such special procedures as central line placement and extensive dressing changes.
- Supporting nursing staff whenever a number of patients were returning from the operating room.
- Assisting in cardiac arrests or other emergencies.
- Transferring unstable patients to the intensive care units.

This program has enabled the hospital to better meet the staffing needs of units whenever workload increases. Since the resource acuity nurse position's establishment, nurses' morale has improved because the nurses know that short-term help is more readily available and will be more equitably distributed among units.[28]

Flexible Hours.   Other flexible hours programs are used at the following:

- Metropolitan Life—90 percent of 28,000 administrative employees can begin work between 7:30 a.m. and 10:00 a.m.
- American Express's travel group—employees benefit from job sharing, shorter workweek, compressed workweeks, and telecommuting.
- Federal Express's treasury and credit departments—one-third of the employees work at home.

Clerical personnel tend to opt for working at home, whereas professionals fear that doing so will make their job less critical.[29]

Negative Aspects

The following are some of the disadvantages of ten- and twelve-hour days:[30]

1. Minimum weekend staffing (or excess staff on weekends).
2. Unsafe travel times.
3. Shift overlaps that decrease total number of personnel on duty.
4. Costs for overtime.
5. Fatigue.
6. Strain on family life.
7. Increased staffing from loss of shifts if schedule is not carefully planned.
8. Possible requirement by state law to pay overtime pay for hours worked in excess of eight in a day and forty in a week.

9. Less continuity of care.
10. Less communication among staff.
11. Developing, maintaining, and explaining the master schedule.
12. Modification of primary assessing.

Working night shifts, split shifts, or extended shifts may create such problems as sleeping on the job, conflicts with family members on other shifts, muddy thinking, or poor memory. Experts suggest the following ways to better handle working late or rotating shifts:[31]

- Use consistency in working shifts—work one shift all the time if possible.
- Rotate shifts clockwise, one shift for a week, forty-eight hours between changing shifts.
- Avoid caffeine, alcohol, nicotine, or other sleep-disturbing chemicals for several hours before bedtime.
- Follow the workday routine on days off as much as possible.
- Prepare for a new shift by splitting time between sleep and wakefulness.
- Shade eyes on long drives to and from work.

Cross-Training

Cross-training of nursing personnel can improve flexible scheduling. Nurses can be prepared through cross-training to function effectively in more than one area of expertise. They can be kept in similar clinical specialties or in families of clinical specialties. During cross-training, they require complete orientation and ongoing staff development to prevent errors and increase job satisfaction. This can be done for both unit-assigned nurses and pool nurses. Nurses should be provided with policies, job descriptions, and performance evaluations. Nurse pools can be in-house supplemental staffing agencies that use full-time and part-time nurses. Benefits can be prorated, or employees can choose between increased pay and benefits.

TEMPORARY WORKERS

Nurses have been working as temporary employees for two decades or more. They have gone to staffing agencies because they want control over their lives, personal and professional. Temporary work was the only way they could get such control until nurse managers and hospital administrators realized the need to apply the science of behavioral technology, including human resource management, to nursing. Many organizations are downsizing to make themselves more productive by decreasing overhead. One result of this downsizing is the use of contract or external workers.

Some analysts predict that by the year 2000, one-half of all working Americans, some 60 million people, will have joined the ranks of freelance providers of skills and services. Others say temporary employees will be reduced.

Trial work periods are effective in hiring the right person for the job. A trial work period allows both employer and the temporary employee to decide whether to make the position permanent. On the negative side, trial employees receive few fringe benefits.

Potential temporaries should become informed about the temporary agency they are going through by asking others about it who have used it, screening the agency by telephone to determine customer treatment, visiting the agency on a busy Monday morning, and then interviewing with the agency.[32]

PART-TIME WORKERS

Today, 21 million Americans work part-time; 6.4 million of them would rather have full-time jobs. Part-timers fill slots at every level of the organization. Twenty percent of 18 million jobs created since 1983 are part-time. Part-timers provide security for full-timers, as they work for lower pay. Nurse leaders should consider whether a part-time or disposable workforce that is not empowered will continue to be motivated, creative, or independent.[33]

SCHEDULING WITH NMIS

Planning the duty schedule does not always match personnel with preferences. This is one major dissatisfaction among clinical nurses. Satisfaction with the schedule can be improved by posting the number of nurses needed by time slot and allowing nurses to put colored pins in slots to select their own times. (Refer to the staffing board in Exhibit 7–7.)

Staffing is a major reason for having an NMIS. A microcomputer can be used to show, via menus and printouts, the number of nurses required by time slot, restrictions, off-duty policy, continual rather than intermittent days-off and cyclical schedule as well as single rotation.[34]

Hanson defines a management information system (MIS) as "an array of components designed to transform a collective set of data into knowledge that is directly useful and applicable in the process of directing and controlling resources and their application to the achievement of specific objectives."[35]

Information stimulates action through management decision making. Data do not; they must be processed to be useful. Information must be timely to be useful. The following is the process for establishing any MIS:[36]

1. State the management objective clearly.
2. Identify the actions required to meet the objective.
3. Identify the responsible position in the organization.
4. Identify the information required to meet the objective.
5. Determine the data required to produce the needed information.
6. Determine the system's requirement for processing the data.
7. Develop a flowchart.

Refer to chapter 21, "Nursing Informatics," for a more detailed discussion.

Group Exercise

1. Form groups of five to eight persons. This can be your permanent seminar group. You may want to consult with a larger representative group of nursing personnel to gain their insights and ideas and to incorporate their beliefs and values into the staffing philosophy.
2. Elect a leader to move the group to completion.
3. Elect a recorder to keep a written record of the group's accomplishments.
4. Prepare to write a staffing philosophy, a statement of beliefs about staffing. The statement should be representative of the beliefs that professional nurses hold about staffing and scheduling. Refer to the exhibits in Chapter 6 on mission, philosophy, vision and values, and objective statements and to Appendix 7–1. Also refer to Appendix 8–2, "Identification of Factors Causing Job Dissatisfaction."
5. Make a list of those key words or statements that you believe should be addressed in a staffing philosophy.
6. Prepare an outline.
7. Write the staffing philosophy.

Keep in mind that a hospital or other health-care institution exists to provide health care to people—to patients or clients. Also, an institution has to make a profit to stay in business. This applies as well to a not-for-profit institution in which the profits go to improving the facility and its human and material resources. Patients must be cared for twenty-four hours a day by nurses satisfied with their work conditions. Prepare a rationale for your final document.

PRODUCTIVITY

Definition

Productivity is commonly defined as $\dfrac{\text{Outputs}}{\text{Inputs}}$. Hanson translates this definition into the following:

$$\frac{\text{Required Staff Hours}}{\text{Provided Staff Hours}} \times 100 = \text{Percent Productivity}$$

To illustrate,

$$\frac{380.50 \text{ Required Staff Hours}}{402.00 \text{ Provided Staff Hours}} \times 100 = 94.7\% \text{ Productivity}$$

Productivity can be increased by decreasing the provided staff hours while holding the required staff hours constant or increasing them. These data become information when related to an objective that indicates variances.[37] Since resources for health care are limited, the nurse manager is faced with the task of motivating clinical nurses to increase productivity.

Productivity in nursing is related both to efficiency of use of clinical nursing in delivering nursing care to avoid waste and to the effectiveness of that care relative to its quality and appropriateness. Brown indicates that productivity in the United States has declined, citing as evidence of this claim increased labor costs without corresponding increases in performance. This decline is due to such factors as inexperienced workers, technological slowdown from outdated equipment and lessened research and development, government regulations, a diminished work ethic, increased size and bureaucracy in business and industry, and erosion of the managerial ethic.[38]

Measuring Productivity

In developing a model for an MIS, Hanson indicates several formulas for translating data into information. He indicates that in addition to the productivity formula, hours per patient day (HPPD) is data element that can provide meaningful information when provided for an extended period of time. HPPD is determined by the formula

$$\frac{\text{Staff Hours}}{\text{Patient Days}} = \text{HPPD}$$

For example,

$$\frac{52,000 \text{ Staff Hours}}{2,883.5 \text{ Patient Days}} = 18.03 \text{ HPPD}$$

52,000 Staff Hours = 25 FTEs × 2,080 work hours per year
2,883.5 Patient Days = 7.9 average daily census (ADC) × 365 days per year

No allowance is made for personal time such as coffee breaks, meals, vacations, holidays, sick time, or decreased census time. The figure of 18.03 HPPD may be a high provision of HPPD even for intensive care.

Another useful formula is

$$\frac{\text{Provided HPPD}}{\text{Budgeted HPPD}} \times 100 = \text{Budget Utilization}$$

$$\frac{18.03 \text{ Provided HPPD}}{16.0 \text{ Budgeted HPPD}} \times 100 = 112.7\% \text{ Budget Utilization}$$

This would be over budget if the provided hours had been net of personal time. Since they were not, the HPPD provided may be highly productive. The adequacy of the budget is determined as

$$\frac{\text{Budgeted HPPD}}{\text{Required HPPD}} \times 100 = \text{Budget Adequacy}$$

$$\frac{16.0 \text{ Budgeted HPPD}}{18.03 \text{ Required HPPD}} \times 100 = 88.74\% \text{ Budget Adequacy}$$

Obviously, if the required HPPD is equal to the provided HPPD and exceeds the budgeted HPPD, productivity is high because of the budget inadequacy. According to Hanson, all data become information when related to the objective.[39] Staffing should be defined in terms of the goal of HPPD to be provided. This will relate to productivity, budget utilization, and budget adequacy. Whether it will be effective or not depends upon measurement of quality of outcomes.

Exercise 7–3   Use Hanson's formula to determine productivity on each nursing unit for a division or department of nursing.

$$\frac{\text{Required Staff Hours}}{\text{Provided Staff Hours}} \times 100 = \text{Percent Productivity}$$

Since high input for low output produces low productivity and high output for low input produces high productivity, the objective of a nursing model of productivity is low input for high output.

Differences Among Productivity Models

Producers of services do not fit the same productivity models as do producers of material goods. There is marked discretion in determining both expected and actual role performances of nurses who do not produce physical outputs. For this reason, such nursing prescriptions as "emotional support" are difficult to measure. Patient output or outcomes can be measured by client satisfaction as well as by client condition upon discharge.

A greater emphasis has been placed upon nursing process than upon nursing outcome. Haas defines efficiency as the relationship of personnel assigned and time spent to materials expended, as well as capital and management employed, for the greatest economy in use. Productive nurses must balance their personal energies and their institution's resources with their effectiveness.[40]

Curtin proposes that productivity in nursing is related to the application of knowledge. Professional productivity must be measured by means of efficacy, effectiveness, and efficiency in applying knowledge. Curtin indicates that these processes can be objectively measured by using the following:[41]

1. Objective measures of efficacy: years of formal education, levels of academic achievement, evidence of continuing education and skill development, and years of experience.
2. Objective measures of effectiveness: demonstrated ability to execute job-related procedures, correctly prioritized activities, performance according to professional and legal standards, appropriate information clearly and concisely recorded, and cooperative working with others.
3. Objective measures of efficiency: promptitude, attendance, reliability, precision, adaptability, and economical disposition of resources.

Curtin and Zurlage acknowledge that human services such as nursing are difficult to test, return, or exchange if unsatisfactory. They propose a system for measuring nursing productivity that includes a nursing productivity equation, an equation relating nursing productivity ratio to hospital revenue, and a nursing productivity index.[42]

A nursing intensity index has been developed and tested in all departments at Johns Hopkins Hospital. A pilot study was done in which records of eight major services were examined. These records were scored by three raters each for average agreement, which varied from 82 percent to 95 percent. Modifications were made in the index as a result of the pilot study. A full study was then done using 784 records, each scored by two nurses. The results are as follows:[43]

1. Nursing intensity levels varied widely within every clinical department and nursing unit.
2. The full study sample included 239 diagnostic-related groups (DRGs). Of these, 64 percent consist of only one level of nursing intensity, 31 percent contain two levels of nursing intensity, 4 percent contain three levels of nursing intensity, and 1 percent contains four levels of nursing intensity.
3. A weighted average coefficient of variation for total charges across all clinical departments was computed.
4. Average interraters' agreement across all clinical departments was 84 percent.
5. The nursing intensity index is both a valid and a reliable instrument for patient classification.
6. The nursing intensity index correlates strongly (0.61) with the severity of illness index.
7. The nursing intensity index can be used to systematize cost allocation for nursing and do variable billing, establish sound nurse staffing systems, monitor quality of patient care delivery, trace patient population trends, and do case mix analysis.

Improving Nursing Productivity

Nursing productivity is being improved, and the reported knowledge and skills are adding to the theory of nursing management. Rabin indicates that professionals can impose productivity values upon themselves. Managers should develop managerial goals and values. They need a standard of performance for themselves. Professionals can commit themselves to fostering innovative attitudes and technologies, stimulating performance by commitment to constructive action and follow-ups, living up to standards of practice, keeping up-to-date, and being receptive to public review. Almost any profession can develop measurable standards of performance and productivity.[44]

Employers should measure nursing output objectively and pay for it accordingly in salary, benefits, and promotions. Some progress has been made in nursing in the form of standards of practice, clinical ladders, and models of peer review, among others. These, along with respect for the individual dignity of nurses, support for their personal commitment to professional goals, and support for the integrity of their professional judgments, need to be supported in the workplace.[45]

Productivity can be managed and improved through the following:[46]

1. Planning that increases the variations between inputs and outputs by
   a. outputs increasing, inputs decreasing.
   b. outputs increasing, inputs remaining constant.
   c. outputs increasing faster than inputs.
   d. outputs remaining constant, inputs decreasing.
   e. outputs decreasing more slowly than inputs.
2. Soliciting staff's ideas and recommendations.
3. Creating challenges.
4. Managers showing interest in staff's achievement and concerns.
5. Praising and rewarding good performances.
6. Involving staff.
7. Having a meaningful set or family of easily understood outcome measures for which data are available or easy to gather and over which workers have some control.
8. Selecting measures compatible with white-collar functions and corporate measures.
9. Monitoring workload changes in staffing requirements with established standards.
10. Combining support with employees' understanding, motivation, and recognition.
11. Increasing ratio of professional to nonprofessional staff.
12. Placing admitted patients based on resource availability.
13. Improving skill, energy, and motivation through such incentives as staff development, books, tuition reimbursement, paid meals, yoga lessons, bonuses, and vacation days.
14. Using such approaches as work simplification and work flow analysis.
15. Making an organizational diagnosis of problems, resources, and realities.
16. Setting the climate for productivity by asking nurses what makes them productive, then doing it, and measuring the before and after.
17. Decreasing waiting and standby time, coffee klatches, social breaks, and mealtimes.
18. Stimulating nurse managers and clinical nurses to want to achieve excellence.
19. Setting targets for increasing output on an annual basis without additional capital or employees.
20. Having personnel keep and analyze time diaries to determine personal improvement actions.
21. Setting personal objectives and measuring performance against them.
22. Making a commitment to improved productivity, effectiveness (doing the right things), and efficiency (doing things right).
23. Seeking new products and services and new ways of producing them.
24. Seeking new and useful approaches to old problems.
25. Improving quality of nursing products, emphasizing such ideas as consistency, longevity, riskiness, perfectibility, and value.

26. Maintaining concern with the process and method of producing nursing care.
27. Improving use of time.
28. Reducing the cost of what nurses do by returning unused budgeted funds.
29. Improving esthetics: the quality of work life and the pleasantness and beauty of the environment.
30. Applying the ethical policy statements of professional nursing organizations.
31. Gaining the confidence of peers.
32. Recognizing the need to do better.

Personnel working in service areas can improve productivity by doing the following:[47]

- Focusing on organizational strategy, customer service, mission, and results rather than methodology.
- Using self-directed work teams to break jobs into observable tasks and responsibilities. Possible breakdowns are step to step, person to person, machine to person, and unit to client or division and then to organization.
- Observing, then making changes or providing training to correct deficiencies.
- Watching for problems such as repetition, duplication, recurring delays, and waste of resources.
- Observing the outcome of the person's work by splitting the person's job into four main areas: managing self, resources, and activities and working with others. What are the key skills? Suggestions include analytical thinking, ability to learn, adaptability, positive self-image, emphasis on results, time management, concern for standards, knowing how to influence others, and independence.
- Providing feedback that is specific, constructive, and frequent.

Case Study.   At the Presbyterian Hospital of Dallas, a study revealed that more time was spent on clerical functions, telephone calls, and reporting patient conditions to other caregivers than on direct patient care. Several actions were taken that changed this and greatly improved productivity:[48]

- A FAX machine network was instituted between nursing units and pharmacy, reducing telephone calls and medication errors.
- A keyless narcotics system was installed that included personal pass codes. The main control system was in the pharmacy, but nurses could enter their personal pass code at the narcotics cabinet. This reduced time wasted to search for keys and produced an audit trail.
- A unit beeper system with eight beepers was purchased at a local store for $375. Beepers given to every staff member at the beginning of each shift made nursing assistants feel valued.

Exercise 7–4   Identify at least twelve activities that could be undertaken to improve productivity in a division or department of nursing in which you work or are assigned as a student.

WEB ACTIVITIES

- Visit www.jbpub.com/swansburg, this text's companion website on the Internet, for further information on Staffing and Scheduling.
- What resources are available on the Internet for staffing and scheduling?
- What can you learn about the staffing industry for nurses from the Internet?

SUMMARY

Staffing and scheduling are major components of nursing management. Traditional patterns have been slavishly adhered to until recent years. A nursing division needs a practical and written philosophy that guides all staffing and scheduling activities and that is acceptable to the staff.

Staffing studies can be used to determine staffing needs related to personnel skills, numbers of personnel, and time/workload requirements. Staffing can be planned by using computer models that calculate workload requirements from patient classification data or patient classification systems (PCSs). Many modified approaches can be taken to nurse staffing and scheduling, including game theory, modified workweeks, team rotation, permanent shifts, and permanent weekends. While some consultants advise against mixing modified workweeks, in practice, such workweeks are frequently mixed.

Productivity, the unit of output of nursing, is a focus of increasing interest to nurse managers. It must include quality care indicators that can be observed and measured. Productivity is commonly defined as the outputs of production divided by the inputs of production. Research needs to be undertaken to determine the key to increased productivity by professional nurses. Is it money or some other aspect of job satisfaction? One theory is that a combination of work, environment, and rewards will maintain or increase productivity.

NOTES

1. M. K. Aydelotte, *Nurse Staffing Methodology: A Review and Critique of Selected Literature* (Washington, D.C.: U.S. Government Printing Office, January 1973), 3.
2. Ibid., 26.
3. M. E. West, "Implementing Effective Nurse Staffing Systems in the Managed Hospital," *Topics in Health Care Financing*, Summer 1980, 11–25.

4. J. N. Althaus, N. M. Hardyck, P. B. Pierce, and M. S. Rodgers, "Nurse Staffing in a Decentralized Organization: Part I," *Journal of Nursing Administration,* March 1982, 34–39.

5. R. C. Minetti, "Computerized Nurse Staffing," *Hospitals,* 16 July 1983, 90, 92; P. P. Shaheen, "Staffing and Scheduling: Reconcile Practical Means with the Real Goal," *Nursing Management,* October 1985, 64–69.

6. M. K. Aydelotte, op. cit., 26–31.

7. M. E. West, op. cit., 16.

8. Ibid., 17.

9. P. J. Schroder and K. L. McKeon, "What Is a Safe Staffing Pattern for Locked Long-Term and Acute Care Units for Adults?" *Journal of Psychosocial Nursing* 28, no. 12 (1990): 36–37.

10. E. M. Price, *Staffing for Patient Care* (New York: Springer, 1970), 12.

11. "Study Questions All-RN Staffing," *RN,* November 1983, 15–16.

12. M. E. Warstler, "Some Management Techniques for Nursing Service Administrators," *Journal of Nursing Administration,* November–December 1972, 25–34.

13. K. V. Rondeau, "Self-Scheduling Can Increase Job Satisfaction," *Medical Laboratory Observer,* November 1990, 22–24.

14. T. P. Herzog, "Productivity: Fighting the Battle of the Budget," *Nursing Management,* January 1985, 30–34; T. Porter-O'Grady, "Strategic Planning: Nursing Practice in the PPS," *Nursing Management,* October 1985, 53–56; K. Johnson, "A Practical Approach to Patient Classification," *Nursing Management,* June 1984, 39–41, 44, 46; R. E. Schroeder, A. M. Rhodes, and R. E. Shields, "Nurse Acuity Systems: CASH vs. GRASP," *Nursing Forum,* February 1984, 72–77; R. R. Alward, "Patient Classification Systems: The Ideal vs. Reality," *Journal of Nursing Administration,* February 1983, 14–18; J. Nyberg and N. Wolff, "DRG Panic," *Journal of Nursing Administration,* April 1984, 17–21.

15. E. J. Halloran and M. Kiley, "Case Mix Management," *Nursing Management,* February 1984, 39–41, 44–45.

16. R. E. Schroeder, A. M. Rhodes, and R. E. Shields, op. cit.

17. K. Johnson, op. cit.

18. Ibid., 41.

19. R. E. Schroeder, A. M. Rhodes, and R. E. Shields, op. cit.

20. R. R. Alward, op. cit.

21. L. O'Brien-Pallas, P. Leatt, R. Deber, and J. Till, "A Comparison of Workload Estimates Using Three Methods of Patient Classification," *Canadian Journal of Nursing Administration,* September/October 1989, 16–23.

22. P. Giovannetti and G. G. Mayer, "Building Confidence In Patient Classification Systems," *Nursing Management,* August 1984, 31–34; R. R. Alward, op. cit.

23. American Hospital Association, "Strategies: Flexible Scheduling," 1985, 12 pages.

24. J. A. Ricci, "10-Hour Night Shift: Cost vs. Savings," *Nursing Management,* January 1984, 34–35, 38–42.

25. C. M. Fagin, "The Economic Value of Nursing Research," *American Journal of Nursing,* December 1982, 1844–1849.

26. M. S. Washburn, "Fatigue and Critical Thinking on Eight- and Twelve-Hour Shifts," *Nursing Management,* September 1991, 80A–CC, 80D–CC, 80 F–H–CC

27. S. I. Imig, J. A. Powell, K. Thorman, "Primary Nursing and Flexi-Staffing: Do They Mix?" *Nursing Management,* August 1984, 39–42.

28. K. O'Donnell, "A Flexible Role: Resource Acuity Nurse," *Nursing Management,* March 1992, 75–76.

29. K. B. Salwea, "Flexible Work Arrangements," *The Wall Street Journal*, 19 January 1993, A1.

30. American Hospital Association, op. cit.; B. Arnold and E. Mills, "Care-12: Implementation of Flexible Scheduling," *Journal of Nursing Administration*, July–August 1983, 9–14; A. Mech, M. E. Mills, and B. Arnold, "Wage and Hour Laws: Their Impact on 12-hour Scheduling," *Journal of Nursing Administration*, (March 1984, 24–25; M. L. Metcalf, op. cit.

31. P. Ancona, "Working Shifts Can Be Dangerous to Your Health, Experts Say," *San Antonio Express-News*, 19 February 1994, 1F–2F.

32. A. Bruzzese, "Companies Turning to Temps to Fill Voids in Workplace," *San Antonio Express-News*, 19 April 1994, 1C, 7C.

33. J. Fierman, "The Contingency Work Force," *Fortune*, 24 January 1994, 30–34, 36.

34. B. Moores and A. Murphy, "Planning the Duty Rota, One, Computerized Duty Rotas," *Nursing Times*, 4 July 1984, 47–48; D. Canter, "Planning the Duty Rota, Two, Back to Basics," *Nursing Times*, 4 July 1984, 49–50.

35. R. L. Hanson, "Applying Management Information Systems to Staffing," *Journal of Nursing Administration*, October 1982, 5–9.

36. Ibid.

37. R. L. Hanson, "Staffing Statistics: Their Use and Usefulness," *Journal of Nursing Administration*, November 1982, 29–35.

38. D. S. Brown, "The Managerial Ethic and Productivity Improvement," *Public Productivity Review*, September 1983, 223–250.

39. R. L. Hanson, "Staffing Statistics: Their Use and Usefulness," op. cit. The formulas are Hanson's; applications are the author's.

40. S. A. W. Haas, Sorting Out Nursing Productivity, *Nursing Management*, April 1984, 37–40.

41. L. Curtin, "Reconciling Pay with Productivity," *Nursing Management*, February 1984, 7–8.

42. L. L. Curtin and C. L. Zurlage, "Nursing Productivity: From Data to Definition," *Nursing Management*, June 1986, 32–34, 38–41.

43. J. A. Reitz, "Toward a Comprehensive Nursing Intensity Index: Part I, Development," *Nursing Management*, August 1985, 21–24, 26, 28–30; J. A. Reitz, "Toward a Comprehensive Intensity Index: Part II, Testing," *Nursing Management*, September 1985, 31–32, 34, 36–40, 42.

44. J. Rabin, "Professionalism and Productivity," *Public Productivity Review*, September 1983, 217–222.

45. L. Curtin, op. cit.

46. M. F. Fralic, "The Modern Professional and Productivity," Annual Meeting of the Alabama Society for Nursing Service Administrators, Huntsville, Ala., 1982; R. L. Hanson, "Managing Human Resources," *Journal of Nursing Administration*, December 1982, 17–23; G. H. Kaye and J. Utenner, "Productivity: Managing for the Long Term," *Nursing Management*, September 1985, 12–13, 15; S. A. W. Haas, op. cit; D. L. Davis, op. cit; D. S. Brown, op. cit.

47. P. Ancona, "How to Measure Productivity and Improve Effectiveness Among Workers," *San Antonio Express-News,* 24 July 1993, 1 B.
48. M. Gilliland, V. S. Crane, and D. G. Jones, "Productivity: Electronics Saves Steps— and Builds Networks," *Nursing Management,* July 1991, 56–59.

Appendix 7–1   University of South Alabama Medical Center Hospital
Department of Nursing Staffing and Assignment Guidelines

SUBJECT: Staffing and Assignment

I. Policy Statement
II. Purpose
   To provide a uniform system for:
   1. Adequate staffing mix to meet acuity needs of patients.
   2. Maintain equitable and consistent staffing for all professional and support groups within nursing.
III. General Information
   A. Appropriate resources are provided to meet patient needs. Indicators for patient outcomes are monitored on an ongoing basis through the Quality Assessment and Improvement Plan. These results are reviewed as part of the budget review process to determine if the same patient care needs are being met throughout the hospital. If outcomes are not acceptable and/or do not demonstrate improvement and if insufficient information exists related to staffing, further investigation may be required.
   B. Staffing requirements are projected by each Nurse Manager and weekly schedules are submitted to the Staffing Office. If there are vacancies, the Staffing Coordinators utilize in-house PRN personnel as well as other staff to provide coverage.
   C. Daily staffing needs are determined by the skill level of employee, acuity measurement, census and anticipated changes in activity. Adjustments are made each shift to meet the staffing requirement, as well as during the shift.
   D. The staffing office is staffed by Staffing Coordinators on the 7–3 and 3–11 shifts, 7 days a week. Staffing for the 11–7 shift is provided by the 3–11 Shift Coordinator. Adjustments to increased acuity of patients or census variations are made by the Staffing Coordinator or Clinical Administrator providing house supervision.
   E. Staffing is individualized and the acuity of patients is the primary concern when assignments are made. Consideration is given to the special needs of selected patients.
   F. Support personnel, which includes ward clerks, telemetry technicians, wound care technicians, guest relation aides, and students, are considered when staffing the unit.
   G. The staffing is adjusted to meet patient needs as effectively as possible. At times it is necessary to reassign nursing personnel on a daily or temporary basis to meet these needs. Whenever possible nursing personnel will be reassigned to a unit within their nursing division, or to a like unit. PRN staff are expected to work where assigned. If scheduled for any Med/Surg Unit, they may be required to work any Med/Surg Unit.
   H. Personnel will be clinically cross-oriented within each division to the individual nursing units.
   I. If staff are reassigned to a unit outside of their division they are assigned as support working with regular unit staff. Licensed personnel reassigned out of their division are not assigned charge duties.
   J. Nursing personnel will be floated based on their qualifications. Refusal to accept reassignment will be handled individually by the Director of Nursing or Assistant Administrator for Nursing. Negotiations between personnel is encouraged.
   K. Regular scheduled staff members cannot be floated in lieu of overtime, PRN, or float staff. Regular staff may be floated only when no other (overtime, PRN, or float) staff is available.
   L. When personnel are requested to work overtime, they can be offered the option to work overtime only within their division, e.g., Med/Surg or Critical Care. No agreement for overtime will be made that specifies one particular unit.
   M. All scheduled overtime work will be approved by the Nurse Manager or Director of Nursing. Directors and Nurse Managers are ultimately responsible for monitoring overtime.
   N. Mandatory meetings of nursing personnel are an extreme inconvenience to off-duty personnel. Personnel will be paid for hours worked when mandated to return for a meeting. Meetings must be approved by the Assistant Administrator prior to announcement.

Source: Courtesy University of South Alabama Medical Center, Mobile, Alabama.

HUMAN RESOURCE MANAGEMENT

OBJECTIVES

- Discuss demographic implications for recruitment of students into nursing. You may profile applicants for a local program.
- Develop a list of strategies to use in recruiting students into nursing education programs.
- Develop an effective nurse recruitment advertisement.
- Conduct an effective simulated interview of a nurse applicant.
- Conduct an effective simulated interview as a nurse applicant.
- Discuss the nurse credentialing process of an employing agency.
- Determine turnover rates for an agency.
- Make a career development plan for self.
- Discuss the promotion and termination policies of an employing organization.

KEY CONCEPTS

recruiting
selecting
credentialing
assigning
retaining
promoting
terminating

Manager Behavior: Oversees development of human resource activities to recruit, select, credential, assign, retain, promote, and terminate personnel.

Leader Behavior: Assures that human resource activities to recruit, select, credential, assign, retain, promote, and terminate personnel are based on up-to-date research of the field and of the results of personnel satisfaction surveys.

INTRODUCTION

The theory of nursing management includes knowledge of personnel management related to recruiting, selecting, credentialing, assigning, retaining, promoting, and terminating personnel. Recruiting has two facets, recruiting students into generic programs and recruiting RNs into service institutions and agencies. Credentialing includes licensing.

RECRUITING

Recruiting Students into Nursing

In 1980, there was a national shortage of 100,000 hospital nurses.[1] A flood of publicity on this shortage led to the formation of a National Commission on Nursing. This commission listed "eight top themes in descending order of importance" that it considered significant in reducing the shortage:[2]

1. Nursing leadership should be an integral part of senior management.
2. Nursing should be more involved in all levels of hospital decision making.
3. Nurses' management skills should be developed, and nurses should be provided more opportunities for leadership positions.
4. The organizational structure should be decentralized to facilitate communication and decision making.
5. Collaborative or joint practice programs between nurses and physicians should be established.
6. The nursing educational system needs to be rationalized in terms of entry-level requirements and clinical practice preparation.
7. Career development programs for clinical practice and administrative positions should continue to be developed and implemented.
8. Nursing leaders should be appointed to key committees to foster and strengthen nurses' interaction with medical staff and the board of directors of the agency.

The Job Market.   More jobs were being created and filled in 1994 than predicted—267,000 versus 170,000 for the month of April.[3] Whether this will translate into more jobs in the health-care system and nursing depends upon whether health insurance benefits are a part of the benefits package of these 267,000 workers. The health-care system has been an "enormous job-generating machine," creating 29,000 new jobs each month in 1992. More than 10 million people, almost 10 percent of employed America, work in the health-care system.[4]

One of the new strategies of employment is job expansion. Predictions are that "advanced practice nurses will be increasingly called upon to perform physical exams and treat minor illnesses," a strategy to increase access to health care while containing costs.[5] Richman indicated that the greatest demand will be for managers of health-care networks, nurses, home health aides, and outpatient therapists. He goes on to state:

> Leading the growth will be demand for so-called "nurse practitioners," diagnostic specialists in HMOs, inner cities, and rural areas. The training they need to serve as patient care managers lasts six years—half as long as it takes to train a doctor and at just one-fifth the cost. More than 100,000 nurses now provide some form of primary care and another 300,000 could join them with a couple of years of training. Salaries for experienced specialists reach $80,000 a year.[6]

Woods projects registered nurses to increase from 1,727,000 jobs in 1990 by 35 percent or more between 1990 and 2005. Registered nurses head the list of professionals for projected job growth.[7]

Another positive job indicator is that earnings increase for employees with degrees. While noncollege graduate workers had an earnings plunge during the past fifteen years, college-educated workers' earnings rose. During the next thirteen years, 25 million of 26 million jobs created will be in service industries. "Of the 10 occupations expected to add the most jobs in the next 20 years, only two require a college degree, registered nurses and systems analysts."[8] Exhibit 8–1 illustrates the earnings differences between full-time workers with a high school diploma and those with a college degree.

Exhibit 8–1   Coping Without a College Degree

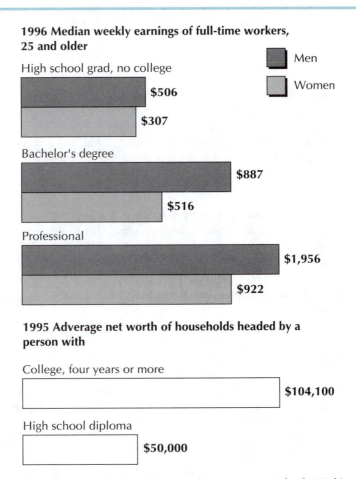

1996 Median weekly earnings of full-time workers, 25 and older

- Men
- Women

High school grad, no college
$506
$307

Bachelor's degree
$887
$516

Professional
$1,956
$922

1995 Adverage net worth of households headed by a person with

College, four years or more
$104,100

High school diploma
$50,000

Source: U.S. Bureau of the Census, Statistical Abstract of the United States 1997, 117th ed. (Washington, DC, 1997: 160, 480.

Nurse practitioners will be competing with physician assistants, whose growth will expand in the next decade. Physician assistant jobs are predicted to grow 44 percent between 1990 and 2005.[9]

Progress and job destruction go hand in hand: 400,000 U.S. workers lose jobs and another 400,000 gain jobs weekly. This process is called "churning." It advances the quality of life. For example, in 1900 it took forty of every one hundred Americans to feed the country. Today it takes three. The other thirty-seven are producing new homes, appliances, computers, and a whole array of goods and services.[10]

Workers are this country's national resource. They have or get the advanced education and training to work in more advanced industries with better jobs as less-skilled jobs migrate to other countries. Workers in those jobs remaining produce goods and services of higher value. Emerging new jobs will relate to technologies associated with discoveries of DNA, lasers, fiberoptics, high-tech ceramics, hard plastics, holography, photonics, and micro-machines. American workers displaced from old jobs will be retrained and learn to enter the new job market.[11]

Exercise 8–1   Check the current nursing enrollments in registered nurse preparation programs for baccalaureate degree, associate degree, diploma, and graduate programs. Are they increasing or decreasing? Which segments of the health-care job market are increasing for professional nurses? Which are decreasing? What are the implications for nurses? For patients?

Job Sharing.   An option for nursing is job sharing, two persons filling one FTE at a ratio of work agreed upon by them. This is convenient for nurses who want to work part-time, can afford to, but need personal time. Less acceptable to nurses is mandatory sharing of available work in a world in which high-tech and organizational restructuring may be reducing the amount of labor for pay available. This may lead to less work and less income or a guaranteed income as an option.[12]

Job Retention and Employee Retention   To retain jobs, people should make themselves more valuable at work by gaining new skills and experiences, and taking on new responsibilities. This can include volunteering for interdepartmental project teams, maintaining a reputation as a helpful, resourceful coworker, and keeping a success folder or journal and using it to build a resume of major accomplishments or new skills.[13]

Of late, women have been entering other career fields, such as medicine, law, business administration, and dentistry, that have traditionally been predominantly male fields with higher pay and better working conditions than nursing. Although numerous studies exist of dissatisfaction among nurses, there appears to be sporadic progress in improving nurses' pay and working conditions.

Nurse managers are not the only people who can change the work environment. An all-RN staff may not be financially possible. The professional nurse practitioner is highly qualified in terms of knowledge and skills and is the decision maker in the nursing process. She or he can direct the work of others without continual direct involvement in such procedures as bathing, making beds, and feeding patients. The professional nurse should do the history, make the nursing diagnosis, direct the application of nursing care, evaluate the results, and make changes as needed. The debate on entry into practice needs to be redesigned and realigned to focus upon the professional nurse as the clinical decision maker. Requirements of the baccalaureate degree in nursing for certification programs will advance this notion.

Every major agency or institution employing nurses should have a committee that focuses on the recruitment of students into nursing education programs. Small organizations can form recruitment consortiums. Clinical nurses should be well represented. They will provide ideas that will give an authentic and positive image of professional nursing practice. The focus should be realistic but positive for men and women, for minorities, and for a cross-section of high-school students; the latter will come from backgrounds in which the number

- below the poverty line increased.
- of white, suburban, middle-class decreased.
- of nonwhites increased.
- of single parents increased.
- of non-English-speaking or bilingual increased.
- of physical and emotional handicaps increased.
- of working mothers increased.[14]

Exercise 8–2   Exhibit 8–2 lists activities to pursue in recruiting students into nursing education programs. Use the list to determine the strategies being used in your community by education programs, employers, and nursing organizations. Summarize your conclusions.

The business of recruiting students into nursing will require long-term strategies for all educators and providers. Recruitment will be more effective if potential consumers of nursing services are involved. Professional nurses can work through community organizations to involve the community in changing the image of nursing and in the recruitment effort. The profession tends to lose sight of this source of support.

Efforts should be made to provide education at times convenient to students, most of whom have to work. More is being done to provide evening and weekend courses for basic or generic students. This could be a major area of breakthrough in recruitment, particularly for older adults. Few reasons exist for the lack of evening and weekend courses, including Sundays, except the will and efforts of faculty and clinical facility personnel.

Exhibit 8–2   Strategies for Recruiting Students into Nursing Education Programs

1. Form committee to make plan.
   (1) Include clinical nurses.
   (2) Set goals.
   (3) Make management plan for each goal.
2. Obtain recruitment materials from organizations.
   (1) National League for Nursing (NLN)
   (2) American Nurses Association (ANA)
   (3) American Organization of Nurse Executives (AONE)/American Hospital Association (AHA)
   (4) National Student Nurses Association (NSNA)
   (5) American Association of Colleges of Nursing (AACN)
   (6) State
   (7) Local
3. Prepare additional recruitment materials.
   (1) News stories for newspapers, TV, and radio
   (2) Posters for schools
   (3) Speakers bureau
   (4) Model speeches
   (5) Tours
4. Coordinate with other nurse education programs and prospective employers of nurses.
   (1) Associate degree programs
   (2) Diploma programs
   (3) BSN programs
   (4) Hospitals
   (5) Public health
   (6) Staffing agencies
   (7) Ambulatory care facilities
   (8) Nursing homes
   (9) LPN programs
   (10) Other

5. Prepare and offer consultation programs for junior and senior high schools.
   (1) Administrators
   (2) Teachers
   (3) Guidance counselors
   (4) Students
6. Coordinate activities of recruiters in schools of nursing.
   (1) Sources of information by telephone and mail
7. Involve community agencies in recruitment efforts.
   (1) Professional organizations
   (2) Social organizations
   (3) Service organizations
   (4) Others
8. Evaluate results accomplished.
   (1) Number and locations of programs presented
   (2) Number of students counseled
   (3) Number of follow-ups
   (4) Number of applicants to local or other programs
   (5) Homerooms visited
   (6) Career days held by high schools
   (7) Career days held by schools of nursing
   (8) Career days held by employers
   (9) Inquiries to source persons by telephone or letter
9. Do work/study programs.
   (1) High schools with employer
   (2) High schools with schools of nursing
   (3) Schools of nursing with employers
   (4) Cooperative education

Research Study.   The number of new entrants into baccalaureate nursing programs needs to be maintained or increased to keep pace with the demand for professional nurses. Using a descriptive design, 641 college-bound high-school seniors were surveyed to determine why nursing is not selected more frequently as a career. The survey was taken to obtain data helpful to nurse educators in developing strategies to increase the number of high-school seniors choosing a career in nursing. Although a majority of the sample had grade point averages between 3.00 and 3.99, 92.3 percent did not choose nursing as a career.

Questions measuring knowledge regarding nursing education, hours, salaries, and work settings indicated that the overall knowledge of these areas of nursing among respondents was fairly accurate. Students were relatively uninformed, however, about the roles and tasks of nurses, and 91.8 percent were unaware that nurses worked with computers.

The overall opinion about nursing was favorable. Although a large percentage (86 percent) of students believed that nurses mainly followed doctors' orders, many students (72.5 percent) believed that nurses made a lot of money, and many (81.1 percent) believed that nursing was a career only for smart people. Very few believed that nurses did important work (5.4 percent), that nursing was challenging (9.4 percent), that it was a real profession (9.3 percent), that it was an important profession (5.4 percent), or that it provided a good opportunity to help people (3 percent).

Neither knowledge nor opinion of nursing was significantly associated with students' choosing or not choosing nursing as a career. Significant differences existed between students who chose nursing and those who did not in gender, ethnicity, and age. Students who chose nursing as a career were significantly more likely to be African-American, female, and 16 to 17 years of age. No significant difference existed between choosers and nonchoosers in religion, socioeconomic status, or grade point average.

Knowing a nurse personally, caring for someone who was seriously ill, having a family member who was a nurse, and living with someone who was seriously ill were significantly associated with the decision to become a nurse. The reason cited most frequently for choosing nursing was the desire to help people. Those who did not choose nursing indicated disliking being around dying people and the salary as the main reasons.

These findings are important to nurse educators as they plan recruitment strategies aimed at increasing the enrollment of high-school students in baccalaureate nursing programs.[15]

Exercise 8–3   Using Exhibit 8–2, "Strategies for Recruiting Students into Nursing Education Programs," identify the strategies you wish to pursue and prepare a management plan to accomplish them. This may be done as a group exercise. You may use the following format for management plans.

Management Plan

Objective:

Actions	*Target Dates*	*Assigned To*	*Accomplishments*

Recruiting Nurses into Employment

Employers of registered nurses are competing for available personnel through such channels as newspaper and journal ads, professional placement agencies, placement bureaus at universities, and special publications. Professional nurses seeking jobs may have personal contacts and can obtain information at job fairs, career days, professional meetings, and conventions. The business of recruiting clinical nurses into jobs should be managed using planning, an organization, direction, and a method of evaluating its effectiveness.

The Recruiter.   Many large organizations employ a nursing recruiter, who could be a professional nurse or a personnel recruitment specialist. Either employee should work from a management plan that includes input from clinical nurses working within the organization.

The objective of the recruiter is to get qualified professional nurses to apply for jobs. First, information about the organization's job openings is made known to the target population. This is done through advertisements in Sunday newspapers and in nursing journals. The ads should be broad enough to give potential applicants knowledge of particular positions, salaries and fringe benefits, and the organizational climate. Results of studies of factors that attract nurses can be used as a basis for developing job advertisements.

In 1983, an American Academy of Nursing study depicted both nurse administrators and staff nurses as agreeing on what factors attracted nurses to come to hospitals and stay there. Among those factors are "adequate and competent colleagues, flexibility in scheduling, educational programs that allow for professional growth, and recognition as individuals."[16] These were labelled magnet hospitals.

During 1985–86, Kramer and Schmalenberg resurveyed sixteen of these magnet hospitals, comparing them with the best-run corporate communities as described by Peters and Waterman in their book *In Search of Excellence*. They found many similarities. Magnet hospitals "are infused with values of quality care, nurse autonomy, informal, nonrigid verbal communication, innovation, bringing out the best in each individual, value of education, respect and caring for the individual, and striving for excellence."[17]

A well-thought-out ad can be a successful method for recruiting nurses. It is better to spend money to develop an effective advertisement than to save money on an ineffective one. A successful ad will get attention when it focuses upon its subject: the professional nurse. It will obtain results when it piques the interest of the professional nurse in seeking more information. Exhibit 8–3 lists criteria for developing an effective newspaper or nursing journal advertisement.

A formal nurse recruitment plan is suggested for each fiscal year, since objectives will be influenced by such factors as structural reorganizations, turnover and retention, and vacant positions.

The following are six steps of a formal plan:[18]

1. Gathering a database through situational scanning, forecasting, and variance audits comparing demand with supply data.
2. Setting desirable objectives.
3. Designing strategies to accomplish the objectives.
4. Establishing the annual nurse recruitment budget.
5. Implementing the strategies through operational plans.
6. Evaluating and using feedback to make corrective action.

Exhibit 8–3   Criteria for Developing an Effective Nurse Recruitment Advertisement

1. Target the population.
2. Catch the reader's attention.
3. Consider a picture that depicts a professional nurse in action, the kind of action nurses say they want.
4. List several factors that attract nurses. These may include the following:
   (1) Opportunity for self-fulfillment
   (2) Knowledge of helping others
   (3) Intellectual stimulation
   (4) Educational opportunity
   (5) Fellowship with colleagues
   (6) Adequate income
   (7) Opportunity for innovation
   (8) Opportunity to choose hours
   (9) Opportunity for advancement
   (10) Chance to be a leader
   (11) Adequate support systems
   (12) Child-care facilities
   (13) Good fringe benefits
5. Involve clinical nurses in developing the advertisement.
6. Test the advertisement on the clinical nurse staff.
7. Run the ad in the Sunday newspapers that are read by the target population.
8. Run the ad in nursing journals that are read by the target population.
9. Provide for telephone and mail replies from applicants.
   (1) Free telephone numbers
   (2) Specific address
   (3) FAX number and e-mail address
10. Provide for effective telephone and mail replies to be returned from organization.
    (1) The phone should be answered with positive responses that elicit interviews. It can be effective if clinical nurses make immediate follow-up calls to prospective applicants.
    (2) Effective packages of recruitment materials mailed to prospective applicants. (Depict and detail factors listed under number 4.)
11. Arrange for interview, including a visit to the organization.
    (1) Contact person and sponsor
    (2) Travel reimbursement
    (3) Paid room and meals
    (4) Interviews with person doing hiring; personnel specialists, including recruiter; and clinical nurses.
12. Follow-up offer in writing.

Marketing.   Several authors recommend a marketing approach to recruitment of nurses. Such an approach would focus upon the nurse as the consumer of employment. These authors advocate a marketing audit of the nursing environment. Exhibit 8–4 presents a scheme for a marketing survey for recruiting and retaining nurses that includes some of these ideas. The marketing plan would be a management plan that would determine what needs to be done to sell employment to prospective professional nurses. Data would be analyzed, objectives set, a plan made and promoted, and the objectives evaluated.[19]

Exercise 8–4   Using Exhibit 8–3, "Criteria for Developing an Effective Nurse Recruitment Advertisement," prepare a management plan. Prepare the advertisement. Make it a marketing rather than a selling ad. This may be done as a group exercise.

Exhibit 8–4 Marketing Survey for Recruiting and Retaining Nurses

1. Number of vacant positions.
   (1) Current
   (2) Previous month
   (3) Percent increase (or decrease)
2. Turnover rate by month and unit.
3. Exit interview results.
   (1) Number of interviews performed
   (2) Number of negative comments (list separately) (See Appendix 8–3)
4. New-hire demographics.
   (1) Diploma graduates
   (2) AD graduates
   (3) BSN graduates
   (4) Average years of experience
   (5) Males
   (6) Females
   (7) Average age
   (8) Percent married
   (9) Percent with children of preschool age
   (10) Percent with children in school
   (11) Percent minorities
   (12) Other
5. Demographics of employed nurses. Profile the "stayers" and target similar recruits.
   (1) Diploma graduates
   (2) AD graduates.
   (3) BSN graduates
   (4) Average years of experience
   (5) Males
   (6) Females
   (7) Average age
   (8) Percent married
   (9) Percent with children of preschool age
   (10) Percent with children in school
   (11) Percent minorities
   (12) Other
6. Attitude survey (list results separately).
7. Audit of meeting minutes.
   (1) Staff nurses
   (2) Others (list results separately)
8. Audit of performance evaluations (list results separately).
9. Salary levels (list by clinical level and by longevity).
10. Overtime.
    (1) Hours by month and unit
    (2) Costs
11. Absenteeism data.
    (1) Daily average
    (2) Cause
    (3) Monthly total
12. Agency nurse use.
    (1) Hours by month and unit
    (2) Costs
13. Monthly budget variances by unit.
14. Utilization of productivity reports (refer to Chapter 5).
15. Acuity data by category and unit.
16. Average daily census by day of week and by month (report trends).
17. Recruiting expenses.
18. Major competitors for prospective hires.
19. Analysis of professional literature on recruitment and availability.
20. Analysis of patient relations reports.
21. Reputation and visibility of the organization and division.
    (1) Community
    (2) Employees
    (3) Organizational culture
    (4) Location of employment
22. Factors causing nurses to avoid organization.
23. Factors that would attract nurses to organization because it is a superior place to work.
24. Sources for recruiting nurses.

SELECTING, CREDENTIALING, AND ASSIGNING

Selecting, credentialing, and assigning are all part of the hiring process. While assigning has sometimes been done after the professional nurse was hired, it is unsatisfactory to applicants, who want to know where they will work before reporting for duty and orientation. The professional nurse does not want surprises and will begin work dissatisfied if they occur.

Selecting

Selecting includes the interview, the employer's offer, the applicant's acceptance of the offer, and the signing of a contract or written offer. While in small organizations, the chief nurse executive may interview and hire prospective applicants, it is best for the nurse manager who will directly supervise the employee to do the hiring. This person may elect to elicit the input of clinical nurses with whom the prospective employee will be working.

The Interview

The nurse recruiter or a human resource specialist will have completed a personnel folder containing a completed application form, a resume or curriculum vitae, references, and any documents required by policy or law, such as a current valid license to practice nursing and school transcripts.

The interviewer should prepare for the interview by reading the information in the applicant's folder. Exhibit 8–5 is a checklist to use in reviewing this folder. The interviewer should make notes of questions to ask about the information contained in the folder.

Adequate time should be set aside for the interview, which should take place in a private office where there will be no interruptions. An interview guide will be helpful in conducting an interview satisfactory to both the nurse manager and the applicant (see Exhibit 8–6).

Thompson defines an interview as "an equal level, face-to-face discussion between a job seeker and a person with full authority to fill the position under discussion."[20] Nurses are the job seekers and want a face-to-face discussion with

---

Exhibit 8–5   Checklist for Reviewing Job Applicant's Personnel Folder

1. The application form
   (1) Completed as directed
   (2) Written statements are positive
   (3) Contains no blanks
   (4) Contains no gaps in employment data
2. References
   (1) Listed
   (2) Have been checked
   (3) Are satisfactory
   (4) Need further checking
3. RN licensure
   (1) Has been verified
   (2) Is current and valid
   (3) No legal suits are pending
4. Transcripts
   (1) Have been verified
   (2) Are available

5. Forms signed
6. Curriculum vitae or resume
   (1) Up-to-date
   (2) Lists career goals
7. Job description provided, including blank performance contract
   (1) Clinical level established as_____
   (2) Years of longevity established as_____
8. Salary information available
   (1) Base salary: $_____
   (2) Clinical level pay: $_____
   (3) Longevity pay: $_____
   (4) Differential: $_____
   (5) Credentialing (certification): $_____
   (6) Total pay: $_____
   (7) Paydays made known

Exhibit 8–6   Interview Guide

Candidate:

Date and time of interview:

1. Make introductions and establish rapport.
2. Arrange seating.
3. Ask prepared questions.
   (1) Tell me about yourself.
   (2) What is your present job?
   (3) What are your three most outstanding accomplishments?
   (4) What is the extent of your formal education?
   (5) What three things are most important to you in your job?
   (6) What is your strongest qualification for this job?
   (7) What other jobs have you held in this or a similar field?
   (8) What were your responsibilities?
   (9) Do you mind irregular working hours? Explain.

(10) Would you be willing to relocate? To travel?
(11) What minimum salary are you willing to accept?
(12) Are you more comfortable working alone or with other people?

4. Answer candidate's questions.
5. Note the following: Candidate was
   (1) On time
   (2) Well-dressed
   (3) Well-mannered
   (4) Positive about self
6. Maintain eye contact.
7. Note candidate's personal values.
8. Close the interview.
   (1) Make an offer
   (2) Obtain acceptance
   (3) Set timetable for making offer or receiving response to offer

---

the person with hiring authority. They may be looking at several jobs, having narrowed the field down to those that specifically fit their career goals. They know how to make contacts and now want interviews to create opportunities to sell themselves.

The Introduction.   The interviewer should step from behind the desk, shake hands with the applicant, call the applicant by name, introduce him- or herself, and ask the applicant to be seated. This is done to put the applicant at ease. The interviewer should then seat the applicant so that she or he will not be blinded by sunlight and will be facing the interviewer.

Questions.   Questions, which should be prepared beforehand, may include those listed in Exhibit 8–6. Any others specifically desired by the interviewer should be added to the list. The answers should not be written down, as this is distracting and time-consuming. Written notes should be made immediately following the interview.

All candidates for nurse jobs should be treated as professionals. It is illegal to ask them certain questions, such as those listed in Exhibit 8–7. Since information about age and date of birth may be necessary for insurance or other fringe benefits, it can be obtained once the candidate is hired.

Candidates will have their own questions they want answered. If complete information cannot be given, the interviewer should make notes and communicate the information to the candidate as quickly as possible. Exhibit 8–8 lists questions that candidates might ask and that the interviewer should be prepared to answer.

Exhibit 8–7   Questions That Are Illegal to Ask

Employment interviewers are forbidden by law to ask the following questions:

1. Age
2. Date of birth
3. The length of time residing at present address
4. Previous address
5. Religion; church attended; spiritual adviser's name
6. Father's surname
7. Maiden name (of women)
8. Marital status
9. Residence mates
10. The number and ages of children; who will care for them while applicant works
11. Transportation to work, unless a car is a job requirement
12. Residence of spouse or parent
13. Whether residence is owned or rented
14. Name of bank; information on outstanding loans
15. Whether wages were ever garnished
16. Whether bankruptcy was ever declared
17. Whether ever arrested
18. Hobbies, off-duty interests, clubs

The objective of both interviewer and candidate at the outset of an interview is to create a positive, amicable relationship that results in a job offer. The interview is the most important factor in obtaining this result, as it allows expression of personal ideas, abilities, and accomplishments. It adds individual personality to the resume and completed application forms.

To prepare for a job interview, nurse managers should do the following:

1. Decide beforehand that they want the interview to end in a job offer.
2. Know the specific qualifications needed by the organization. Relating them to the candidate will help to identify a fit between candidate and job.
3. Decide to win the candidate's favor. The interviewer should come across as someone who respects and values employees. It is important for both interviewer and interviewee to have self-confidence, optimism, good manners, charm, and enthusiasm.

Exhibit 8–8   Possible Questions from Candidates

1. How much job security does this job have?
2. What previous experience does this type of job require?
3. What is the future of this type of job?
4. What is the growth potential for this particular job?
5. Where will the most significant growth for this type of job in the health care industry occur?
6. What is the starting salary for this job?
7. How do pay raises occur?
8. How does one find out when other job openings occur?
9. What are the fringe benefits of this job?
10. What are the requirements for working shifts and weekends?
11. What is the floating policy?
12. What are the opportunities for continuing education?
13. What are the opportunities for promotion?
14. What child-care facilities are available?
15. What are the staffing and scheduling policies?

4. Gain a feeling for the values of the candidate. Are they compatible with the organization's mission, philosophy, and objectives?

5. Have expectations about the dress, mannerisms, and other personal characteristics of the candidate. (These will, of course, be objective.) A serious candidate will dress conservatively for the interview. If the applicant is a man, he should be clean-shaven, have neatly cut and styled hair, be dressed in a business suit and tie, and wear appropriate footwear. Beards can be acceptable but should be neatly trimmed. If the applicant is a woman, she should have a neat hairdo, be dressed in a business suit or dress, wear hosiery, and wear appropriate jewelry. Makeup should be in good taste, and perfume or cologne, if any, should be discreet. One's appearance should be interpreted as an indication of one's good judgment and impeccable taste. Candidates thus tell the prospective employer that they regard the interview as important. The interviewer also should dress, act, look, and smell like the right person to be the candidate's manager.

The candidate should come across as a thoroughly pleasant, cooperative, and competent person, who can tactfully, objectively, and successfully deal with the most difficult people problems. The candidate should be neither blustery nor flamboyant or mouselike and servile. The interviewer should meet the same personal standards as those of the person being interviewed. Candidates who disagree with the interviewer's tastes or values should not be rejected unless the disagreement is related to the welfare of the organization. They should not be made to feel intimidated. Exhibit 8–9 summarizes what happens during an interview.

Exhibit 8–9   What Happens During an Interview

The Hiring Executive	The Candidate
1. Gives information about job and institution.	1. Gives information about self.
2. Assesses the competencies the candidate possesses in relation to the job opening.	2. Assesses the opportunity for developing and using competencies on the job.
3. Evaluates the candidate's personal characteristics in relation to the staff members with whom candidate will work (fit to staff).	3. Assesses ability to relate to the employees with whom candidate will work.
4. Assesses candidate's potential to move organization toward its goals.	4. Assesses potential for achieving personal career goals.
5. Assesses candidate's enthusiasm and state of health.	5. Assesses the institution's climate and the morale of the employees.
6. Forms impressions about candidate—behavior, appearance, ability to communicate, confidence, intelligence, personality.	6. Assesses opportunities for promotion and success.
7. Assesses candidate's ability to do the job.	7. Assesses own ability to do the job.
8. Determines facts about candidate.	8. Determines facts about the organization and working conditions.

Exercise 8–5 Using Exhibit 8–6, "Interview Guide," simulate the job interview of an applicant by interviewing one of your group members. Discuss the results with your group.

The Assessment Center Process

An assessment center is a method for screening candidates for jobs. It is specific to the job for which candidates are applying. Sullivan, Decker, and Hailstone describe an assessment center for the selection of a nurse manager that has the following seventeen job dimensions,[21] each being subdivided into abilities that are observed and scored.

1. Clinical nursing background.
2. Development of subordinates.
3. Delegation/management control.
4. Planning and organization.
5. Perception/sensitivity.
6. Problem analysis.
7. Problem solving/decision making.
8. Risk taking.
9. Initiation/leadership.
10. Communication skills.
11. Listening skills.
12. Energy level.
13. Stress tolerance.
14. Resilience.
15. Assertiveness.
16. Behavioral flexibility.
17. Accessibility.

The following are some other characteristics of this process:[22]

1. Exercises are developed to measure job dimensions.
2. Assessors from the supervisor group are selected and trained to rate the candidates.
3. The Head Nurse Assessment Center (HNAC) is conducted for one day. Each candidate is assessed by at least two persons.
4. Reliability and validity of assessment centers are high. The HNAC has many benefits, including selection of competent nurse managers, objectivity, broader applicant support, consistency, qualified applicants, nurse manager development, and improved management reputation.
5. Among the drawbacks of the HNAC are that it is stressful, time-consuming, and tiring for assessors, it favors outsiders, and it intimidates.
6. The process is job-specific.
7. The process is equitable to minorities and women.
8. Supervisors who will work with applicants select them.

9. The process has self-development value for participants.
10. The process is expensive, is stressful, may favor conformists, and may create self-fulfilling prophesies.
11. The process diminishes the risk for hiring or promoting inappropriate candidates.
12. The process is used in over 2,000 companies.

Peter's recommendations support the principles underlying the assessment center process:[23]

- Applicants should have multiple lengthy interviews over one or two days.
- Applicants should be interviewed by senior line people, peers, and potential subordinates.
- Interviews should unequivocally stress the attitudes and skills necessary to thrive in an ever more ambiguous and fast-changing world.

Credentialing

Credentialing is the process by which selected professionals are granted privileges to practice within an organization. In health-care organizations, this process has been largely confined to physicians. Limited privileges have been granted to psychologists, social workers, and selected categories of nurses, such as nurse anesthetists, surgical nurses, and midwives. Generally, these categories have been restricted by physician credentialing policies and fall into the category of allied professional staff.

Requirements of the Joint Commission on Accreditation of Healthcare Organizations (JCAHO) are that hospitals investigate, develop recommendations, reach conclusions, and be responsible for their actions in credentialing the medical staff. Licensing and certification provide data to consider in the process.

Components of Credentialing.   As they are for physicians, the components of a credentialing system for nurses would be as follows:[24]

1. *Appointment*—evaluation and selection for nursing staff membership.
2. *Clinical privileges*—delineation of the specific nursing specialties that may be performed and the types of illness or patients that may be managed within the institution for each member of the nursing staff.
3. *Periodic reappraisal*—continuing review and evaluation of each member of the nursing staff to assure that competence is maintained and consistent with privileges.

Criteria for Appointment.   Criteria for appointments would include proof of licensure, education and training, specialty board certification, previous experience, and recommendations. Clinical privileges criteria would include proof of specialty training and of performance of nursing procedures or specialty care during training and previous appointments.

During the credentialing process the committee should look for red flags of high mobility, graduation from foreign schools, professional liability suits, and professional disciplinary actions. Each red flag is a reason for exercising extra care in reviewing the applicant.

While professional nurses have mostly been hired through personnel offices, nurse managers should give consideration to increasing the professional status of nursing through the credentialing process. (See Appendix 8–1.)

The American Nurses Association (ANA).   A report of the Committee for the Study of Credentialing in Nursing, made in 1979, included fourteen principles of credentialing related to the following:[25]

1. Those credentialed.
2. Legitimate interests of involved occupation, institution, and general public.
3. Accountability.
4. A system of checks and balances.
5. Periodic assessments.
6. Objective standards and criteria and persons competent in their use.
7. Representation of the community of interests.
8. Professional identity and responsibility.
9. An effective system of role delineation.
10. An effective system of program identification.
11. Coordination of credentialing mechanisms.
12. Geographic mobility.
13. Definitions and terminology.
14. Communications and understanding.

Credentialing in a hospital relates to appointing health professionals to the staff. Credentialing by professional organizations such as the ANA's certification/recertification programs can be a qualification for such appointments:

> The American Nurses Association, Inc. established the ANA Certification Program in 1973 to provide tangible recognition of professional achievement in a defined functional or clinical area of nursing. Based on the 1989 recommendation from the ANA Commission on Organizational Assessment and Renewal (COAR), the American Nurses Credentialing Center (ANCC) has been established as a separately incorporated center through which ANA would serve its own credentialing programs. The ANCC bases its credentialing programs on the standards set by the ANA Congress for Nursing Practice. Goals of the ANCC include promoting and enhancing public health by certifying nurses and accrediting organizations using ANA standards of nursing practice, nursing services, and continuing education. Primary responsibility for the ANCC certification and recertification programs rests with the Boards on Certification whose members are nominated by the respective peer group. These Boards are: Community Health Nursing Practice, Maternal-Child Nursing Practice, Medical-Surgical Nursing Practice, Primary Care in Adult and Family/Health Nursing Practice, Gerontological Nursing Practice, Nursing Administration Practice, General Nursing Practice, and Nursing Continuation Education/Staff Development Nursing Practice.[26]

Over 90,000 registered nurses have been certified by the American Nurses Credentialing Center. Beginning in 1998, all generalist programs require a baccalaureate in nursing for the initial certification process.

Credentialing at Carondelet St. Mary's Hospital and Health Center in Tucson, Arizona, focuses on patient care, leadership, and education. Benefits to the nurses include clinical ladder promotions, compensation, paid education time, tuition reimbursement, and a paid day monthly for meetings and research. Patients benefit from improved infection control, reduced numbers and increased healing of pressure ulcers, new product introduction, and improved teaching. The employer benefits from retention of satisfied customers, nurses, and patients.[27]

Exercise 8–6	Review Appendix 8–1, "USAMC Department of Nursing Credentialing Process." Credentialing is a process requiring top management decisions and support for implementation. What changes would you make in the process? Note them. Make an appointment to explore this process with the chief nurse executive of the agency in which you work or are assigned as a student. Plan your interview.

Assigning

Assigning professional nurses to jobs is the third part of the hiring process. During the assignment period, the new nurse is oriented to the job description and its use. While assignment to a specific position may not be possible during the selecting and credentialing processes, candidates should know the possible units to which they will be assigned.

Where can a candidate who wants to work in the operating room, but there are no vacant positions, be assigned? Offer the candidate a choice of vacant positions. Make a verbal or written contract to transfer the individual to a vacated operating room position when one becomes available. If others are waiting for a similar assignment, indicate the order in which they will be assigned to the operating room.

Candidates should not receive assignment surprises when they arrive for orientation. Assignment policies should be fair, reasonable, and acceptable to candidates, who will then start work with a positive attitude. A principle for a nurse manager or leader to follow is to provide necessary orientation and training to nursing employees to ensure competency, job satisfaction, and high productivity in the particular assignments they are accepting.

RETAINING

The retention of competent, professional nurses in jobs is a major problem of the U.S. health-care industry, particularly for hospitals. Most Americans change jobs about fifteen times by age 35, and nurses are no exception. Nurses change and achieve major career goals four or five times in their lifetime, including changing their specialty or the role they play in the profession.[28] Many do both. Some even retire from two or more systems.

Turnover

The annual turnover rate among hospital nurses nationally appears to be between 20 percent and 70 percent. An organization should determine its turnover rate by unit as well as by organization. Such determination should be done monthly to keep abreast of trends. Leavers should be profiled and defined by average age, marital status, type of program from which graduated, additional education, years of experience, specialty, sex, race, and any other characteristic that will give clues that could decrease turnover and increase retention of competent nurses. Nurse managers should review the performance of the leavers and do exit interviews.

The crude turnover rate depicts the volume of turnover. It is not a very selective index. An example is given in Exhibit 8–10. Other data that will provide information about turnover and retention are the mean and median service of stayers. These data provide the average tenure of employees. Examples of these data are illustrated in Exhibit 8–10, as are mean and median service of leavers, instability rate, wastage rate, and survival curve of leavers.[29]

The sum of the number of months of employment of each nurse as well as other data can be determined by having a good nursing management information system (NMIS), which will accumulate the data on electronic spreadsheets.

The Leadership, Evaluation and Awareness Process (LEAP), developed by DeBerry as a common preselection process for first-line managers, consists of the following:

- A one-day program called "Is Management for Me?" covering the realities of management; 60 percent of the takers are self-selected out of competition.
- A developmental session with current managers, covering such skills as charisma, individual consideration, intellectual stimulation, courage, dependability, flexibility, integrity, judgment, and respect for others.
- A three-way evaluation of manager as coach, peers, and self-profile of leadership on nine skills.
- A panel of executives using in-basket exercises and oral and written tests on nine skills; 75 percent of candidates were endorsed.
- Application.

The outcome of LEAP has been an 80 percent reduction in turnover of first-line managers at an average turnover cost of $125,000 each and a positive cost/-benefit analysis.[30]

Since 70 percent of families are headed by a single working parent or by two wage earners, vanguard companies are changing their corporate culture to accomplish goals of workforce dedication, focus, and productivity. Vanguard companies consider it good business to make it easier for employees to come to work. To do this, they are changing corporate culture to

- Make it family friendly.
- Provide child care around the clock.
- Foster candor, assertiveness, and commitment.

Exhibit 8–10 Turnover Data

1.

$$\text{Crude turnover rate} = \left[\frac{\text{Number } (N) \text{ of Leavers}}{\left(\dfrac{N \text{ at start} + n \text{ at end}}{2} \right)} \right] \times 100$$

Number (N) of leavers = number of nurses who left during a year
N at start = number of nurses employed at beginning of year
n at end = number of nurses employed at end of year

Example: $(N) = 189$
$N = 543$
$n = 529$

$$\frac{189}{\left(\dfrac{543 + 529}{2} \right)} \times 100 = \frac{189}{536} \times 100 = 35.26 \text{ percent}$$

2.

$$\text{Mean service of stayers} = \frac{\text{Sum of the number of months of employment of each nurse}}{\text{Number of nurses employed}}$$

Example:

$$\frac{10,563 \text{ months}}{529 \text{ nurses}} = 19.97 \text{ months}$$

3. Median service of stayers
   Rank currently employed nurses by the number of months of employment from the shortest to the longest and choose middle ranking value.

Example:

Months	1–6	7–12	13–18	19–24	25–30	31–36	37–42	43–48	49–54	55–60+
No. of Employees	73	61	55	50	41	39	40	27	39	104
Total	73	134	189	239	280	319	359	386	425	529

Total nurses (stayers) = 529

$$\text{Median} = \frac{529}{2} = 265.5$$

Median occurs at 25 to 30 months, indicating that more than one-half of the nurses have been employed 30 months or less. The median is considered a better measure of central tendency than the mean.

Exhibit 8–10 *Turnover Data (Continued)*

4.

$$\text{Mean services of leavers} = \frac{\text{Sum of the number of months of employment of each nurse who left}}{\text{Number of nurses who left}}$$

$$\frac{2417 \text{ months}}{189 \text{ nurses}} = 12.79 \text{ months}$$

5. Median service of leavers

Months	1–6	7–12	13–18	19–24	25–30	31–36	37–42	43–48	49–54	55–60+	61+
No. of Employees	49	35	27	19	14	9	9	10	7	6	4
Total	49	84	111	130	144	153	162	172	179	185	189

$$\text{Total nurses (leavers)} = 189$$
$$\text{Median} = \frac{189}{2} = 94.5$$

The median occurs at 13 to 18 months. Since the mean and median of leavers are both low, short-term employees are leaving.

6.

$$\text{Instability rate} = \frac{\text{Number of leavers who had been employed at beginning of year}}{\text{Number of nurses employed at beginning of year}} \times 100$$

Example:

$$\frac{151}{529} \times 100 = 28.54 \text{ percent}$$

Of nurses employed at the beginning of the year, 28.54 percent left during the year.

7.

$$\text{Wastage rate} = \frac{\text{Number of newly hired nurses who leave during first year}}{\text{Number of nurses newly hired during year}} \times 100$$

Example:

$$\frac{40}{113} \times 100 = 35.4 \text{ percent}$$

Among newly hired nurses, over one-third, or 35.4 percent, leave before the end of one year.

Exhibit 8–10 Turnover Data *(Continued)*

8. Survival curve of leavers

Example:

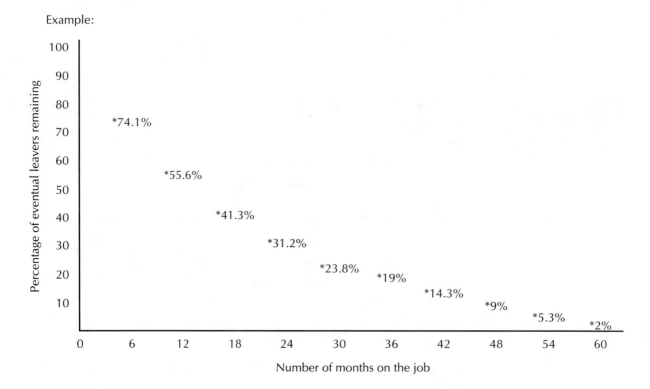

Using data from item 5, 100 percent of 189 leavers were employed at beginning of 12 months period.

$$\frac{189 - 49}{189} = \frac{140}{189} = 74.1 \text{ percent of leavers were employed 6–12 months.}$$

$$\frac{140 - 35}{189} = \frac{105}{189} = 55.6 \text{ percent of leavers were employed 13–18 months.}$$

Since the curve drops sharply and then gradually, it shows that the turnover concentration is among new employees. A straight line would indicate turnover to be independent of length of service.

Source: Adapted from M. L. Duxbury and G. D. Armstrong, "Calculating Nurse Turnover Indices," *Journal of Nursing Administration,* March 1982, 18–24. Reprinted with permission of J. B. Lippincott.

■ Focus on managers bringing about cultural change through a common collaborative management style and a human resource philosophy, the bedrocks of which are equity and flexibility.
■ Provide eldercare referral.
■ Provide professional counseling for coping with stress.
■ Provide paid days off for taking care of personal obligations.
■ Empower managers and workforce.
■ Provide resources.
■ Tailor the culture to the individual's need.

The outcome has been loyalty, dedication, and team spirit.[31] Since nursing is a workforce with many of the same working-parent characteristics, the objectives of staffing should be staff retention by making it easier for nursing personnel to come to work.

Turnover causes increased costs of hiring and orienting as well as staff instability and decreased quality of care. Exhibit 8–10 presents a conceptual framework for nursing turnover. Among the causes of turnover are job stress, lack of autonomy, job dissatisfaction, and a poor overall health-care environment (regulatory, political, economic, and social factors). These factors include the political factor of resource allocation and economic factors such as profit margins, policy, organizational diagnosis involving structures, interaction, and competition.

Turnover includes both replacement and transfer employees. The direct costs of turnover are attributed to recruitment of replacements. The cost of turnover ranges from $1,280 to $50,000 per RN turnover. Turnover benefits include savings on salaries and benefits and infusion of new knowledge and ideas. Incentives for retention include financial benefits, flexible scheduling, and participative management.[32]

Job Expectations and Satisfactions

The author contends that the high turnover rate in nursing is a result of job dissatisfactions (see Appendix 8–2). In a survey of nurse job and career satisfaction and dissatisfaction, 6,277 surveys were mailed to nurses in a five-county area around Jacksonville, Florida. There were 1,921 responses, with the following results:[33]

■ *Money was the number one concern and the preferred remedy.*
■ Recognition was the second most serious concern; hours and scheduling were third; too much responsibility for the money fourth; and stress fifth.

A study to determine why new graduates select particular settings and why many leave in a short time surveyed 279 nursing seniors in five schools in northern Alabama. These new graduates had the following expectations:

1. Work full-time.
2. Work days or a desired shift (46 percent of single nurses and 36.5 percent of married nurses would work evenings).
3. Work in a medium-sized to large hospital.

4. Earn a good salary.
5. Have pleasant working conditions.
6. Gain self-fulfillment and a sense of achievement from giving adequate and complete care.
7. Have educational opportunities, intellectual stimulation, and opportunity to develop new skills.
8. Receive satisfactory supervision by nurse managers.
9. Be recognized and encouraged.
10. Have professional autonomy and power.
11. Work in a community that offered higher education opportunities and a good place to raise a family. Factors considered important included good schools, a low crime rate, an economically stable region, a low tax structure, and low cost of living.

In addition, more baccalaureate degree nurses expected to become head nurses, supervisors, and public health nurses than did associate degree nurses. Many would *not* consider working in small hospitals (17.2 percent), veterans administration or federally owned hospitals (19.5 percent), investor-owned hospitals (18.8 percent), nursing homes (65.7 percent), doctor's office or clinic (18.6 percent), temporary or private-duty agency (41 percent), or psychiatric or mental health clinic (45.5 percent).[34]

Drucker states that salaries are not the basic problem with nurse retention and recruitment, a position in opposition to most surveys. He states, "The basic problem is that nurses aren't allowed to do nursing. I've been saying that now for 20 years. The doctors still treat nurses as if they were scullery maids, and that's just not going to work any longer." Drucker believes that hospital administrators must change the attitudes of doctors. Also, focusing nurses' responsibilities on their professional role and increasing their salaries will improve job retention.[35]

Exercise 8–7	Using Exhibit 8–10, "Turnover Data," collect turnover data to establish the following for a unit, department, or division of nursing.

1. Crude turnover rate
2. Mean service of stayers
3. Median service of stayers
4. Mean service of leavers
5. Median service of leavers
6. Instability rate
7. Wastage rate
8. Survival curve of leavers

Career Planning

Nurse managers will recognize the results of nurse satisfaction surveys. They must now learn to manage professional nurses so that they will achieve career and job satisfaction. The first step is to establish a career plan for them within the nursing organization.

To be successful in their careers, professional nurses need a sense of personal fulfillment and job significance, indicating that they are growing as persons. Nurse managers create these conditions by determining and correcting the causes of the following:

- Anxiety and uncertainty.
- Inability to meet personal and organizational goals.
- Lack of clarity about roles played.
- Contradictory demands.
- Dissatisfaction with human relations.
- Rebellion against rules, policies, and regulations.
- The inherent nature of the tasks of the job.
- Competition.
- Being overworked and underutilized.
- Lack of personal and professional growth.
- Dissatisfaction with the quality of associates.

A professional nurse is a reasonable person, and reasonable people can accommodate to reality, accept themselves, be interested in others, learn from experience, and be self-actualized.[36]

Nurse managers should restructure nursing services to link assignments and responsibilities to education, experience, and competence. This should be a part of a career program that provides more promotions and pay for clinical nurses, more pay for increased competence, and increased participation. It should provide for continuing education to upgrade knowledge and skills. It should provide clinical rotation policies that prevent burnout, and it should meet professional nurses' scheduling and salary preferences.[37]

When a career structure has been established, it will provide for upward mobility for clinical nurses, nurse managers, nursing teachers, and nursing researchers. Professional nurses will decide to take advantage of career advancement opportunities. Jobs for those advancing will be identified and will require advanced knowledge and skills, particularly those related to decision making. Registered nurses who do not want promotions will be rewarded by merit pay increases for doing their jobs well. Advancing nurses will be rewarded for increased responsibility and accountability. Nurses will finally have a career rather than just a job.

Sovie labels the career development functions of the staff development department as professional identification, professional maturation, and professional mastery. These areas can be related to a career ladder program where competencies have been identified for the nurse practicing at several rungs of the ladder. The competencies are stated in the form of job descriptions and increase in complexity. Policies and procedures exist for the process of climbing the ladder. The process is facilitated by a program of staff development for career advancement.

Sovie's model could educate nurses to gain advanced specialized knowledge and skills through individual plans, with staff development educators acting as counselors and teachers. Nurses could learn to provide the leadership in solving the health-care problems of patients and families. They could develop materials for patient and family education. They could learn to be a primary nurse in practicing the nursing process, not just within the nursing modality. They could learn to engage in professional nursing dialogue with colleagues. Their training could include the competencies of consulting, participation in quality assurance activities, processing and applying reports of research findings, participation in research, and involvement in committee functions. This training could be part of a personal career plan.[38]

Nurses in an organization that has a career development program should be moving up the ladder of their choice. The career development program should also provide an opportunity for moving laterally into clinical practice, management, teaching, or research. It should provide job satisfaction and a salary that increases with development and mastery.

If such a career development program does not exist in the organization, nurses can stimulate it. They can first learn about it through research and study, master the knowledge of career development, and then present it to their supervisors and get their support. If attempts to move up fail, nurses may want to move out, but they should not give up easily.

Career Ladders.   Clinical nursing offers the most diverse kinds of opportunities. Clinical nursing was largely a nonpromotable area until recent years. Numerous interesting clinical areas had been expanded with advanced technology, but nurses seldom could be promoted within a clinical area. This is changing fast with the development of clinical career ladders and levels of increasing competence to mastery.

A career ladder requires individual effort, assisted by organizational support and reward. It results in career satisfaction to the nurses who participate and in increased productivity for the employer if the program is appropriately conceived and implemented. More results must occur than title changes and increased wages or salaries.

A clinical career ladder is a horizontal development system based on specific criteria used to develop, evaluate, and promote nurses desiring and intending to remain at the bedside. Clinical ladders apply to nurses who want to remain in the clinical setting, whereas career ladders are for those who leave the clinical realm in pursuit of a future in administration, teaching, or research.

If the pay differential between levels is not significant, that also will impede motivation to change. Salary increases should be enough to further motivate the nurses to improve their skills (competence). Responsibility should increase with promotion. If nurses are still performing the same tasks with the same supervision and no additional responsibility after advancement, they cannot be said to have really advanced professionally.

Performance criteria in any clinical ladder system should be clearly differentiated and specific at each level. The evaluation process must be measurable. Salary differentials must be significant enough to provide motivation. Any system should involve evaluation of educational and leadership criteria as well as skill performance.

Finally, the evaluation of each individual should include input from the direct supervisor and the individuals themselves. A board or panel of three or more nurses may be assembled to review all eligible personnel for promotion.

The advantages of such a system are that it increases job satisfaction, improves clinical skills, offers positive motivation for acceptance of continued leadership and educational responsibility, and provides an opportunity for career advancement while remaining in clinical nursing. The disadvantage is that positions may not always be available at higher levels.

Management promotes the system to the end that productivity will be increased. Also, management must assure the maintenance of quality of nursing care.

Exhibit 8–11 is a basic clinical ladder model that can be added to or fleshed out by management.

Exhibit 8–11   Basic Clinical Ladder Model

A.   Clinical/Staff Nurse I (beginner/novice)

1. Experience and Education
   Current state licensure with less than one year of experience.
2. Description
   a. Needs close supervision.
   b. Performs basic nursing skills/routine patient care.
   c. Begins to develop patient assessment skills/communication skills.

B. Clinical/Staff Nurse II (advanced beginner)

1. Experience and Education
   a. Current state licensure with more than one year of experience.
   b. BSN with more than six months of experience.
   c. MSN without experience.
2. Description
   a. Demonstrates adequate/acceptable performance.
   b. Can differentiate importance of situations and set priorities.
   c. Requires less supervision.
   d. Demonstrates interest in continuing education.

C. Clinical/Staff Nurse III (competent)

1. Experience and Education
   a. Current licensure with two or more years of experience.
   b. BSN with more than one year of experience.
   c. MSN with more than six months of experience.
2. Description
   a. Demonstrates unsupervised competency using nursing process.

b. Is able to plan and organize in terms of short-range and long-range goals.
   c. Demonstrates direction in actions.
   d. Accepts leadership responsibility readily.
   e. Demonstrates well-developed communication skills.
   f. Shares ideas and knowledge with peers.

D. Clinical/Staff Nurse IV (proficient)

1. Experience and Education
   a. Current licensure with three years of clinical experience and pursuit of BSN.
   b. BSN with more than two years of experience.
   c. MSN with more than one year of experience.
2. Description
   a. Demonstrates specialized knowledge and skills.
   b. Continues professional education.
   c. Assumes leadership/supervisory responsibility.
   d. Recognizes and adjusts to situations that vary from the norm.
   e. Delegates responsibility appropriately; uses wide range of alternatives in solving problems.

E. Clinical/Staff Nurse V (expert)

1. Experience and Education
   a. MSN with more than two years of appropriate clinical experience.
   b. BSN required with more than three years of experience; pursuing MSN.
2. Description
   a. Demonstrates expertise in clinical practice.
   b. Assumes/delegates personnel and management responsibility.

PROMOTING

Professional nurses have had to turn to management, education, or research for promotion. The development of professional nurse clinical ladders is making some headway, albeit not quickly enough. Many professional nurses want to stay in clinical nursing and will do so if they can be rewarded with promotions that increase their pay and standing within the organization.

One way for nurse managers to assure that all professional nurses have promotion opportunities is to develop a promotion system that indicates all promotion categories within the organization (see Exhibit 8–12). Nurse managers should develop specific promotion policies with input from all categories of professional nurses and the human resource department. These policies should include the following:

1. All vacant positions will be posted. This should be true even though change in pay and rank does not occur. Some nurses will want to change units, specialty, shifts, and so on.

Exhibit 8–12   Promotion System

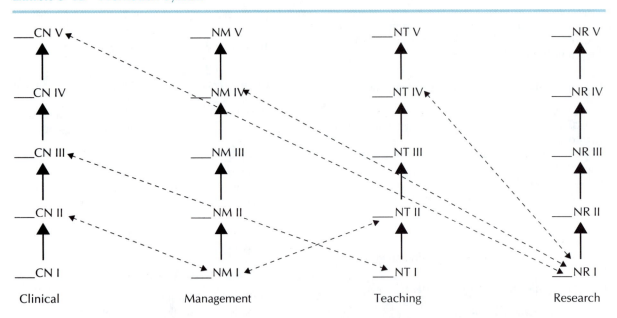

This is a model. Each level would require specific and increasing education, experience, and performance accomplishments. The arrows indicate the levels at which nurses from each group could advance. The clinical nurse II (CN II) could advance to nurse manager (NM I), or vice versa. The nurse teacher IV (NT IV) could advance to nurse researcher I (NR I), or vice versa. The number of budgeted positions would be entered in the blanks in front of each group. For nurse researchers, this could be only one position but would allow for appointment at or promotion to higher levels.

2. All interested applicants should file applications for promotion in the human resource department.
3. Human resource department personnel should prepare promotion rosters that rank all candidates by such objective criteria as education, experience, and performance. The best-qualified candidate should be at the top of the list.
4. Applicants should be interviewed and rated by the same set of criteria, a process described previously in this chapter under "Selecting."
5. The best-qualified candidates should be selected for promotion.
6. The results of the promotion process should be announced. Those not selected should be notified and counseled individually rather than learn that they were passed over from a third party or from seeing the list of those promoted.
7. The promotion system must be fair and be perceived as fair by professional nurses.

An effective promotion policy will provide the same opportunity for people of equal ability to apply and will treat such people equitably during interviews. Nonpromoted employees should be allowed to ventilate their disappointment. Managers may expect a temporary performance dropoff from them.[39]

Promotions are becoming more competitive because of increased numbers of qualified competitors and because downsizing has eliminated tens of thousands of middle-management jobs across all sectors of the economy. This potential lack of a future causes great individual stress.

Employees are starting their own businesses by buying franchises and turning hobbies that use special skills into profit makers. Some make lateral moves within a company to learn new skills. Others return to school, retire early, or do community work to increase their self-satisfaction. Employers are granting long-term, unpaid sabbaticals to employees to return to school or work for noncompetitive organizations. Some loan out executives to charitable organizations. Many have moved authority to lower levels to increase autonomy and job satisfaction.[40]

TERMINATING

Employees cannot be terminated at will. They are protected by public policy set forth in the National Labor Relations Act, the Civil Rights Act of 1964, the Discrimination in Employment Act, the Vocational Rehabilitation Act, and the Occupational Safety and Health Act. Also, laws protect whistle blowers.

Employees should be terminated only after all efforts to retain them have been exhausted. The theory of management includes concepts and principles that, when learned and applied by nurse managers, will assist employees to be competent and productive. Punishment or disciplinary action should be a last resort and should be progressive, moving from verbal conference, to a recorded conference, to suspension, to discharge. Such action should be covered by written policies and procedures.

First-line nurse managers should have firing authority. They should consult with superior managers and human resource personnel when terminating staff to make sure the action will stand up in court. All policies must be legal, and they must be consistently and correctly enforced. Any employee is entitled to a fair hearing and review. The process allows for appropriate representatives at investigating interviews. Terminated employees should be paid all benefits they have accrued.[41] Exhibit 8–13 is a checklist for assessing a legally supportable discharge. The checklist applies to the discharge of both hourly and salaried employees of union employers.

Firing an employee is an unpleasant job. It is done for the following reasons:

- Economic downturns when employees are surplus.
- Personality mismatches—everything has been tried, including transfers, but the employee does not fit anywhere.
- Progressive discipline in which the employee fails to meet agreed-upon performance.
- Incorrigibles—serious mistakes, stealing, other gross failures.

The nurse manager needs to plan the session well ahead and be well-prepared to do the following:[42]

- Coordinate with personnel office, superiors, unions, outplacement people, and others.
- Keep the firing from the grapevine.
- Time the session for the end of the day and the middle of the week to keep it confidential and to rebuild the organization.
- Be straightforward and up-front.
- Have all documentation ready.
- Deal with four stages of employee reaction: shock with physical symptoms, rejection, emotion, and withdrawal. Be quiet during the shock and emotion stages. Confirm the message during rejection. Provide information during withdrawal and terminate the meeting.

Exercise 8–8   Design a questionnaire and take a random survey of clinical personnel in the organization where you work or are assigned as a student.

1. Identify problems in the areas of recruitment, selection, credentialing, assignment, staffing, retention, promotion, and termination.

2. Tabulate and analyze the results. What are the problems?

3. What are the possible solutions to these problems?

4. How would the assessment center improve nurse selection or promotion? Support your decision.

5. How can the productivity of professional nurses be improved in this setting?

Exhibit 8–13   A Quick Test to Assess the Legality of Firing an At-Will Employee

1. Has the employee been terminated with one of the reasons being
   a. Race
   b. Religion
   c. Sex
   d. Age (over 40)
   e. National origin
   f. Children or childbirth
   g. Pregnancy
   h. Handicap
2. Did the discharged employee engage in union activity immediately before the discharge or did the employee act in concert (and this is the reason for the discharge) with other employees to
   a. Organize collectively
   b. Push for a raise or shorter hours
   c. Ask for changes in other working conditions
   d. Support another employee in a protest?
3. Will the discharge violate any type of contract?
   a. Does your employee handbook provide for warnings before an employee may be discharged or say that an employee may be discharged only for cause?
   b. Do you have written employee policies that promise "fair treatment"?
   c. Is there a written, signed employment contract?
4. Will the discharge violate any state tort laws?
   a. Have you committed the tort of "outrage"—has the company been abusive in discharging the employee, either through high-handed interrogation methods or through flagrant misrepresentations as to why the employee is being discharged?
   b. Has the company been negligent in not following its own policies, which has thus resulted in the employee's discharge?
5. Are you terminating the employee for any of the following reasons?
   a. Refusing to do an illegal act.
   b. Filing a workers' compensation claim.
   c. Reporting violations of such federal statutes as the Equal Employment Opportunity Act, the Occupational Safety and Health Act, or the Employee Retirement Income Security Act?
   d. Whistle-blowing over the company's possible violations of state laws, such as antitrust laws?
6. Is the employee being discharged for refusing to do a job the employee considers unsafe (giving rise to a possible OSHA violation)?

a. Would doing the job *reasonably* place the employee in imminent danger?
b. The key to safety cases is: if this job has been performed safely many times in the past, why is it now considered unsafe? Has there been an accident on this job within a short time period giving the employee reason to be concerned about safety?
7. Did you provide a hearing (with company witnesses present) to provide the employee an opportunity to admit or deny the charges?
8. Was the employee given an oral or written warning to correct the conduct?
9. Have you let other employees pass undisciplined for the same conduct for which you are discharging this employee?
10. Did you promise the employee, when hiring or subsequently, that the job was there for as long as the employee wanted? Alternatively, did you promise the employee an annual contract?
11. Under state and federal disability laws, is the employee being discharged for a physical condition (e.g., high blood pressure, diabetes, or back conditions)? Have you tried to make reasonable accommodations for the employee to work at another, less strenuous job?
12. Do you have any evidence in writing covering the wrongful conduct (e.g., prior written reprimands) for which the employee is being terminated?
13. Did the employee give up another job or sell a home in another city to work for you, and were promises made to secure that employee for having done so?
14. Are you calling the termination a reduction-in-force (RIF), when in fact you selected this particular employee for reasons of unsatisfactory work performance?
15. If the employee, in the investigatory interview held by the company (if any) to determine the facts, requested a union representative or other employee to represent him or her at the interview, did the company deny the request and proceed with the interview in spite of the request?

Source: Reprinted from *Hospitals* 58, no. 14, by permission, July 16, 1984. Copyright 1984, American Hospital Publishing, Inc.

SUMMARY

A major focus of a theory of nursing management is that personnel should be managed for productivity, for achieving the mission and objectives of the organization. This involves recruiting, selecting, credentialing, and assigning nurses, first into the educational program, then into the division or department of nursing.

Since nursing, a predominantly female occupation, must now compete with all other professions for students, nurse managers should create conditions of work that are attractive, including competitive salaries and fringe benefits, optional schedules, and satisfying conditions of work such as autonomy and recognition.

The population from which all occupations will recruit will change greatly during the next decade. Its demographic makeup will shift, causing recruitment goals to change. Nurse managers should plan student recruitment at early stages of the secondary education process. The poor, minorities, children of single parents, and those with physical and emotional disabilities must be prepared now for careers, including careers in nursing. Equal career opportunity is the promise of America.

Each nurse manager should work with other health-care system managers and with secondary school teachers and counselors to prepare young men and women for careers in nursing. Once nurses are recruited, selected, credentialed, and assigned, nurse managers should develop strategies to retain them. For high-level positions, search committees are frequently used to recruit. The implication is that professional workers will have input into selecting those with whom they will work and who will give them leadership.

Nurse managers should consider a credentialing process for professional nurses similar to that used for physicians. It is essential that career planning be a major personnel management program within each nursing organization. Employees are not motivated by dead-end jobs. They desire the opportunity to qualify for promotion in clinical, management, education, and research positions. There should be clear communication of job vacancies, which should be filled by the best-qualified individuals.

Personnel who do not meet acceptable standards of performance should be counseled, warned in writing, and suspended without pay. When all else fails, they should be terminated.

Exercise 8–9   Conduct an exit interview using the format of Appendix 8–3. Discuss the results with your peer group.

NOTES

1. American Hospital Association, "Background on the National Nursing Shortage," *Hospital Nurse Recruitment and Retention: A Source Book for Executive Management* (Chicago: American Hospital Association, November 1980).
2. National Commission on Nursing, *Nursing in Transition: Models for Successful Organizational Change* (Chicago: American Hospital Association, Hospital Research and Educational Trust and American Hospital Supply Corporation, 1982), 41–42.
3. Associated Press, "U.S. Jobless Rate Slips to 6.4 Percent," *San Antonio Express-News,* 7 May 1994, 1B.
4. Associated Press, "Health-Care Job Machine May Shift into Low Gear," *Mobile Register,* 19 September 1993, 4F.
5. Ibid.
6. L. S. Richman, "Jobs That Are Growing and Slowing," *Fortune* 12 July 1993, 52–53.
7. W. Woods, "The Jobs Americans Hold," *Fortune,* 12 July 1993, 54–55.
8. Gannett Service, "Earnings Chasm Widens for Employees with Degrees," *San Antonio Express-News,* 20 February 1994, 3G.
9. Knight-Ridder Service, "Physician-Assistant Training Draws Many," *San Antonio Express-News,* 15 August 1993, 3J.
10. D. Hendricks, "Jobs Don't Die; They Move Up," *San Antonio Express-News,* 4 June 1993, 1B.
11. Ibid.
12. Editorial, *Times-Colonist* (Victoria, British Columbia, Canada), 12 July 1993, A4.
13. P. Ancona, "Make Yourself More Valuable at Work," *San Antonio Express-News,* 4 September 1993, 1 B.
14. H. L. Hodgkinson, "Reform? Higher Education? Don't Be Absurd!" *Phi Delta Kappan,* December 1986, 271–274.
15. K. A. Stevens and E. A. Walker, "Choosing a Career: Why Not Nursing for More High School Seniors?" *Journal of Nursing Education,* January 1993, 13–17.
16. American Academy of Nursing Task Force on Nursing Practice in Hospitals, *Magnet Hospitals: Attraction and Retention of Professional Nurses* (Kansas City, Mo.: American Nurses Association, 1983), 99.
17. M. Kramer and C. Schmalenberg, "Magnet Hospitals: Part II Institutions of Excellence," *Journal of Nursing Administration,* February 1988, 17.
18. J. E. Pattan, "Developing a Nurse Recruitment Plan," *Journal of Nursing Administration,* January 1992, 33–39.

19. J. A. Connelly and K. S. Strauser, "Managing Recruitment and Retention Problems: An Application of the Marketing Process," *Journal of Nursing Administration,* October 1983, 17–22.

20. M. R. Thompson, *Why Should I Hire You?* (New York: Jove Publications, 1975), 94.

21. E. J. Sullivan, P. J. Decker, and S. Hailstone, "Assessment Center Technology: Selecting Head Nurses," *Journal of Nursing Administration,* May 1985, 14.

22. Ibid.

23. T. Peters, *Thriving on Chaos* (New York: Harper & Row, 1987), 378–385.

24. H. S. Rowland and B. L. Rowland, *Hospital Legal Forms, Checklists, & Guidelines* (Rockville, Md.: Aspen, 1987), 17:1.

25. Committee for the Study of Credentialing in Nursing, "Credentialing in Nursing: A New Approach," *American Journal of Nursing,* April 1979, 674–683.

26. American Nurses Credentialing Center, *Recertification Catalog* (Washington, D.C.: American Nurses Credentialing Center, 1994).

27. C. Richelson, "Update on Credentialing," *Nursing Management* October 1991, 101–102.

28. P. E. Norris, *How to Find a Job* (Fairhope, Ala.: National Job Search Training Laboratories, 1982), 1.

29. M. L. Duxbury and G. D. Armstrong, "Calculating Nurse Turnover Indices," *Journal of Nursing Administration,* March 1982, 18–24.

30. L. DeBerry, "Preselection Process for First Line Managers Cuts Turnover," *Training,* July 1992, 80.

31. P. Berns and J. Berns, "Good for Business: Corporations Adopt the Family," *Management Review* 81, no. 9 (1992): 34–38.

32. C. B. Jones, "Staff Nurse Turnover Costs: Part 1, A Conceptual Model," *Journal of Nursing Administration,* April 1990, 18–23.

33. E. Ginsberg, J. Patray, M. Ostow, and E. A. Brann, "Nurse Discontent: The Search for Realistic Solutions," *Journal of Nursing Administration,* November 1982, 7–11.

34. C. E. Burton and D. T. Burton, "Job Expectations of Senior Nursing Students," *Journal of Nursing Administration,* March 1982, 11–17.

35. "Peter F. Drucker and Karl D. Bays Discuss the Toughest Job—Running a Hospital, Part 2." *HMQ,* summer 1982, 2–5.

36. A. Levenstein, "Career Dissatisfaction," *Nursing Management,* November 1985, 61–62.

37. E. Ginsberg, J. Patray, M. Ostow, and E. A. Brann, op. cit.

38. M. D. Sovie, "Fostering Professional Nursing Careers in Hospitals: The Role of Staff Development, Part 1," *Journal of Nursing Administration,* December 1982, 5–10.

39. "Who Gets the Promotion?" *Small Business Reports* 17, no. 10 (1992): 28.

40. Cox News Service, "Chances for Moving Up at Work Going Down," *San Antonio Express-News,* 12 December 1993, 6H.

41. B. C. Rutkowski and A. D. Rutkowski, "Employee Discharge: It Depends . . . ." *Nursing Management,* December 1984, 39–42.

42. J. C. Dumville, "Delivering the Mortal Blow," *Supervision* 54, no. 4 (1993): 6–7.

Appendix 8–1   USAMC Department of Nursing Credentialing Process

Definitions

Credentialing: Those degrees, licenses, skill checklists, and certificates that allow a nurse to practice nursing at USAMC.

Clinical Privileges: Permission given to an individual professional nurse by USAMC to practice specific skills based on credentials, experience, and demonstrated competence/performance.

Clinical privileges will be delineated for each member of the professional registered nursing staff. According to this standard, privileges are granted based on demonstrated competence, performance, and results of care.

When patient-care problems arise in areas that require qualification or certification, the nurse's credentials are checked first. If the nurse is credentialed for that activity, counseling may reveal the need for remediation; if the nurse is not credentialed, immediate steps are taken to correct the deficiency.

1. The first step is to complete application for entry. In completing this form, please do not leave *any* blanks. Indicate information that does not apply as N/A. Submit this completed form to the Nurse Manager of the designated area for which application is made.

2. Secondly, general nursing orientation must be completed as scheduled. Demonstrating entry-level requirements at six months credentials nurses to practice as a nurse at this institution.

3. The third step, meeting the requirements criteria for distinct specialty areas, allows nurses working in these specialty areas to practice advanced skills. These nurses must complete critical care or other specialty care skills and a preceptorship with a senior staff member. We identify skills on particular specialty units that require training beyond that encompassed in the basic orientation.

Review of departmental and/or individual practice and results of care will be an ongoing process through the hospitals Quality Assessment & Improvement Program. Professional Nursing Practice is expected to assist the Department of Nursing in meeting Standards of Practice. It is further expected that results of nursing care reveal patients' attaining desirable outcomes and without any adverse effects related to individual performance.

In summary, prior to privileges, professional nurses must meet all credentialing requirements for their designated level of expected practice. Advanced practice at USAMC requires completion of: orientation, appropriate courses, demonstrated skills, and preceptorship. Successful performance of required skills will be verified annually for recredentialing by the Clinical Nurse Specialist, Clinical Coordinator, Clinical Consultant, or a preceptor. This process is the responsibility of the Nurse Manager, CNS, and individual involved.

(Continued)

Appendix 8–1 USAMC Department of Nursing Credentialing Process *(Continued)*

APPLICATION FOR ENTRY

AREA FOR WHICH YOU ARE APPLYING _____

I. DEMOGRAPHICS

Name _____ SSN _____

Address _____ Phone(s) _____

_____

Emergency notification (Name) _____ Phone _____

Languages spoken (other than English/include sign language) _____

_____

Military Status _____ Branch _____ Rank _____

II. PROFESSIONAL EDUCATION

ADN/YR _____ Diploma/YR _____ BSN/YR _____ MSN/YR _____ PHD/YR _____

Other Degrees _____

III. PRACTICE

Have you ever been on probation with a State Board of Nursing? YES/NO (Circle)

Certification Type	Organization	Expiration	Cert. Initials
1. _____	_____	_____	_____
2. _____	_____	_____	_____
3. _____	_____	_____	_____

Areas of nursing experience beginning with most current: Date From To

_____	_____	_____
_____	_____	_____
_____	_____	_____
_____	_____	_____
_____	_____	_____

IV. VERIFICATION

I have read the credentialing process information.   ____Yes   ____No

I have read the standards of practice expected of me.   ____Yes   ____No

I have read standards of care that my patients expect.   ____Yes   ____No

SIGNATURE _____ Date _____

Applicant

ACCEPTED _____ Date _____

Nurse Manager

Source: Courtesy of the University of South Alabama Medical Center, Mobile, AL.

Appendix 8–2 Identification of Factors Causing Job Dissatisfaction

Item	Not at All → A Great Deal				
1. Factor: Salaries and fringe benefits					
(1) Pay is satisfactory.	1	2	3	4	5
(2) Education and experience are recognized and used.	1	2	3	4	5
(3) Opportunities exist for career advancement.	1	2	3	4	5
(4) The pay system rewards my years of experience.	1	2	3	4	5
(5) The pay is adequate for shifts, weekends, and holidays.	1	2	3	4	5
(6) Fringe benefits are known.	1	2	3	4	5
(7) Employees are satisfied with fringe benefits.	1	2	3	4	5
(8) Child-care services are satisfactory.	1	2	3	4	5
(9) The retirement program is a strong one.	1	2	3	4	5
2. Factor: Staffing philosophy; clerical work; floating; rotating shifts					
(1) The staffing philosophy is fair.	1	2	3	4	5
(2) A float pool covers absences and supplemental staffing.	1	2	3	4	5
(3) Clinical nurses have input into staffing policies and procedures.	1	2	3	4	5
(4) Opportunities exist for flexible work schedules.	1	2	3	4	5
(5) Clerical duties are performed by clerical personnel.	1	2	3	4	5
(6) Appropriate activities are performed by other departments, such as pharmacy, medical laboratory, and dietary.	1	2	3	4	5
3. Factor: Professionalism; interdisciplinary relationships; public relations					
(1) Clinical nurses serve on all organizational committees.	1	2	3	4	5
(2) Administrators promote cooperative interdisciplinary relationships.	1	2	3	4	5
(3) Clinical nurses spend their time giving care to patients.	1	2	3	4	5
(4) Clinical nurses make decisions about patient care.	1	2	3	4	5
(5) Clinical nurses participate in nursing management.	1	2	3	4	5
(6) Clinical nurses are recognized and rewarded for nursing excellence.	1	2	3	4	5
(7) Clinical nurses participate in quality assurance.	1	2	3	4	5
(8) Clinical nurses receive awards for merit.	1	2	3	4	5
(9) The communication system is informative, provides for clinical nursing input, and gives feedback.	1	2	3	4	5
(10) Job vacancies are posted.	1	2	3	4	5
(11) Clinical nurses participate in public relations functions.	1	2	3	4	5
4. Factor: Staff development					
(1) A career development program exists.	1	2	3	4	5
(2) Good opportunities for continuing education are available.	1	2	3	4	5
(3) A good orientation program is in force.	1	2	3	4	5
(4) Personnel are reimbursed for staff development activities.	1	2	3	4	5
(5) Refresher courses are available.	1	2	3	4	5
(6) Staff development programs are marketed.	1	2	3	4	5
(7) Incompetent nurses are identified and handled appropriately.	1	2	3	4	5
(8) Good leadership training courses are available.	1	2	3	4	5
(9) Clinical nurses participate in staff development planning.	1	2	3	4	5

(Continued)

Appendix 8–2   Identification of Factors Causing Job Dissatisfaction *(Continued)*

5. Factor: Administration support

(1) Clinical nurses can follow through on beliefs and values.	1	2	3	4	5
(2) Clinical nurses are not subjected to punitive action by supervisors.	1	2	3	4	5
(3) Productivity standards are known.	1	2	3	4	5
(4) Employees have access to senior management.	1	2	3	4	5
(5) Nursing service and nursing education are in harmony.	1	2	3	4	5
(6) Patient safety is emphasized.	1	2	3	4	5
(7) An up-to-date nursing management information system is available.	1	2	3	4	5
(8) Managers are visible to nursing staff and patients.	1	2	3	4	5

Compiled from

1. Mabel A. Wandelt et al., "Why Nurses Leave Nursing and What Can Be Done About It," *American Journal of Nursing,* January 1981, 72–77.
2. Alabama Hospital Association, *Report from the Task Force to Study Nurse Shortage Situation in State of Alabama,* December 1981.
3. National Commission on Nursing, *Summary of the Public Hearings,* 1981, and *Nursing in Transition: Models for Successful Organizational Change,* August 1982 (Chicago: American Hospital Association, Hospital Research and Educational Trust, and American Hospital Supply Corporation).
4. American Academy of Nursing, Task Force on Nursing Practice in Hospitals, *Magnet Hospitals: Attraction and Retention of Professional Nurses* (Kansas City: American Nurses Association, 1983).
5. Alabama Hospital Association, *The Alabama Nurse Study: A Survey of Registered Nurses' Attitudes About Their Profession* (Montgomery, Ala., 1983).
6. Committee on Nursing and Nursing Education, Institute of Medicine, *"Recommendations: Meeting Current and Future Needs for Nurses"* (Washington, D.C.).

Appendix 8–3   University of South Alabama Medical Center Employee Exit Interview

Date _____

Name _____ Date Hired _____ Shift _____

Position Title _____ Department _____

Supervisor's Name _____ Date Separated _____

CHECKLIST:

_____ ID card returned to personnel department
_____ Final payroll check form completed
_____ State retirement refund form completed
_____ Received insurance conversion information
_____ Locker keys returned

I. REASON FOR SEPARATION (CHECK APPROPRIATE BOX)

VOLUNTARY RESIGNATION   INVOLUNTARY TERMINATION

_____ New position   _____ Retirement (mandatory)
_____ Retirement (voluntary)   _____ Reduction of staff
_____ Relocation   _____ Other (specify)
_____ Illness   _____
_____ Pregnancy
_____ Job dissatisfaction
_____ Return to school
_____ Other (specify)
_____

II. INTERVIEW

A. SELECTION

What kind of work have you been doing in our hospital? _____

_____

_____

_____

What kind of work did you do prior to joining our hospital? _____

_____

_____

_____

What type of work do you like best? _____

_____

_____

What type of work do you like least? _____

_____

(Continued)

Appendix 8–3   University of South Alabama Medical Center Employee Exit Interview *(Continued)*

Why? _____

_____

B. ORIENTATION

Who explained your job to you? _____

Describe your orientation. _____

_____

_____

Length of time? _____

What did your orientation lack? _____

_____

_____

Were in-service education programs sufficient for your needs? _____

If not, how could programs be improved? _____

_____

C. SUPERVISION

How do you feel about your supervisor? _____

_____

_____

_____

Did you take any complaints to your supervisor? _____ Yes _____ No

If yes, how were they handled? _____

_____

Have you had any problems with your supervisor? _____ Yes _____ No

If yes, describe. _____

_____

_____

What kind of working relationship did you have with the staff in your department? _____

_____

_____

Appendix 8–3   University of South Alabama Medical Center Employee Exit Interview *(Continued)*

Was there ample opportunity for communication with co-workers, your supervisor, and your department head?

_____

_____

How could communication be improved? _____

_____

_____

Have you felt administrative support by hospital administrators? _____

_____

_____

D. FINANCIAL

How do you feel about your pay? _____

_____

_____

How do you feel about your progress within this hospital? _____

_____

_____

E. FOR NURSES

Was your unit adequately staffed? _____

_____

How do you feel about being pulled to other units? _____

_____

How often were you pulled? _____

_____

F. SUMMARY

What did you like best about your job? _____

_____

_____

What did you like least about your job? _____

_____

_____

(Continued)

Appendix 8–3 University of South Alabama Medical Center Employee Exit Interview *(Continued)*

What did you like best about our hospital? _____

_____

_____

What did you like least about our hospital? _____

_____

_____

Why are you really leaving? _____

_____

_____

Would you be willing to stay with our hospital under a more satisfactory arrangement? _____ Yes _____ No

What changes would be required? _____

Would you return to this hospital if the opportunity existed? _____

_____

G. COMPLETE FOR RESIGNATION

New employer _____ Location _____

Position _____ Pay _____

Hours _____

III. INTERVIEWER COMMENTS _____

_____

_____

Source: Courtesy University of South Alabama Medical Center, Mobile, Alabama.

INTRODUCTION TO COLLECTIVE BARGAINING

OBJECTIVES

- Discuss the meaning of collective bargaining.
- Discuss the history of collective bargaining in nursing.
- Identify the characteristics of a profession and their relationship to collective bargaining.
- Identify and discuss the issues that lead to unions and collective bargaining.
- Describe the process of collective bargaining.
- Describe a grievance procedure and illustrate how it should work.
- Discuss the processes of arbitration and mediation.
- Discuss the benefits of collective bargaining.
- Discuss the ills of collective bargaining.

KEY CONCEPTS

collective bargaining
grievance
mediation
arbitration

Manager Behavior: Directs human resource personnel to develop and implement policies and procedures to curtail issues leading to collective bargaining.

Leader Behavior: Shares decision-making power with nursing employees through clearly stated policies and procedures that boost their morale, maintain their trust, and result in cooperative efforts for greater productivity.

INTRODUCTION

Collective bargaining is the "process by which organized employees participate with their employers in decisions about their rates of pay, hours of work, and other terms and conditions of employment."[1] Representatives of the employer and its employees meet at reasonable times, confer in good faith about wages, hours, and other matters, and put into writing any agreements reached. The duty to bargain is required of both the employer and the union.[2]

Collective bargaining is the professional nurse's means of influencing hospital nursing care delivery systems and labor-management relations through a united voice.[3] It is often viewed as a power relationship, either adversarial or cooperative.[4] During recent years, executives of firms have learned that empowerment and autonomy of employees is good for business. As productivity increases, this knowledge has led to increased training of employees at the production level, elimination of middle management, decentralization of decision making with participatory management at the production level, and an upsurge in the success of the firm. This commitment to sharing power with employees gives employees less reason to resort to collective bargaining.

HISTORY OF COLLECTIVE BARGAINING IN NURSING

Laws

The following is a summary of the chronology of collective bargaining related to nursing in the United States:

> 1935—National Labor Relations Act (NLRA), or the Wagner Act, noted that hospitals were "employers." It protected employees of *private, for-profit* health-care institutions.
>
> 1947—Amendment to NLRA (called the Taft-Hartley Act). Congress excepted not-for-profit hospitals from coverage, from the right to organize and bargain collectively.
>
> 1960—National Labor Relations Board (NLRB) excepted proprietary hospitals from coverage of the NLRA.
>
> 1974—NLRA amendments repealed exceptions and subjected all acute-care hospitals to coverage by the Act. They made no change in the NLRB's authority to determine the appropriate bargaining unit in each case.
>
> 1989—NLRB ruled eight bargaining units appropriate for each hospital. One such unit would be solely for registered nurses. Ruling was challenged by the American Hospital Association.
>
> 1991—U.S. Supreme Court upheld ruling for eight bargaining units, which included separate units for RNs, physicians, other professionals, technical employees, skilled maintenance employees, clerical employees, guards, and other nonprofessional employees. The exception is units with fewer than six employees.[5]
>
> 1994—Supreme Court decision indicates that in any business in which supervisory duties are necessary to the provision of services, personnel who use independent judgments to direct the work of less-skilled employees are supervisors and are not protected by the NLRA. Already employers of nurses are using the decision to challenge unions, decrease licensed personnel, and increase unlicensed personnel.[6]

The National Labor Relations Act (NLRA) defines a professional employee as

> (a) any employee engaged in work (i) predominantly intellectual and varied in character as opposed to routine mental, manual, mechanical, or physical work;

(ii) involving the consistent exercise of discretion and judgment in its performance; (iii) of such a character that the output produced or result accomplished cannot be standardized in relation to a given period of time; (iv) requiring knowledge of an advanced type in a field of science or learning customarily acquired by a prolonged course of specialized intellectual instruction and study in an institution of higher learning or a hospital, as distinguished from a general academic education or from an apprenticeship or from training in the performance of routine mental, manual, or physical processes; or (b) any employee who (i) has completed the courses of specialized intellectual instruction and study described in clause (iv) of paragraph (a), and (ii) is performing related work under the supervision of a professional person to qualify himself to become a professional employee as defined in paragraph (a). (Labor Management Relations Act, 1947).[7]

Strauss summarizes the following characteristics of professional behaviors:[8]

1. Specialized education and expertise.
2. Autonomy.
3. Commitment.
4. Societal responsibility for maintenance of standards of work.

Pavolka differentiates between professionals and other workers by stating that professionals have the following:[9]

1. A systematic body of knowledge and theory as a base for work and expertise.
2. Social ability in times of crisis (during such times are sought out by the public).
3. Specified training, including transmission of ideas, symbols, and skills.
4. Motivation for service to clients.
5. Autonomy, self-regulation, and control by individual practitioners.
6. A sense of long-term commitment.
7. A need for common identity and destiny with shared values and norms.
8. A code of ethics.

Nurses have noted these characteristics through the actions of professionals. Their professional organizations have supported the development of nursing theory and the goal of self-regulation and have long had a code for nurses (see Exhibit 9–1). When unable as individuals to attain their goals, professional nurses pursue them through collective bargaining.

Nursing Organizations and Unions

The American Nurses Association (ANA) historically views itself as the professional organization for nurses. The history of collective bargaining by nursing organizations is outlined as follows:

1946—ANA became active.
1970—One-third of U.S. workforce is organized.
1977—Twenty percent of hospital workers are represented by labor unions.
1980—Twenty-three percent of U.S. workforce is organized.

Exhibit 9–1 ANA Code for Nurses

1. The nurse provides services with respect for human dignity and the uniqueness of the client, unrestricted by considerations of social or economic status, personal attributes, or the nature of health problems.
2. The nurse safeguards the client's right to privacy by judiciously protecting information of a confidential nature.
3. The nurse acts to safeguard the client and the public when health care and safety are affected by the incompetent, unethical, or illegal practice of any person.
4. The nurse assumes responsibility and accountability for individual nursing judgments and actions.
5. The nurse maintains competence in nursing.
6. The nurse exercises informed judgment and uses individual competence and qualifications as criteria in seeking consultation, accepting responsibilities, and delegating nursing activities to others.

7. The nurse participates in activities that contribute to the ongoing development of the profession's body of knowledge.
8. The nurse participates in the profession's efforts to implement and improve standards of nursing.
9. The nurse participates in the profession's efforts to establish and maintain conditions of employment conducive to high quality nursing care.
10. The nurse participates in the profession's effort to protect the public from misinformation and misrepresentation and to maintain the integrity of nursing.
11. The nurse collaborates with members of the health professions and other citizens in promoting community and national efforts to meet the health needs of the public.

Source: Reprinted with permission from *Code for Nurses with Interpretative Statements,* © 1985, American Nurses Association, Washington, D.C.

1982—ANA represented 110,000 nurses, the goal being the control and protection of nursing practice.

1985—Ohio Nurses Association represented nurses in twenty-nine facilities. The Michigan Nurses Association represented 4,000 nurses in sixty bargaining units.

1989—Seventeen percent of U.S. workforce is organized, a decline of six percent since 1980.

1990—State nurses associations (SNAs) represented 139,000 registered nurses, with 841 bargaining units in twenty-seven states. Other unions represented 102,000 RNs. Twelve percent of U.S. workforce is organized (according to T. Porter-O'Grady).

1991—Within three months of the Supreme Court decision allowing all-RN bargaining units, twenty petitions for union elections were filed by nurses in seven states. An estimated 1.12 million nurses do not belong to unions.

1992—According to Joel, 20 percent of health-care workers are now organized, an increase of 6 percent of health-care workers since 1980. Approximately 3.6 million hospital employees are protected by collective bargaining.

The difference between the 1977 version and the 1992 version of percentages of union members may relate to hospital workers versus the entire health-care industry. An additional ten petitions for RN bargaining units brought the total to thirty petitions, twenty-three of which were filed by constituent members of the ANA.

Of 1.6 million practicing registered nurses, with 67.9 percent working in hospitals, about 250,000 are represented by collective bargaining. Collective bargaining by the California Nurses Association is over fifty years old. The pioneers were Shirley Titus, RN, a nurse leader, and J. St. Sure, a labor lawyer, who together built a good public relations image and a solid database. Their work promoted a sense of self-confidence among nurses. Their interest preceded that of the ANA.[10]

The ANA Institute of Constituent Member Collective Bargaining Programs is an elective, deliberative body of the American Nurses Association. It comprises one member from each SNA with a collective bargaining program and meets twice annually at ANA headquarters. It focuses on collective bargaining issues of concern to SNAs.[11]

Many nurses are represented by trade unions. The ANA would rather it represented these nurses.

ISSUES

Issues develop between employers and employees that lead to petition for unions. Usually issues develop because employers do not want to share power with employees. Historically, the chief executive officers of firms built bureaucratic organizations to retain power in the management structure. This has been costly for firms and has resulted in their restructuring to eliminate layers of management, empower employees with management knowledge and skills, and improve productivity and profits.

The following are among the major issues leading to unions and collective bargaining:[12]

1. Absence of procedures for reporting unsafe or poor patient care. Quality of patient care is the number one issue.
2. Short staffing and improper skills mix to complement patient acuity.
3. Floating without orientation and training.
4. Lack of promotion opportunities.
5. Lack of professional practice committees.
6. Resistance of employers to accept joint decision making.
7. Use of temporary personnel and unlicensed assistant personnel.
8. Lack of staff development and continuing education.
9. Poor differentials for shift work, education, and experience.
10. Pension portability.
11. Child care.
12. Elder care.
13. Lack of respect for employees.
14. Lack of autonomy: incursions by management into scope of practice.
15. Lack of involvement in leadership activities

16. Adversarial relationships.
17. Exploitation.
18. Poor management.
19. Low wages.
20. Poor compensation packages.
21. Poor communication.
22. Limited benefits.
23. Overwork.
24. Low morale.
25. Patient classification systems.
26. On-call arrangements.
27. Mandatory overtime.
28. Nonnursing duties.
29. Flexible scheduling.
30. Employee assistance programs.
31. Health insurance.
32. Seniority.
33. Shift rotation.
34. Dismissals.
35. Standards.
36. Policies.
37. Procedures.
38. Breaks.
39. Discipline.
40. Posting vacancies.
41. Peer review.
42. Career ladders.

The professional nurse works in an environment where human resources are not always valued but are viewed as a commodity. To do their jobs as taught, professional nurses might get fired. Thus, they often work in a climate of fear that results in poor morale, poor productivity, stifling of creativity, reluctance to take risks, ineffective communication, and reduced motivation.[13]

Exercise 9–1   Take a survey of personnel with whom you work. How many issues are evident in their perceptions of their workplace? How can these issues be resolved?

PROCESS OF COLLECTIVE BARGAINING

Once nurses have decided to pursue collective bargaining because they believe they have no alternative, the general process is as follows:

1. An organizing committee is formed. It should be broad-based in structure and representative of the major issues so as to represent all

prospective members on all shifts and in all practice areas. Members should be well-known and respected.

2. The major campaign issues are identified and discussed.

3. The organizing committee does research to obtain extensive knowledge of all facets of the institution, including history, structure, organization, finances, administration, and culture.

4. A timetable is prepared delineating the specific organizing activities.

5. Possible employer tactics are identified and discussed, and specific strategies are developed to manage them.

6. A system is established for keeping constant communication with nurses.

7. A structural plan is made, including adoption of a set of bylaws and election of officers.

8. Recognition occurs by employer or NLRB certification. Voluntary recognition requires authorization cards signed by a majority of nurses. If the employer will not recognize the action, NLRB certification requires that at least 30 percent of the nurses sign cards. A majority is best.

9. An election is held in which nurses vote for or against a collective-bargaining unit. The NLRB sets the election date by mutual agreement. Notices are posted on employee bulletin boards that include date, hours, and places of election; payroll period for voter eligibility; description of the voting unit; a sample of the ballot; and general rules for conduct of the election. With a majority (50 percent plus one) of voting nurses voting for it, the NLRB certifies the petitioners as the exclusive bargaining unit. Otherwise the NLRB will not accept another petition for one year.

10. A bargaining committee is elected by the nurses to negotiate a contract.[14]

11. A contract is negotiated. Members of the bargaining committee should survey the membership to gather data for contract proposals. They should know the composition of the bargaining team. At the first meeting, proposals are made. The easiest ones should be settled first. Management strategy will be to set the tone of the sessions and package proposals to be able to slip some past the nurses. Their strategies will include flattery, conciliation, anger, astonishment, and total silence. For this reason, nurse members should track all proposals using their minutes of meetings and making index cards listing each side's proposals. Debriefings at the end of each session are helpful; they should respond to management with care, spirit, and no unconditional concessions.[15]

12. When all proposals have been fully discussed and agreed upon, the contract is written.

13. The contract is then presented to union members, who vote to ratify it or reject it. If ratified, it is signed by both sides.

14. The contract is enforced through grievance and arbitration procedures and is reviewed or amended on a regular basis.[16]

Exercise 9–2   Interview a union official in the community. Prepare a list of questions to ask him/her regarding the process of collective bargaining as it occurs within that union.

Grievance Procedure

Because a strong grievance procedure increases employee satisfaction, it represents good human resource management both with and without a union. Potential trouble spots can be identified early and may include claims for higher wages when jobs are modified. Grievance procedures must be perceived as fair. Their contents should be presented to all employees, and managers should be trained to follow them. Such training allays managers' fears that grievances will be formalized or that unions will be established.[17]

Grievance policy should be communicated as an employee benefit and included in the personnel handbook (see Exhibit 9–2). Peer review should be used in employee appraisals involving grievances and final decisions. Some courts have equated peer review to due process. Peer review builds values of conflict resolution, teamwork, decision making at lower levels, employee empowerment, and ownership.[18]

Exhibit 9–2   Sample Employee Grievance Procedure

Grievances and Discipline

8.1 General Policy

I. It is the policy of the University of South Alabama to maintain the highest level of academic standards and to provide the highest quality in health care delivery as efficiently as possible. To further this policy, the University has established policies and procedures to enable employees to contribute their ideas and suggestions to meet these goals and to provide a framework to discipline employees whose actions are contrary to achieving these goals.

II. In order to insure that all employees are treated fairly, the University has established a grievance and appeal procedure to provide a means for employees who have completed the probationary period and who feel that they are or have been treated unfairly to have an impartial review of their complaint without fear of reprisal or prejudice.

III. Employees who feel that they have been discriminated against specifically because of race, color, creed, sex, age, religion, national origin, or non-job-related physical or mental disability may avail themselves of this policy.

8.2 Disciplinary Guidelines, Table of Penalties

I. Policy:

A. In any organization it is necessary that employees of the organization conduct themselves in accordance with the rules set forth by that organization to ensure that it is a safe and productive place to work.

B. The University of South Alabama, in its desire to provide a safe and productive environment, has established disciplinary guidelines for its employees.

C. The following list of guidelines is provided to assure the equitable treatment of employees. The list is not all inclusive. The University reserves the right to disci-

Exhibit 9–2 Sample Employee Grievance Procedure *(Continued)*

pline its employees for any other behavior, not listed, which it finds contrary to making the University a safe and productive place to work.

D. In all cases the chosen penalty will be appropriate to the offense. Discipline will be administered in a progressive manner if at all possible and shall be supported by written documentation.

E. In some cases the offenses may be so flagrant in first or second occurrences that dismissal may be warranted rather than the lesser penalties shown in the Table of Penalties.

F. Supervisors are authorized to take disciplinary action, including official warnings, suspensions, and dismissals.

G. Since it is the policy of the University of South Alabama to provide employees who are not performing adequately an opportunity to overcome their deficiencies, these employees may be counselled prior to any disciplinary action when circumstances permit.

H. In all cases of disciplinary action, other than an oral or written warning, affected employees will be informed in writing by the Supervisor of the reasons for the disciplinary action taken and their rights to appeal in writing by the Supervisor.

I. The guidelines that follow are recommended to assist the Supervisor in fairly disciplining an employee if and when it is necessary to correct certain types of behavior. All offenses are not listed and the severity of the discipline should be appropriate to the offense and administered in a progressive manner. The University may elect to discipline an employee for reasons other than those listed in the guideline and where appropriate.

II. Policy:

A. A permanent employee who is charged with a felony offense shall be suspended without pay pending the outcome of the trial.

B. Employees suspended without pay because of a felony charge, who are otherwise eligible for benefits, may continue to participate in the group medical and life insurance programs for the duration of the suspension. The employee is responsible for making arrangements with the Payroll Office to pay the total monthly premium costs for these benefits.

C. Upon conviction of a felony offense, the employee shall be immediately dismissed.

D. Should an employee be found not guilty of a felony offense as charged, he or she shall be reinstated with back pay for the period during which he or she was suspended without pay pending outcome of the trial. An employee so reinstated shall have no break in service to the University and shall retain accrued vacation and illness benefits.

III. Procedure

A. Upon notification by an employee who has been officially charged with a felony offense, the Supervisor will complete a Personnel Action Recommendation (PR Form 126) placing the employee on suspension without pay pending outcome of the trial.

B. An employee who wishes to continue to participate in the group medical and life insurance programs should contact the Payroll Office to make arrangements to pay the monthly premiums.

C. An employee who wishes to resign due to a felony charge should do so, in writing, to the immediate Supervisor.

D. Upon a verdict by the Court, a Personnel Action Recommendation should be submitted by the Supervisor indicating reinstatement or termination of the employee and the effective date.

Source: Courtesy University of South Alabama Medical Center, Mobile, Alabama. Reprinted with permission.

Eldridge suggests the following points for effective settlement of grievances:[19]

1. Accurate definition of the problem: Does it violate the contract or the law? It is timely? Is it documented?
2. Timely presentation: Does it follow the time limits and steps of the grievance procedure and for notifying appropriate persons?
3. Documentation: Are the facts accurate? Is the claim adjustment desired? Is the form signed and dated and given to appropriate persons?
4. Is the procedure carried out with a businesslike attitude to facilitate objectivity and communication?

Exercise 9–3 Discuss the grievance procedure with a member of your human resource department where you work or are assigned as a student. How many times has the procedure been used within the past year? What have the issues been? How have they been resolved?

Mediation

"Mediation is a process under which an impartial person, the mediator, facilitates communication between the parties to promote reconciliation, settlement or understanding among them. The mediator may suggest better ways of resolving the dispute, but may not impose his own judgment on the issues for that of the parties."[20]

Mediation is assisted negotiation. When the negotiating parties cannot reach agreement on an issue during contract negotiations or during a labor dispute unresolved by grievance procedure, the issue is referred to a mediator trained to resolve such disputes.

The mediator assists the parties in defining the issues, dissolving obstacles to communication, exploring alternatives, facilitating the negotiations, and reaching an agreement. In law cases, mediation works 80 percent of the time or better. The mechanics of mediation are: good faith is evident; all parties are present during the entire mediation session; adequate time is allowed; mediator lays ground rules, describes the process, and answers questions; session is private; parties are separated into "caucuses," where their conversations are private; and mediator shuttles between parties until a settlement is reached. The parties negotiate the settlement.[21]

Arbitration

Whereas the mediator works with the parties to a dispute to have them resolve their differences, the arbitrator examines the facts and makes a decision that is binding. Arbitration uses as the source of law the express provisions of the contract, past practices of the industry, and the shop (health care and nursing). Past practice must

1. Be unequivocal (clarity, consistency, acceptability)—the practice must be accepted by the people involved as the normal and proper response to the underlying circumstances presented.
2. Have longevity—the practice must have existed for a sufficient length of time to have developed a "pattern."
3. Have mutuality—both parties must regard the conduct as correct and customary in handling the situation.

Practices that have been long-standing and accepted by both parties are as binding as those that are written. Subjects not covered in the agreement remain the residual rights of management. They include methods of operation and direction of the workforce. Union rights include areas of benefits, wages, and working conditions. Unchallenged customs and practices are considered accepted as part of the agreement by both parties. Arbitrators should effectuate the agreement and contain conflict.[22]

Supervisory Influence

With the power of unions declining in general, goals for unions of professional nurses are best met by multipurpose organizations that can respond and adapt to nurses' particular concerns. One of these concerns is supervisory influence. Generally, employers raise these concerns relative to who will represent professional nurses. Rank-and-file nurses may be concerned that nurse managers will dominate the bargaining unit through membership in the SNA. The bargaining unit needs some insulation from SNA members who are managers. The issue usually extends beyond legal characterizations to political overtones of power and control within the organization. The legal standard on the issue of supervisory influence was established by the California Nurses Association in the *Sierra Vista* decision in 1979. This standard is best met by an integrated, multipurpose professional association as a bargaining agent.[23] This agent would include and meet the needs of clinical nurses of all specialities and of nurse managers, educators, and researchers who are members of the SNA.

BENEFITS

Unions view the health-care field as a potential pool for membership. This is a threat to hospital leaders, even though concrete evidence shows "that collective bargaining, when used effectively, actually facilitates delivery of the best care and services."[24]

Collective bargaining has contributed to the high standard of living by the working people of Western countries. Employee compensation levels are higher when determined at the bargaining table.[25]

Collective bargaining is viewed by employees as the means for securing justice in the workplace, as a means of enforceable right, as a means for employees to share power with employers. It provides a fundamental protection against arbitrary or unfair treatment in the matter of promotions, remuneration, dismissal, and retirement. The bargaining agreement or contract balances management power with the combined might of all the employees. Protection under collective bargaining is greater than the contract itself. Unfair management authority can be challenged through a grievance system.[26]

Research indicates that nurses have been reluctant to exercise collective power. Involvement peaks during organizing activity and in times of crisis of conflict. Nurses are more involved with committees related to the nursing product than those related to bargaining unit affairs.[27]

The Michigan Nurses Association views nurses who choose it as their exclusive labor representative to have combined the philosophies of professional nursing care and collective bargaining. Its goal is protection of patients through protection of nurses' professional and economic rights.[28] Contracts give nurses input on nursing care standards, policies, and procedures. Unions improve working conditions related to shift rotation, floating, nonnursing duties, flexible staffing, meal breaks, rest periods, time away from work, continuing education, tuition reimbursement, educational leave, grievance and arbitration procedures, maternity/paternity leave, discipline, posting of vacancies, recall from layoffs, peer review, career ladders, joint committees to improve safety and quality of patient care, and adherence to the Code for Nurses (refer to Exhibit 9–1).[29]

The success of unions depends upon the quality of the work environment and the credibility and effectiveness of the organization as a bargaining agent and workplace advocate.[30] Outcomes of labor negotiations will depend upon employee and employer relationships, attitudes, and philosophies.[31] Estimates are that union members average six percent higher salaries than nonunion workers.[32]

Collective bargaining environments can be suitable for a professional practice model of nursing that provides for career mobility, advancement, and wage increases using criteria beyond mere seniority.[33]

The purposes of collective bargaining include facilitating communication between the parties to the contract; establishing and maintaining mutually satisfactory salaries, hours of work, and working conditions; prompt disposition of differences of opinion or grievances; resolution of disputes. The goal is collaboration. A fully implemented nursing information system (NIS) provides clinical data quickly and improves nurses' work. A fully operational NIS will coordinate management activities, physician-delegated tasks, and professional nursing practice. Decision support systems are information systems designed as sources of information needed to make clinical decisions about patient care. Input of data such as history and test results is processed against stored data to give decision outputs such as differential nursing diagnosis and suggested therapeutic recommendations.[34]

Source data entry should be from bedside terminals or two-way radio transmission of data. Patient discharge abstracts should be expanded to include nursing care delivery information. A Nursing Minimum Data Set is being tested. The collective bargaining unit can be a powerful ally to nursing management in nursing integration of a professional practice model of nursing informatics.[35]

ILLS OF COLLECTIVE BARGAINING

Unions cost money and create adversarial relationships. They focus on seniority rather than merit. Before joining a union, a nurse should study its experience or history and track record. The nurse should talk to union members, tally the annual costs for dues and fees, and read the union's financial statement.[36]

A former union member claims that unionism is a lopsided religion, with management as the devil. Because, like politicians, they are elected, union officials have a vested interest in maintaining a combative relationship with management. Unions discourage hard work and personal ambition while encouraging dependence on them.[37]

Once nurses gain collective-bargaining status, they indicate low participation in related activities. A survey of 261 registered nurses employed in voluntary hospitals in New York state and represented by the New York State Nurses Association for collective bargaining indicated the following:

1. Few nurses attended union meetings regularly, although more did than do blue-collar workers.
2. Only 10.3 percent of respondents attended union conventions. Excuses included family responsibilities, location, expense, time off, and lack of interest.
3. Members read literature from bargaining agent.
4. Few nurses submit bargaining demands.
5. Forty-five percent of respondents voted in the most recent local bargaining unit election; 35 percent in statewide election.
6. Sixty-two and one-half percent read the bargaining agreement.
7. Few file formal grievances. Sixty percent who did were for professional concerns, and 37.5 percent were for economic concerns. One-third knew little about the grievance procedure. They did informal handling of grievance first.
8. Nurses do not appear prepared to assume leadership roles in bargaining units.
9. College-educated nurses were more militant about work stoppage and picketing.

Beletz concluded that "nurses who have adopted collective bargaining and who fail to exercise their responsibilities are responsible for the abridgement of their own rights and the success or failure of collective bargaining in their institutions."[38]

Strikes

Firing striking workers is illegal, but companies threaten to hire permanent replacements as standard management strategy. They are then obligated only to hire former strikers as future openings occur. In 1989, approximately 21,000 workers in U.S. companies lost their jobs through permanent replacement policies. Organized labor has been unable to get congressional legislation banning striker replacement. The Supreme Court ruled permanent replacements legal in 1938.[39]

Exercise 9–4 Interview a professional nurse or other person who is a member of a union. Determine the person's perceptions of the benefits and weaknesses of collective bargaining.

COLLECTIVE BARGAINING VULNERABILITY

An increased interest in collective bargaining among health-care workers has taken place since the Supreme Court decision of 1991. The long-term goal of the ANA is to "enable the country's two million nurses to achieve control over their own practice and work environment."[40] If nurse administrators wish to avoid dealing with collective-bargaining units, they should create the conditions in which nurses have such control.

The following signs and symptoms indicate increased vulnerability to collective-bargaining activity and are significant of an unhealthy environment:[41]

1. Increased nursing staff turnover.
2. Increased employee-generated incidents.
3. Increased grievances filed.
4. Breakdown in communication.
5. Sudden changes in staff behavior.
6. Increased inquiries about personnel policies and practices.
7. Changes in behavior of "problem children."
8. Pro-union, collective-bargaining, or professional organization literature, posters, or graffiti.
9. Organization of and invitation to any off-site meetings for staff members only.
10. Formation and submission of petitions.
11. Manager's solid gut feeling.

Nurse administrators should make a formal assessment of collective bargaining and a plan for action that prevents it. Some of the activities to consider in this plan of action are training of front-line management in communications, counseling, mentoring, participatory management, and shared governance and immediate addressing of quality-of-care issues.[42] Other actions to take include the following:[43]

1. Make the nurses feel like stakeholders. This is especially important with the need for advanced technically trained nurse specialists.
2. Make nurses feel connected and invested in the work so they will be creative and productive.
3. Prepare nurses to increase role functions as members of interdisciplinary teams.
4. Examine possibility of new partnership models with nurses: shared ownership, gainsharing, bonuses, pay for performance, outcome pay, per-diem contracting, caseload payment structures, benefits smorgasbords, increased autonomy of work, participation, self-managed teams, and roles performed by several occupations.

5. Work can be redesigned as a result of union leadership and manager partnership, with mutually formed mission, goals, and planning for the future.

Exercise 9–5   Prepare a plan to evaluate the vulnerability of a health-care organization for collective bargaining. Use it to assess the organization. Prepare a list of recommendations for decreasing the vulnerability of the organization to collective bargaining. Present the results to the nurse administrator. This exercise may be done by a small group of nurse managers or students.

Collective bargaining is unnecessary when nurses and management have good communication and participate in decision making and when nurses receive adequate support and appropriate recognition. Nurses should be provided with a voice in decision making for practice, resources to do the job, safeguarding of standards of practice, protection of employment rights, and attractive terms and conditions of employment.[44] These are all aspects of a model of human resource management that works and that keeps nurse employees happy.

One of the most important benefits of collective bargaining is increased job security. While nurses can be fired for economic reasons and for incompetence, management should be sure that terminations are done only for good and just causes. Laws prevent discrimination on the basis of sex, race, religion, national origin, age, and handicap, and some for whistle blowing. The NLRA prevents discrimination because of union activity. Termination should never be related to public policy or requirement to perform illegal practice.[45]

The employer is considered to have the absolute right to determine staffing patterns, ratios, and other personnel requirements. Employers should consider consulting nurses in formulating standards of nursing practice and strong education benefits, ridding nurses of nonnursing work, and giving input into hiring, promotions, and transfers.[46]

Exercise 9–6   Good management prevents the need for collective bargaining by nurses. Poor management promotes collective bargaining. Analyze the case study in Exhibit 9–3. Identify the issues and make a management plan for preventing the confrontation indicated.

WEB ACTIVITIES

- Visit www.jbpub.com/swansburg, this text's companion website on the Internet, for further information on Collective Bargaining.
- Is there any information available from the government concerning collective bargaining?
- Explore the Internet to locate various discussions on the benefits and downsides of collective bargaining.

Nurses at the county-owned University Hospital were unilaterally told they would no longer be paid time-and-a-half for overtime. In the past they had been subjected to other unfavorable "adjustments."

The American Federation of State, County, and Municipal Employees, Local No. 2399, took out a large ad in the *Medical Gazette,* a weekly newspaper distributed free at area hospitals. The ad announced three union organization meetings at a hotel near the hospital. Nurses reported rumors of newspapers being confiscated and nurses being told they would be fired if caught reading the paper while on duty. A personnel director at one of the larger nonprofit hospitals called the *Medical Gazette* editor to complain about the ad, saying "This is Texas, and we don't have much use for unions here."[1]

A subsequent column in the city newspaper, written by a registered nurse who was president of AFGE Local 4032, stated that registered nurses were burdened by low wages, understaffing, and increasing workload. The nurse further stated that registered nurses are routinely excluded from hospital policy decisions that directly affect their care of patients. This nurse went on to state that "since 1978, TNA has refused to support collective bargaining for registered nurses."[2]

The problem issues that led to efforts for unionization at University/Medical Center Hospital were

- The elimination of time-and-a-half overtime pay for RNs.
- A 50 percent reduction in merit-pay scales for RNs.
- No rollover of merit pay into base pay, resulting in a de facto salary cap.
- No change in mandatory overtime policy.
- Implementation of policy before additional staff were brought on-line.[3]

A series of additional letters to the editor supported the union and indicated that nurses were told to take compensatory time off rather than be paid time-and-a-half for overtime. This occurred even though nurses could not get vacation requests honored.[4]

The overtime pay was restored at $8 per hour in excess of their regular pay for overtime.[5] Apparently, this action terminated efforts to establish the union.

1. R. Casey, "Indicted by SAC Prof, My Plea Is 'Not Innocent," *San Antonio Express-News,* 15 February 1994, 2A.
2. V. C. Barrera, "Besieged Nurses Opted to Unionize," *San Antonio Express-News,* 25 February 1994, 5C.
3. Ibid.
4. M. Barrera, "Hospital Can't Run Without Nurses," *San Antonio Express-News,* 28 April 1994, 5B.
5. "Nurses' Overtime Pay Restored," *San Antonio Express-News,* 30 April 1994, 3C.

SUMMARY

Collective bargaining through unionization is a process whereby employees join together to gain collective power that somewhat neutralizes the power of management. The collective-bargaining process has been used in the nursing profession for approximately fifty years. In 1991, the U.S. Supreme Court affirmed the ruling of the 1989 NLRB that professional nurses could form a distinctly separate bargaining unit within hospitals.

Issues related to collective bargaining include pay, fringe benefits, and conditions of work related to provision of quality care to patients. Many professional nurses are reluctant to use the process of collective bargaining. Those who do, put the safety of patients above their own concerns.

The theories of human resource management that put trust in employees by training them to manage themselves is the best management strategy to deter collective bargaining. Nurse and health-care leaders who work collaboratively with practicing clinical nurses through decentralization and participatory management can prevent collective bargaining. It has been proven time and time again that people who manage their own work and make professional decisions about their practice increase the productivity and profitability of the organization.

NOTES

1. B. White, "An Introduction to Collective Bargaining," *Oregon Nurse,* May 1984, 23, 27.
2. "Common Questions About Union Organizing and Representation," *The Michigan Nurse,* March/April 1985, 3; W. E. Fulmer, *Union Organizing: Management and Labor Conflicts* (New York: Praeger, 1982).
3. K. J. Hannah and J. Shamian, "Integrating a Nursing Professional Model and Nursing Informatics in a Collective Bargaining Environment," *Nursing Clinics of North America,* March 1992, 31–45.
4. E. E. Beletz, "Nurses Participation in Bargaining Units," *Nursing Management,* October 1982, 48–50, 52–53, 56–58.
5. V. S. Cleland, "A New Model of Collective Bargaining," *Nursing Outlook,* September/October 1988, 228–230; "Supreme Court Affirms 8 Bargaining Units Per Hospital," *The Regan Report on Nursing Law,* June 1991, 1; J. F. Easterling, "Autonomy, Professionalism, and Collective Bargaining," *The Michigan Nurse,* March/April 1983, 86–87; L. G. Acord, "Protection of Nursing Practice Through Collective Bargaining," *International Nursing Review* 29, no. 5 (1982): 150–152; K. B. Stickler, "Union Organizing Will Be Divisive and Costly," *Hospitals,* 5 July 1990, 68–70; P. S. Brenner, "Labor Relations in Nursing," *The Michigan Nurse,* July/August 1983, 2–4; L. Flanagan, "How the Bargaining Process Works," *The American Nurse,* October 1991, 11–12; H. Lippman, "Expect to Hear About Unions," *RN,* October 1991, 67–72; "Nurses Hail Crucial Supreme Court Ruling," *California Nurse,* June 1991, 1.
6. K. Markus, "Ruling May Change Labor Relations," *NURSEweek,* 2 December 1994, 5, 12.
7. P. S. Brenner, op. cit.
8. G. Strauss, "Professionalism and Occupational Associations," *Industrial Relations* 2, no. 3 (1968): 7–31.
9. R. Pavalko, *Sociology of Occupations and Professions* (Itasca, Ill.: F. E. Peacock, 1971).
10. J. F. Easterling, op. cit.; P. S. Brenner, op. cit.; L. G. Acord, op. cit; L. D. MacLachlan, "Meeting the Challenges of Collective Bargaining," *California Nurse,* March 1990, 1, 4–5; T. Porter-O'Grady, "Of Rabbits and Turtles: A Time of Change for Unions," *Nursing Economics,* May–June 1992, 177–182; L. Joel, "Collective Bargaining: A Positive Force in the Workplace," *The Missouri Nurse,* September–October 1992, 18–20; H. Lippman, op. cit; L. J. Shinn, "NLRB Rulemaking Upheld: What's Next for Hospitals?" *Aspen's Advisor for Nurse Executives,* March 1992, 7–8; "Nurses Hail Crucial Supreme Court ruling," op. cit; "Beyond Collective Action: Individuals Can Protect Their Jobs," *Ohio Nurses Review* March 1985, 5–6; "Steps to Organize and Obtain a Collective Bargaining Contract," *The Michigan Nurse,* March/April 1985, 2; J. O. Hepner and S. E. Zinner, "Nurses and the New NLRB Rules," *Health Progress,* October 1991, 20–22; J. Stanley, "Collective Bargaining Turns 40," *California Nurse,* December 1986/January 1987, 1, 3.
11. A. Reynolds, "ANA Institute Makes Great Strides for Collective Bargaining," *Pennsylvania Nurse,* May 1992, 17.
12. P. S. Brenner, op. cit; H. Lippman, op. cit; L. J. Shinn, op. cit; K. M. Fenner, "Unionization: Boon or Bane?" *Journal of Nursing Administration,* June 1991, 7–8; "Nurses Hail Crucial Supreme Court Ruling," op. cit; J. O. Hepner and S. E. Zinner, op. cit; T. Benton, "Union Negotiating." *Nursing Management* 23, no. 3 (1992): 70, 72; J. A. Krasnansky, "Time to Stop the Debate," *RN,* May 1992, 116; L. Holmsted, "E & GW Annual Business Meeting," *The Maine Nurse,* winter 1991, 5.

13. D. Wheaton, "Collective Bargaining—Confronting the Conflicts," *The Maine Nurse,* winter 1991, 10.

14. "Steps to Organize and Obtain a Collective Bargaining Contract," op. cit; E. E. Beletz, op. cit.

15. M. K. Friedheim, "Negotiating a Union Contract," *Medical Laboratory Observer,* December 1982, 58–63.

16. "Steps to Organize and Obtain a Collective Bargaining Contract," op. cit.

17. P. Eubanks, "Employee Grievance Policy: Don't Discourage Complaints," *Hospitals,* 20 December 1990, 36–37.

18. Ibid.

19. I. Eldridge, "Some Techniques and Strategies of Collective Bargaining," *Washington Nurse,* April 1986, 13.

20. S. Brutsche, "Mediation Cross-Examined," *Texas Bar Journal,* June 1990, 584.

21. Ibid.

22. J. M. Dvorak, "Past Practice Concepts in Collective Bargaining," *The Michigan Nurse,* July/August 1983, 5–7.

23. L. D. McLachlan, op. cit.

24. L. Flanagan, op. cit.

25. L. G. Acord, op. cit.

26. B. White, op. cit.

27. E. E. Beletz, op. cit.

28. "Steps to Organize and Obtain a Collective Bargaining Contract," op. cit.

29. Ibid; L. G. Acord, op. cit.

30. L. Joel, op. cit.

31. L. J. Shinn, op. cit.

32. J. O. Hepner and S. E. Zinner, op. cit.

33. K. J. Hannah and J. Shamian, op. cit.

34. Ibid.

35. Ibid.

36. H. Lippman, op. cit.

37. R. Worsler, "Still Fighting Yesterday's Battle," *Newsweek,* 27 September 1993, 12.

38. E. E. Beletz, op. cit.

39. M. Levinson and F. Chideya, "One for the Rank and File," *Newsweek,* 19 July 1993, 38–39.

40. "Sparks of Union Activity," *Journal of Nursing Administration,* September 1991, 4.

41. K. M. Tenner, op. cit.

42. Ibid.

43. T. Porter-O'Grady, op. cit.

44. L. Joel, op. cit.

45. "Beyond Collective Action: Individuals Can Protect Their Jobs," op. cit.

46. A. Cohen, "The Management Rights Clause in Collective Bargaining," *Nursing Management,* November 1989, 24–26, 28–30.

BUDGETING BASICS

OBJECTIVES

- Discuss concepts of budgeting.
- Identify examples of budget-planning steps.
- Identify examples of stages of the budget.
- Define selected terms related to budgeting.
- Differentiate between direct and indirect costs.
- Differentiate among fixed, variable, and sunk costs.
- Describe various budgets: operating or cash budget, personnel budget, supplies and equipment budget, capital budget.
- Discuss the budget as a controlling process.
- Discuss monitoring of the budget.
- Discuss motivational aspects of the budget.
- Discuss cutting the budget.
- Observe preparation of the budget for an agency or a cost center.

KEY CONCEPTS

budgeting
cost center
revenue budgeting
expense budgeting
operating budget
cost-to-charge ratio
zero-base budgeting
personnel budget
supplies and equipment budget
capital budget

Manager behavior: Develops budgets for personnel, supplies, equipment, and capital expenditures for one or more cost centers.

Leader behavior: Guides nursing personnel by decentralization of budget development for personnel, supplies, equipment, and capital expenditures for one or more cost centers.

INTRODUCTION

Because the amount and quality of nursing services depend on budgetary plans, nurses should become proficient in related procedures. This proficiency will provide the resources necessary for safe and effective nursing care. With limited resources and a competitive market, personnel and material resources need to be used wisely and efficiently. The enlightened nurse knows that the person who controls the budget is the person who controls nursing services. The costs of nursing services have been identified for many years, but the income earned from nursing services has been included in "bed and board" on the budget sheets. To achieve reimbursement for nursing services will mean that many government regulations and third-party payer policies will change to allow for direct payment to nursing providers, based on the amount of care given and the skills of the persons giving it.

Budgeting is an ongoing activity in which revenues and expenses are managed to maintain fiscal responsibility and fiscal health. The nurse manager has financial responsibility and is accountable for managing the nursing budget and makes all of the decisions about how to adjust the nursing budget to manage programs and costs. These decisions include adding and dropping programs, expanding and contracting programs, and making all modifications of revenues and expenses within the nursing unit.

BASIC PLANNING FOR BUDGETING

Planning yields forecasts for one year and for several years. The budget is an annual plan, intended to guide effective use of human and material resources, products or services, and managing the environment to improve productivity. Budgetary planning ensures that the best methods are used to achieve financial objectives. It should be based on valid objectives to provide a product or service that the community needs and for which it will pay. In nursing, budgetary planning helps assure that clients or patients receive the nursing services they want and need from satisfied nursing workers. A good budget is based on objectives, is simple, flexible, and balanced, has standards, and uses available resources first to avoid increasing cost.

No formula exists for the form, detail, or periods covered by budgets. Each budget system is designed for the situation at hand, bearing in mind the character of the company, the company's position, and the nature of the plans involved. Ordinarily, the budget system is most detailed in aspects of operations most important to the firm's success. Furthermore, the period covered by the budget varies with the nature of the plans and with the degree of accuracy possible in the preparation of estimates.[1]

A nursing budget is a systematic plan that is an informed best estimate by nurse administrators of revenues and nursing expenses. It projects how revenues will meet expenses and projects a return on equity—profit. It should be stated in terms of attainable objectives so as to maintain motivation of nurses at unit or cost-center levels. The nursing budget serves three purposes: (1) to plan the objectives, programs, and activities of nursing services and the fiscal resources needed to accomplish them; (2) to motivate nursing workers through analysis of actual experiences; and (3) to serve as a standard to evaluate the performance of nurse administrators and managers and increase awareness of costs. These purposes should include the group's mission, strategic plans, new programs or projects, and goals.

Managing the financial end of nursing through an operational budget obviously can create a new dimension for nurses. The budget can be a strong support for developing written objectives for the nursing division and for each of its units. It can provide strong motivation for effective planning, and it can certainly provide standards by which to evaluate the performance of nurses.[2] Effective planning provides for contingencies by indicating which programs or activities can be reduced or eliminated if budget goals are not met.

Revenues and costs, or expenses, and operating and capital budgets should all be projected for the long term. Possible problems in future years should be flagged. Every planning decision, whether long- or short-term, should be accounted for in the budget.[3]

BUDGETING PROCEDURES

Decentralized budgeting involves the nursing unit managers and their staff in the process. Nursing service is labor-intensive, reflected in the fact that the first six budget-planning steps pertain to labor. Note that only steps 7 and 8 are concerned with nonlabor expenses. The steps are as follows:

1. *Determine the productivity goal.* The director of nursing services and the nurse manager determine the unit's productivity goal for the coming fiscal year.
2. *Forecast workload.* The number of patient days expected on each nursing unit for the coming fiscal year are calculated.
3. *Budget patient-care hours.* The expected number of hours devoted to patient care for the forecasted patient days are calculated.
4. *Budget patient-care hours and staffing schedules.* The budgeted patient-care hours are reflected in recommended staffing schedules by shift and by day of the week.
5. *Plan nonproductive hours.* Vacation, holiday, education leave, sick leave, and similar hours are budgeted for the coming year.
6. *Chart productive and nonproductive time.* To aid in the planning process, a graph is used to show nurses how the level of forecasted patient days, and therefore the staffing requirements, are expected to increase and decrease during the year. Productive time is the time spent on the job in patient care, administration of the unit, conferences, educational activities, and orientation.
7. *Estimate costs of supplies and services.* The supplies and services to be purchased for the year are budgeted.
8. *Anticipate capital expenses.* The expected capital investments for the coming year are figured into the budget.

These eight steps result in a proposed budget that goes to the nursing administrator for review. After preliminary acceptance, this budget is sent to the accounting department, where the forecasted patient days are turned into expected revenue. The budgeted productive and nonproductive time is converted into dollars, as are the costs for supplies, services, and other operating expenses that will be allocated to a given nursing unit for the coming year. A pro forma operating statement is then returned to the director of nursing for review with the nurse manager. When the director of nursing and the nurse manager accept the budget, it is returned to the accounting department and forwarded with the rest of the agency managers' budgets to administration and the board of directors.[4]

People who pay high prices for health care want accountability of both costs and quality of service. The nursing budget can be a shared responsibility, with unit budgets being prepared with staff involvement at the clinical level. The planning and controlling processes are ongoing. Through their participation, clinical nurses enhance their professional stature. A budget prepared and executed as a shared experience becomes an object of ownership to a staff who will put forth effort to work within its framework.

According to Osborne and Gaebler, budgets should be developed without line items, based on the idea that funds can be moved around to fit shifting needs. Many health-care organizations follow this policy. In one instance, a new cardiac rehabilitation program was developed and budgeted based on this policy. Cost-center managers agreed to shift funds because they could see the advantages of the program and had been led to believe that they owned their budgets. All unused funds should be carried over into the new budget. This policy reduces the wasteful practice of spending money to keep budgets constant or to prevent reduction.[5]

Managing Cost Centers

A cost center is a given area of assigned accountability for both direct and indirect expenditures. A department of nursing is a cost center, as are each of its units, each clinic, in-service education, surgical suites, long-term care, home-health care, and any other section with a nursing mission in which nurses provide services to clients. Each cost center is assigned a code. A reference (Seawell) is available for a uniform accounting and reporting system for hospitals. An organization may use this coding system, usually referred to as the patient-care system. Workload measurements, sometimes referred to as performance classifications or units of measure, are necessary. The unit of measure for each cost center is identified as a specific, quantitative statistic, such as inpatient days or relative value units (RVUs). The number of RVUs defines the tangible things done as evidence of production and to measure quantity, quality, and cost.

Each cost center is an internal department dealing with distribution of services and products. The cost-center manager is responsible for determining the cost of such service or product and how these services or products are distributed within the organization. Two types of cost centers are mission, or revenue-producing, and service cost centers. Examples of mission, or revenue-producing, centers are radiology and laboratory departments. Such centers have monetary income related to the purpose of the organization. Service centers are support centers that provide a service to other units and charge for that service; no exchange of revenue takes place. The unit served adds the costs of these support services to its costs of output.[6] Examples of service centers are communication, purchasing, and laundry.

Each cost center has a manager, called the cost-center manager or the responsibility-center manager, who is responsible for identifying needs for equipment and programs to maintain progress at the current level of technology in the unit.

Budgeted costs within the cost center are broken down into subcodes. This promotes better budgetary planning and control, because items are specifically identified during the budget planning process. Also, each item purchased is charged to (deleted from) the balance shown for that specific subcode.

Relationship of Budget and Objectives

One of the chief planning activities is to identify the objectives of the nursing division and each of its units. This includes developing a management plan with a budget for each objective. One of the first sources of budgetary information is the nursing objectives. By using these objectives, nurse managers see the benefit of developing pertinent, specific, practical budgeting objectives.

Stages of the Budget

For practical purposes, the nursing budget follows three stages of development: (1) the formulation stage, (2) the review and enactment stage, and (3) the execution stage. These stages are sometimes labeled forecasting, preparation, and control.[7]

Formulation Stage.   The formulation stage is usually a set number of months (six or seven) prior to the beginning of the fiscal year for the budget. During this period, procedures are used to obtain an estimate of the funds needed, funds available, expenses, and revenues.

Financial reports of expenses and revenues of the previous fiscal year and the year to date will be analyzed by the chief nurse executive, department heads, and cost-center managers.

One of the first steps in writing a budget is gathering data for accurate prediction of expenses (costs) and revenues (income). This task can be developed into a system. Primary sources of data are the objectives for the division of nursing and for each cost center. Each program and activity needs to have an estimated cost placed on it. If in-service educators want new audiovisual equipment, they should not walk into the nurse administrator's office and expect to have it next week or next month. Such equipment should be planned for six to seven months before the next fiscal year begins, and it may be budgeted for any quarter or month within that fiscal year. In surveying the objectives, nurse administrators and managers evaluate the previous year, review the philosophy, and rewrite the objectives for the future.

Other data include programs from other departments that will require use or expansion of nursing resources, expansion of nursing clinics and client-teaching programs, travel costs for attendance at professional and educational meetings, incentive awards, library requirements, clinical and office supplies and equipment, investment equipment and facilities modification on a five-year plan, and contracts for such items as intravenous pumps and oxygen equipment. Data can be obtained from historical financial records of the organization.

Among the cost-center reports that will assist the nurse manager are the following:

- daily staffing reports
- monthly staffing reports
- payroll summaries
- daily lists of financial categories of patients
- biometric reports of occupancy
- biometric reports of workload
- monthly financial summaries of revenues and expenses

Review and Enactment Stage.   Review and enactment are budget development processes that put all the pieces together for approval of a final budget. Once the cost-center managers present their budgets to the budget council, the chief nurse executive will consolidate the nursing budget. The budget will then be further consolidated into an organizational budget by the budget officer. The chief executive officer of the organization and the governing board will then give their approval. During this entire process, conferences will be held at which budget adjustments are made. The budget can be sold by nurses using a marketing strategy, anticipating challenges, being persuasive without being emotional, and working for win/win situations.[8]

Execution Stage.   Both the formulation and the review and enactment stages of the budget are planning activities. Execution of the budget involves directing and evaluating activities. The budget is executed by the nurse administrators and managers who planned it. Revisions in execution of the budget are scheduled at stated intervals, frequently once or twice during the fiscal year. Certain procedures are followed for evaluating the budget at cost-center levels. Budgets are prepared for either fiscal years or calendar years, depending on the policy of the organization.

The entire budgeting process is given a specific time frame, with target dates assigned for each step (see Exhibit 10–1). During the fiscal year of the execution stage of budgeting, the formulation and review and enactment stages for the next fiscal year are being carried out.

Exhibit 10–1   The Budget Calendar

Formulation Stage
1. Develop objectives and management plans.
2. Gather all financial, historical, and statistical data and distribute to cost center managers.
3. Analyze data.

Review and Enactment Stage
4. Prepare unit budgets.
5. Present unit budgets for approval.

6. Revise and combine into organizational budget.
7. Present to budget council.
8. Revise and present to governing board.
9. Revise and distribute to cost center managers.

Execution Stage
10. Direct and evaluate expenses and receipts.
11. Revise budget if indicated.

Exercise 10–1   Identify the budget cycle of the organization in which you work or are assigned as a student. List the major events for the entire cycle. How are clinical nurses involved in the budgeting process?

COST FACTORS

Cost is money expended for all resources used, including personnel, supplies, and equipment. The volume of service provided is the greatest factor affecting costs. Other factors include length of patients' stay, salaries, prices of material, case mix, seasonal factors, and efficiencies such as simplification of procedures and quality management to prevent errors that increase patient complications (morbidities and mortalities) and increase costs. Still other factors that have an impact on costs are regulation and competition, third-party payers, the age and size of the agency, type and amount of services provided, the agency's mission, and relationships among nurses, physicians, and other personnel.

Fixed, Variable, and Sunk Costs

Fixed costs are not related to volume. They remain constant as volume increases and decreases over a period of time. Among fixed costs are depreciation of equipment and buildings, salaries, fringe benefits, utilities, interest on loans or bonds, and taxes.

Variable costs do relate to volume and to census (patient days). They include such items as meals and linen. Supplies are usually volume-responsive, meaning that total costs increase or decrease according to use. For example, supplies vary by patient census, physician orders, and diagnosis. Surgical dressings increase in cost when a patient's wound has drainage and dressings must be changed frequently. As census varies, the cost of supplies also varies, increasing or decreasing with the census. For this reason, every cost center should have an established unit of measure for productivity. This unit may be numbers of tests, procedures, patients of a specific acuity type, hours or minutes of service, discharges, or relative value units (RVUs). Most activities include elements of both fixed and variable costs. For example, personnel costs and utility costs can be both fixed and variable, since a minimum number or amount is required for each.

Sunk costs are fixed expenses that cannot be recovered even if a program is cancelled. Advertising is a good example.[9]

Direct and Indirect Costs

Direct costs are the costs of providing the product or service and are often considered to be those directly related to patient care. They include personnel costs and the variable cost of supplies. The definition of direct costs varies by department. In areas removed from direct patient care, each department incurs its own category of direct costs.

Indirect costs are those incurred in supporting the provision of the product or service. These costs are not directly related to patient care, and include utilities, administration, housekeeping, and building maintenance. However, as previously mentioned, they are direct costs for the source department. Some indirect costs are fixed, such as depreciation and administration. Others, such as laundry and accounting, are variable. All indirect costs are allocated or transferred by a specific method to the departments that use the service.

Every hospital has a method of establishing costs, including the *Hospital and Hospital Health Care Complex Cost Report Certification and Settlement Summary,* commonly known as the *Medicare Cost Report.* In a few agencies, the method is more refined. Nurse administrators should become informed about this activity.

Cost Accounting

A cost-accounting system assigns all costs to cost centers. Periodically, usually monthly, reports of costs are provided to cost-center managers, but they do not reflect all costs. Many indirect costs are allocated only once a year in the *Medicare Cost Report.* They include the costs of such items as utilities, accounting, administration, data processing, and admitting. Informed and influential nurse managers use these cost allocations when preparing budgets. Such allocations are usually hidden in the operational budget under the category of "room costs."

Cost assignments to cost centers are made on the basis of direct costing if they are direct costs of patient care. Otherwise they are made by transfer costing from a patient-care support department or by cost allocation if not related to direct patient care or support. Job-order sheets are used to account for all services to patients. Direct overhead costs that cannot be identified with specific services rendered are allocated based on some other measurement, such as square feet of floor space.

Service Units

Service units are measurable units of productivity or volume for identifying and counting costs. They must be measurable, known to managers, and affected by volume. Productivity is measured by service units produced.

With the increased sophistication of information systems, it is easier for nurse managers to become involved in identifying and costing service units. This can be done by hours of nursing care per category of acuity of illness. To make this an RVU, all other direct and indirect costs must be allocated on the basis of hours of nursing care per category of acuity of illness.

Chart of Accounts

A chart of accounts that includes a number and table for each cost center (see Seawell in references section of this chapter) is subdivided into major classifications and subcodes, such as salaries and wages, employee benefits, medical and surgical supplies, professional fees, nonmedical and nonsurgical supplies, purchased services, utilities, other direct expenses, depreciation, and rent. These classifications are further subclassified.

To be assigned to the correct cost center, all movement of labor and materials between cost centers must be recorded. All fringe benefits must be charged to the appropriate cost center by some established method. So must all purchases, including those shared. This is usually done using allocated shares of service units.

Amortized expenses are deferred charges allocated to units over a specified period of time. They include depreciation charges for aging plant and equipment in addition to prepaid items. Usually the prepaid items are charged monthly as service units. Other deferred expenses include unamortized borrowing costs and costs incurred for capital expansion or renovation programs.

Inventory and Cost Transfer

Identifying actual costs of any service unit is improved through an accurate system of inventory control. Based on the number of orders or requisitions for any item, the appropriate proportion of the item's costs can be transferred to the cost center that ordered the item.

Financial Accountability

In being assigned and accepting financial accountability, nurses have a first duty to their patients, who have given them their trust. They should be accountable to themselves for their work, to their professional peers, to their employers, and, in publicly funded institutions, to taxpayers.

One way or another, patients pay the costs of health care. It may be through insurance premiums, taxes, or fringe benefits or from their own pockets. Financial accountability means that nurses and others can account for the efficient spending of the money paid for health care.

Nurse managers need information on the costs of all services provided by their own and competing institutions. This information will, in turn, be provided to clinical nurses, who should know what it costs to do their work. Cost-consciousness leads to reduction of waste and to effective cost management.

Some managers mistakenly believe that overspending can be controlled by controlling nursing labor power and expenditure. This misconception can be rectified by holding nurses accountable for their budgets, both revenues and expenses. Nurse managers have to justify the cost/benefit ratio of services provided and devise new methods to increase cost-effectiveness.

The Cost of Nursing Care

To determine the cost of nursing care, several factors should be considered. Nursing charges should be quantifiable. A patient-acuity system would serve this purpose. The patient-acuity system usually separates patients into four or five levels of nursing care and enumerates nursing requirements for each level.

Charges could be set by level and negotiated with third-party payers. These costs could be separated from the cost of nonnursing requirements. Nonnursing tasks would be reassigned to assure that the charges for nursing care reflect the actual cost of providing such care.

A second method of costing nursing services is determining what share of total agency cost is attributable to nursing. This will vary by DRG or patient acuity. An industrywide effort for each region could produce standards for nursing costs and charges. Otherwise, a majority of the health-care institutions in the United States would need to undertake research to determine nursing costs and charges on an agency-specific basis. Multinational corporations, of course, can apply research studies across member institutions.

Exercise 10–2   Determine whether and how nursing services are unbundled and costed out from other services in the agency in which you work or are assigned as a student. If nursing services are costed out, how is this information used? If nursing services are not costed out, determine the reason.

DEFINITIONS

Budget

According to *Webster's New Twentieth Century Dictionary, Unabridged,* Second Edition, a budget is "a plan or schedule adjusting expenses during a certain period to the estimated or fixed income for that period." Herkimer has stated that "an effective budget is the systematic documentation of one or more carefully developed plans for all individually supervised activities, programs, or sections. . . . The budget is a tool which can aid decision makers in evaluating operating performance and projecting what future operations might produce."[10]

A budget is an operational management plan, stated in terms of income and expense, covering all phases of activity for a future division of time. It is a financial document that expresses an operations plan of action. In the division of nursing, it sets the limits of financial support, thereby controlling the extent and quality of nursing programs. The budget will determine the number of kinds of personnel, materials, and financial resources available to care for patients and to achieve the stated nursing objectives. It is a financial statement of policy. Budgeting is the process whereby objectives and plans are translated into financial terms and evaluated using financial and statistical criteria.

Unit of Service

The unit of service is a measurement of the output of agency services consumed by the patient. In the surgical suite and recovery room, it is minutes or hours; in the emergency room, it is visits or time and procedures; and in the nursing units, it is the acuity category of patients and hours per day expressed in

RVUs. Types of measurement include procedures, patient days, patient visits, and cases.

Revenue

Revenue is the income from sale of products and services. Traditionally, nursing revenue has been included with room charges. Increasingly, it is being unbundled from the room rate as a separate charge per patient-acuity category and per visit, day, or procedure.

Revenue can include assets, such as accounts receivable and income-producing endowments. The latter can be restricted to specific purposes. Buildings, land, and other items can be assets if they produce income or are capable of producing income. Total income is frequently termed *gross income,* with the excess of revenues over expenses being known as *net income* or *profit.*

Revenues also come from such sources as research grants, gift shops, donations, gifts, rentals of cots and televisions, parking fees, telephone charges, and vending machines. Many may be elements of product lines, such as orthopedic services that include orthopedic nursing, traction equipment, and prostheses.

Revenue Budgeting

Revenue budgeting, or rate setting, is the process by which an agency determines revenues required to cover anticipated costs and to establish prices sufficient to generate those revenues. Complicating the process is the fact that patients (purchasers) don't all pay an equal, fair share of an agency's costs.

To remain viable, any business must generate sufficient revenues to cover operating costs and make a profit. These costs include increases in working capital, capital replacements, and inflation adjustments. Nonprofit agencies are identified as such for tax status only! Nonprofits use profits to improve plants and services; profits do not go to shareholders or owners. Profit appears as positive balance on account ledgers.

Fundamental to the rate-setting process are adequate statistical data, historical and projected, for implementing the rate-setting method to be employed. These data include, on a departmental basis, volume of services, current rate, allocated costs, and rate increase constraints. The goal is to obtain the greatest impact from a minimum cumulative rate increase in today's cost-management environment. This is done by increasing rates in high-profit departments while instituting rate reductions in low-profit departments so that they offset each other.

In today's reimbursement milieu, revenues are often budgeted before expenses. This is necessary to determine how much revenue will be available.

Exercise 10–3   Determine whether and how nursing revenues are budgeted in the agency in which you work or are assigned as a student.

Expenses

Expenses are the costs of providing services to patients. They are frequently called *overhead,* and they include wages and salaries, fringe benefits, food service, utilities, and office and medical supplies. As part of the budget, they are a collection or summary of forecasts for each cost center's account.

Full costs include both direct and indirect expenses. While direct costs such as nursing can be traced to the source, indirect costs such as utilities, telephones, or purchasing services are allocated to the source department by a standard formula.

Expense Budgeting

Expense budgeting is the "process of forecasting, recording, and monitoring the manpower, materials and supplies, and monetary needs of an organization in such a manner that the operation of the various components of the organization can be controlled."[11] The components of expense budgeting are cost centers. Purposes of expense budgeting include the following:

- To predict labor hours, materials, supplies, and cash flow needs for future time periods.
- To establish procedures for making comparative studies.
- To provide a mechanism for determining when changes in procedures need to be made, providing gross information on the kinds of changes needed, and providing evidence that control has been established or reestablished.

Historical trends are the single best inexpensive indicator available to the institution. They are valid most of the time for the prediction of present and future trends.

Patient Days

Patient days are used to project revenues. They are commonly used as units of service to compute staffing. Patient-day statistics are usually derived from census reports that are done daily at midnight and summarized monthly for the year to date and annually. A patient admitted on May 2 and discharged May 10 is charged for nine patient days. Exhibit 10–2 illustrates patient days per unit for one month.

Fiscal Year

The *fiscal year* (FY) is the budgetary or financial year. It may be the calendar year in some organizations, beginning on January 1 and ending on December 31. Many organizations use October 1 to September 30 as the fiscal year. Some use July 1 to June 30 to coincide with budget decisions of state legislatures and the U.S. Congress. In the latter examples, the fiscal year obviously overlaps two calendar years.

Exhibit 10–2   A Patient-Day Census

	Current Year			Year to Date		
	July	*OCC (%)*	*June*	*Current Year*	*OCC (%)*	*Previous Year*
Nursing Station						
3rd Floor	1,014	79.8	833	9,792	78.6	8,650
4th Floor	811	76.9	718	7,834	75.8	7,255
5th Floor North	526	65.3	524	5,300	67.1	4,838
5th Floor South	622	77.2	592	5,587	70.7	5,603
6th Floor	792	71.0	866	8,730	79.8	8,176
7th Floor	850	68.5	895	9,086	74.7	8,885
8th Floor	0	0.0	0	0	0.0	4,403
8th Floor North	376	60.6	383	4,624	76.1	2,393
8th Floor South	303	69.8	274	3,253	76.4	1,729
9th Floor	0	0.0	0	0	0.0	5,138
9th Floor North	526	84.8	501	5,332	87.7	2,690
9th Floor South	481	77.6	506	5,118	84.2	2,617
MINU	104	83.9	89	1,041	85.6	432
SINU	73	58.9	84	964	79.3	471
Burn Unit	173	79.7	188	1,723	81.0	1,912
Labor and Delivery	138	37.1	99	1,228	33.7	1,258
CCU	206	83.1	148	1,848	76.0	1,937
Clinical Research Unit	137	73.7	132	1,342	73.6	1,361
EAU	23	0.0	7	390	0.0	634
MICU	213	85.9	191	2,099	86.3	2,291
PICU	169	54.5	112	1,612	53.0	1,834
SICU	229	92.3	207	2,175	89.4	2,302
NTICU	209	84.3	87	1,891	77.8	2,277
Total	7,975	73.1	7,436	80,969	75.7	79,086
Nursery						
Newborn	832	103.2	632	7,666	97.0	7,307
Intermediate	577	103.4	457	4,761	87.0	3,991
Intensive Care	955	110.0	716	8,526	100.2	7,022
Total	2,364	105.9	1,805	20,953	95.7	18,320

Source: Reprinted with permission of University of South Alabama Medical Center, Mobile, Alabama.

Year to Date

The term *year to date* (YTD) describes the accumulated units of service at a particular point in the fiscal year. If the fiscal year begins October 1, the year-to-date patient days for December 31 would be the summary for 92 days. Exhibit 10–2 illustrates year-to-date statistics.

Average Daily Census

The census is summarized for a specific number of days and divided by that number of days. For example, the average daily census (ADC) for the month of June would be the total patient days for June divided by 30. From Exhibit 10–2, the number of patient days for June was 7,436. When this is divided by 30, the average daily census is 248.

Hours of Care

From the nursing viewpoint, hours of care have traditionally been the number of hours of care allocated per patient per day (24 hours) on a unit. With the use of patient-acuity rating systems, hours of care can be determined to the hour or even fraction of an hour. Usually patients fall into one of four or five patient-acuity categories, each of which is assigned a specific number of hours of care per patient day.

Caregiver

Each nurse who works with patients is labeled a "caregiver." In nursing, the three common types of caregivers are registered nurses, licensed practical nurses, and nurse aides or extenders. Most personnel budgets have a ratio of registered nurses to other caregivers. Considerable research support an all-RN caregiver staff. The current cost-management environment often alters this goal.

Operating Budget

The overall plan identifying expected revenues and expenses, both fixed and variable, for the forthcoming fiscal year is termed the *operating budget,* an annual budget that includes the cash budget and the capital budget. In addition, the operating budget identifies the source and nature of expected revenues and expenses. The operating budget determines the per-diem and other charges to be made to the patient. A cost-to-charge ratio is used.

Cost-to-Charge Ratios

Cost-to-charge ratios are convenient tools for computing the cost of providing a service. For example, if the charge to a patient for fiberoptic laboratory services was $1,000 and the cost-to-charge ratio was 0.815626, one would know that the cost to the hospital for these services was approximately $815.63 (see Exhibit 10–3). This cost includes the expense of running the fiberoptic laboratory and a portion of the hospital's overhead cost. In some instances, the cost-to-charge ratio is greater than one, which means that the cost of operating these cost centers is greater than the charges.

The hospital has two types of cost centers. The first is the revenue-producing cost center, such as the fiberoptic laboratory, which bills patients for services provided. The second type is the overhead cost center, such as the accounting

Exhibit 10–3   Cost-to-Charge Ratios

Cost Center	Cost-to-Charge Ratio
Operating room	1.072993
Recovery room	0.731813
Delivery room	0.920547
Radiology	0.846045
Laboratory	0.502010
Respiratory therapy	0.288370
Physical therapy	1.261435
EKG-EEG-CVL	0.698327
Fiberoptic lab	0.815626
Medical supplies	0.303416
Drugs	0.275234
Cast room	0.238285
Emergency room	1.131543
Routine inpatient	1.321196
Surgical ICU	1.044988
Coronary care	0.892522
Burn unit	2.054106
Pediatric ICU	1.153027
Medical ICU	1.038597
Nursery ICU	0.756198
Nursery	1.138131

Source: Reprinted with permission of University of South Alabama Medical Center, Mobile, Alabama.

department, which exists to support the revenue-producing centers. The cost of the overhead cost centers is allocated to the revenue-producing centers by various statistical methods. For example, utility costs are allocated to the revenue-producing departments based on the square foot of space they occupy. However, the accounting department costs are allocated based on the size of the operating budget of each revenue-producing cost center. The cost-to-charge ratio is computed by dividing the total cost of the cost center, direct and overhead, by the total charges for the same department.

Exercise 10–4   Identify the cost-to-charge ratios in the agency in which you work or are assigned as a student. Which centers are profitable, and which are losing money?

Cost/Benefit Analysis

Cost/benefit analysis is a planning technique[12] that answers the following questions: What are the costs of pursuing a goal, an objective, a program, or a specific nursing intervention? How do costs compare with the benefits? Is the project worthwhile? Comparison of different nursing interventions for the same nursing diagnosis or problem results in using the least costly intervention to achieve similar or better results. The intervention used is then cost-effective.

Zero-Base Budgeting

Zero-base budgeting is a method of budgeting used to control costs. In a zero-base budget, the budgeting process starts from zero, and everything must be justified by each new budget cycle. A previous activity can be included in the budget, but funding for it must be justified by its relation to the current organizational objectives. In theory, each function in a zero-base budget must stand on its own merits, and the merits of each function are reviewed annually. All labor power and costs are recalculated, and decisions are made as to whether to continue the function and at what levels.

Program Budgeting

Program budgeting is a part of budget planning. Such items as continuing education programs, employee benefits fairs, and health promotion programs should be incorporated into the annual budget. The budget for each program should enumerate fixed expenses, such as rent, advertising, fixed speaker fees, and department overhead, and variable expenses, such as food, handouts, and per-person honorarium speaker fees. Some costs, such as advertising, are unrecoverable even if the program is cancelled. They are referred to as *sunk costs* and should be in the cost center as well as in the individual program's budget.

Program budgets should include a break-even analysis. If the cost of the program is $2,000 and the reasonable charge is $50 per participant, the break-even point is forty paid participants. A break-even chart may be made for each program (see Exhibit 10–4). Income above the break-even point is profit; below it is loss.

The point at which the cost to carry out a program is equal to the cost to cancel it is called the least-loss point. If enough people have registered to pay the sunk costs, the net loss will be the same whether the program is cancelled or held. It may be good public relations to carry out a program at the least-loss point.[13]

OPERATING OR CASH BUDGET

The cash budget is the actual operating budget in detail, usually excluding the capital budget. A cash budget indicates whether cash flow will be adequate to meet anticipated payments such as debt obligations, including replacement and expansion of facilities, unanticipated requirements, payroll, payment for supplies and services, and a prudent investment program. Cash receipts come from third-party payers, tuition, endowment fund earnings, and sales of food, gifts, and services.

The cash budget is the day-to-day budget and represents money coming in and going out. It is advisable to have cash reserves so that cash flow, the money

Exhibit 10–4   Break-Even Analysis

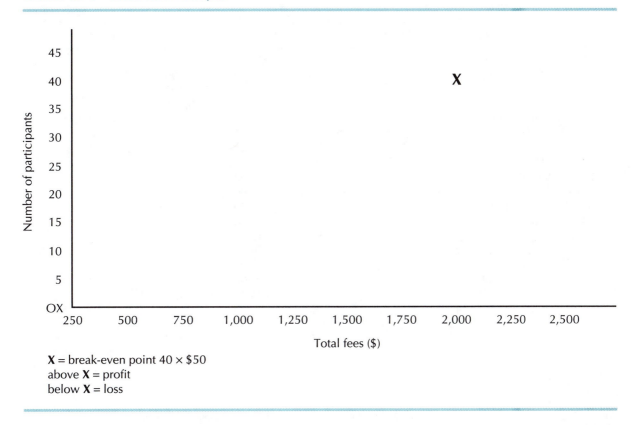

X = break-even point 40 × $50
above **X** = profit
below **X** = loss

coming in, will pay the bills. Otherwise, revenues must be speeded up or pay-ment of bills slowed down. Cash reserves should not be excessive; they may rep-resent money that should be working for the organization. Cash budgets show revenues and expenses, while operating budgets show plans. They are usually considered integrated entities.[14]

Developing the Operating Budget

Operating budget information supplied to the chief nurse executive (CNE), department heads, and cost-center managers includes a budget worksheet (Exhibit 10–5) and a worksheet that explains budget adjustments (Exhibit 10–6). The budget worksheet depicts information by each cost center's account number and subcode. It lists prior-year expense, original budget, and annualized expense. Usually, this form is provided during the new budget formulation stage, and the annualized expense is the projected total expense if current rates con-tinue to the end of the fiscal year. The columns headed "Budget Detail" and "Budget Pool" are empty so that the cost-center manager can fill in the budget expenses for the projected fiscal year. Note in Exhibit 10–5 that the cost-center

Exhibit 10–5 Budget Worksheet

Subcode	Description	ABR	Prior-Year Expense	Original Budget	Annualized Expense	Budget Detail	Budget Pool
200	Pool-Med/Surg Supply	0	.00	10,975.00		$10,780	$ 8,985
211	Med & Surg Supplies	4	10,893.80	.00	8,790	$ 8,790	
213	Drugs	4	129.59	.00	195	$ 195	
Pool Total			11,023.39	10,975.00	8,985		
220	Pool-General Supply	0	.00	2,705.00			$ 2,848
232	Office Supplies	4	303.34	.00	672	$ 810	−320
234	Printing	4	37.75	.00	3	$ 3	
240	Housekeeping Supply	4	1,404.06	.00	1,482	$ 1,482	
270	Food Expense	4	913.73	.00	523	$ 523	
Pool Total			2,658.88	2,705.00	2,680		
300	Pool-Travel/Entertain	0	.00	110.00			$ 50
314	Local Travel	4	13.80	.00	18	$ 50	
Pool Total			13.80	110.00	18		
320	Pool-Other Expenses	0	.00	130.00			$ 660
336	Equip Maint & Repair	4	66.60	.00	123	$ 610	
372	Books & Subscription	4	25.00	.00		$ 50	
Pool Total			91.60	130.00	123		
501	Minor Equipment	0	.00	.00	72	−53	$ 465
Pool Total			.00	.00	72		
Acct Total			13,787.67	13,920.00	11,878		
						Total	$14,968
							−373
							$14,595

Source: Reprinted with permission of University of South Alabama Medical Center, Mobile, Alabama.

manager had projected an increased budget of $10,975 for subcode 200, the pool for medical and surgical supplies and drugs. This was reduced to an annualized projection of $8,985 (subcodes 211 and 213, Budget Detail and Budget Pool columns) at the budget council hearings when hospital administration decided *not* to project inflation.

Also in Exhibit 10–5, note that subcode 232, office supplies, was increased by $138 (from $672 to $810). This was justified on the adjustment explanation (Exhibit 10–6). However, information available to the administrator indicated that $320 had been budgeted and expended in the current year for new chartholders. Since this was a one-time expense, it was taken out of the budget (−$320 in the Budget Pool column). A similar transaction for $53 was taken out of subcode 501 (−$53 in the Budget Detail column, minor equipment). Overall, increases were approved for subcodes 501 and 372 (books). The total budget for supplies and minor equipment for this cost center was approved for $14,595. (Exhibit 10–6 shows the adjustment explanation for both subcodes 232 and 372.)

Exhibit 10–6   Adjustment Explanation, for calendar year —————-

DEPARTMENT NAME _____ 9th floor _____

DEPARTMENT NUMBER _____ 60686 _____

Subcode Number	Subcode Description	Adjustment Amount	Adjustment Explanation
		$ 30.00	2 lg blue policy binders 15.00 ea
		6.00	1 sm blue policy binder
		32.00	2 large red 4″ (8 1/2 × 11) 3-ring binders— normal wear and tear, 2 yrs old
232	Office Supplies	$ 25.00	4 black 3-ring binders (MAR & Kardex)— normal wear and tear
		28.00	48″ × 36″ cork and wood-frame bulletin boards—↑ appearance ↓ clutter
		17.00	25″ × 25″ 1/4″ thick Plexiglas—↑ appearance
		$138	
		$	
		$ 30.00	Tabers Medical Dictionary—ref. book needed to ↑ professionalism
372	Books	$ 20.00	Websters Ninth New Collegiate Dictonary— ↑ learning
		$ 50.00	

Source: Reprinted with permission of University of South Alabama Medical Center, Mobile, Alabama.

In the formulation stage described here, the assistant administrator for finance distributes the worksheets to the other assistant administrators and department heads, who develop budgets with their cost-center managers and defend them before the budget council.

PERSONNEL BUDGET

Most budgets for nursing personnel are based upon quantitative workload measurements, such as a patient-acuity system. Usually a computer software program produces staffing requirements by shift and by day. It produces an acuity index for each patient, and the formula indicates needed staff by level of quali-fication (RN, LPN, NA) and by shift. It also compares actual staffing with that required and can be summarized by month and year. Each day at a given time, a clerk enters each patient's acuity rating, as determined by a licensed nurse, into a computer terminal. To promote objectivity of the ratings, nurses should be trained to use the same procedures when evaluating each patient. Quality checks can compare the trainer's ratings with those made by licensed nurses.

Exhibit 10–7 is a nursing personnel budget based on a patient-acuity rat-ing system. The average daily census (ADC) is obtained from records produced in the admissions office. It is the result of dividing the total patient days for a unit for one year by 365 days. Census reports are computer-generated on a daily, monthly, and annual basis.

Exhibit 10–7   Nursing Personnel Budget

Nursing Budget

1. The attached personnel budget for all nursing units is based on a patient-acuity rating system purchased from Medicus Systems. The standard is

Acuity	Nursing Hours per Patient Needed During 24-hour Period
0.5	0–2 hours
1.0	2–4 hours
2.5	4–10 hours
5.0	10–24 hours

2. The staffing formula is

$$\frac{\text{Average census} \times \text{nursing hours} \times 1.4 \times 1.14}{7.5}$$

3. The total nursing personnel needed includes ward clerks and units not using a patient acuity rating system:

Maternal Child

Unit	ADC	Acuity	NSG/HRS	RN	LPN	NA	Other	Total
3rd	31.8	0.9	4.0	14	9	4	5	32
Peds	22.0	1.3	4.5	16	5	0	4	25
PICU	4.4	3.4	12.0	11	0	0	2	13
ICN	21.7	2.9	12.0	41	7	6	4	58
Inter.	11.9	2.3	4.5	6	4	1	1	12
NBN	19.7	1.0	4.0	9	6	1	3	19
Del. Rm.	—	—	—	20	3	1	4	28
Play Rm.	—	—	—	—	—	—	1	1
Total				117	34	13	24	188

Exhibit 10–7   Nursing Personnel Budget *(Continued)*

Medical

Unit	ADC	Acuity	NSG/HRS	RN	LPN	NA	Other	Total
5 No.	14.3	1.3	4.5	11	3	0	3	17
5 So.	22.1	1.3	4.5	12	5	4	3	24
CRU	3.6	—	4.5	6	—	1	1	8
8th	25.1	1.7	4.5	15	7	2	3	27
MICU	7.2	4.0	12.0	18	0	0	3.5	21.5
CCU	6.5	3.0	12.0	16	0	0	1	17
Telemetry	—	—	—	—	1	5	0	6
Total				78	16	12	14.5	120.5

Surgical

Unit	ADC	Acuity	NSG/HRS	RN	LPN	NA	Other	Total
9th	16.2	1.2	4.5	11	2	2	3	18
6 Surg.	26.5	1.6	4.5	16	6	3	3	28
6 Ortho.	23.5	1.5	4.5	15	4	4	3	26
SICU	6.4	3.8	12.0	17	0	0	2	19
B.U.	3.7	2.8	12.0	8	2	0	1	11
Ortho Tech	—	—	—	—	—	—	1	1
Total				67	14	9	13	103

Psychiatry

Unit	ADC	Acuity	NSG/HRS	RN	LPN	NA	Other	Total
7th	23.5	—	5.5	11	4	11	6	32

OR/RR/EAU/ED

Unit	ADC	Acuity	NSG/HRS	RN	LPN	NA	Other	Total
OR	—	—	—	21	13	4	2	40
RR/EAU	—	—	—	16	0	1	2	19
ED	—	—	—	25	0	7	8	40

Administration

Unit	ADC	Acuity	NSG/HRS	RN	LPN	NA	Other	Total
N/S Adm.	—	—	—	13.0	0	0	3.5	16.5
Staff Dev.	—	—	—	8.5	0	0	1.0	9.5
Health Nurse	—	—	—	1.0	—	—	—	1
CVICU								
Pool	—	—	—	4.5	12	18	2	36.5
Total				362	93	75	76	606

Note: The formulary budget is based on actual ADC for 12 months (July–June). All positions above formula calculations are placed in CVICU budgeted cost center and held vacant.

Source: Reprinted with permission of University of South Alabama Medical Center, Mobile, Alabama.

Exhibit 10–8   Calculating the Nursing Personnel Budget

The staffing formula is

$$\frac{\text{Average daily census} \times \text{nursing hours} \times 1.4 \times 1.14}{7.5}$$

Example: 3rd Floor
Average daily census = 31.8
Nursing hours = 4 (per 24 hours)
1.4 is a constant representing 7 days in a week with a full-time worker working 5 days in a week: 7 ÷ 5 = 1.4
1.14 is a constant representing an allowance of 0.14 FTE for vacation, illness, etc. for each 1.0 FTE
7.5 represents one workday

$$\frac{31.8 \times 4 \times 1.4 \times 1.14}{7.5} = 27 \text{ FTEs}$$

There are 14 RNs, 9 LPNs, and 4 NAs (27 FTEs) budgeted for 3rd floor. The Others column represents ward clerks or other nonnursing personnel not included in the formula. While quantitative measurements justify a full complement of nursing personnel, the budget committee can reduce this number. Note in Exhibit 8–4 that ICN has been reduced from the formula calculation by 1.0 FTE.

Acuity is the result of the sum of all acuities for one year divided by 365 days. This figure is also computer-generated daily, monthly, and annually. The nursing hours are generated from the acuity standard listed in item 1 of Exhibit 10–7. Application of a staffing formula for preparing the personnel budget for a specific unit is illustrated in Exhibit 10–8.

In planning the personnel budget, the nurse has quantitative information related to staffing and can accurately predict the number of full-time equivalents (FTEs) needed for patient care. Other considerations must be weighed at the same time. Will there be a pay increase next year? If so, it must be calculated and budgeted. Will fringe benefits increase or decrease? They must also be budgeted. If new programs are being implemented, do they require additional labor power? Will this labor power come from cutbacks in other programs or from added FTEs? See Exhibit 10–9 for adding new positions to the budget.

In the budgeting process, personnel account for the largest portion of the nursing budget. When one is preparing budgets for clinics, emergency departments, recovery rooms, operating rooms, delivery rooms, and home care, it is important to have quantitative data, such as number of visits, procedures, and deliveries. Records of length of time required for each activity can be taken by using management engineering techniques in which visits, procedures, or other activities are charted over a period of time.

Exhibit 10–9   New Position Questionnaire, Budget Year ————-

1. Department _____   Department number _____

2. Position class, title _____   Position FTE _____

3. Minimum starting salary _____   Expected starting date _____

4. Permanent _____   Temporary _____   If temporary, ending date _____

5. Describe briefly the new position responsibilities:

_____

_____

_____

_____

Need for new position

6. New service _____   Increased volume _____
   If new service, complete question 7.
   If increased volume, complete question 8.

7. Describe the new service to be provided and estimate new revenues.

_____

_____

_____

_____

_____

8. Document increased volume and provide staffing analysis for your department.

_____

_____

_____

_____

(Attach additional pages if necessary) _____

_____

Source: Reprinted with permission of University of South Alabama Medical Center, Mobile, Alabama.

Nonproductive FTEs

Nonproductive FTEs are hours for which an employee is paid but does not work. Nonproductive FTEs include vacation days, holidays, sick days, education and training time, jury duty, funerals, and military leave. These nonproductive hours must be determined and added to personnel expenditures as replacement

FTEs. A full-time equivalent is based on 2,080 hours per year. If the nonproductive FTE average is to be used for personnel budgeting, it will be provided by the human resource department payroll section. For example:

Average vacation FTE	12.5 days
Average holiday FTE	7.0 days
Average sick days FTE	3.5 days
Average training and education FTE	3.0 days
Average other leave FTE	1.5 days
Total	27.5 days, or 220.0 hours

The total work time is 2,080 hours less 220 hours, and the actual work time is 1,860 hours. The percentage of nonworked to total hours paid is 10.6 percent. The percentage of nonworked to worked hours is 11.8 percent.

A cost-center manager prepares the budget according to management rules. The budget should include a budget for replacement FTEs to cover nonproductive FTEs by assigning a fixed amount to each person's paid time off. An option is to determine percentage of nonproductive FTEs and add this total to the budget. This information is then used for staffing determination, taking into consideration seasonal fluctuations for vacations, census, and other pertinent factors.[15]

SUPPLIES AND EQUIPMENT BUDGET

The supplies and equipment budget is part of the operating or cash budget. It includes all supplies and equipment used in provision of services, except capital equipment and supplies charged directly to patients. Examples of supplies to be budgeted are office supplies, medical and surgical supplies, and pharmaceutical supplies. (Refer to Exhibits 10–5 and 10–6.)

Minor equipment includes such items as sphygmomanometers, otoscopes, and ophthalmoscopes. It is equipment that costs less than the base amount set for capital equipment. If the base amount is $500, all equipment under $500 appears as minor equipment in the supplies and equipment budget.

Generally, the director of materials management furnishes the total cost of supplies and equipment per cost center to the accounting office, which generates a cost per patient day. This is used for budgeting purposes, increases for inflation being a decision of top management. Based on projected patient days and revenues, decisions can be made to increase or decrease the supplies and equipment budget.

Costs can be decreased by controlling the amounts of supplies and equipment kept in inventory. Nurse managers should look at inventories they control and reduce them according to usage.

Factors that might influence the supply and equipment aspects of the budget include new program development in the institution, new physicians, and product upgrades. A product evaluation committee may be very cost-effective.

PRODUCT EVALUATION

Product Evaluation Committee

A product evaluation committee usually has as its members representatives of nursing, medical staff, central supply, and purchasing (see Exhibit 10–10). It is headed by a products and equipment specialist or medical materials manager,

Exhibit 10–10   Product Evaluation and Standardization Committee

I. *Purpose*
1. To bring about cost containment in supply and equipment utilization through the review of the quality and cost of products utilized.
2. To review product utilization or special problems in order to maintain standards on the products throughout the hospital system and eliminate needless duplication.
3. To maintain communication among Hospitals, Nursing Service Departments, Medical Staff, and the Purchasing Department concerning product utilization and quality.
4. To evaluate items presented to Purchasing on which formal bids will be obtained.
5. To evaluate items not on bid as recommended by the Purchasing Department, a member of the committee, Administration, or individual departments through requests for evaluation or for addition to inventory.
6. To review performance of in-house products to determine if they fit present needs.

II. *Membership.* Membership of the committee shall consist of

1. Manager of Hospital Resource Analysis
2. Hospital Resource Analyst
3. Budget Director
4. Purchasing Agent
5. Nursing representative from each hospital
6. Ancillary representative from each hospital

Nursing and Ancillary representatives from each hospital shall be appointed by the Administrator on a rotating basis. The infection control nurses will serve in an ex-officio capacity when a product has infection control implications. Additional rep-

resentatives from a facility will be used when a product is to be evaluated that has a distinctive group involved (e.g., OR representatives when OR equipment is involved).

III. *Operations/Meetings.* The Manager of Hospital Resource Analysis shall call and conduct the meeting and shall have voting privileges only in the case of a tie. The Committee shall meet on the third Friday of each month with the location rotating among the facilities. Meetings will usually be one hour long and shall not exceed two hours. A written agenda will be issued to each member prior to the meeting. The agenda will be strictly adhered to unless the committee votes to change it. The chairperson will provide time at the end of each meeting to discuss general information. If a problem arises, the Chairperson may appoint a subcommittee or member to investigate and resolve the problem and to report back to the committee at the next meeting.

Everyone will be given a chance to express his or her ideas before voting. The majority vote shall rule in all cases unless otherwise overridden by Administration. Visiting guests shall have no voting power.

Routine minutes shall be taken at each meeting and will be distributed at the following meeting.

Established July 1989, Policy 949-14, by authority of _____.

Reviewed: July 1990, July 1992
Revised: August 1993, October 1994

Source: Courtesy University of South Alabama Medical Center, Mobile, Alabama.

who can be a nurse. This committee is responsible for evaluation and purchase of supplies and equipment. The following are among its goals:

1. Standardization, with all units using the same products.
2. Lower prices through higher volume.
3. Removal of contract negotiations between vendors and individual nursing units, allowing valuable time to be spent on nursing functions.
4. Addition of a clinical perspective to purchase of all products; the purchasing department does not "just make changes" in products or purchases without appropriate assessment. All clinical implications are considered!

Thus, systematic control of the introduction of patient-care products into the institution is achieved. Exhibits 10–11 and 10–12 present a product information checklist and minutes of a product evaluation meeting respectively.

Exhibit 10–11   Product Information and Justification Checklist

The goal of product evaluation is to provide optimal patient care while managing costs. Therefore, please provide all information requested on this checklist to the department of Hospital Resource Analysis for consideration by the Product Evaluation and Standardization Committee. This report must be reviewed and signed by your Assistant Administrator before it can be evaluated by the committee.

1. Name and function of the product.
2. Is this a new product or a replacement?
3. How will the product be paid for (departmental budget, patient chargeable, etc.)?
4. Why is this product necessary or preferable to the current or other products, in your own words? Please discuss at least two other similar products.
5. What products are currently being used to perform this function in other departments and at all three hospitals?
6. What is the expected utilization of this product throughout the USA System?
7. What is the current utilization of the products that are performing this or a similar function throughout the USA System?
8. If this product is used to treat or prevent a specific ailment or range of ailments, what is the inci-

dence of this ailment that is seen in the USA System?
9. What are the following costs, if applicable, for this product as compared to other similar products and how can these costs be justified?
   • purchase price
   • installation
   • training
   • personnel
   • support
   • maintenance (Also include who is responsible for maintenance.)
10. If cost savings are anticipated with the use of this product, how will those "savings" be utilized?
11. Who will control the use of the product?
12. If applicable, please provide a sample protocol for the use of this product that will be used to ensure proper use of this product.
13. What are the long-term implications of this product?

If you need assistance, please contact _____ or _____ at _____.

Source: Courtesy University of South Alabama Medical Center, Mobile, Alabama.

Exhibit 10–12   Product Evaluation and Standardization Committee Meeting

December 9, 1994
8:30 A.M., Board Room, USA Knollwood

Members Present
Chairman, Hospital Resource Analyst, USAMC
Director of Nursing, USAKPH
Director of Respiratory Therapy, USADH
Nurse Manager, Surgical Services, USADH
Director of Radiology, USAMC
SPD Supervisor, USAKPH
Nurse Manager, High Risk/Antenatal Obstetrics, USAMC
Director of Budgets, USAMC

Members Absent
Purchasing Agent, USAMC
Hospital Resource Analyst, USAMC

Guests
Trauma Coordinator, USAMC

Product Evaluation

Closed Arterial Line System
The Director of Respiratory Therapy and the Trauma Coordinator presented their findings from the evaluation of the closed arterial line system. In their discussion with Nursing and Respiratory Care providers, there were many issues raised regarding the practicality of such a system. These issues revolved around tubing size, heparinization and sampling through the ports available on the SafeSite system. In general, they concluded that the issue of blood waste could be solved without purchasing such a system and that there was no documentation present which could prove that contamination with the current stopcock system was a problem. They therefore recommended that we not pursue this system any further at this time. However, they did recommend that we evaluate such systems again when it is time to bid our current system again.

The committee unanimously agreed to not recommend the addition of a Closed Arterial Line System.

Old Business

Gloves
The data provided regarding glove usage was determined to have been helpful to managers in evaluating their departments. _____ requested that _____ provide comparable information for the current fiscal year to date.

_____ addressed the quality issue with our current stock gloves. None of the other committee members have been made aware of a major quality problem with the gloves. It is unclear whether the problem has not been apparent in other departments or is just not being reported. _____ was not present at the meeting to answer how the company has responded to his inquiry regarding the quality issue.

After much discussion, it was decided that _____ would send a memo to all managers asking them to address specific quality issues to the committee representatives in their respective facilities.

Communication Issues
_____ brought up the problem that managers have in being informed of bid item changes in advance. Although it may not be possible to evaluate every item that is on bid, the committee determined that it would be helpful if the Purchasing Department could announce upcoming bids 3 to 6 months ahead of time. This would allow managers the opportunity to provide information regarding specific products. It was also suggested that bids be posted in all three facilities, rather than just at USAMC; this problem seems to be most apparent at USADH and USAKPH. _____ will discuss this with _____.

Presentation of Committee's Purpose to Managers
This presentation has not yet been accomplished. _____ agreed to have a proposal for this purpose ready for the January meeting. It was suggested that it might be helpful to have each facility's representatives make the presentation at their facility.

(Continued)

Exhibit 10–12   Product Evaluation and Standardization Committee Meeting *(Continued)*

New Business

None.

The next regularly scheduled meeting will be held at USAMC on Friday, January 20, 199x at 8:30 A.M. in the USAMC Board Room.

The meeting was adjourned at 9:30 A.M.

Respectfully submitted,

Chairman

Source: Courtesy of University of South Alabama Medical Center, Mobile, Alabama.

The following is a suggested process for product evaluation by a committee:[16]

1. Determine objectives of product evaluation.
2. Define use of the product with input from potential users.
3. Define objectives for each evaluation project.
4. Do initial review of various products: features, techniques for use, and prices.
5. Select products for evaluation and evaluate techniques for use, staff acceptance, and problems.
6. Conduct in-service tests to use products.
7. Use simple closed-ended questions, open-ended questions, and rating scales to evaluate the product.
8. Compile and analyze data, including costs, cost savings, conversion cost, and reimbursement potential. The Deming theory of working with one supplier to improve products is noted in chapter 25.
9. Make decision for purchase.

Exercise 10–5   Examine the supplies and equipment budget for the institution in which you work or are assigned for clinical experience. What input did clinical nurses have in preparing it? Are the nurses informed about this aspect of the budget? Do they want to be? What would be the advantages?

CAPITAL BUDGET

A capital budget is usually separate from the operating budget (see Exhibit 10–13). A capital budget projects the planned costs of major purchases. Each item of a capital budget is defined in terms of dollar value and is an item of

Exhibit 10–13 Capital Budget Requested FY 19xx–19xx:
University of South Alabama Medical Center

Dept.	Item	Quantity	Amount
7th & 8th	Beds & misc. pat. furn.	85	$ 200,000.00
Admin	Pneumatic tube system	1	75,000.00
Anest	Capnograph-portable	1	4,200.00
Anest	Trans. Mon.- inc NIPB & O_2 Sat	1	9,200.00
Anest	Ventilators	2	5,050.00
Aero Med	Pro Pac 106	1	13,790.00
Bio Med	Safety tester	1	1,695.00
Blood Bk	Table top centrifuge	1	2,000.00
Blood Bk	Automated cell washer	1	6,250.00
Cath Lab	Pulse oximetry	1	2,600.00
Cath Lab	Dynamap	1	3,800.00
Clin. Lab	Miscellaneous equipment	1	250,000.00
Dialysis	Dialysis machine	1	25,000.00
Dietary	Refrigerator-bakery	1	3,500.00
Dietary	Refrigerator-bakery	1	6,950.00
Dietary	Refrigerator-cook area	1	3,500.00
Dietary	Refrigerator-PFS	1	3,100.00
Dietary	Meat slicer	1	3,500.00
ED	New monitoring system	1	160,000.00
ED	Propak monitor	1	3,500.00
Envir	High-speed burnisher	4	8,000.00
Envir	Slow-speed buffers	2	1,600.00
GI Lab	Video processor CV-100	1	20,000.00
HStation	Blood pressure monitor	1	4,500.00
HStation	Stress test system	1	20,000.00
HStation	ECG management system	1	70,000.00
MICU/CCU	Faceplates-central monitors	12	4,920.00
Nursing	Medication carts	17	25,000.00
Nutri	Computer & printer	1	2,011.00
OR	Laparoscopic video system	1	30,165.00
OR	Electrosurgical cautery	2	17,200.00
PACU	RR stretchers	10	20,000.00
Plant Op	4000-watt portable generator	1	1,495.00
Plant Op	8 ch. OPS card for telephone swi	1	1,337.00
Radio	Rebuilt film processor	1	12,000.00
Res. Th	Sterile pass-through drier	1	12,567.00
SPD	Washer decontaminator	1	75,000.00
Staff Dev	Overhead projector	1	700.00
Staff Dev	CPR mannikin	1	5,641.00
Total requested USA Medical Center			$1,114,771.00

Source: Courtesy University of South Alabama Medical Center, Mobile, Alabama.

equipment that is used over a period of time. The budget provides for depreciation of each item in the capital budget, sets aside the amount of depreciation in an escrow account, and uses this account to finance new capital purchases (see Exhibit 10–14). Depreciation records the declining value of a physical asset. In addition, department heads are required to justify and set priorities on capital budget items (see Exhibit 10–15). The exact definition as to what constitutes a capital budget item with regard to dollar amount and life expectancy varies among hospitals.

Capital budgets also deal with maintenance, renovations, remodeling, improvements, expansion, land acquisition, and new buildings (see Exhibits 10–14 and 10–16). The financial manager for nursing is the nurse manager, who should evaluate past decisions and advise the nurse administrator whether they were good or bad.

Exhibit 10–14   Investment in Plant Assets for the Ten Months Ended July 31,———

Plant assets consisting of land, buildings, and equipment are stated at cost or, if contributed, at fair market value at date of gift. No provision is made in the accounts for depreciation of plant assets. Investment in plant is reduced for disposal of plant assets.

All hospital equipment purchases are funded by the renewals and replacements fund. The hospital also uses plant assets purchased by the University. These assets are not presented in the hospital's financial statements.

Depreciation expense is included in Medicare, Medicaid, and Blue Cross cost reports. This information is presented below.

	Cost	Depreciation Expense 07-31-xx	Accum. Depreciation 07-31-xx	Net Book Value 07-31-xx
Hospital-Designated Funds				
Land	$ 186,096	$ 0	$ 0	$ 186,096
Buildings	8,070,647	184,063	3,942,812	4,127,835
Fixed Equipment	10,386,318	605,671	5,878,008	4,508,310
Major Movable Equipment	15,079,892	1,235,052	8,971,493	6,108,399
Minor Equipment	186,757	0	186,757	0
Construction in Progress	762,874	0	0	762,874
Total	$34,672,584	$2,024,786	$18,979,070	$15,693,514
University-Designated Funds				
Buildings	$ 1,544,927	$ 39,481	$ 581,958	$ 962,969
Fixed Equipment	2,564,683	158,533	1,914,366	650,317
Major Movable Equipment	5,315,499	0	5,315,499	0
Total	$ 9,425,109	$ 198,014	$ 7,811,823	$ 1,613,286
Total equipment used for patient care	$44,097,693	$2,222,800	$26,790,893	$17,306,800

Source: Reprinted with permission of University of South Alabama Medical Center, Mobile, Alabama.

Exhibit 10–15   Capital Equipment Request Form

Hospital: ___USA Medical Center___

Dept: ___Department of Nursing___   **Dept no.** ___60601___

Equipment requested: ___85 electric beds/7th–8th floor___

Equipment description: Give a simple description of the device and its use.

85 electric beds with high-low features, ability for trendelenburg/reverse trendelenburg positions; instant CPR

emergency lever; head of bed frame removable to facilitate cervical traction and emergency procedures; side

arm control for patient use.

_____

_____

_____

$210,000.00	**Equipment costs**	None	**Training costs**
Minimal	**Maintenance costs**	Incl in Eqpt.	**Shipping costs**
None	**Personnel costs**	None	**Supply costs**
None	**Installation/renovation costs**		

Expected useful life: ___15___ **yrs**

1	List priority (1-2-3-4) of equipment with regard to the other requests submitted by your department.
Yes	(Y/N) Will this item be a replacement for an existing piece of equipment? If "Y," what is to become of the existing equipment? Equipment to be evaluated by the Hospital Committee to determine.
No	(Y/N) Is this new technology or a new procedure? If "Y," how will the expense be recuperated (e.g., through revenue)?

Manager: _____, RN, MSN Director, Nursing Resources_____

Assistant administrator: _____

Apr # _____

Source: Courtesy University of South Alabama Medical Center, Mobile, Alabama. Reprinted with permission.

Exhibit 10–16 Statement of Changes in Fund Balance
Renewals and Replacements Fund for the Ten Months Ended July 31, _____

Account Number	Description	Balances Prior Year	Funded Depreciation	Other Additions Deductions	Expended for Plant Facilities	Intrafund Transfers	Balances Current Year
79008	Unallocated—USAMC	$9,915,392.38	$2,222,800.29	$78,134.71	$.00	$159,538.18–	$12,056,789.20
79030	Defects—Joint Commis	65,818.19	.00	.00	.00	65,818.19–	.00
79039	Information System	92,709.68	.00	.00	.00	.00	92,709.68
79050	Helicopter—USAMC	712,120.33	.00	127,667.94	.00	.00	839,788.27
79057	USAMC Emer Generator	48,562.09	.00	.00	.00	.00	48,562.09
79063	Donated Eq—Others	2,313.49	.00	153.00	1,928.70–	384.79–	153.00
79064	USAMC Aux Purch Eq	.00	.00	688.08–	538.08	150.00	.00
79068	Hosp Adm Purch Eq	.00	.00	33,809.52	33,809.52–	.00	.00
79075	HVAC System—Surgery	74,475.00	.00	.00	.00	74,475.00–	.00
79077	Labor Deliv Unit 3FL	291,990.72	.00	.00	.00	.00	291,990.72
79083	H.A.S. Telephone Sym	13,007.00	.00	.00	.00	13,007.00–	.00
79092	Capital Budget previous	364,110.78	.00	5,208.00–	334,654.47–	.00	24,248.31
79093	Xray Silver Recovery	49,944.03	.00	12,678.45	.00	.00	62,622.48
79095	Capital Exp <$10,000	75,414.38	.00	.00	146,864.18–	150,000.00	78,550.20
79097	Linear Accelerator	.00	.00	.00	45,994.26	45,994.26–	.00
79098	Mini Van	1,606.48	.00	2,847.51	.00	.00	4,453.99
79099	O/P Surg Cap Equip	161,720.27	.00	.00	225,718.54	64,324.93	326.66
79101	O/P Surg Renov	37,425.00	.00	.00	1,316.60–	.00	36,108.40
79102	Angiograph Lab Eqmnt	1,000,000.00	.00	.00	189,259.00–	.00	810,741.00
79103	Nuclear Medical Eqmnt	284,000.00	.00	.00	246,035.68–	.00	37,964.32
79104	Telethon Purch Equip	.00	.00	40,185.00	40,185.00–	.00	.00
79105	Medical Rec Dict Sys	.00	.00	.00	.00	86,288.00	86,288.00
79106	Renal Transplant Prg	.00	.00	.00	.00	96,000.00	96,000.00
79110	ELENA-USAMC Damage	31,916.36	.00	5,629.15	.00	37,545.51–	.00
	Final Totals	$13,222,526.18	$2,222,800.29	$295,209.20	$1,173,239.35–	$.00	$14,567,296.32

Source: University of South Alabama Medical Center, Mobile, Alabama. Reprinted with permission.

All proposals for capital equipment must be fully evaluated for amount of use, method of payment, safety, replacement, duplication of service, and every conceivable other factor, including the need for space, personnel, and renovation. The needs and desires of the medical staff should be considered. Staff involvement in planning helps ensure wise purchases of capital equipment.

The capital budget must address increased forms of competition, dwindling financial resources, and regulatory constraints. Management should enhance conditions under which effective planning and capital budgeting increase the agency's chance of long-term survival. Capital budgeting is a part of the overall budget planning process for the organization and not an entity unto itself.

When each entry or item in the capital budget list has been analyzed and reduced to the amount available, the budget is again tabulated. It is now ready to present to the board of directors (refer to Exhibit 10–13). With the board's approval, the list is distributed to cost-center managers, who prepare requisitions for purchase. The purchasing department prepares bid specifications, with input from cost-center managers. Purchases are finalized based on results of bids submitted by vendors who meet the required specifications. Exhibit 10–17 is a status report of a capital budget in which all remaining dollars are committed. Purchases are finally entered into the depreciation budget schedule. The latter is published by the American Hospital Association and is considered the standard for the industry (see Exhibit 10–18).

Capital equipment accounts for approximately 10.4 percent of a hospital's annual expenditures.[17]

When evaluating capital equipment, one should evaluate similar products one at a time. When purchasing capital equipment, one should determine whether it can be upgraded or must be replaced when technology improves. One should consider construction, durability, modularity, warranty, availability of parts, and service agreements as part of the total cost of equipment. One might consider leasing versus buying.[18]

Part of the capital equipment budgeting process includes estimating the use of each item. For revenue budgeting purposes, a price or charge should be put on each item's use. The cost-center manager can then determine the break-even point at which the item will be paid for.

Exercise 10–6

1. Examine a health-care business's capital budget for the previous year. What was the total dollar amount requested? Approved? What process was used to produce the capital budget? What was the degree of nurse participation?

2. Prepare a capital equipment budget request using the format of Exhibit 10–15 (or use a form from the institution in which you work or are assigned for clinical experience).

Exhibit 10–17 Capital Budget, as of June 30, _____

Department	Dept. No.	Item Description	Budget	Paid 06-30-xx	Encumbrances	Total Committed	Budget Balance
Nursing Services							
Nursing Services—Admin	60601	Software License	$ 0.00	$ 18,135.00	$2,000.00	$ 0.00	$0.00
		External Modem		527.12			
		Electric & Manual Beds—6		31,704.72			
		Cardio System Special Care Beds		13,725.00			
		Telemetry Monitoring System		113,080.12			
		COMPAQ Computer		9,842.70			
		Department Total	$189,014.66	$187,014.66	$2,000.00	$189,014.66	$0.00
Private U. 6th Floor	60609	Lifepack 7 Defibrillator		5,500.00			
		Facsimile Machine		1,600.00			
		Lifepack 7 Defibrillator		5,208.00			
		Department Total	$ 12,308.00	$ 12,308.00	0.00	$ 12,308.00	0.00
Coronary Care	60615	Lifepack 6 Defibrillator		7,621.32			
		Department Total	$ 7,621.32	$ 7,621.32	0.00	$ 7,621.32	0.00
5th Fl—Shared Supplies	60619	Facsimile Machine		1,550.00			
		Department Total	$ 1,550.00	$ 1,550.00	0.00	$ 1,550.00	0.00
Fifth Floor—North	60622	Lifepack 7 Defibrillator		5,500.00			
		Department Total	$ 5,500.00	$ 5,500.00	0.00	$ 5,500.00	0.00
CCU	60626	Telemetry Transmitters		3,300.00			
		Department Total	$ 3,300.00	$ 3,300.00	0.00	$ 3,300.00	0.00
Pediatric Unit	60630	Lifepack 7 Defibrillator		5,500.00			
		Facsimile Machine		1,550.00			
		Department Total	$ 7,050.00	$ 7,050.00	0.00	$ 7,050.00	$0.00

Source: University of South Alabama Medical Center, Mobile, Alabama. Reprinted with permission.

Exhibit 10–18   Composite Estimated Useful Lives of Depreciable Hospital Assets

Building Components, Buildings, and Fixed Equipment

Item	Years
Boiler house	15–25
Masonry building, reinforced concrete frame	25–30
Masonry building, steel frame	
Fireproofed	25–30
Not fireproofed	20–25
Masonry building, wood frame	20–25
Multilevel parking structure, masonry	20–25
Reinforced concrete building, common design	25–30
Residence	
Masonry	20–25
Wood frame	15–20
Storage building	
Masonry	20–25
Wood frame	15–20

Movable Equipment

Item	Years
Major movable equipment	7–12
Minor movable equipment	2–5

Source: Reproduced with permission from *Estimated Useful Lives of Depreciable Hospital Assets,* published by American Hospital Publishing, Inc., copyright 1993. All rights reserved.

REVENUES

The sources of nursing revenue or for securing a financial base for nursing include grants, continuing education, private practice, community visibility, health care for students and staff, HMOs, city health departments, industry, unions, third-party payments, professional corporations, and nurse-managed centers.

Operating room nursing is an example of a cost that can be billed as a source of revenue. This can be done by determining the level of care needed for different procedures and the room charges, based on use of supplies and equipment, and billing the services separately. In computing the nursing charges, the cost of nursing personnel per case can be determined from the records. To this can be added cost for preparation time for assembling supplies and equipment and setting up the room, preoperative and postoperative patient visits, nursing administration, and staff development. Room costs would include environmental services and maintenance.[19]

Using product-line strategy, nursing divisions can sell a number of product lines, such as staff development programs, consultation services, home health care, wellness programs, and computer software.

Many items and services have been used to generate revenues for hospitals, including drugs, supplies, respiratory therapy, and physical therapy. In most instances, the charges have been excessive, and areas exist where cost shifting has accounted for revenues (and profits) to cover services delivered and charged at a price below costs. As the hospital bill is unbundled, charges will eventually reduce to costs at a 1:1 ratio. Not-for-profit hospitals are not allowed a return on equity or credit for bad debts as a cost of doing business; they carry these items as cash or ledger balances.[20]

While in business and industry, technology is used to reduce costs by increasing output, the opposite has been encouraged in the health-care industry by charge-based reimbursement schemes. Increases in equipment costs and types and numbers of procedures were paid for by third-party payers. That has changed somewhat with the prospective payment system (PPS). With control of reimbursement, less expense is best. The old revenue producers such as drugs, respiratory therapies, laboratory tests, and x-rays are being reimbursed at their true costs. Nursing care is the source of revenue for the future. Nurses must identify the relative value units of care by which they will be reimbursed. They must learn to use information systems to process data and to select and use the supply item that does the best job for the least money. They must standardize procedures and practices and review and revise jobs.

Because of their relatively high fixed costs, hospitals must maintain high productivity. If productivity declines, costs must be decreased. This is done by decreasing staff and the use of supplies and by making other reductions in use of resources.

THE CONTROLLING PROCESS

Now that the nursing budget has been viewed from its planning and directing aspects, it will be looked at from its controlling or evaluating aspect. The budget establishes financial standards for the division of nursing and through the division's cost center for each nursing unit. Feedback on a daily, weekly, monthly, and quarterly basis supplies information to compare managerial performance with the established standards. The results are used to make adjustments. What kind of feedback is needed by nurses relative to their budgets and cost control? Nurses need information to tell whether their goals are being met. Are they exceeding the budget? Is the excess both for cost and for revenues? Are the supplies and expenses of the quantity and quality planned? Is the equipment being purchased and installed as scheduled? Are employees being recruited and utilized effectively to produce the expected quality and quantity of nursing services? Is employee morale good? What adjustments need to be made? Where are the problems, and who is responsible for them?

Budget processes should be flexible to allow for increased and decreased volume of business. The hospital business office provides cost-center managers with needed biometric information to make adjustments in staffing and in use of supplies.

It should be remembered that a budget is a plan based on the best estimates of the costs of running an organization. It cannot be inflexible, but neither can it hide waste and inefficiency.

The nurse administrator should be sure that nurses will not be penalized when budgetary objectives are not met as a result of events beyond their control. Nurses are working within the confines of an organizational environment that is affected by both internal and external constraints. One of the external constraints facing them is federally mandated cost control or cost containment, which is seen by some administrators as reimbursement control.

The colossal mistakes of budgeting are made in the control area. Top management should view variations in budget as a tool for decision making, not an instance to make arbitrary cuts resulting in unrealistic operating budgets for line managers. One way to overcome this problem is through employee education about the budget process. Such knowledge helps employees view the budget as an aid rather than an obstacle.[21]

Decentralization of the Budget

Cost-center managers, usually nurse managers and supervisors of units, are capable of planning and controlling their own budgets. The nurse administrator, assisted by financial managers, should prepare them to do so. Through decentralized budgeting, cost-center managers propose innovative objectives and gather data to defend their objectives and operating plans. The unit budget becomes their responsibility, and they zealously guard its integrity. They sense when adaptations have to be made because of increased costs or decreased revenues, and they make or recommend immediate remedies. Decentralized budgeting provides for internal controls.

Monitoring the Budget

Various techniques have been described and defined for monitoring the budget, although all budget objectives should contain procedures for quality review, including identification of a team to perform such a review. If a program is not successful—is not meeting objectives or is running above predicted costs and below predicted revenues—a decision should be made whether to rework or cancel it. This is very difficult, but it is essential to good control. The technique of cancelling budgeted programs is sometimes referred to as *sunsetting*. A nurse manager should accept the responsibility for sunsetting programs that are costly and unprofitable.

In developing the nursing budget, it is necessary that the unit structures for nursing administration are comparable in type and quantity of workload. This can be ensured by developing and providing financial policies and guidelines. This is most successful when the top administrative team works with the budget monitor to develop such financial policies. The nurse administrator is part of this team and brings to its meetings standards of service that are defensible, such as data on workload, including numbers and types of procedures, patients, surgical operations, and visits. These policies should reflect the long-range plans of the governing board.

Part of the information furnished to nurse administrators and managers is in the form of reports, which include statistical reports of revenues and expenditures for the current year. Exhibit 10–19 illustrates financial information

Exhibit 10–19 Accounting System Report

Account statement in whole dollars for fiscal year ending _____
83% of fiscal year elapsed
Distribution code = 700
Medical Intensive Care Unit—Expense

Computer Date _____
Time of Day _____
Acct: 4-60680
Dept: 60680

		Budget		Actual		Open	Balance	Percent
Subcode	Description	Original	Revised	Current Month	Fiscal Year	Encumbrances	Available	Used
100	Pool—Salary & Wages	948,742	901,053				901,053	0
130	Professional Salry			72,533	775,790		775,790–	***
135	Tech Salry & Wages			4,085	50,947		50,947–	***
140	Office Salaries			4,347	53,168		53,168–	***
155	Service Empl Wages			3,936	52,195		52,195–	***
160	Student Wages		14,898	1,518	14,898			100
166	Accrued Salaries		32,791	11,462	32,791			100
	Salaries	948,742	948,742	97,880	979,789		31,047–	103
170	Pool—Empl Benefits	254,683	55,722				55,722	0
182	Employers FICA		112		112			100
183	Group Life Ins		2,569	264	2,569			100
184	Disability Ins		4,869	526	4,869			100
185	Teachers Retirement		134		134			100
188	Group Health Ins		59,973	5,887	59,973			100
198	State Paid Retiremnt		62,158	5,591	62,158			100
199	State Paid FICA		69,146	6,313	69,146			100
	Employee Benefits	254,683	254,683	18,581	198,961		55,722	78
200	Pool—Med/Surg Supply	75,000	23,920				23,920	0
211	Med & Surg Supplies		128,235	14,846	128,235			100
213	Drugs		1,317	140	1,317			100
214	Solutions		36,091	4,389	36,091			100
	Med/Surg Supplies	75,000	189,563	19,375	165,643		23,920	87
220	Pool-General Supply	5,789	2,553–				2,553–	0
232	Office Supplies		1,070	19	1,069	1		100

Exhibit 10–19 Accounting System Report *(Continued)*

Subcode	Description	Budget		Actual		Open Encumbrances	Balance Available	Percent Used
		Original	Revised	Current Month	Fiscal Year			
233	Copying & Binding		36	30	36			100
234	Printing		1,494	115	1,494			100
235	Printing Paper		633	83	633			100
240	Housekeeping Supply		1,880	323	1,880			100
243	Housekeeping Furnish		1,395		1,395			100
244	Linen Replacement		214		214			100
250	Maintenance Supplies		1,001		1,001			100
270	Food Expense		619	49	619			100
	General Supplies	5,789	5,789	620	8,341	1	2,553–	144
300	Pool—Travel/Entrtain		1,005				1,005	0
316	Workshop & Training		425		425			100
	Travel/Entertainment	1,430	1,430		425		1,005	30
320	Pool—Other Expenses		12,624				12,624	0
324	Contract Service		140,390	16,720	140,390			100
336	Equip Maint & Repair		3,700		2,950	750		100
372	Books & Subscription		286		286			100
	Other Expenses	157,000	157,000	16,720	143,626	750	12,624	92
501	Minor Equipment	4,000	4,000				4,000	0
	Total Expenses	1,446,644	1,561,207	153,176	1,496,785	751	63,671	96
	Account Total	1,446,644	1,561,207	153,176	1,496,785	751	63,671	96

Open Encumbrance Status

Account	P.O. Number	P.O. Date	Description	Liquidating Expenditures	Adjustments	Original Enc	Current Enc	Last Act Date
4-60680-232	H01764	10/06/xx	Waller Brothers			.85	.85	10/18
4-60680-336	H07584	07/24/xx	Scaletronix Inc			750.00	750.00	08/01
			**Account Total			750.85	750.85	

Source: Courtesy University of South Alabama Medical Center, Mobile, Alabama. Reprinted with permission.

that is needed by the cost-center manager and the nursing service administrator.

Note that the account number at the head of the table in Exhibit 10–19 is 4-60680. The prefix 4 denotes that the account balance does *not* turn over at the end of the fiscal year. The cost center or department is 60680. Financial transactions, including purchase orders for supplies and minor equipment as well as the payroll, are identified with this cost-center number and are charged by the purchasing and accounting departments to this number and to the appropriate subcodes 100 through 501. Table columns indicate the operational budget, the actual expenditures for the current month and for the fiscal year, open encumbrances, and the balance available. Because 83 percent of the fiscal year (which begins October 1) has elapsed, this has some relationship to the Percent Used column. Although 103 percent of the budgeted salary has been used, indicating a variance of 20 percent, only 78 percent of employee benefits have been used, which indicates a use of overtime plus part-time employees working less than the 0.5 FTE required to qualify for fringe benefits. Zero percent of the budgeted money for minor equipment has been spent to date. Total budget expenses were 96 percent, indicating a variance of 13 percent overspending. While this report serves as a control for nurse managers, the expenditure of budgeted money for any one subcode could cause the total expenses to date to be greater than the percentage of fiscal year elapsed without creating an alarm. In this instance, overspending should be related to increased census and revenue.

Exhibit 10–20 informs the nurse managers of the specific financial transactions that took place during the month of July. These transactions can be checked against Exhibit 10–19.

Information on revenues is reported in a similar manner. Exhibit 10–21 illustrates the inpatient revenue for the Medical Intensive Care Unit, which includes nursing and hotel services. It is all credited to nursing. The revenue account is 4-30815, while the cost center is the same as for expenses, 60680. The budgeted revenues for the year are listed, as are the revenues for the month and for the fiscal year. Note that although 83 percent of the fiscal year has elapsed, only 76 percent of the budgeted revenues have been charged, a variance of –7 percent. Also, Exhibit 10–22 indicates that 76 percent of budgeted equipment revenues have been billed.

Since the amount billed (that is, the unit's revenues), 76 percent, is less than the 83 percent of fiscal year elapsed, the nurse managers can note that revenues are currently lower than expenses, a negative financial report. The manager's goal is to maintain or improve this financial status to the end of the fiscal year.

Additional financial information can be furnished to each nurse manager, including summary reports in whole dollars and for all cost centers supervised. This can be done by subcode (see Exhibit 10–23), by subcode and cost center (see Exhibit 10–24), and by any unit or department (see Exhibits 10–25 and 10–26).

Exhibit 10–20 Accounting System Report

Computer Date _____
Time of Day _____
PGM = AM091

Acct: 4-60680
Dept: 60680

Report of transactions for fiscal year ending _____
Distribution code = 700
Medical Intensive Care Unit—Expense

Subcode	Description	Date	EC	Ref.	2nd Ref.	J.E. Offset Account	Budget Entries	Current Rev/Exp	Encumbrances	Batch Ref.	Date
130	Payroll Expense	07/07	64	900001		0-10080-118CR		35,017.03		PPS584	07/07
130	Payroll Expenses	07/21	64	900001		0-10080-118CR		37,516.33		PPS588	07/21
130	CM Total Professional Salry							72,533.36			
135	Payroll Expense	07/07	64	900001		0-10080-118CR		1,630.89		PPS584	07/07
135	Payroll Expense	07/21	64	900001		0-10080-118CR		2,454.11		PPS588	07/21
135	CM Total Tech Salry & Wages							4085.00			
140	Payroll Expense	07/07	64	900001		0-10080-118CR		2,082.44		PPS584	07/07
140	Payroll Expense	07/21	64	900001		0-10080-118CR		2,264.26		PPS588	07/21
140	CM Total Office Salaries							4,346.70			
155	Payroll Expense	07/07	64	900001		0-10080-118CR		1,884.26		PPS584	07/07
155	Payroll Expense	07/21	64	900001		0-10080-118CR		2,051.29		PPS588	07/21
155	CM Total Service Empl Wages							3,935.55			
160	Payroll Expense	07/07	64	900001		0-10080-118CR		494.83		PPS584	07/07
160	Payroll Expense	07/21	64	900001		0-10080-118CR		1,022.81		PPS588	07/21
160	CM Total Student Wages							1,517.64			
166	Susp Corr/Accr Sal	06/30	60		S01544	0-13000-160CR		65.00		HJV002	07/10
166	Susp Corr/Accr Sal	06/30	60		S01543	0-13000-160CR		45.00		HJV002	07/10
166	RVS Accrd Sal & Wage	07/01	60		075101	0-15300-220DR		40,318.00–		HJV001	07/10
166	RVS Accrd Sal & Wage	07/01	60		075101	0-15300-220DR		65.00–		HJV001	07/10

(Continued)

Exhibit 10–20 Accounting System Report *(Continued)*

Subcode	Description	Date	EC	Ref.	2nd Ref.	J.E. Offset Account	Budget Entries	Current Rev/Exp	Encumbrances	Batch Ref.	Batch Date
	RVS Accrd Sal & Wage	07/01	60		075101	0-15300-220DR		45.00–		HJV001	07/10
	Accrued Sal & Wages	07/31	60		075100	0-15300-220CR		51,780.00		HJV019	07/31
166	CM Total Accrued Salaries							11,462.00			
183	Payroll Expense	07/21	64	900001		2-77000-180CR		264.04		PPS588	07/21
183	CM Total Group Life Ins							264.04			
184	Payroll Expense	07/21	64	900001		2-77000-180CR		526.48		PPS588	07/21
184	CM Total Disability Ins							526.48			
188	Payroll Expense	07/07	64	900001		2-77000-180CR		65.81		PPS584	07/07
188	Payroll Expense	07/21	64	900001		2-77000-180CR		5,821.12		PPS588	07/21
188	CM Total Group Health Ins							5,886.93			
198	Payroll Expense	07/07	64	900001		2-77000-180CR		2,659.96		PPS584	07/07
198	Payroll Expense	07/21	64	900001		2-77000-180CR		2,930.66		PPS588	07/21
198	CM Total State Paid Retiremnt							5,590.62			
199	Payroll Expense	07/07	64	900001		2-77000-180CR		3,019.55		PPS584	07/07
199	Payroll Expense	07/21	64	900001		2-77000-180CR		3,293.55		PPS588	07/21
199	CM Total State Paid FICA							6,313.10			
211	Inventory Exp Alloc	07/31	60		075264	0-12100-140CR		14,845.75		HJV027	07/31
211	CM Total Med & Surg Supplies							14,845.75			
213	Pharmacy Distrib—Jul	07/31	60		075006	4-60730-213CR		140.34		HJV033	07/31
213	CM Total Drugs							140.34			
214	Inventory Exp Alloc	07/31	60		075264	0-12100-140CR		4,389.27		HJV027	07/31
214	CM Total Solutions							4,389.27			
232	Inventory Exp Alloc	07/31	60		075264	0-12100-140CR		19.49		HJV027	07/31
232	CM Total Office Supplies							19.49			

Exhibit 10–20 Accounting System Report *(Continued)*

Subcode	Description	Date	EC	Ref.	2nd Ref.	J.E. Offset Account	Budget Entries	Current Rev/Exp	Encumbrances	Batch Ref.	Batch Date
233	Xerox Expense-J/J 89	07/31	60		075008	4-60960-965CR		30.21		HJV026	07/31
233	CM Total Copying & Binding							30.21			
234	Print Shop Chrgs—Jul	07/26	60		075011	4-60960-960CR		115.20		HJV013	07/27
234	CM Total Printing							115.20			
235	Inventory Exp Alloc	07/31	60		075264	0-12100-140CR		82.69		HJV027	07/31
235	CM Total Printing Paper							82.69			
240	Inventory Exp Alloc	07/31	60		075264	0-12100-140CR		323.42		HJV027	07/31
240	CM Total Housekeeping Supply							323.42			
270	Inventory Exp Alloc	07/31	60		075264	0-12100-140CR		48.61		HJV027	07/31
270	CM Total Food Expense							48.61			
324	Nephrology Applicati Accure Jly	07/26	68		563631	0-15030-211CR		3,520.00		HPD850	07/26
324		07/31	60		075259	0-15030-210CR		13,200.00		HJV024	07/31
324	CM Total Contract Service							16,720.00			
336	Scaletronix Inc	07/24	50	H07584					750.00	HEN010	07/31
336	CM Total Equip Maint & Repair								750.00		
	Account Total							153,176.40	750.00		

Source: Courtesy University of South Alabama Medical Center, Mobile, Alabama. Reprinted with permission.

Exhibit 10–21 Accounting System Report

Computer Date _____
Time of Day _____
PGM = AM090-B1

Account statement in whole dollars for fiscal year ending _____
83% of fiscal year elapsed
Distribution code = 700
Medical Intensive Care Unit—Revenue

Acct: 4-30815
Dept: 60680

Tab Code	Description	Budgets		Actual			Balance Available	Percent Used
		Original	Revised	Current Month	Fiscal Year	Open Encumbrances		
040								
0/0	Inpatient Revenue	1,511,400–	1,511,400–	115,500–	1,146,600–		364,800–	76
	Total Revenues	1,511,400–	1,511,400–	115,500–	1,146,600–		364,800–	76
	Account Total	1,511,400–	1,511,400–	115,500–	1,146,600–		364,800–	76

Source: Courtesy University of South Alabama Medical Center, Mobile, Alabama. Reprinted with permission.

Exhibit 10-22 Accounting System Report

Account statement in whole dollars for fiscal year ending _____
83% of fiscal year elapsed
Distribution code = 700
Medical Intensive Care Unit—SP&D—Revenue

Computer Date _____
Time of Day _____
PGM = AM090-B1

Acct: 4-30818
Dept: 60680

		Budgets		Actual				
SubCode	Description	Original	Revised	Current Month	Fiscal Year	Open Encumbrances	Balance Available	Percent Used
040	Inpatient Revenue		1,080,088–	101,637–	818,031–		262,057–	76
	Total Revenues		1,080,088–	101,637–	818,031–		262,057–	76
	Account Total		1,080,088–	101,637–	818,031–		262,057–	76

Source: Courtesy University of South Alabama Medical Center, Mobile, Alabama. Reprinted with permission.

Exhibit 10–23 Accounting System Report

Computer Date _____
Time of Day _____
PGM = AM095-B1

Summary report in whole dollars for fiscal year ending _____
Distribution code = 750

SubCode	Description	Budgets		Actual			Open Commitments	Balance Available	Percent Used
		Original	Revised	Current Month	Fiscal Year	Project Year			
001	Prior Year Balance		302,976					302,978	0
002	Transfers								0
010	Income	16,419,272–	16,419,272–	1,342,529–	13,782,618–	13,782,618–		2,636,654–	84
020	Income			13,078–	127,981–	127,981–		127,981	0
023	Interest Income			1,353–	11,022–	11,022–		11,022	0
025	Original Budget	600,000–	600,000–	77,740–	1,236,565–	1,236,565–		636,565	206
026				191–	210–	210–		210	0
028	Bad Debt Recovery				169,932	169,932		169,932–	0
030									0
040	Inpatient Revenue			1,852–	29,682–	29,682–		29,682	0
041	Outpatient RF								0
042	Outpatient ED								0
050	Ded/Gross Revenue	75,009,000	75,009,000	8,904,127	72,586,402	72,586,402		2,422,598	97
099	State Paid Benefits								0
	Total Revenues	57,989,728	58,292,706	7,467,383	57,568,256	57,568,256		724,450	99
100	Pool—Salary & Wages	1,416,748							
110	Exec & Adm Salaries		82,157					82,157	0
120	Instruction Salaries		170,518	23,443	170,518	170,518			100
130	Professional Salary		210,392	15,839	210,592	210,592			0
131	Interns Salaries							200–	100
135	Tech Salary & Wages		11,906	1,195	11,906	11,906			100
140	Office Salaries		840,893	79,028	840,893	843,866		2,973–	100

Exhibit 10–23 Accounting System Report *(Continued)*

SubCode	Description	Budgets		Actual			Open Commitments	Balance Available	Percent Used
		Original	Revised	Current Month	Fiscal Year	Project Year			
150	Craft/Trade Wages				143	808		808–	0
155	Service Empl Wages					154		154–	0
159	Temp Craft/Trade Wge					2,431		2,431–	0
160	Student Wages		20,975	2,678	20,975	20,975			100
164									0
166	Accrued Salaries		41,158	10,264	41,158	41,158			100
167									0
168	Tuition Reimbursement		6,971	2,756	6,971	6,971			100
169	Budget Correction								0
	Salaries	1,416,748	1,384,969	135,202	1,303,156	1,309,378		75,591	95
170	Pool—Empl Benefits	340,007	116,982					116,982	0
180	Employee Benefits	187,747	205,413	3,318	421,300	421,300		215,888–	205
181	Unemployment Ins	41,307	41,307	7,722	22,717	22,717		18,590	55
182	Employers FICA	266	266	54	266	1,871		1,605–	703
183	Group Life Ins	91,969–	91,969–	435	91,969–	91,967–		3–	100
184	Disability Ins	9,090	9,090	1,015	9,106	9,110		20–	100
185	Teachers Retirement								100
186	Meal Books	4	4		4	4			0
187	TIAA-CREF Retirement	2,068	2,068	259	2,068	2,068			100
188	Group Health Ins	96,262	96,262	12,650	116,322	116,342		20,080–	121
190	Tuition Reimbursement	56,911	56,911	7,955	49,916	49,916		6,996	88

Source: Courtesy University of South Alabama Medical Center, Mobile, Alabama. Reprinted with permission.

Exhibit 10–24 Accounting System Report

Computer Date _____
Time of Day _____
PGM = AM095-B1

Subcode summary audit report for fiscal year ending _____
Distribution code = 750

Subcode	Subcode Description	Original Budget	Revised Budget	Current Month	Year to Date	Project to Date	Open Commitments	Balance Available
001								
364100	General Hospital Fnd	0.00	30,653.57	0.00	0.00	0.00	0.00	30,653.57
364105	Burn Unit	0.00	22,495.81	0.00	0.00	0.00	0.00	22,495.81
364110	Intensv Care Nursery	0.00	4,438.37	0.00	0.00	0.00	0.00	4,438.37
364120	J Erwin Ped Surgery	0.00	942.96–	0.00	0.00	0.00	0.00	942.96–
364127	Heart Statn—Holters	0.00	14,205.00	0.00	0.00	0.00	0.00	14,205.00
364173	Helping Hands/3&4 Fl	0.00	3,618.70	0.00	0.00	0.00	0.00	3,618.70
364174	Telethon—C&W USAMC	0.00	32,797.51	0.00	0.00	0.00	0.00	32,797.51
364175	Heart Fund Donations	0.00	864.10	0.00	0.00	0.00	0.00	864.10
364176	Telethon—C&W	0.00	71,327.96	0.00	0.00	0.00	0.00	71,827.96
364178	WOCD/Palmer Mem Fund	0.00	1,403.81	0.00	0.00	0.00	0.00	1,403.81
364179	Telethon—C&W	0.00	122,923.92	0.00	0.00	0.00	0.00	122,923.92
364197	Payroll Inserter	0.00	1,308.00–	0.00	0.00	0.00	0.00	1,308.00–
	Subcode Total	0.00	302,977.79	0.00	0.00	0.00	0.00	302,977.79

Source: University of South Alabama Medical Center, Mobile, Alabama. Reprinted with permission.

Exhibit 10–25 Accounting System Report

Time of Day _____
PGM = AM047-H1

Responsibility roll-up report as of fiscal year ending _____
Revenue

Cost-Center 9-82301
Reports to: 9-81000

Responsibility Units	Budgets		Actual			Open Commitments C	Balance Available A–B–C	Percent Used (B + C)/A
	Original	Revised A	Current Month	Fiscal Year	Project Year B			
Responsibility Units								
Cardiovas Rehab	790–	790–		869–	869–		79	110
Revenue-Enter Thpy	3,968–	3,968–	2,960–	39,582–	39,582–		35,614	997
Chemothrapy-O/P Revn	90,729–	90,729–	15,107–	110,452–	110,452–		19,723	121
Clinical Research Un	268,800–	482,051–	34,340–	346,521–	346,521–		135,530–	71
Cardiac ICU	1,524,600–	3,254,816–	252,996–	2,426,084–	2,426,084–		828,732–	74
Orthopedic Cast Room	108,459–	108,459–	8,128–	91,765–	91,765–		16,696–	84
5th Floor North/Reve	31,592–	31,592–	4,013–	39,076–	39,076–		7,484	123
5th Floor South/Reve	2,054,000–	2,977,320–	236,359–	2,331,656–	2,331,656–		645,664–	78
Psychiatric Unit/Rev	1,701,300–	1,725,507–	137,906–	1,463,792–	1,463,792–		261,715–	84
8th Flr Medical/Reve	2,315,220–	2,959,584–	216,324–	2,456,181–	2,456,181–		503,403–	82
Medical ICU/Revenue	1,773,840–	2,853,928–	244,778–	2,232,035–	2,232,035–		621,893–	78
Coronary Care/Revenu	2,148,888–	2,148,888–	167,130–	1,801,879–	1,801,879–		347,010–	83
6th Flr Surgical/Rev	1,787,100–	2,409,563–	172,079–	1,930,916–	1,930,916–		478,648–	80
Burn Center/Revenue	1,254,000–	3,090,809–	193,436–	2,155,646–	2,155,646–		935,163–	69
9th Flr Surgical/Rev	2,029,260–	3,122,028–	230,728–	2,446,790–	2,446,790–		675,238–	78
Neuro/Trauma ICU/Rev	1,504,800–	1,504,800–	111,100–	1,035,650–	1,035,650–		469,150–	68
Newborn Nursery/Reve	804,600–	896,817–	87,603–	794,535–	794,535–		102,282–	88
Premature Nursy/Reve	615,672–	615,672–	71,803–	596,432–	596,432–		19,240–	96
Neonatal Nursy/Reven	4,692,600–	5,468,373–	580,112–	5,178,067–	5,178,067–		290,306–	94
Obstetric Unit/Reven	1,930,440–	2,379,997–	217,489–	2,091,217–	2,091,217–		288,781–	87
Pediatric Unit/Reven	1,438,080–	2,013,282–	171,673–	1,658,513–	1,658,513–		354,769–	82
Pediatric ICU/Revenu	1,141,800–	1,915,268–	115,489–	1,208,778–	1,208,778–		706,490–	63
Delivery Room/Reven	3,396,552–	3,396,552–	410,192–	3,553,291–	3,553,291–		156,738	104
Emergency Room	4,922,867–	4,922,867–	446,310–	4,716,353–	4,716,353–		206,514–	95
Total	37,539,957–	48,373,660–	4,128,055–	40,706,080–	40,706,080–		7,667,586–	84

(Continued)

Exhibit 10–25 Accounting System Report *(Continued)*

| | Budgets | | Actual | | | Open Commitments | Balance Available | Percent Used |
	Original	Revised A	Current Month	Fiscal Year	Project Year B	C	A–B–C	(B + C)/A
Rev/Exp by Fund								
Operating Revenues	37,539,957–	48,373,660–	4,128,055–	40,706,080–	40,706,080–		7,667,586–	84
Total	37,539,957–	48,373,660–	4,128,055–	40,706,080–	40,706,080–		7,667,586–	84
Rev/Exp by Type								
Revenues	37,539,957	48,373,660	4,128,055	40,706,080	40,706,080		7,667,586	84
Expenses								
Salaries								
Employee Benefits								
Med/Sur Supply								
Office/Other Suply								
Travel/Entertain								
Other Expenses								
Minor Equipment								
Cost Offsets								
Total Expenses								

Source: Courtesy University of South Alabama Medical Center, Mobile, Alabama. Reprinted with permission.

Exhibit 10–26 Accounting System Report

Responsibility roll-up report as of fiscal year ending _____
Expense

| Responsibility Units | Budgets | | Actual | | | Open Commitments | Balance Available | Percent Used |
	Original	Revised A	Current Month	Fiscal Year	Project Year B	C	A–B–C	(B + C)/A
Medical Nursing	1,446,644	1,561,207	153,176	1,496,785	1,496,785	751	63,671	95
Psychiatric Nursing	659,186	661,552	63,520	590,664	590,664	566	70,323	89
Staff Development	274,449	274,748	17,680	295,828	295,828	2	21,082–	107
Nursing Svcs-Admin	869,036	880,078	91,347	779,791	779,791	6,242	94,044	89
Clinical Resch Unit	211,846	222,854	17,962	250,545	250,545	16	27,707–	112
Cardiac ICU	429,808	429,807	3,424	53,440	53,440		376,367	12
Float Nurses Pool			110	2,589	2,589		2,589–	
Orthopedic Cast Room	27,195	27,196		12,461	12,461	1,172	13,563	50
Employee Health Nurs	155,423	155,423	18,779	149,601	149,601	5	5,817	96
9th Floor-North	527,221	527,222	46,442	496,133	496,133	98	30,991	94
9th Floor-South	521,411	521,412	40,785	461,240	461,240	2	60,170	88
8th Floor-Medical	810,508	894,965	109,696	1,131,504	1,131,504	1,557	238,095–	126
5th Floor-Shrd Supp	66,529	157,455	25,770	185,295	185,295	862	28,702–	118
Burn Center	546,449	940,030	77,567	836,022	836,022	3,353	100,656	89
6th Floor-Surgical	1,222,187	1,363,087	117,908	1,278,709	1,278,709	2,101	82,276	93
Surgical ICU	1,074,332	1,332,394	138,564	1,309,157	1,309,157	338	22,899	98
7th Floor-Shrd Supp	626,522	696,032	72,802	833,026	833,026	787	137,781–	119
Newborn Nursery	667,925	939,910	81,197	892,992	892,992	868	46,051	95
Intermediate Nursery	236,612							
Intensive Care Nursy	1,810,927	1,944,960	202,179	1,749,864	1,749,864	1,241	193,856	90
Obstetric Unit	628,047	668,254	64,748	632,055	632,055	226	35,974	94
Pediatric Unit	923,577	998,643	91,105	895,375	895,375	263	103,005	89
Pediatric ICU	560,288	645,410	48,874	568,314	568,314	50	77,045	88
Delivery Room	1,113,286	1,208,604	134,770	1,107,944	1,107,944	20,154	80,506	93

(Continued)

Exhibit 10–26 Accounting System Report *(Continued)*

	Budgets		Actual			Open Commitments	Balance Available	Percent Used
	Original	Revised A	Current Month	Fiscal Year	Project Year B	C	A–B–C	(B + C)/A
Emergency Room	1,613,253	1,691,149	160,935	1,524,713	1,524,713	13,885	152,550	90
Patient Transport	220,377	220,377	18,889	186,146	186,146	40	34,191	84
Total	17,243,038	18,962,769	1,798,229	17,720,193	17,720,193	54,579	1,187,999	93
Rev/Exp by Fund								
Nursing Division	17,060,420	18,750,317	1,771,862	17,527,171	17,527,171	53,402	1,169,746	93
Professional Division	27,195	57,029	7,588	43,421	43,421	1,172	12,436	78
Administrative Divis	155,423	155,423	18,779	149,601	149,601	5	5,817	96
Total	17,243,038	18,962,769	1,798,229	17,720,193	17,720,193	54,579	1,187,999	93
Rev/Exp by Type								
Revenues								
Expenses								
Salaries	12,382,495	12,461,654	1,256,095	12,391,869	12,391,869		69,785	99
Employee Benefits	3,031,241	3,033,250	239,363	2,487,863	2,487,863		545,387	82
Med/Sur Supply	1,502,492	3,020,154	262,420	2,447,985	2,447,985	30,781	541,387	82
Office/Other Suply		109,306	9,788	107,656	107,656	1,652		100
Travel/Entertain	43,989	45,788	2,209	27,555	27,555		18,233	60
Other Expenses	212,976	211,676	19,555	196,765	196,765	4,019	10,891	94
Minor Equipment	55,585	66,681	7,590	21,443	21,443	18,127	27,113	59
Cost Offsets	14,060	14,060	1,209	39,057	39,057		24,797–	273
Total Expenses	17,243,038	18,962,769	1,798,229	17,720,193	17,720,193	54,579	1,187,999	93
Net Revenue/Expense	17,243,038	18,962,769	1,798,229	17,720,193	17,720,193	54,579	1,187,999	93
Total	**17,243,038**	**18,962,769**	**1,798,229**	**17,720,193**	**17,720,193**	**54,579**	**1,187,999**	**93**

Source: Courtesy University of South Alabama Medical Center, Mobile, Alabama. Reprinted with permission.

Exhibit 10–27 Accounting System Report

Account statement in whole dollars for fiscal year ending _____

Computer Date _____

Time of Day _____

PGM = AM090-B1

83% of fiscal year elapsed

Distribution code = 700

Maternal Child Health

Education Fund

Acct: 3-64155

Dept: 64155

		Budgets		Actual				
Subcode	Description	Original	Revised	Current Month	Fiscal Year	Open Encumbrances	Balance Available	Percent Used
001	Prior Year Balance		3,624				3,624	0
020	Income				5,285–		5,285	***
021	Refunds				55–		55–	***
	Total Revenues		3,624		5,230–		8,854	144–
224	Recreation Supplies				60		60–	***
231	Postage				60		60–	***
234	Printing				257		257–	***
	General Supplies				377		377–	***
311	Travel			459	1,463		1,463–	***
314	Local Travel				27		27–	***
316	Workshop & Training			3,338	3,498	2,500	5,998–	***
	Travel/Entertainment			3,796	4,989	2,500	7,489–	***
422	Honorarium				425		425–	***
450	Expense Offset				1,000–		1,000	***
	Total Expenses			3,796	4,790	2,500	7,290–	***
	Account Total		3,624	3,796	440–	2,500	1,563	57

Open Encumbrance Status

Account	P.O. Number	P.O. Date	Description	Original Enc	Liquidating Expenditures	Adjustments	Current Enc	Last Act Date
3-64155-316	H04118	01/26/XX	Perdido Hilton Hotel	2,500			2,500	03/22/XX
			Account Total	2,500			2,500	

Source: Reprinted with permission of University of South Alabama Medical Center, Mobile, Alabama.

Exhibit 10–28 Accounting System Report

Computer Date _____
Time of Day _____
PGM = AM090

Report of transactions for fiscal year ending _____
Distribution code = 700
Maternal Child Health Education Fund

Acct: 3-64155
Dept: 64155

Subcode	Description	Date	EC	Ref.	2nd Ref.	J.E. Offset Account	Budget Entries	Current Rev/Exp	Encumbrances	Batch Ref.	Date
311	Dorothy May	07/11	48		218418			458.65		HPC804	07/11
311	CM Total Travel							458.65			
316	Perdido Beach Hilton	07/19	48		220893			3,337.73		HPC832	07/19
316	CM Total Workshop & Training							3,337.73			
	Account Total							3,796.38			

Source: Courtesy University of South Alabama Medical Center, Mobile, Alabama. Reprinted with permission.

Rollover funds, designated by prefix 3, are also included in the financial reports that can be provided to the chief nurse executive and nurse managers. Balances in these funds are carried over into the next fiscal year to be spent at any future date. An example of a rollover fund is account 3-64155, the maternal child health education fund. Exhibit 10–27 shows activities for this fund for the month, and Exhibit 10–28 shows how the debits were spent. Rollover funds can be managed by the chief nurse executive, a department head, or a cost-center manager.

Exercise 10–7	Examine the system used for monitoring the budget for a cost center in the agency in which you work or are assigned as a student. Where is the cost-center manager overspending or underspending? Determine why.

MOTIVATIONAL ASPECTS OF BUDGETING

Budgeting can be a motivating force for personnel if current programs must increase in effectiveness and efficiency to remain, if decentralization and staff involvement provides an increased sense of responsibility and satisfaction, and if merit increases, promotions, and bonuses are tied or linked to budgetary performance.

Budgeting facilitates communication within interdependent departments, thus increasing knowledge and understanding of other areas. It provides learning opportunities for future nurse managers.

CUTTING THE BUDGET

When the budget has to be cut, planning is a vital aspect of the process. This is happening today as hospital admissions and stays decrease and reimbursement takes on a new character. The form and the process of nursing management can determine the course of events when the budget has to be cut.

A nursing administration that delegates decision making to the lowest level and encourages participative management is an effective administration. When clinical nurses are informed at the unit level and invited to offer their input, they can help with suggestions for cutting costs. They will gladly implement and support the activities they recognize as resulting partly from their input. A nursing organization that promote self-direction at the clinical nurse level, nurse manager level, clinical consultant level, and executive nurse level will support direction to reduce cost and to increase productivity and profit. As an example, when a hospital CEO discovered that self-pay patient care was the only category not reviewed for use of resources, a review process was established by a clinical nurse. This process was supported by physicians and other health-care professionals.

Nursing budgets are enormous, with budgets for a single unit running into hundreds of thousands of dollars per year. Pay awards or increases have to be met by budget cuts (personnel cutbacks), use of less expensive supplies and techniques, or increased productivity. The latter requires more paying patients, shorter stays, and increased sales of all paying services. When personnel cuts are to be made, numbers make nursing vulnerable. Some cuts can come from all services, but nursing has greater numbers. The nurse manager who controls these numbers daily, weekly, and yearly has greater credibility. Many sources indicate that turnover is costly. The cost of turnover of personnel low on the salary scale is sometimes weighed against the higher cost of employees who are at the top of the salary scale. An assumption is made that long-time employees are better satisfied with their jobs and do better work, an assumption that needs to be validated through research.

As workload data indicate shifts from one unit to another, resources must be shifted. This can be done by asking for volunteers, moving vacated positions, and using PRN pools. A shift is taking place today from inpatient procedures in hospitals to outpatient procedures, either in hospitals or at ambulatory surgery centers. Also, many more diagnostic procedures are done on an outpatient basis. As a result, inpatients are often a sicker group, requiring more nursing care.

Because nurse administrators control multimillion-dollar budgets, they are powerful people. They are also vulnerable to personnel cuts. Much of this vulnerability stems from external controls imposed by the state and federal governments and health insurance companies. Power comes from the ability of nurse administrators to use knowledge and skills in defending, directing, and controlling their budgets. They learn to hold the line on staffing, on overtime, and on appropriate use for supplies and equipment.

WEB ACTIVITIES

- Visit www.jbpub.com/swansburg, this text's companion website on the Internet, for further information on Budgeting Basics.
- Search for offices of planning and budgeting on the Internet. What information can you find?
- Can you find separate sites that give examples of the stages of a budget?

SUMMARY

It is important for nurses to have a working knowledge of the objectives of budgeting and of component costs. Every activity that takes place in a health-care agency costs money. There must be a standard for assigning costs to user departments. The nursing department should pay its user share and no more. Knowledge of the cost accounting system will provide accurate information for budgeting and for cost management.

Efficient nurse managers use a budget calendar that covers formulation, review and enactment, and execution stages of the total budget process.

Major elements of nursing budgets include those for personnel, supplies and equipment (minor), and capital equipment. Generally, equipment costing below a fixed dollar amount are included in the supplies and equipment budget. A product evaluation committee is a useful process for assuring that supplies and equipment will promote effective and efficient patient care. The capital equipment budget includes equipment costing above a fixed dollar amount. It is prepared separate from the supplies and equipment budget.

Evaluation is an administrative aspect of budgeting that in itself serves as a controlling process. Decentralization vests control at the lowest competent level of decision making. Good budget feedback is essential if the budget is to be an effective controlling process. This includes information about revenues and expenses and internal comparisons of projected and actual budgets. The budget can motivate professional nurses to facilitate their development of innovations.

The belief of nurses that budgets are beyond comprehension can effectively sabotage the nurses' effectiveness. Spiraling health-care costs, cost-management efforts, and increasing accountability from individual cost centers should serve as an impetus for nurses to learn at least the fundamentals of budgets and the budget process. To assume the responsibility of budget work increases the nurse's potential realm of planning, predicting, and reviewing programs within the nurse's jurisdiction.

Similar to a nursing care plan, the budget is an activity guidance tool. It is a plan expressed in monetary terms, carried out within a time frame. To be an effective caregiver, the nurse knows how to develop and use a nursing care plan. Similarly, to be most effective as a manager, the nurse manager knows how to develop and use a budget.

Exercise 10–8   Every hospital prepares the *Hospital and Hospital Health Care Complex Cost Report Certification and Settlement Summary,* commonly known as the Medicare Cost Report. Obtain the latest copy for your employing or clinical experience hospital. Select a nursing cost center and complete Exhibit 10–29, "Preparing a Budget for a Unit or Project."

This exercise has acquainted you with the Medicare Cost Report. You can use projected medical inflation rates to prepare a budget for the following year. If they are projected to be 8 percent, multiply all costs by 1.08 to project and budget costs. You will note that intensive care units are budgeted separately. All other inpatient units are grouped as "Adults and Pediatrics (General and Routine Care)." To separate these units for revenue and expenditures, make the following calculations:

1. Select a patient-care unit of a hospital.
2. Determine the number of patient days of occupancy for this unit (from the biometric records): _____

(continued)

Exhibit 10–29   Preparing a Budget for a Unit or Project

Unit _____ Revenue Center Number _____

Direct Expenses (Directly Assigned)
   Salaries (attach position questionnaire for new ones) $_____._____
   Employee benefits $_____._____
   Personnel services $_____._____
   Supplies $_____._____
   Other $_____._____

Total Direct $_____._____

Indirect Expenses
   Depreciation of capital buildings and fixtures $_____._____
   Capital equipment (movable) $_____._____
     (attach requests for new items) $_____._____
   Worker's compensation $_____._____
   Life insurance $_____._____
   Communications $_____._____
   Data processing $_____._____
   Purchasing $_____._____
   Admitting $_____._____
   Patient accounts $_____._____
   General administration $_____._____
   Plant operations $_____._____
   Biomedical $_____._____
   Laundry $_____._____
   Housekeeping $_____._____
   Nursing administration $_____._____
   Patient transport $_____._____
   Preparation $_____._____
   Central supply $_____._____
   Pharmacy $_____._____
   College of nursing (or other college) $_____._____
   Interns and residents $_____._____
   Other $_____._____

Total Indirect $_____._____

Total Costs (Direct + Indirect) $_____._____
Total Charges or Revenues $_____._____
Cost-to-Charge Ratio (Divide total costs
   by total charges or revenues.) $_____._____
   divided by $_____._____
   minus $_____._____
   or _____%

Exercise 10–8
(continued)

3. From the Medicare Cost Report determine
  a. Total direct and indirect costs $_____
  b. Total patient days _____
4. Divide total direct and indirect costs $ _____ by total
  patient days _____ = $ _____ cost per
  patient day
5. Patient days for unit (from no. 3b) _____ × cost per patient
  day (from no. 4) _____ = $_____, or approxi-
  mate expenses for the nursing unit for this year.

Exercise 10–9

Exhibit 10–28 is an excerpt from a prime source document—an operational or
management plan for achieving the objectives for a social services department. Using this management plan format, construct a prime source document that budgets an objective for a nursing division, department, service, or
unit.

NOTES

1. R. W. Johnson and R. W. Melicher, *Financial Planning* (Boston: Allyn & Bacon, 1982).
2. J. D. Baker, "The Operating Expense Budget, One Part of a Manager's Arsenal," *AORN Journal* 54, no. 4 (1991): 837–841; S. Klann, "Mastering the OR Budgeting Process Is Key to Success," *OR Manager,* October 1989, 10–11.
3. D. Osborne and T. Gaebler, *Reinventing Government* (New York: Plume, 1992), 237, 241.
4. J. N. Althaus, N. M. Hardyck, P. B. Pierce, and M. S. Rodgers, *Nursing Decentral- ization: The El Camino Experience* (Gaithersburg, Md.: 1981); G. R. Whitman, "Analyzing and Forecasting Budgets," in *Management Issues in Critical Care,* ed. C. Birdsall (St. Louis, Mo.: Mosby, 1991), 287–307.
5. D. Osborne and T. Gaebler, op. cit., 3.
6. R. N. Anthony and D. W. Young, *Management Control in Nonprofit Organizations,* 4th ed. (Chicago: Irwin, 1988).
7. S. Klann, op. cit.
8. B. Huttman, "Taking Charge: Selling Your Budget," *RN,* April 1964, 25–26.
9. G. J. Talbot, "Key for Successful Program Budgeting," *Journal of Continuing Edu- cation in Nursing* 14, no. 3 (1983): 8–10.
10. A. G. Herkimer, Jr., *Understanding Hospital Financial Management* (Rockville, Md.: Aspen, 1978), 132.
11. R. P. Covert, "Expense Budgeting," in *Handbook of Health Care Accounting and Finance,* ed. W. O. Cleverly (Rockville, Md.: Aspen, 1982), 261–278.
12. J. Buchan, "Cost-Effective Caring," *International Nursing Review* 39, no. 4 (1992): 117–120.
13. G. J. Talbot, op. cit.
14. R. K. Campbell, "Understanding the Management Process and Financial and Man- agerial Accounting," Part IV. "Cash Flow Analysis and Budgeting," *Diabetes Educa- tion,* February-March 1989, 126–127, 129.

15. "Planning Your Replacement Budget," *Journal of Nursing Administration,* November 1990, 3, 17, 24.
16. M. Dickerson, "Product Evaluation: A Strategy for Controlling a Supply and Equipment Budget," In Patients and Purse Strings, ed. H. C. Scherubel (New York, National League for Nursing, 1988). NLN Publication #20-2192, 2, 465–468.
17. C. Tokarsi, "Creative Proposal Plays to Tough Crowd," *Modern Health Care,* 4 March 1991, 53–56.
18. B. Aronsohn and N. Deal, "Navigating the Maze of Capital Equipment Acquisition," *Nursing Management,* November 1992, 46–48.
19. P. N. Palmer, "Why Hide the Revenue Produced by Perioperative Nursing Care?" *AORN Journal,* June 1984, 1122–1123.
20. In business and industry, bad debts are considered an expense of doing business. In hospitals, bad debt is subtracted from revenue. It becomes a reduction of revenue rather than a cost of doing business. Profit or return on equity is not allowed by Medicare or Medicaid except for for-profit hospitals. A few third-party payers allow a return on equity.
21. G. R. McGrail, "Budgets: An Underused Resource," *Journal of Nursing Administration,"* November 1988, 25–31.

MANAGING A CLINICAL PRACTICE DISCIPLINE

OBJECTIVES

▪ Discuss the use of nursing theory.
▪ Discuss differences among the modalities of nursing practice, including functional nursing, team nursing, primary nursing, case method, joint practice, and case management.
▪ Identify selected ethical concerns and ethical issues and make plans for resolving them.
▪ Confirm the assessment of cultural needs in patient assessment.

KEY CONCEPTS

nursing theory
nursing modality
functional nursing
team nursing
primary nursing
case method
joint practice
case management
autonomy
nonmalficence
beneficence
justice
advance directives

Manager behavior: Uses effective human resource policies and procedures to manage a group of clinical nursing personnel to achieve the outcomes of the nursing process.

Leader behavior: Supports the application of a theory of nursing by a group of nursing personnel. Provides a conduit for ethical deliberations by nursing personnel. Furthers the inclusion of cultural needs assessment of individual patients.

INTRODUCTION

Nursing is a clinical practice discipline. Professional nurses want autonomy in their own practice. They want to apply their nursing knowledge and skills without interference from nurse managers, physicians, or persons in other disciplines. The effective nurse manager trusts the professional nurse to apply knowledge and skills correctly in caring for a group of patients. In turn, the clinical nurse trusts the nurse manager to coordinate supplies, equipment, and support systems with personnel of other departments. Clinical nurses trust a human relations management in which they participate rather than one in which they have rules and regulations imposed upon them. They use the body of nursing knowledge (theory) gained in nursing school and maintained through continuing education and staff development to practice nursing as they determine it should be practiced. In doing so, they adhere to management policies regarding such things as documentation or quality improvement, because these requirements are also part of clinical nursing practice.

USE OF NURSING THEORY

In developing nursing as a scientific discipline, nursing educators and researchers have developed theoretical frameworks for the clinical practice of nursing that are used by clinical nurses as models for testing and validating applications of nursing knowledge and skills. The results are added to the body of knowledge commonly called the theory of nursing. Theory gives practicing nurses professional identity. It is based on scientific inquiry: nursing research. Each result of nursing research adds tested facts to nursing theory that can be learned by nursing students and active practitioners.

Models and Examples

Models are frequently used in the development of nursing theory. A model usually communicates in graphic format an abstract entity, structure, or process that cannot be directly observed. Models depict behavioral processes that cannot be directly observed except as indirect behaviors of those engaged in the process. They order, clarify, and systematize selected components of the phenomenon they serve to depict. Models illustrate and clarify theories. Because nursing theories have not been widely applied, they are frequently described as models.[1]

Orem's and Kinlein's Theories.   Dickson and Lee-Villasenor report testing of Orem's self-care nursing theory as modified by Kinlein. As independent generalist nurses, they did their research in a private nursing practice setting. They used grounded theory methodology to systematically obtain and analyze data from clients. As the clients spoke, the researchers recorded data, identifying self-care assets, self-care demand, and self-care measures with their clients.

In performing a content analysis, Dickson and Lee-Villasenor classified events as expressions of need, self-care assets, self-care demands, and self-care measures. They catalogued events by numbers of expressions of need—a perception of self, an action taken, a want, a wish, or a question—and by perception of self according to mind-body combinations. Events were also catalogued according to evidence of patterns of self-care actions that contributed positively to a client's state of health and number of self-care assets: action, motivation, knowledge, and potential.[2]

Roy's Theory.   Roy advocates adaptation-level theory to nursing intervention. She notes that a person adapts to the environment through four modes: physiologic needs and processes, self-concept (beliefs and feelings about oneself), role mastery (behavior among people who each occupy a different position within society), and interdependence (giving and receiving nurturance).[3] Just as the individual patient adapts to changes in the environment, so does the nursing worker.

According to Roy, the goal of nursing is to assist the patient to adapt to illness so as to be able to respond to other stimuli. The patient is assessed for positive or negative behavior in the four adaptive modes. Once the assessment is made at the necessary (first or second) level, intervention is established by a nursing care plan of goals and approaches. The approach is selected to match the goal.[4] According to Mastal and Hammond, Roy's views are "that the developing body of nursing knowledge now contains verifiable theories and general laws related to: (1) persons as holistic beings, and (2) the role of nursing in promoting the person's maximum potential health and harmonious interaction with the environment."[5]

Frederickson illustrates application of the Roy adaptation model to the nursing diagnosis of anxiety. He describes or defines anxiety from the nursing perspective as exhibited by "poor nutritional status, reduction in unusual physical activity, and lowered self-esteem, in addition to concern for job security." The nurse diagnoses the symptoms of anxiety through assessment via the four modes and then designs and implements intervention that promotes client adaptation.[6]

Evaluation criteria for empirical testing of nursing theory were developed by Silva and expanded by others. Theory testing includes processes to verify whether what was purported or experienced is true or solves problems in one's discipline or practice. Silva and Sorrell define nursing theory as "a tentative body of diverse but purposeful, creative, and logically interrelated perspectives that help nurses to redefine nursing and to understand, explain, raise questions about, and seek clarification of nursing phenomena in their research and practice."[7] They list three alternative approaches of testing to verify nursing theory:

1. Through critical reasoning.
2. Through description of personal experiences.
3. Through application to nursing practice. (This concept has been applied at the National Hospital for Orthopedics and Rehabilitation, Arlington, Virginia, where the Roy Adaptation Model has been implemented throughout the hospital.)

Newman's Theory.   Engle tested Margaret Newman's conceptual framework of health in a sample of older women. She indicates that Newman uses Rogers's concept of the life process and the relationship of the individual within the environment. In this model, aging is considered a natural process, the person's individual state being a fusion of health and disease. Movement is a correlation of health measured by a basic time factor and tempo.[8] Engle indicates tempo to be the characteristic rate of performing a task. Time is the second correlation of health. Tempo and time occur in a succession of events, rhythmic patterns of temperatures and movement, and patterns within the environment. Time perception and tempo are hypothesized to be altered by age and illness. The patient does self-assessment of his or her health as a criterion measure. Self-assessment and physician assessment of health have been shown to correlate. Self-assessment of health is altered by ability to perform everyday activities, by age self-concept, and by movement and time.[9]

In her study, Engle measured personal tempo, time perception, and self-assessment of health by using the Cantril ladder in 114 females age 60 or older. She found no age effect for time perception in this study, nor did Newman and Tompkins in similar studies. Nor was there any age effect for personal tempo.[10]

A significant relationship existed between time perception and personal tempo that could have significance for the patient and the clinical nurse. The patient or nurse with a physical or mental condition that alters personal tempo may have an altered perception of time. This could be true in older nurses in whom physical and mental states are more often altered. Further research in this area is needed, particularly as the population ages.

Levine's Theory. Levine indicates that nursing practice has mirrored prevailing theories of health and disease. Nursing has created an environment for healing: cleanliness, safety, and physical and emotional comfort. Nursing enhances the reparative process. It became disease-oriented when diseases, not patients, were the focus of treatment. As nurses became concerned with the multiple factors impacting the course of disease, they developed the total-patient-care concept.[11]

People respond to illness in individual ways. Nursing intervention should match the individual response, which is identified from observation and data analysis. Assessment reveals unique needs requiring unique nursing measures. Nursing supports repair and maintenance of a person's integrated self-homeostasis and equilibrium. Equilibrium is maintained by adaptation. The nurse intervenes to support successful adaptation to achieve a therapeutic or supportive role.[12]

Johnson's Theory. The Johnson behavioral system model is a theory of nursing practice. Johnson incorporated the nursing process (assessment, planning-diagnosis, intervention, and evaluation) into a general systems model. Rawls applied it to care of a patient for the purpose of testing, evaluating, and determining its utility for predicting the effect of nursing care on a patient. Rawls indicates that the model has disadvantages but is a tool that can be used "to accurately predict the results of nursing interventions prior to care, formulate standards of care, and most importantly administer truly holistic empathic nursing care."[13]

Derdiarian sampled 223 cancer patients to verify the relationship among the eight subsystems of Johnson's behavioral system model. These eight subsystems (aggressive/protective, sexual, eliminative, ingestive, achievement, dependence, affiliative, and restorative) function through behavior to meet a person's demands (see Exhibit 11–1). Illness disrupts and changes behavior sustained in the subsystems, resulting in negative effects on the behavioral systems. Changes in one subsystem initiate changes in others. Findings of this research indicated "fairly large, statistically significant ($P<.001$) direct relationships between the aggressive/protective subsystems and each of the other subsystems." The research presents a model for continued research of Johnson's behavioral system model with "implications for comprehensive assessment, early intervention, prevention of patients' potential problems, and ultimately for efficient care."[14]

Exhibit 11–1   Elements of the Eight Subsystems

Drives	Goals
Aggressive/Protective	Protection of person, property, ideas, beliefs, and emotional and cognitive well-being
Sexual	Demand for libido, relief of sexual tension, and procreation
Eliminative	Expulsion of biologic wastes
Ingestive	Satisfaction of hunger, thirst
Achievement	Ego gratification, mastery
Dependence	Succor
Affiliative	Belonging
Restorative	Relief of fatigue

Source: Compiled from A. K. Derdiarian, "The Relationships Among the Subsystems of Johnson's Behavioral System Model," *Image,* Winter 1990, 219–225. Reprinted with permission.

Peplau's Theory.   Peplau's theory defines nursing as a "significant, therapeutic, interpersonal process."[15] Peplau's theory involves such concepts as communication techniques, assessment, definition of problems and goals, direction, and role clarification.

Peplau states that four components make up the main elements of the nurse-patient relationship: nurse, patient, professional expertise, and client need. The nurse-patient relationship has three phases: the orientation phase, the working phase, and the resolution phase. During encounters with patients, the nurse observes, interprets what she or he observes, and then decides what needs to be done. Interpersonal relations uses the theoretical constructs of concepts, processes, and patterns:

- A *concept* is a small, circumscribed set of behaviors pertaining to a particular phenomenon, such as conflict.
- A *process* is more complicated—more comprehensive and lasting longer.
- A *pattern* is made up of separate acts that may have variations but share the same theme, aim, or intention.

Interpersonal theory is especially useful in psychiatric nursing and is useful in relation to psychosocial problems and nurse-patient relationships in all clinical areas of nursing. The joint effort of the nurse-patient relationship "includes identification of the presenting problems, understanding the problems and their variation in pattern, and appreciating, applying, and testing remedial measures in order to produce beneficial outcomes for patients."[16]

Orlando's Theory.   Orlando's theory of nursing develops three basic concepts:

1. Professional nursing has as its function the identification and meeting of patients' immediate needs for help.

2. Professional nursing has as its outcome or product both verbal and nonverbal improvement in the patient's behavior.
3. Regardless of its form, the patient's presenting or initial behavior may be a plea for help.

Schmieding applied Orlando's theory to solving problems in managing the behavior of clinical nurses. She recommends that the work of one theorist be used as the practice model within a given organization. This application of Orlando's model has helped nurses apply common concepts and a framework for nursing. The model could be adapted if the nursing staff synthesized the concepts of several theories.[17]

Other Theories.   Wiens presents Meyer's model of patient autonomy in care as a theoretical framework for nursing (see Exhibit 11–2). With laws for advance directives and increased emphasis on patients' rights, the right to patient self-determination has increasing implications for care providers. Historically, patients have been perceived by providers to be dependent and compliant.

Exhibit 11–2   Patient Control in the Nurse-Patient Relationship

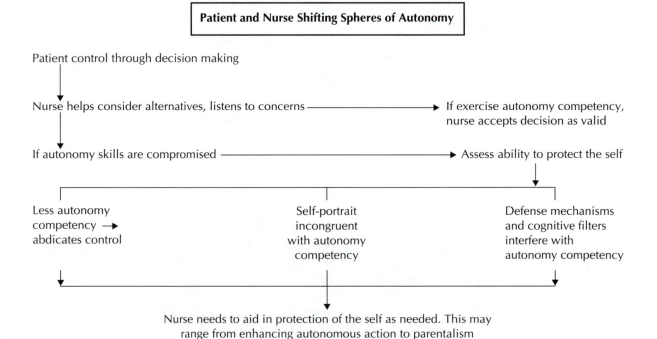

Source: A. G. Wiens, "Patient Autonomy in Care: A Theoretical Framework for Nursing," *Journal of Professional Nursing*, March/April 1993, 102. Reprinted with permission.

Autonomy competency includes a repertory of the following skills or abilities that contribute to an individual's life plan of value, emotional ties, and personal ideals:

- Self-reference, where a person recognizes his or her response to life situations.
- Self-direction, where a person expresses himself or herself in ways considered fitting and worthy of self.
- Self-definition, where a person knows and acts as his or her true self.
- Self-discovery, where a person examines his or her socialization for self-understanding and future self-control.
- Self-portrait or self-concept.

Patients need to be encouraged to be autonomous, to ask questions and make decisions about their care. Nurses will have to change their nurse-patient relationships to accommodate autonomy competency in patients.

Illness decreases the patient's autonomy competency. To accomplish autonomy competency requires that patients be encouraged to make decisions regarding their care. Frequently, as patients become increasingly autonomy-competent, they are viewed as noncompliant troublemakers. Informed consent requires decision making and truth telling. In the case of truth telling, providers need to be kind and caring.[18]

Sociotechnical systems theory views an organization as an open and living system in interaction with the environment. The components of this system are social, technological, physical design, and work setting. The system produces products or services. Employers participate in designing and redesigning work and jobs to achieve a high-quality work life. More studies are needed to test the assumption that the work environment is important to care delivery.[19]

| Exercise 11–1 | Use your student group or form an ad hoc committee of nurses to plan for needed implementation of nursing theory in a nursing unit. Make a management plan. The following format may be used for all management plans. |

Management Plan

Problem:

Objective:

| Actions | Target Dates | Assigned To | Accomplishments |

MODALITIES OF NURSING PRACTICE

Several modalities or methods of nursing practice have evolved during the past fifty years, including functional nursing, team nursing, primary nursing, case method, joint practice, and case management. All are practiced in various forms in health-care institutions in the United States.

Functional Nursing

Functional nursing is the oldest nursing practice modality. It can best be described as a task-oriented method in which a particular nursing function is assigned to each staff member. One registered nurse is responsible for administering medications, one for treatments, one for managing intravenous administration; one licensed practical nurse is assigned admissions and discharges, another gives bed baths; a nurse's aide makes beds and passes meal trays. No nurse is responsible for total care of any patient. The method divides the tasks to be done, with each person being responsible to the nurse manager. It is efficient and the best system for a nursing staff confronted with a large patient load and a shortage of professional nurses.

The advantage of functional nursing is that it accomplishes the most work in the shortest amount of time. Its disadvantages are that

- It fragments nursing care.
- It decreases the nurse's accountability and responsibility.
- It makes the nurse-client relationship difficult to establish, if it is ever achieved.
- It gives professional nursing low status in terms of responsibility for patient care.

Team Nursing

Team nursing developed in the early 1950s when various nursing leaders decided that a team approach could unify the different categories of nursing workers. Under the leadership of a professional nurse, a group of nurses work together to fulfill the full functions of professional nurses. Assignment of patients is made to a team consisting of a registered nurse as a team leader and other staff—RNs, LPNs, and aides—as team members. The team leader has the responsibility for coordinating the total care of a block of patients and is the leadership figure.

The intent of team nursing is to provide patient-centered care. The patient's nursing care needs are identified and met through nursing diagnosis and prescription. Ward clerks and unit managers perform the nonnursing functions of the unit. The process requires planning with the objective of taking nursing personnel to the bedside so that they can focus upon nursing care of patients.

Implementing team nursing requires study of the literature on the team plan, development of a philosophy of team nursing, planning for appropriate utilization of all categories of nursing workers, and planning for team conferences, nursing care plans, and development of team leadership. Exhibit 11–3 depicts schema for a team nursing organization, with team members performing different but coordinated roles in self-managed work teams. The following is a summary of the team plan:

> The team plan gives priorities to the development of leadership potential—leadership in the practice of nursing—leadership that is creative and that encourages improvement of communications among team members, patients, and leaders. It gives priority to emphasis on democratic leadership, the nurturing of cooperative effort and free expression of ideas of all team members. It gives priority to motivation of people to grow to this self-approved or maximum level of performance. Through the team plan the contributions of all team members in improving patient care are recognized. Priority is given to the strengthening of their weaknesses.
>
> Patient-centered care employs effective supervision and recognizes that personnel are the media by which the objectives are met in a cooperative effort between team leaders and team members. Through supervision the team leader identifies nursing care goals; identifies team members' needs; focuses on fulfilling goals and needs; motivates team members to grow as workers and citizens; guides team members to help set and meet high standards of patient care and job performance—all of them supporting the priority of *practicing nursing.*[20]

The advantages of team nursing are that

- It involves all team members in planning patients' nursing care through team conferences and written nursing care plans.
- It provides the best care at the lowest cost, according to some advocates.

Disadvantages of team nursing include the following:

- It can lead to fragmentation of care if the concept is not implemented totally.
- It can be difficult to find time for team conferences and care plans.
- It allows the RN who is the team leader to have the only significant responsibility and authority.

The disadvantages of team nursing can be overcome by educating competent team leaders in the principles of nursing team leadership.

Primary Nursing

Primary nursing is an extension of the principle of decentralization of authority with the primary authority for all decisions about the nursing process being centered in the person of the professional nurse. The primary nurse is assigned to care for the patient's total needs for the duration of the hospital stay. Responsibility covers a twenty-four-hour period, with associate nurses providing care when the primary nurse is not available. The care given is planned and prescribed totally by the primary nurse.

Marram, Schlegel, and Bevis state that "primary nursing . . . is the distribution of nursing so that the total care of an individual is the responsibility of one nurse, not many nurses."[21] They indicate autonomy to be the key to the

Exhibit 11–3   Team Nursing Organization

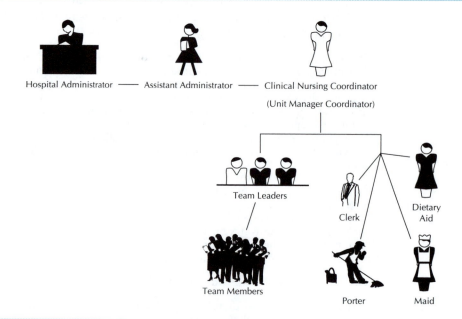

Hospital Administrator ——— Assistant Administrator ——— Clinical Nursing Coordinator

(Unit Manager Coordinator)

Team Leaders

Team Members

Clerk

Porter

Dietary Aid

Maid

development of professional nursing. The following are characteristics of the primary nursing modality:[22]

1. The primary nurse has responsibility for the nursing care of the patient 24 hours a day from admission through discharge.
2. Assessment of nursing care needs, collaboration with patient and other health professionals, and formulation of the plan of care are all in the hands of the primary nurse.
3. Execution of the nursing care plan is delegated by the primary nurse to a secondary nurse during other shifts.
4. The primary nurse consults with nurse managers.
5. Authority, accountability, and autonomy rest with the primary nurse.

Fagin states that research studies on primary nursing showed that it reduced hospital stays and complications of renal transplant patients at the University of Michigan Medical Center in Ann Arbor. The hospital saved $51,000 in one year. Primary nursing at Evanston (Illinois) Hospital near Chicago resulted in fewer nursing hours and less salary expense per patient during a five-year period. Nurses aides had 27 percent unoccupied time per day, while RNs had 8 percent at Rush Presbyterian. Also, turnover was decreased in the operating room, with an increased RN-to-operating-room technician ratio. Other studies indicate that primary nursing saves money; increases job satisfaction, group adhesion, and patient satisfaction; and decreases costs of overtime, sick time, and compensatory time.[23]

The following are advantages of primary nursing:

- It provides for increased autonomy on the part of the nurse, thus increasing motivation, responsibility, and accountability.
- It assures more continuity of care as the primary nurse gives or directs care throughout hospitalization.
- It makes available increased knowledge of the patient's psychosocial and physical needs, because the primary nurse does the history and physical assessment, develops the care plan, and acts as liaison between the patient and other health workers.
- It leads to increased rapport and trust between nurse and patient that will allow formation of a therapeutic relationship.
- It improves communication of information to physicians.
- It eliminates nurses aides from the administration of direct patient care.
- It frees the charge nurse to assume the role of operational manager to deal with staff problems and assignments and motivate and support the staff.

The main disadvantage of primary nursing is that it is said to require that the entire staff be RNs, which increases staffing costs. However, this has been disputed in cost studies. For example, money is saved when nonnursing duties are performed by other categories of personnel and are not taken over by RNs.[24]

In recent years, primary nursing has been modified to employ nurse extenders as technical assistants to RNs. The RNs assess the patients, develop care plans, and direct others. Modifications of team nursing and primary nursing to merge the advantages of each will result in more efficient and effective outcomes. This is particularly true in the new health-care environment.

Case Method

The case method of nursing provides for one-to-one RN-to-client ratio and constant care for a specified period of time. Examples are private duty, intensive care, and community health nurses. This method is similar to that of primary nursing, except that relief nurses on other shifts are not associate RNs.

Joint Practice

Joint practice is more than a modality. It entails nurses and physicians collaborating as colleagues to provide patient care. Nurses and physicians work together to define their roles within the joint practice setting, such goals being reciprocal and complementary rather than mutually exclusive. They may use mutually agreed-upon protocols to manage care within a primary setting.[25]

The primary nursing modality is preferred for joint practice, or collaborative practice. There must be an adequate number of professional nurses who are freed from nonnursing tasks. Decision making is decentralized, and in-service education and certification are used to upgrade the nurse's scope of practice. Compensation is increased to match increased responsibility and accountability.

Physicians are required to accept responsibility for their part in joint collaborative practice. Administration includes joint practice nurses on every committee within the hospital. It takes as long as a year to establish truly functional relationships, because both physicians and nurses have to modify their behaviors.

The following elements are needed to establish successful joint practice in a hospital setting:

1. A committee of physicians and nurses with equal representation and equal voice in establishing the objectives and ground rules of operation.
2. An integrated patient record system.
3. Primary nursing and case management.
4. Collaborative practice with honest communication and encouragement of clinical decision making by nurses.
5. Joint education of physicians and nurses.
6. Joint nurse-physician evaluation of patient care.
7. Trust.

Results of a joint practice demonstration project at four hospitals concluded the following:[26]

- Patients receive better nursing care and are highly satisfied with their care.
- Doctor-nurse communications are better, and there is increased mutual respect and trust between nurses and physicians.
- Both doctors' and nurses' job satisfaction is increased.

Case Management

Case management is more than a modality of nursing. It has been described as a clinical system that focuses on the accountability of an identified individual or group for conditioning a patient's care (or care for a group of patients) across a continuum of care; insuring and facilitating the achievement of quality, and clinical and cost outcomes; negotiating, procuring, and coordinating services and resources needed by the patient/family; intervening at busy points (and/or when significant variance occurs) for individual patients; addressing and resolving patterns in aggregate variances that have a negative quality-cost impact; and creating opportunities and systems to enhance outcomes.[27]

"Simply stated, case management is a process of coordinating services and the case manager is the person who does the coordinating."[28]

The Center for Case Management's model of case management was designed as a clinical one. The model's underlying assumption was that caregivers of each discipline needed to have management skills, better patient care management tools, and more responsible administrative support to create quality clinical outcomes within a new cost-conscious milieu. The organizational structure is flat, with attending level physician and "selected primary care nurses expanded into case managers to produce the integration of processes, aided by critical paths."[29] Critical paths have been integrated into CareMaps™ (see Exhibit 11–4). It should be noted that *a CareMap™ is used as the nursing care plan and for documentation.*

A collaborative team approach is used when integration of care occurs across geographic care units such as ER, CCU, step down, and ambulatory clinic. Formally oriented primary nurses from these units join the team.[30]

Personnel of the Center for Case Management believe that 100 percent of patients need their care managed by a CareMap™. Approximately 20 percent of patients need a case manager in addition to or instead of a CareMap™ system.[31]

In the restructuring of nursing care, Zander places increased emphasis on accountability, as demonstrated in Exhibit 11–5. It should be noted that case management is not a care delivery system.

Quality improvement is an integral part of the case management system. Quality management is operationalized by the use of critical paths, CareMaps™, and case management, all of which provide the tools for accomplishing the nursing process.[32] When interventions and goals are recorded that are different from those planned, they are termed *variances.* Variances show how the CareMaps™ and reality differ, both positively and negatively. CareMaps™ present problems by defining quality as a product.[33] A variance indicates deviations from a norm or standard. Variance indicates intervention that works or does not work. Variances alter discharge dates, expected costs, and expected outcomes[34] (see Exhibits 11–6 and 11–7).

Variance that shows negative outcomes requires action to improve quality. Variance data are collected, totaled, analyzed, and reported and then result in decisions that revise CareMaps™, critical paths, procedures, and other elements of the Plan-Do-Check Act (PDCA) cycle (see Exhibit 11–8). Since CareMaps™ can be used to document nursing care, are outcome-based, and have been found to be effective and efficient, nurses may want to use a computerized version for documentation.

Exercise 11–2   Evaluate case management as practiced in the agency in which you are employed or assigned as a student. Do this by gathering and analyzing data that

1. Describe the model of case management being used.
2. Identify the standards used to trigger the case management process.
3. Trace the continuum of case management from patient's entry through discharge.
4. Measure the achievement of stated outcomes.
5. Relate the nursing modality to case management.

(text continues on p. 291)

Exhibit 11–4   CareMaps™: The Core of Cost/Quality Care

CareMaps™ are the newest breakthrough in cost/quality outcomes management. They have evolved from their longer version, Case Management Plans, and their condensed version, Critical Paths, into "user friendly" documents which:

- *replace nursing care plans* as patient care plans[1]
- describe the contributions of every department
- show standards of care and standards of practice, and the timed, sequenced relationship between the two for a given case type, DRG, ICD9, or *constellation of problems*
- individualize care through analyzing and acting upon variances
- provide a data base for Continuous Quality Improvement (CQI)
- integrate with *acuity* systems, *costing* systems, and *research.*

CareMaps™ are cause and effect grids; i.e., staff actions should result in patient/family reactions or responses, which over time are "transformed" into desired outcomes. Staff actions are equivalent to Standards of Practice; patient reactions are equivalent to Standards of Care. CareMaps™ are built on a basic formula:

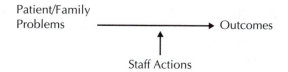

This basic formula describes very complex practice patterns, which themselves have many sources. *To build a CareMap™ requires deep respect for the knowledge, concern, and tradition that the clinicians of each discipline use in the care of their patients.* They reflect good practice, and can never replace good judgement.

Format

CareMaps™, like their Critical Path predecessors, are simplistic charts which graph phenomena associated with a homogeneous patient population on two axes: action vs. time. Critical Paths graph multidisciplinary staffs' actions in terms of interventions against the timeline most appropriate for the phase of treatment of a specific population. CareMaps™ go an additional step by including patient/family actions in terms of responses to staffs' interventions.

Classic Critical Path			Time →
	Patient/Family Actions	problems	
	Multidisciplinary Staff Actions	categories	

Patient/Family actions are categorized by problem statements which transform into intermediate goals and, by the last time frame, outcomes. Patient/Family actions are measurable and behavioral, and may include responses in the realms of physiological, self-care, activities of daily living, follow-up plans, psychological, and absence of complications often related to their medical diagnoses. In 1987, Stetler and DeZell suggested four generic categories that should always be considered for inclusion in problem outcome statements:[2]

1. **Potential for Complications Selfcare.** Presence of risk factors that may limit a patient's ability to manage his or her own disease and/or engage in health promoting activities in the home environment.
2. **Potential for Injury Unrelated to Treatment.** Presence of risk factors related primarily to the person's general state of health and/or to the specific disease symptom that could lead to physical injury within the institutional setting.
3. **Potential for Complications Related to Treatment.** Presence of risk factors, at times inherent in the inhospital treatment, that endanger the health and safety of the patient if (a) appropriate preventive measures are not instituted and maintained, and/or (b) on-going observations and monitoring are not instituted.
4. **Potential for Extension of the Disease Process.** Presence of a specific condition or pathological process that carries with it a risk that endangers the recovery of the patient; i.e., presence of a risk that will be increased if a treatable extension or sequela are undetected. Multidisciplinary staff actions can be categorized in a variety of ways. Over the last five years, eight classic categories have emerged:

1. Consults/Assessments
2. Treatments
3. Nutrition
4. Meds (IV, other)

Exhibit 11–4   CareMaps™: The Core of Cost/Quality Care *(Continued)*

5. Activity/Safety
6. Teaching (Patient, Significant Other)
7. Discharge Planning/Coordination
8. Specimens/Tests

Additional Categories such as "Chest-tube Management" or "Psychosocial" may be desired depending on the case type. Some institutions have incorporated their intermediate patient/family goals and outcomes into the traditional (staff action) Critical Path. Others have written the staff's actions into the patient/family outcomes section. Yet others have integrated actions and outcomes into their current data flow sheets. *Anytime both the staff's and patient/families' behaviors are graphed against a timeline, the concept of a CareMap™—by whatever name—is being used.*

A CareMap™ System
A CareMap™ System includes the use of CareMaps™ twenty-four hours a day. The heart of the system is the written CareMap™ and the variances that arise from the standard interventions and outcomes. In a CareMap™ System, variances are not bad, they are real and reflect the way staff are responding to individual patient needs. Variances can be categorized per patient using standard codes, and when aggregated retrospectively for groups of similar patient populations, form a data base for continuous quality improvement.

The ultimate result of a CareMap™ system is that unnecessary variance is reduced to a minimum because of an increasingly accurate learning curve that helps clinicians predict, prevent, and manage. It is not unusual for collaborative groups to begin developing CareMaps™ for the more straightforward diagnoses, proceed to several varieties of that map, then combine constellations of problems, and finally map care for the patient populations that were initially felt to be totally unpredictable.

Currently, CareMaps™ are used either on paper as references only, on paper as permanent documentation, on personal computers, or on mainframes. As institutions and clinicians become increasingly comfortable with CareMap™ development, and as computer systems convert to CareMap™ systems, higher percent-

ages of patients will be managed by them (with daily or per visit screens). Similarly, variances are presently being handled differently depending on each agency's goals for implementing the system in the first place. Minimally, patient/family and community variances are recorded in the medical record. A few institutions have decided to also include clinician and hospital-generated variances in the chart as well.

Summary
A complete CareMap™ System includes variance analysis, use of CareMaps™ in change-of-shift report, case consultation, and health care team meetings for patients at more-than-acceptable variance, and continuous quality improvement. The challenge, of course, is creating a dynamic system of complex care management from a static piece of paper. This can be accomplished with a series of CareMaps™ for different phases of treatment (i.e., Acute Myelogenous Leukemia: AML—induction, AML—consolidation, AML—fever and neutropenia, etc.) and the use of blank CareMaps™ for anecdotal documentation or for those patients who require a totally individualized map. Any individualized outcomes and interventions written on a CareMap™ are generally outside the variance field. When a patient's reason for remaining in the hospital changes in a major way (such as a patient having a craniotomy who remains on a vent), the CareMap™ changes as well.

All professional disciplines should be involved in the formation of CareMaps™ and education as to their use. Secretaries, computer and medical records department members, and the "forms" department are all integral to the implementation of a CareMap™ System. Our future issues will address physician involvement in CareMap™ Systems and Case Management, as well as other key development and maintenance factors.

Notes
1. P. Brider, "Who Killed the Nursing Care Plan?" *American Journal of Nursing,* May 1991, 35–39.
2. C. Stetler, and A. DeZell, *Case Management Plans: Designs for Transformation* (Boston: New England Medical Center Hospitals, 1987), 26–32.

Exhibit 11–4 CareMaps™: The Core of Cost/Quality Care *(Continued)*

CareMap™: Congestive Heart Failure

Problem	Day 1 ER 1–4 hours	Day 1 Floor Telemetry or CCU 6–24 hours	Day 2 Floor	Day 3 Floor	Day 4 Floor	Day 5 Floor	Day 6 Floor
Location			Benchmark Quality Criteria				
1) Alteration in gas exchange/profusion and fluid balance due to decreased cardiac output, excess fluid volume	Reduced pain from admission or pain free; Uses pain scale O₂ sat. improved over admission baseline on O₂ therapy	Respirations equal to or less than on admission	O₂ sat = 90 Resp 20–22 Vital signs stable Crackles at lung bases Mild shortness of breath with activity	Does not require O₂ Vital signs stable Crackles at base Respirations 20–22 Mild shortness of breath with activity	Does not require O₂ (O₂ sat. on room air 90%) Vital signs stable Crackles at base Respirations 20–22 Completes activities with no increase in respirations No edema	Can lie in bed at baseline position Chest X-ray clear or at baseline	No dyspnea
2) Potential for shock	No signs/symptoms of shock	No signs/symptoms of shock	No signs/symptoms of shock	No signs/symptoms of shock Normal lab values	No signs/symptoms of shock	No signs/symptoms of shock	No signs/symptoms of shock
3) Potential for consequences of immobility and decreased activity: skin breakdown, DVT	No redness at pressure points No falls	No redness at pressure points No falls	Tolerates chair, washing, eating, and toileting	Has bowel movement Up in room and bathroom with assist	Up ad lib for short periods		
4) Alteration in nutritional intake due to nausea and vomiting, labored		No c/o nausea No vomiting Taking liquids as offered	Eating solids Takes in 50% each meal	Taking 50% each meal	Taking 50% each meal Weight 2 lbs from patient's normal baseline	Taking 75% each meal	Taking 75% each meal
5) Potential for arrhythmias due to decreased cardiac output: decreased irritable foci, valve problems, decreased gas exchange	No evidence of life-threatening dysrhythmias	Normal sinus rhythm with benign ectopy	K(WNL) Benign or no arrhythmias	Digoxin level DNL Benign or no arrhythmias	Digoxin level WNL Benign or no arrhythmias	Digoxin level WNL Benign or no arrhythmias	Digoxin level WNL Benign or no arrhythmias

6) Patient/family response to future treatment & hospitalization	Patient/family expressing concerns Following directions of staff	Patient/family expressing concerns Following directions of staff	Patient/family expressing concerns Following directions of staff	States reasons for and cooperates with rest periods Patient begins to assess own knowledge and ability to care for CHF at home	Patient decides whether he/she wants discussion with physician about advanced directives	States plan for 1–2 days postdischarge as to meds., diet, activity, Follow-up appointments Expresses reaction to having CHF
						Repeats plans States signs and symptoms to notify physician/ER Signs discharge consent
7) Individual problem						
Staff Tasks						
Assessments/ Consults	Vital signs q 15 min Nursing assessments focus on lung sounds, edema, color, skin integrity, jugular vein distention Cardiac monitor Arterial line if needed Swan Ganz Intake & output	Vital signs q 15 min–1 hr Repeat nursing assessments Cardiac monitor Arterial line Swan Ganz Daily weight Intake & output	Vital signs q 4 hrs Repeat nursing assessments D/C cardiac monitor 24 hr D/C arterial and Swan Ganz Daily weight Intake & output	Vital signs q 6 hrs Repeat nursing assessments Daily weight Intake & output	Vital signs q 6 hrs Repeat nursing assessments Daily weight Intake & output Nutrition consult	Vital signs q 6 hrs Repeat nursing assessments Daily weight Intake & output
						Vital signs q 6 hrs Repeat nursing assessments Daily weight Intake & output
Specimens/Tests	Consider TSH studies Chest X-ray EKG CPK q 8 hr × 3 ABG if pulse Ox: (range) Lytes, Na, K, Cl, CO_2 Glucose, BUN, Creatinine Digoxin: (range)	B/G	Evaluate for ECHO Lytes, BUN, Creatinine			Chest X-ray Lytes, BUN, Creatinine
Treatments	O_2 or intubate IV or Heparin lock	O_2 IV or Heparin lock	IV or Heparin lock	DC pulse Ox if stable D/C IV or Heparin lock		
Medications	Evaluate for Digoxin Nitrodrip or paste Diuretics IV Evaluate for antiemetics Evaluate for antiarrhythmics	Evaluate for Digoxin Nitrodrip or paste Diuretics IV Evaluate for pre-load after-load reducers K supplements Stool softeners	D/C Nitrodrip or paste Diuretics IV or PO K supplements Stool softeners Evaluate for nicotine patch	Change to PO Digoxin PO diuretics K supplements Stool softeners Nicotine patch if consent	PO diuretics K supplement Stool softeners Nicotine patch if consent	PO diuretics K supplement Stool softeners Nicotine patch if consent
						PO diuretics K supplement Stool softeners Nicotine patch if consent

(Continued)

Exhibit 11–4 CareMaps™: The Core of Cost/Quality Care *(Continued)*

CareMap™: Congestive Heart Failure

	Day 1	Day 1	Day 2	Day 3	Day 4	Day 5	Day 6
				Benchmark Quality Criteria			
Location	ER 1–4 hours	Floor Telemetry or CCU 6–24 hours	Floor	Floor	Floor	Floor	Floor
Problem							
Nutrition	None	Clear liquids	Cardiac, low-salt diet	Cardiac, low-salt diet	Cardiac, low-salt diet	Cardiac, low-salt diet	
Safety/Activity	Commode Bedrest with head elevated Reposition patient q 2 hrs Bedrails up Call light available	Commode Bedrest with head elevated Dangle Reposition patient q 2 hrs Enforce rest periods Bedrails up Call light available	Commode Enforce rest periods Chair with assist ½ hr with feet elevated Bedrails up Call light available	Bathroom privileges Chair × 3 Bedrails up Call light available	Ambulate in hall × 2 Up ad lib between rest periods Bedrails up Call light available	Encourage ADLs that approximate activities at home Bedrails up Call light available	Encourage ADLs that approximate activities at home Bedrails up Call light available
Teaching	Explain procedures Teach chest pain scale and importance of reporting	Explain course, need for energy conservation Orient to unit and routine	Clarify CHF Dx and future teaching needs Orient to unit and routine Schedule rest periods Begin medication, teaching	Importance of weighing self every day Provide smoking cessation information Review energy conservation schedule	Cardiac rehab level as indicated by consult Provide smoking cessation support Begin medication teaching Dietary teaching	Review CHF education material with patient	Reinforce CHF teaching
Transfer/Discharge Coordination	Assess home situation notify significant other If no arrhythmias or chest pain transfer to floor Otherwise transfer to ICU	Screen for discharge needs Transfer to floor	Consider Home Health Care referral		Evaluate needs for diet and anti-smoking classes Physician offers discussion opportunities for advanced directives	Appointment and arrange-ment for follow-up care with Home Health Care nurses Contact VNA	Reinforce follow-up appointments

Source: Center for Case Management, South Natick, Mass. CareMap is a registered trademark of the Center for Case Management. Reprinted with permission.

Exhibit 11–5 Expanding Scope of Accountability

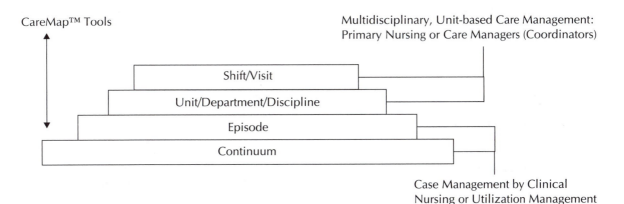

Glossary

Shift or Visit: A typical 8, 10, 12-hour nursing shift, consult, outpatient, or home health visit by any discipline, etc. A "billable" amount of service.

Unit, Department, Discipline: The classic ways in which services are organized, i.e., nursing units, satellite pharmacies, dietary departments, GYN services.

Episode: All services given to a patient and family from the first contact to the last contact for that specific set of symptoms or procedures; i.e., chest pain to cardiac rehab, diagnosis through hospice, MD office through surgery and recuperation.

Continuum: An infinite time frame which includes a person's health and life-style. May include chronic but stable states, such as well-maintained diabetes or handicaps.

Primary Nursing: A unit-based model for the decentralization of accountability for the outcomes of nursing care from the head nurse to designated staff nurses. Usually all staff nurses who work 4–5 shift equivalents per week are included as primary nurses, making a caseload (not shift assignment) number of 2 to 6.

Accountability: The answerability for outcomes and results. Accountability assumes that the necessary underlying authority to act has been acquired.

Care Management: A unit-based model for the decentralization of accountability for the outcomes of nursing care and an acknowledgment of the authority to coordinate all outcomes important to the treatment team. Nurses serve as care coordinators, sometimes in tandem with other professional disciplines. Only several nurses (avg. 1 to 4) are care managers.

Case Management: A clinical system that focuses on the accountability of an identified individual or group for coordinating a patient's care across a continuum of care; insuring and facilitating the achievement of quality, clinical and cost outcomes; negotiating, procuring and coordinating services and resources needed by the patient/family; intervening at key points for individual patients; addressing and resolving patterns in aggregate variances that have a negative quality-cost impact; and creating opportunities and systems to enhance outcomes.

Responsibility: The fulfillment of distinct behaviors and expectations.

Source: Center for Case Management, 1993. Developed by K. Bower; adapted by K. Zander, 1994. Reprinted with permission.

Exhibit 11–6   Sample Variance Sheet

Date	Description	Prob	Path	Source	Action	Initials
1-Feb	Son unavailable: out of town on business		8	A3	Ask ICU to call 2/2	AB
1-Feb	Afib	5	•	A1	Transfer to ICU	CD
	O_2 sat + 85%	1	•	A1	Lasix, O_2 6L	
	glucose 250		•	A1	Diabetic regime	
	no Swan Ganz		1	B6		
2-Feb	Unable to transfer to floor	•		C9	Order to drop pt. to general care rate	EF
	•	5		•		
	Afib—benign			A1	No action needed	
2-Feb	Echo not done		2	C9	Schedule for Monday	EF
	Hct 34, Hgb 13				Begin FeSO4	

Source: K. Zander, ed., "Quantifying, Managing, and Improving Quality. Part III: Using Variance Concurrently," *The New Definition,* Fall 1992, 3. Reprinted with permission.

Exhibit 11–7   Variance Source Codes

A	Patient/Family	
	1 Condition	
	2 Decision	
	3 Availability	
	4 Other	
B	Clinician	
	5 Order	
	6 Decision	
	7 Response Time	
	8 Other	
C	Hospital	
	9 Bed/Appt. Availability	
	10 Info/Data Availability	
	11 Other	
D	Community	
	12 Placement/Home Care	
	13 Transportation	
	14 Other	

Source: K. Zander, ed., "Quantifying, Managing, and Improving Quality. Part III: Using Variance Concurrently," *The New Definition,* Fall 1992, 3. Reprinted with permission.

Exhibit 11–8 Comparison of Generic Steps in Clinical Decision Making

Scientific Method	CareMap™ System Concurrent Use	CareMap™ System Retrospective Use	CQI Technique (PDCA)*
1. Assess	Assess		
2. Plan; using problem/ approach statements	Plan; using a CareMap™ tool with collaboratively determined outcome measures	CareMap™ tool	Plan
3. Intervene	Intervene		Do
4. Evaluate	Evaluate; using variance Compare Consult Analyze Document	Aggregate Variance	Check
5.		Inform Discuss Revise CareMap™ if needed Make other changes	Act

* PDCA Control circle: K. Ishikawa. *What Is Total Quality Control? The Japanese Way* (Englewood Cliffs, N.J.: Prentice-Hall, 1985), 59.

Source: K. Zander, ed., "Quantifying, Managing, and Improving Quality. Part III: Using Variance Concurrently," *The New Definition* (South Natick, Mass.: Center for Case Management, Fall 1992). Reprinted with permission.

ETHICAL CONCERNS

Many ethical issues are directly related to the providing of patient care services. They have become more important during the past decade because of the increased sophistication of medical science and technology, interprofessional relationships, organ donations and transplants, AIDS, the uninsured, the aged, high-risk neonates, concern about practical limits on financial resources for health care, changes in society, and growing emphasis on the autonomy of the individual.[35]

Professional nurses implement the employer's policy concerning the moral responsibility of health care. They have responsibility for supervising and reviewing patient care, meeting quality standards, making certain that decisions about patients are based on sound ethical principles, developing policies and mechanisms that address questions of human values, and responding to social problems and dilemmas that affect the need for health-care services.[36]

To fulfill this responsibility, professional nurses support nurses confronted with ethical dilemmas and help them think through situations by open dialogue. Nurse managers establish the climate for this. Davis recommends ethics rounds as a means of discussing ethical dilemmas. Such discussions can stem from hypothetical cases, case histories, or a case based on a current patient. Ethical reasoning requires participation by a knowledgeable person. Davis describes four ethical principles:[37]

1. *Autonomy.* Personal freedom of action is an ethical principle to be applied by nurse managers toward professional nurses, who in turn apply the principle in the care of the patients. The professional nurse is given autonomy to deliberate about nursing actions and has the capacity to take nursing actions based on this deliberation.

   Hospitalized or ambulatory patients may have diminished autonomy, and the professional nurse becomes an advocate or autonomous agent for these patients' rights. The patient is responsible for making decisions about his or her care, and the patient's family may be involved with the patient's consent.

2. *Nonmalficence.* Avoidance of intentional harm or the risk of inflicting harm on someone is termed *nonmalficence.* The use of restraints is an area that pits the principle of autonomy and self-determination against that of nonmalficence. When risks outweigh costs, one must protect the patient. Side rails, safety vests, tranquilizers, and wrist restraints all have the potential for abuse.

   Discharge planning can prevent negative outcomes and potential errors. When errors do occur, the nurse should acknowledge them to the patient or a surrogate, with full and immediate disclosure to the physician and the institution's administration. Nurses can protect patients from incompetent practitioners yet protect their own rights at the same time.

3. *Beneficence.* Beneficence is the principle of viewing persons as autonomous and not harming them, contributing to their health and welfare.

4. *Justice.* Justice involves giving people what is due or owed, deserved or legitimately claimed.

Many ethical issues relate to nursing and health care, including the issue of the right to health care. However, we do not have a law that says that society is obliged to provide health care. The following are some other ethical issues:

1. The rights of individuals and their surrogates versus the rights of the state or society. This issue creates confrontations among consumers and practitioners and may lead to management efforts to cut costs by cutting services (staff) or closing treatment centers. A survey of the Association of Community Cancer Centers indicated that 84 percent of them staff oncology units higher than other medical/surgical units.[38]

2. The rights of patients unable to make their own decisions versus the rights of their family versus the rights of institutions.

3. The rights of patients to forgo treatment versus the rights of society.

4. Issues related to
   a. Reproductive technology—preselection of desired physical characteristics of children, genetic screening

      b. Organ harvesting and transplants

      c. Research subjects

      d. Confidentiality

      e. Restraints

      f. Disclosure

      g. Informed consent

      h. Patient incapacity

      i. Court intervention

5. Reporting of ethical abuse of patients and staff.

The American Nurses Association Committee on Ethics has published several position statements and guidelines that seek to assist nurses in making ethical decisions in their practice. These guidelines are based on ethical theory and the ANA Code for Nurses, an expression of "nursing's moral concerns, goals, and values." They are designed to provide nurses with guidance on a range of ethical issues, including the withdrawing or withholding of food or fluid; risk versus responsibility in providing care; safeguarding client health and safety from illegal, incompetent, or unethical practices; nurses' participation in capital punishment; and nurses' participation and leadership in ethical review practices.[39]

Nurse managers need to know the legal framework for their actions. They should help clinical nurses to balance teaching, research, clinical investigation, and patient care. All should work for social justice to ensure a quality of life and health-care services that is desirable. Nurses may promote compassion and sensitivity through protest of public policies that reduce quality of or access to health care for the poor. They pursue human values, wholeness, and health values.[40] This does not mean that nurses must subsidize health care by working for lower salaries; rather they should work to have the cost shared by all of society.

A study of ethical issues and problems encountered by fifty-two nurses in their work in one hospital used a thirty-two-item ethical issues in nursing instrument. Results indicated that nurses encountered few ethical issues. The five most common issues were inadequate staffing patterns, prolonging life with heroic measures, inappropriate resource allocations, dealing with situations where patients are being discussed inappropriately, and dealing with irresponsible activity of colleagues. Ethical issues were more frequent in critical care than in medical or surgical units. Since the frequency was not increasing, the study group recommended institutional ethics committees and nursing ethics rounds to sensitize nurses to ethical issues.[41]

A 1988 survey of institutions in the metropolitan New York area was done to determine how nurses were addressing ethical concerns in their practice; 71 of 116 hospitals responded. Topics addressed by hospital ethics committees are listed in Exhibit 11–9, the formats for addressing these issues are listed in Exhibit 11–10, and the ethical issues in nursing practice are listed in Exhibit 11–11. All ethics committees had nursing representatives, mostly from administrative and management positions. It was concluded that a majority of institutions do not adequately address nursing issues and concerns.[42]

Exhibit 11–9   Topics Addressed By Ethics Committees (*N* = **41**)

Topic	Number	%
Do-not-resuscitate (DNR)	29	70
Withholding/withdrawing treatment	10	24
AIDS	9	22
Allocation of resources	9	22
Patient's rights	8	19
Death and dying	7	17
Minors	4	9
Professional practice issues	3	7
Abortion	1	2
Prison health	1	2
Institutional issues	1	2

Source: C. Scanlon and C. Fleming, "Confronting Ethical Issues: A Nursing Survey," *Nursing Management,* May 1990, 64. Reprinted with permission.

Exhibit 11–10   Formats for Addressing Ethics Issues (*N* = **44**)

Format	Number	%
Nursing meetings	29	66
Inservice education	8	18
Hospital committees	4	9
Individual discussion/consultation	4	9
Hospital Ethics Committee	4	9
Interdisciplinary rounds	2	4

Source: C. Scanlon and C. Fleming, "Confronting Ethical Issues: A Nursing Survey," *Nursing Management,* May 1990, 64. Reprinted with permission.

Among the ethical dilemmas seldom addressed by nurse managers are ethical boundaries, particularly those involving sex. Nurse managers and administrators should provide continuing education to increase nurses awareness of improper nurse-patient relationships, including accepting gifts and favors, doing business with patients and their families, being coerced or manipulated by patients, visiting patients at home while off duty, and making nontherapeutic disclosures. Risk environments include inpatient psychiatric services and chemical-dependency treatment programs.[43]

Patients are still being denied pain relief by lazy or policy-adamant providers. While letters to Ann Landers are not scientific, they are revealing. One writer wrote that a physician would not give her father pain medication the

Exhibit 11–11   Ethical Issues in Nursing Practice

Topic	Number	%
Do-not-resuscitate (DNR)	31	44
Patient's rights	25	35
Professional practice issues	22	31
AIDS	15	21
Death and dying	14	20
Allocation of resources	14	20
Withholding/withdrawing treatment	7	10
Institutional issues	6	8
Abortion	3	4
Minors	3	4
Prison health	0	

Source: C. Scanlon and C. Fleming, "Confronting Ethical Issues: A Nursing Survey," *Nursing Management,* May 1990, 64. Reprinted with permission.

night before he died of terminal cancer. Reason: The physician would have had to walk to another unit for a small needle. In another letter, the wife of a terminal cancer patient requesting relief of intense pain was told by a nurse, "He has to wait another 30 minutes."[44] The ethical and professional answer to such incidences is for assertive nurses to obtain adequate pain medication orders and implement them.

One of the leading experts in nursing ethics, Leah Curtin, advocates creation of moral space for nurses to preserve their integrity. A nurse who believes an action to be wrong should not be forced to take that action.[45] Curtin states that since ethics deals with values as well as with facts and interests, answers to ethical questions do not fall strictly within the bounds of any one discipline. Because ethical questions are complex, they are puzzling, even bewildering. Since any answer we frame has inflections that touch many areas of concern, we cannot foresee all the consequences of the answers we choose. To solve an ethical problem, Curtin recommends that we

1. Gather as much information as possible to understand precisely what the problem is.
2. Determine as many possible ways to resolve the problem as present themselves.
3. Consider the arguments for and against each alternative we can discover or imagine.

The nurse has an obligation to protect the welfare of patients and clients by virtue of her legal duties, the code for nurses, and the nurse's social role. From a moral perspective, one cannot knowingly harm another person. Any freely chosen human act is right insofar as it protects and promotes the human rights of individual nurses. Professionals have duties to guide their young members, and nurses on all levels have mutual duties to support and guide one another.[46]

Values-based management stems from the actions of CEOs who set the stage for using a values credo of shared beliefs that govern the decisions and actions of top management. Two companies that do this are Levi Strauss and Holt Cos. Their values include openness, teamwork, diversity, ethical behavior, and honest communication. Their priority is on ethics, human dignity, and self-fulfillment. The employees believe they make important contributions to the company, customers, and the community. Such companies find that productivity and products increase.[47]

Nursing ethics committees should be established to prevent burnout. Their goals would include providing a forum expressing concerns, promotion of awareness and education, participation in clinical decision making, policy and procedure development, professional identity, and linkage to other committees.[48]

Advance Directives

An advance directive is "a written instruction, such as a living will or a durable power of attorney for health care, recognized under state law (whether statutory or as recognized by the courts of the state) and relating to the provision of such care when the individual is incapacitated." Advance directives are mandated by the Patient Self-Determination Act (a provision of the Omnibus Budget Reconciliation Act of 1990).[49]

The advance directive is a directive to physicians and other health-care providers given in advance of incapacity with regard to a person's wishes about medical treatment. As an example, the Texas Natural Death Act gives the person the right to provide instructions about care when faced with a terminal condition. It covers such procedures as cardiopulmonary resuscitation (CPR), tube feeding, respirators, IV therapy, or kidney dialysis.

A directive to physicians may be called a living will. The attending physician and another physician certify that a person has a terminal condition that will result in death in a relatively short time and is comatose, incompetent, or otherwise unable to communicate.

A durable power of attorney for health care allows a person to name another person to make medical decisions for an incapacitated person.

An advance directive is a legal document. In Texas it does not have to be drawn up by a lawyer or notarized, but it does have to be witnessed. An oral statement suffices when done in the presence of two witnesses and the attending physician. Witnesses cannot be physicians, nurses, or hospital personnel, fellow patients, or persons who will have claim against a person's estate.[50]

Under Texas law (Consent to Medical Treatment Act), the following people have the option to make medical decisions for an incompetent person: spouse, sole child who has written permission from the other children to act alone, majority of children, parents, a person whom the patient clearly identified before becoming ill, any living relative, or a member of the clergy (surrogate).[51]

Ethics in Business

Lee indicates that all organizations should develop a policy on ethics. Business ethics helps people find the best way to satisfy the demands of competing interests. Ethics is part of corporate culture. Ethical organizations try to satisfy all of their shareholders, are dedicated to high purpose, are committed to learning, and try to be the best at whatever they do.

According to Beckstrand, "The aims of practice can be achieved using the knowledge of science and ethics alone."[52] To apply Beckstrand's theory to nursing management, nurse managers would apply their knowledge to change the nursing work environment to realize a greater good where and when needed.

Donley states that a health-care system should be built based on values promoting both the individual and the common good.[53] Current dilemmas in nursing are partly due to limitations in nursing management knowledge. Changes are needed that address values and goals. There could be a hierarchy of values in managing practice. Nurse managers need to determine how much decision-making power clinical nurses want and how much managers can delegate. A theory of ethics should be meshed with a theory of nursing management that is congruent with a theory of ethical conduct for clinical nurses.

Both clinical nurses and managers use scientific knowledge to determine whether conditions support change. The intrinsic value of the management actions should be given careful thought and should be debated by nurse managers who consciously attempt to practice management that realizes the highest good. The manager is more apt to be successful if scientific management knowledge is applied.

Ethics in management translated into nursing theory can be summed up as follows:[54]

1. Nurse managers can influence the ethical behavior of nursing personnel by treating them ethically.
2. Nurse managers have a code of ethics that peers have agreed upon. They enter into ethical dilemmas when they go against that code.
3. Nurse managers fall into moral dilemmas when they go against their internal values.
4. While ethical and moral dilemmas differ, an ethical nurse manager is a moral nurse manager.
5. Ethical functions can be confronted by three questions:
   a. "Is it legal?" Resolves some dilemmas but not nonsensical laws and policies.
   b. "Is it balanced?" The nurse manager should aim for a win-win solution.
   c. "How will it make me feel about myself?" The nurse manager should consider the impact of each action on her/his self-respect.
6. Nurse managers with a positive self-image usually have the internal strength to make the ethical decision.
7. An ethical leader is an effective leader.

8. Nurse managers should apply six principles of ethical power:
   a. The chief nurse executive promotes and ensures pursuit of the stated mission or purpose of the nursing division, since this statement reflects the vision of practicing nurses. While the mission statement should be reviewed periodically, goals or objectives are set for yearly achievement.
   b. Nurse managers should build an organization to win, thereby building up employees through pride in their organization.
   c. Nurse managers should work to sustain patience and continuity through a long-term effect on the organization.
   d. Nurse managers should plan for persistence by spending more time following up on education and activities that build commitment of personnel.
   e. Nurse managers should promote perspective by giving their staff time to think. They should practice good management for the long term.
   f. Nursing service managers should consider developing an organization-specific code of ethics expressed in observable and measurable behaviors.

A code of ethics should be ingrained in employees to create a strong sense of professionalism. Such a code should be the basis of a planned approach to all management functions of planning, organizing, leading, and evaluating. Nursing employees can help develop the code of ethics, implement it, and determine its associated rewards and punishments. A code of ethics should be read and signed by employees and regularly reviewed and revised.

Contents of a code of ethics include definition of ethical and unethical practices, expected ethical behavior, enforcement of ethical practices, and rewards and punishments. To be objective, a code of ethics specifies rules of conduct. To be effective, it should be applied to all persons.[55]

Exercise 11–3   Form a group of six to eight peers. Each group member identifies and describes, orally or in writing, an ethical dilemma. Discuss each from the viewpoints of care for the patient and support for the caregiver. What are the implications for interpersonal relationships among caregivers and care recipients?

Exercise 11–4   Set up two teams to debate the following:

"Professional nurses should intervene in instances where they observe unethical conduct or illegal or unprofessional activities."

VERSUS

"Professional nurses should *not* intervene in instances where they observe unethical conduct or illegal or unprofessional activities."

Exercise 11–4
(continued)

Select a moderator. The two teams may be divided according to viewpoint. First decide on rules for selection of team members and then decide on rules of procedure. For example, each speaker from each side may be allowed to speak to a question for three minutes.

Consider the following questions:

1. What is the individual responsibility of professional nurse employees in instances where they observe unethical conduct or illegal or unprofessional activities by their employer?
2. What is the responsibility of professional nursing organizations when they are made aware of such instances?
3. What is the responsibility of community organizations if they are made aware of such instances?

Consider the following:

- Accreditation action
- Government action (Medicare)
- Publicity (media)
- Prevention

Exercise 11–5

Examine organizational policies related to patients' rights as well as statements made by nursing associations and hospital associations and articles in professional journals. What authority or source would lead one to believe that the patient has a right to know his or her nursing diagnosis, the goals of care related to that diagnosis, and the nursing actions prescribed to meet those goals? What authority or source would lead one to believe that the patient has a right to assist in the planning of his or her nursing care? What authority or source would lead one to believe that the patient has a right to know what to expect as a result of his or her nursing care?

MULTICULTURAL ASPECTS OF NURSING

While nurses have attended to the multicultural aspects of patient care through the decades, the importance of such aspects has received increasing attention during recent years. Multicultural relates to such characteristics as race, gender, religion, cognitive diversity, sexual orientation, age, and class. It also relates to all of the ideas and habits a social or ethnic group learns, practices, shares, and transmits from generation to generation.

An ethnic group can be both a minority and a majority. For example, the French-Canadians are a majority in Quebec province and a minority in other provinces of Canada. Ethnic groups have cultural needs relating to their beliefs, values, and lifestyles. They have distinct *learned* knowledge and skills that are socially inherited. Ethnic groups have distinct eating habits, ways of raising children, political beliefs, and beliefs related to health and illness.[56] Knowledge of a patient's culture assists the caregiver in preventing stress and morbidity in caring for the patient.[57]

Signals of stress are culturally grounded.[58] As an example, persons from different cultures respond to pain differently. Patients from some cultures are stoic about pain and illness, while others are emotional and expressive. Through interview and observation, the professional nurse assesses the cultural needs of the patient as she or he assesses the patient's other needs. Among the needs assessed are the need for an interpreter—sometimes because of language or other communication limitations. Language is sometimes a challenge for political reasons. Some groups want the official U.S. language to be English. The professional nurse transcends the political argument. If a patient cannot speak English, the caregiver obtains a translator from the family or other source to translate for the patient. Communication is enhanced when nurses respect and appreciate diversity of culture.

Since diet is important in treating most diseases and in maintaining health, nurses and other health-care workers should establish which foods and beverages a person from another culture will consume and how the foods should be prepared. National studies on illnesses have used predominantly male subjects. These studies have led to wrong conclusions in treating female patients. Studies have also led to wrong conclusions in treating pain in women. As a result, women may have inadequate pain management.[59]

Nurses may need to do self-examination to identify their personal biases and prejudices regarding cultural issues. Such issues may center around religious differences, superstitions, and customs related to space and colors, and questions related to survival, sharing, protecting the environment, and even intelligence. Educators are exploring the concept of people having multiple (seven) intelligences: linguistic, logical-mathematical, spatial, bodily-kinesthetic, musical, interpersonal, and intrapersonal. A dominant intelligence may become the conduit for developing another or others.[60] This knowledge may help in assessing patients needs.

Cultural goals are defined by nurses to fit the assessed needs of patients, including equity, tolerance, and acceptance. Cultural awareness leads to responsible action and empowerment. Desirable cultural outcomes include being accepted, being valued, being loved, having a sense of belonging, cooperation in reaching decisions, and resolving problems. As caregivers learn the cultural beliefs of other ethnic groups, they become less idealistic and more understanding. Conflict is tempered by conformity and commonality.

Exercise 11–6   Read the work of M. L. Leininger (see references). With a group of your peers, discuss application of Leininger's theory of culture care. Outline the steps to follow in assessing, diagnosing, and identifying outcomes for the cultural needs of patients. Discuss how you would apply these steps in clinical practice.

WEB ACTIVITIES

- Visit www.jbpub.com/swansburg, this text's companion website on the Internet, for further information on Managing a Clinical Practice Discipline.
- On the Internet, which organizations or journals could you search for discussions on ethical concerns and issues regarding this topic?
- What sites would you recommend for more details on various nursing theories?

SUMMARY

Nurse managers work with staff who are clinical practitioners. Educated in nursing management, they can assist these practitioners in their work according to the models of such theorists as Orem, Kinlein, Roy, Newman, Levine, Johnson, Peplau, and Orlando.

Several modalities of nursing have evolved during the past fifty years. Functional nursing, the oldest nursing practice modality, is a method in which each staff member is assigned a particular nursing function, such as administering medications, admitting and discharging patients, and making beds and serving meals. It accomplishes the most work in the shortest period of time. Later, team nursing became the modality of choice for many hospital nursing services. Under the leadership of a professional nurse, a group of nurses work together to provide patient care. Team nursing rests on theoretical knowledge related to philosophy, planning, leadership, interpersonal relationships, and the nursing process.

During the past two decades, the modality of total patient care through primary nursing has evolved. With primary nursing, the total care of a patient and a caseload is the responsibility of one primary nurse.

Joint or collaborative practice by a physician-nurse team has developed as a modality of nursing in a very few hospitals. The latest development is case management, a method of practicing nursing that incorporates any modality but in which the knowledgeable nurse becomes the case manager, making or facilitating all clinical nursing decisions about a caseload of patients during an entire episode of illness.

As new technologies of patient treatment develop and the health-care delivery system evolves around managed care, nurses need avenues to pursue the ensuing ethical dilemmas. Nursing practice is further complicated by the need for multicultural assessments as part of the nursing process and its outcomes.

NOTES

1. H. A. Bush, "Models for Nursing," *Advances in Nursing Science,* January 1979, 13–21.

2. G. L. Dickson and H. Lee-Villasenor, "Nursing Theory and Practice: A Self-Care Approach," *Advances in Nursing Science,* October 1982, 29–40.

3. Sister C. Roy, "Adaptation: A Basis for Nursing Practice," *Nursing Outlook,* April 1971, 254–257; K. Frederickson, "Using a Nursing Model to Manage Symptoms: Anxiety and the Roy Adaptation Model," *Holistic Nursing Practice,* January 1993, 36–43.

4. Ibid.

5. M. F. Mastal and H. Hammond, "Analysis and Expansion of the Roy Adaptation Model: A Contribution to Holistic Nursing," *Advances in Nursing Science,* July 1980, 71.

6. K. Frederickson, op. cit.

7. M. C. Silva and J. M. Sorrell, "Testing a Nursing Theory: Critique and Philosophical Expansion," *Advances in Nursing Science,* June 1992, 14–15.

8. V. F. Engle, "Newman's Conceptual Framework and the Measurement of Older Adults' Health," *Advances in Nursing Science,* October 1984, 24–36.

9. Ibid.

10. Ibid.

11. M. E. Levine, "Adaptation and Assessment: A Rationale for Nursing Intervention," *American Journal of Nursing,* November 1966, 2450–2453.

12. Ibid.

13. A. C. Rawls, "Evaluation of the Johnson Behavioral System Model in Clinical Practice," *Image,* February 1980, 12–16.

14. A. K. Derdiarian, "The Relationships Among the Subsystems of Johnson's Behavioral System Model," *Image,* winter 1990, 219–225.

15. L. Thompson, "Peplau's Theory: An Application to Short-Term Individual Therapy," *Journal of Psychosocial Nursing,* August 1986, 26–31.

16. H. E. Peplau, "Interpersonal Relations: A Theoretical Framework for Application in Nursing Practice," *Nursing Science Quarterly,* spring 1992, 13–18.

17. N. J. Schmieding, "Putting Orlando's Theory into Practice," *American Journal of Nursing,* June 1984, 759–761; I. J. Orlando, *The Discipline and Teaching of Nursing Process: An Evaluative Study* (New York: Putnam, 1972); I. J. Orlando, *The Dynamic Nurse-Patient Relationship: Function, Process, Principles* (New York: Putnam, 1961).

18. A. G. Wiens, "Patient Autonomy in Care: A Theoretical Framework for Nursing," *Journal of Professional Nursing,* March/April 1993, 95–103.

19. M. B. Happ, "Sociotechnical Systems Theory," *Journal of Nursing Administration,* June 1993, 47–54.

20. D. P. Newcomb and R. C. Swansburg, *The Team Plan: A Manual for Nursing Service Administrators,* 2nd ed. (New York: Putnam, 1953, 1971), 56.

21. G. D. Marram, M. W. Schlegel, and E. O. Bevis, *Primary Nursing: A Model for Individualized Care* (St. Louis: Mosby, 1974), 1.

22. Ibid., 16–17.

23. C. M. Fagin, "The Economic Value of Nursing Research," *American Journal of Nursing,* December 1982, 1844–1849.

24. J. C. Lyon, "Models of Nursing Care Delivery and Care Management: Clarification of Terms," *Nursing Economics,* June 1993, 163–169.

25. National Joint Practice Commission, *Guidelines for Establishing Joint or Collaborative Practice in Hospitals* (Chicago: Neely Printing, 1981).

26. Ibid.

27. "Toward a Fully-Integrated CareMap[TM] and Case Management System," *The New Definition,* spring 1993, 1.

28. "Part 1: Rationale for Care-Provider Organizations," *The New Definition,* summer 1994, 1.
29. Ibid.
30. Ibid.
31. Ibid.
32. "Quantifying, Managing, and Improving Quality Part I: How CareMaps™ Link CQI to the Patient," *The New Definition,* spring 1992, 1.
33. Ibid.
34. "Quantifying, Managing and Improving Quality Part III: Using Variance Concurrently," *The New Definition,* fall 1992, 1–2.
35. Report of the Special Committee on Biomedical Ethics, *Values in Conflict: Resolving Ethical Issues in Hospital Care* (Chicago: American Hospital Association, 1985.)
36. Ibid.
37. A. J. Davis, "Helping Your Staff Address Ethical Dilemmas," *Journal of Nursing Administration,* February 1982, 9–13.
38. L. E. Mortenson, "Are Oncology Nurses too Expensive?" *Oncology Nursing Forum,* January/February 1984, 14–15.
39. Committee on Ethics, American Nurses Association, *Ethics in Nursing: Position Statements and Guidelines* (Kansas City, Mo.: American Nurses Association, 1988).
40. J. E. Sauer, "Ethical Problems Facing the Healthcare Industry," *Hospital & Health Services Administration,* September/October 1985, 44–52.
41. M. C. Berger, A. Severson, and R. Chvatal, "Ethical Issues in Nursing," *Western Journal of Nursing Research,* August 1991, 514–521.
42. C. Scanlon and C. Fleming, "Confronting Ethical Issues: A Nursing Survey," *Nursing Management,* May 1990, 63–65.
43. S. Pennington, G. Gafner, R. Schilit, and B. Bechtel, "Addressing Ethical Boundaries Among Nurses," *Nursing Management,* June 1993, 36–39.
44. A. Landers, "Pain-Free Death Is Right Worth Defending," *San Antonio Express-News,* 17 June 1994, 5J.
45. L. L. Curtin, "Creating Moral Space for Nurses," *Nursing Management,* March 1993, 18–19.
46. L. L. Curtin, "When the System Fails," *Nursing Management* August 1992, 21–25.
47. P. Konstam, "Values-Based System Focuses on Ethics," *San Antonio Light,* December 12 1992, D 1.
48. S. Buchanan and L. Cook, "Nursing Ethics Committees: The Time Is Now," *Nursing Management,* August 1992, 40–41.
49. Sec. 4206, "Medicare Provider Agreements Assuring the Implementation of the Patient's Right to Participate in and Direct Health Care Delivery Affecting the Patient," *Congressional Record-House,* 26 October 1990, H12456–H12457.
50. Bexar County Hospital District, "Understanding Advance Directives: Your Rights as a Patient" (San Antonio, Texas, 1991).
51. P. Premack, "Medical—OK Law Has a Key Change," *San Antonio Express-News* 23 July 1993, 11D.
52. J. Beckstrand, "The Need for a Practice Theory as Indicated by the Knowledge Used in the Conduct of Practice," *Research in Nursing and Health,* December 1978, 175–179.
53. Sister R. Donley, "Ethics in the Age of Health Care Reform," *Nursing Economics,* January–February 1993, 19–23.
54. K. C. Fernicola, "Take the High Road . . . to Ethical Management: An Interview with Kenneth Blanchard," *Association Management,* May 1988, 60–66.

55. M. Mizock, "Ethics—The Guiding Light of Professionalism," *Data Management,* August 1986, 16–18, 29.

56. H. A. Robinson, "Weaving the Tapestry of Diversity," *National Forum,* winter 1994, 3–5; S. Dobson, "Bringing Culture into Care," *Nursing Times,* February 1983, 53, 56–57.

57. J. Doku, "Approaches to Cultural Awareness," *Nursing Times,* 26 September 1990, 69–70.

58. C. F. Diaz, "Dimensions of Multicultural Education," *National Forum,* winter 1994, 9–11.

59. A. H. Vallerand, "Gender Differences in Pain," *IMAGE: Journal of Nursing Scholarship,* fall 1995, 235–251.

60. J. H. Gray and J. T. Viens, "The Theory of Multiple Intelligences," *National Forum,* Winter 1994, 22–25.

DECISION MAKING AND PROBLEM SOLVING*

OBJECTIVES

- Define decision making.
- Distinguish among different models of decision making.
- Describe the steps in the decision-making process.
- Apply the decision-making process.
- Identify ways to make decision making more effective.
- Describe the place of intuition in the decision-making process.
- Distinguish between organizational and personal decisions.
- Describe the steps in the problem-solving process.

KEY CONCEPTS

decision making
intuition
problem solving

Manager Behavior: Applies decision-making theory and the problem-solving process in achieving the mission of the nursing agency.

Leader Behavior: Coaches and involves team members and associates when applying decision-making theory and the problem-solving process in achieving the mission of the nursing agency.

INTRODUCTION

Decision making is essential to problem solving. It is doubtful that anyone would argue with that statement. Nurses already know how to make decisions, don't they? They have been doing so since they were small children. Certainly their decisions were not always made after careful deliberation and by consciously following specified steps in a process. Nurses may not have known how they did it; they just did it. Thus, a nurse might be thinking, "I wouldn't be

---

* Material from this chapter first appeared in Russell C. Swansburg, *Management of Patient Care Services* (St. Louis, Mo.: C. V. Mosby, 1976). It was updated and expanded upon by Claudette T. Coleman, EdD, RN, for *Management and Leadership for Nurse Managers* (Boston: Jones and Bartlett, 1990) and for *Student Workbook and Study Guide for Management and Leadership for Nurse Managers* (1991). Further update was made for *Staff Development: A Component of Human Resource Development* (1994) and for succeeding management books.

where I am professionally if I didn't know how to make decisions, so I'll go to the next chapter."

Wait! How often have nurses made bad decisions? Why were the decisions bad? How do nurses avoid making similar errors in future decisions? How do they deal with indecision?

This chapter explores the answers to these questions. Complex decision making is a part of any level of nursing. To function successfully, the nurse must consistently demonstrate the ability to solve problems in rapidly changing and uncertain situations in which indecisiveness or poor decisions are costly. The ability to foster organizational decision making and problem solving is an essential personal skill for nurses. This chapter deals with models and strategies that nurses can use to successfully strengthen personal skills and help further develop the decision-making and problem-solving abilities of staff members.

The theory of decision making, a required competency for all professionals, is an essential component of the nursing process and the management process.

THE DECISION-MAKING PROCESS

Definition

Since everyone is involved at some time in making decisions, it may be assumed that innate abilities, past experience, and intuition form the basis for making successful decisions. Decisions are often made by choosing among known alternatives. But what about unknown alternatives? Making a choice is not the only element of decision making. The process, which usually involves a systematic approach of sequenced steps, should be adaptable to the environment in which it is used. Lancaster and Lancaster define decision making as a systematic, sequential process of choosing among alternatives and putting the choice into action. This definition acknowledges natural and learned abilities while providing order and continuity to the process of decision making.[1]

Empirical evidence shows that speedy decision makers are needed in today's environment. Such decision makers consider more alternatives, more batches of options at one time. They are themselves, or they rely on, older, experienced mentors. Speedy decision makers thoroughly integrate strategies and tactics. They juggle budgets, schedules, and organizational options simultaneously. They constitute the winning culture in decision making.[2]

A review of the literature yields a number of decision-making models. The description model is covered in this chapter, since it has been used extensively in making managerial and clinical decisions.

The Descriptive Model

Simon developed the descriptive model based on the assumption that the decision maker is a rational person looking for acceptable solutions based on known information. This model allows for the fact that many decisions are made with incomplete information because of time, money, or people limitations; it also allows for the fact that people do not always make the best choices. Simon wrote that few decisions would ever be made if people always sought optimal solutions. Instead, he contended, people identify acceptable alternatives. The following are the steps in the descriptive model:[3]

1. Establish acceptable goal.
2. Define subjective perceptions of the problem.
3. Identify acceptable alternatives.
4. Evaluate each alternative.
5. Select alternative.
6. Implement decision.
7. Follow up.

The descriptive model may lend itself well to nurses faced with daily decisions that must be made rapidly and that will have significant consequences. Steps in the model are not unlike those in the familiar nursing process, although the sequencing is different. Readers may readily identify conditions in their own environments similar to those described by Simon and see immediate application of this model.[4] Exhibit 12–1 has been developed by the author after many years of experience using the descriptive model.

Steps in the Process

From these and other models of decision making, seven general steps of the process have been identified. Goals and objectives may be set prior to beginning the general process. They will answer the question, What do we want the outcome or results of this decision to be? When new products or services are the outcome, the goals and objectives are established first, and problems or decisions are then forecast (see step 1 of Exhibit 12–1). (Managers who wish to reverse steps 1 and 2 may do so.)

The problem must be identified (step 2 of Exhibit 12–1). Although this step may seem simple, recognizing and defining the problem is complex because of the diversity of individual perceptions. Because all individuals affected by the problem should be involved in discussing it, authority for decision making should be delegated to individuals at the level of impact. When this is impossible, representatives of various affected groups may provide input. Each representative may have a different perspective as to what the outcome should be. Nurses should make certain that the identified problem is one that requires their attention and cannot be handled alone by those involved. Collecting factual information in addition to subjective perceptions is essential. Logical and systematic fact-finding includes questioning all sources for divergent opinions and objective data. When the difference between desired and present situations or outcomes is significant, it may signal recognition of the problem.

Once the problem has been identified, the nurse must then evaluate the potential for a solution and determine the priority of the problem. Reitz suggests three approaches to setting priorities for problems:[5]

1. Deal with problems in the order in which they appear.
2. Solve the easiest problems first.

Exhibit 12–1   The Decision-Making Process Including Cost/Benefit Analysis

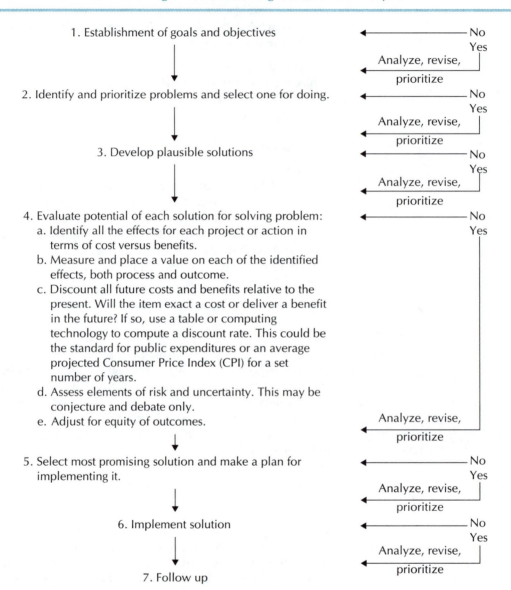

Establishing goals and objectives requires that decisions be made as to how they will be achieved. A first decision may be setting the priority in which they will be carried out. Decisions do not relate only to problems. They relate to development of plans and programs to accomplish nursing goals and objectives. When the best alternative does not work, another decision on whether to start over from step 1 is required, especially if other alternatives have less chance of success. The cost versus the benefit of the solution is introduced at step 4.

3. Solve crisis problems before all others. A decision will depend on the time and energy that can be devoted at that time. When a high-priority problem with limited potential for resolution is identified, the decision maker may be forced to give it lower priority until more information is collected and acceptable alternatives can be found. The fact that needed information is missing may help define the real problem underlying the perceived one.

The third step in decision making is *gathering and analyzing information related to the solution* (step 3 of Exhibit 12–1). This step involves defining, through a series of activities, the specifications to be met by the solution. A thorough information search may be needed to validate that the problem has been correctly identified. This search should include knowledge of organizational policy, prior personal experience or training, or the experience of others. Externally, the nurse begins to identify alternatives, comparing the potential solutions with the desired outcome, and the desired outcome with available resources. In organizational settings, database information systems may provide this information quickly. Establishing goals with measurable objectives helps focus the search for alternatives. Certainly to be considered while comparing potential alternatives is the cost, the time required and available, and the capabilities of those who will be involved in implementing a decision.

Once again, it is essential to involve in these discussions the individuals who will be affected by the choice. Irrelevant, insignificant, and extraneous factors must be eliminated from consideration. Gaining a commitment to implement a decision before the choice is made supports the process. It is possible to reach a point of overload when the searcher has received information too quickly or in too great a quantity to process. Research indicates that the quantity of information sought has a direct, positive correlation with the degree of anticipated risk in the decision to be made. The personal confidence of the decision maker also affects the amount of information required to support decision-making choices. Less searching is required by the nurse who recognizes patterns or similarities to previously encountered problems and confidently makes a choice of alternatives.

The fourth and fifth steps in decision making are *evaluating all alternatives and selecting one for implementation* (steps 4 and 5 of Exhibit 12–1). In the evaluation of alternatives, possible positive and negative consequences and the estimated probability of each choice are identified. A common approach involves identifying the best and worst possible outcomes to an alternative and then the outcomes that fall between the two extremes. As each alternative is evaluated, additional options may become apparent. Disagreement may stimulate the imagination and produce better solutions.

The effects of making no decision must be weighed against the effects of each proposed solution. Each alternative must be systematically evaluated for its efficiency and effectiveness in accomplishing the desired outcome and for the likelihood of achieving it with available or obtainable resources. The advantages and disadvantages of each alternative are identified during these steps to determine risk factors in possible outcomes. Identifying the solution that best satisfies specifications should receive attention before any compromises, concessions, or revisions are made by involved parties. The alternative that provides the greatest probability of an acceptable desired outcome using available resources is most likely to be selected.

A sixth step in the decision-making process is to *act on or implement the selected alternative* (step 6 of Exhibit 12–1). The knowledge and skills of the decision maker transform the alternative into action by completing any necessary plans involving sequencing steps and preparing individuals to implement the solution, all the while effectively communicating the process with all involved.

Orton suggests asking seven questions to increase the success of one's decision choice:[6]

1. Does the quality of the decision really make a difference?
2. Do I have all the information I need to make the decision alone?
3. Do I know what I'm missing? Do I know where to find the information? Will I know what to do with the information I'm given?
4. Do I need anybody's commitment to make sure this succeeds?
5. Can I gain commitments without offering participation in the decision?
6. Do those involved in the decision share the organization's goals?
7. Is there likely to be conflict about the available alternatives?

A final step in the process of decision making is to *monitor the implementation and evaluate outcomes* (step 7 of Exhibit 12–1). The nurse compares actual results with anticipated outcomes and makes modifications as needed to accomplish the desired outcome. Evaluation criteria obtained from measurable objectives provide feedback for testing the validity and effectiveness of the decision against the actual sequence of events in the process. Determination of flaws or gaps in the process may assist the decision maker to monitor the process more closely in the future and prevent the reccurrence of problems. The effective decision maker consciously follows these seven steps in a logical sequence.

Cost/Benefit Analysis

Cost/benefit analysis has a major role to play as a decision-making tool. Is the expenditure justified in terms of the return or benefit on the investment? Figure 12–1 illustrates the addition of cost/benefit analysis to the decision-making process. Additional reference to cost/benefit analysis is found in chapter 10 on budgeting.

Cost/benefit analysis should be as objective as possible. Many actions can be quantified and a value placed on them. Others are qualitative and should be evaluated on a rational basis.[7]

PITFALLS OF DECISION MAKING

Although information technology is having an increasing effect on decision making, pitfalls in the process stem more from individuals than from computers. Individuals are still resistant to change involving risk and new ideas. Such attitudes stifle not only individuals but also groups. When nurses find themselves resisting, they should analyze their behavior toward the goal of becoming more imaginative and creative. It is important that they too move away from becoming authoritarian and controlling. If the nurse chooses to control decision making and omit from the process those affected by the decision, less commitment to implementing the decision is a natural result. When feasible, the nurse may use a team approach to decision making, as in a matrix organization. Group decision making usually produces greater commitment to putting the selected alternative into action and working for success.

Other pitfalls of decision making include inadequate fact-finding, time constraints, and poor communication.

Failing to systematically follow the steps of the decision-making process will likely result in unanticipated outcomes.

IMPROVING DECISION MAKING

Basic precepts other than those already mentioned include educating people so they know how to make decisions, securing top management support for decision making at the lowest possible level, establishing decision-making checkpoints with appropriate time limits, keeping informed of progress by ensuring access to firsthand information, using statistical analysis when possible to pinpoint problems for solution,[8] and staying open to use of new ideas and technologies to analyze problems and identify alternatives. Computers can be used to support decision making through databased management systems. Numerous strategies and tools are available to improve decision-making abilities.

Consensus Building

One of the strong points of decision making by Japanese leaders is consensus building. When a major change is to occur, Japanese leaders may spend months and even years gaining consensus of internal customers and even of some external customers such as suppliers. When the change is initiated, all concerned parties have had input into the decision-making process and so get behind it to make it successful. They are stakeholders with a perception of a shared future. Kanter would probably label this process a synergy, since it encourages cooperation of all groups. Partnerships among groups require consultation and cooperation. Such partnerships are egalitarian, with members talking about work and its tasks. These members search for consensus on goals that lead to successful outcomes for the corporation, the employees, and shareholders.[9]

Group-think and consensus building are somewhat of a paradox. To build consensus, one listens to all parties, uses their ideas, and brings them onto the team by involving them in critical thinking and realistically considering their ideas. Group-think aims for fast solutions with minimal critical thinking and participant input.

THE ROLE OF INTUITION

Intuitive reasoning abilities have a place in the decision-making process. Intuition is a powerful tool for guiding decision making. So-called left-brain activities, such as analytical and logical thinking, mathematics, and sequential information processing, are essential in decision making and problem solving. But right-brain functions allow people to simultaneously process information, conceive and use contradictory ideas, fantasize, and perceive intuitively. Intuition is defined as the power to apprehend the possibilities inherent in a situation. It is a subspecies of logical thinking and integrates information from both sides of the brain—facts and feeling cues.[10] Nurses who can think intuitively have a sense of vision; they generate new ideas and ingenious solutions to old problems. Agor reported research involving 2,000 managers using a Myers-Briggs Type Indicator (MBTI) for measuring intuitive ability. The MBTI is widely used to measure intuition. Initial findings showed intuitive ability varying by managerial level, with higher ability in top-level managers than in middle- or lower-level managers.

Factors cited by middle- and lower-level managers that impeded the use of intuition included lack of confidence, time constraints, stress factors, and projection mechanisms such as dishonesty and attachment. Follow-up of the 200 top executives who scored in the top 10 percent of the first study revealed that all but one used intuitive ability as a tool in guiding decisions. These managers stated that their intuitive ability stemmed from years of knowledge and experience. From this research, Agor identified eight conditions in which intuitive ability seems to function best:[11]

1. When a high level of uncertainty exists.
2. When little previous precedent exists.
3. When variables are less scientifically predictable.
4. When "facts" are limited.
5. When facts don't clearly point the way to go.
6. When analytical data are of little use.
7. When several plausible alternative solutions exist to choose from, with good arguments for each.
8. When time is limited and there is pressure to come up with the right decision.

Nurses can certainly identify with each of these decision-making situations. It should be gratifying to know that research has supported the use of intuition in decision making. However, it is stressed that there are appropriate times for using intuition as an *adjunct* to the logical steps of decision making—*not* where objective data are complete. Because basic nursing education stresses the need for assessing facts and avoiding personal opinions, it may be difficult for some nurses to activate intuition for decision making. Agor has identified techniques and exercises used by executives to activate and expand their intuitive decision-making abilities, including relaxation and mental/analytical techniques. A full account of Agor's research is beyond the scope of this chapter; the reader is referred to Agor's extensive writings on the subject of intuitive decision making.[12]

Intuition is observed in individuals and in groups and is a creative and powerful attribute. Groups use intuition to reach consensus, particularly where information is incomplete. Consensus in a group leads to selection of a solution to a problem or to the making of a decision. Intuition can be developed through group brainstorming sessions, group visualization, and quiet thinking time.[13]

The human brain has a specialized region for making personal and social decisions. This region is located in the frontal lobes at the top of the brain and is connected to deeper brain regions that store emotional memories. Injury or stroke damage to this area causes personality changes, and the person can no longer make moral decisions. This knowledge has implications for behavior related to intuitive versus rational decision making.[14]

Decision making involves critical thinking. As the nurse becomes more expert, the process becomes more intuitive, and the expert nurse automatically processes the decision-making action as a consequence of a high level of knowledge and experience. The decision-making process is fostered by training, feedback, and the expansion of nursing knowledge. Case studies are good vehicles for teaching critical thinking.[15]

Nurses make critical decisions about resources affecting patient care. Resources include staff, equipment, supplies, bed space, time, and patient assignments to staff. Expert nurses make different decisions from those of novice nurses. All nurses make decisions requiring intelligence and judgment, personal and professional values, ethics, law, political reality, organizational culture, norms of classes, and economics.[16]

ORGANIZATIONAL VERSUS PERSONAL DECISIONS

A model for decision making has been identified, and specific steps involved in the process, including the role of intuition, have been described. Now the question is raised of when to make an organizational or a personal decision.

Organizational decisions relate to organizational purpose; constant refinement of organizational purpose is required because the organizational environment changes. This process provides opportunities for participative management styles, thereby giving subordinates the prerogative and responsibility of professional decision making.[17]

When are organizational decisions necessary? It would be easy to say we deal with professionals who are capable of making decisions related to their practice. An effective manager would not make decisions for competent professionals. However, incapacity of subordinates, uncertain instructions, novel conditions, conflicts, or failure of authority to make effective decisions, or to make decisions at all, could cause decisions to be appealed to a higher authority. Effective organizational decisions require collaboration and consultation with those having specialized knowledge.

From an organizational standpoint, decisions may be analyzed on the basis of futurity, impact, qualitative or value factors, and whether the decision is recurrent, rare, or unique. *Futurity* is defined as the length of time over which the decision will affect the organization in the future and the time required to reverse its impact. *Impact* refers to the number of individuals or departments affected and is a determinant of the level at which the decision is made. When philosophy or ethics are involved, decisions must be made at a higher level. The last characteristic refers to the uniqueness of the decision; recurrent decisions are made following a rule or principle already established.[18]

But what about institutional policy? Historically, decision making in nursing has been authoritarian, with minimal input from nursing staff, particularly when it involves institutional policy. Nurses have also been limited in their professional autonomy. Literature on the sociology of professions has indicated that a professional person has an ultimate or independent decision-making authority granted by society on the basis of unique knowledge and skill. This viewpoint gave physicians control over nurses. The traditional definition of autonomy no longer applies: Patients now demand more input in decision making, and increasingly, patient care technology requires nurses to make independent life-or-death decisions. McKay redefined professional autonomy as "both independent and interdependent practice-related decision making based on a complex body of knowledge and skill.[19] Primary nursing promotes nurse accountability, intraprofessional and interprofessional consultation, and an assertive synthesis of nursing and medical care plans. Interdependent decision making promotes professional autonomy.

Since nurse caregivers are functioning with increasing professional autonomy, nurse managers are moving into more executive positions in health-care administration. Nurse managers recognize the advantages of nurses being involved in strategic institutional decisions such as those concerning major programs, policies, promotions, personnel, and budgets. In addition to enhancing professional autonomy, the involvement of nurses in decision making has resulted in higher job satisfaction, better morale, lower turnover, improved communication, improved professional relationships with peers and colleagues from other disciplines, and higher productivity.[20]

Blegen and others at the University of Iowa studied nurses' preferences for decision-making autonomy in Iowa hospitals. They found that nurses wanted a more independent level of authority and accountability in twelve of twenty-one patient-care decisions, including those that concern patient teaching, pain management, preventing complications, clarifying and advancing orders, scheduling and discussing the plan of care with the patient, consulting with other providers, and arranging daily assignments and schedules. They also found that nurses wanted to make group decisions about such matters as setting policies, procedures, unit goals, job descriptions and standards, or quality improvement, and job performance. Nurse managers desired to increase decision making by staff nurses. It would appear that nurse managers should provide the impetus for more involvement in decision making by staff nurses by asking them what they want and actively involving them. The latter would include training and education. Staff nurses may want decision-making autonomy in areas where they are expert and competent.[21]

Many nurses equated decision-making autonomy with nurse professionalism. Most nurses are nonautonomous, since they are not self-employed. Research studies do not always support the premise that decision-making autonomy increases job satisfaction or performance or decreases nurse turnover.[22]

The nurse manager can maximize the opportunity for staff nurses to be involved in interdependent decision making by involving them at all levels of patient-care decision making, especially on interdisciplinary institutionwide committees. Strategies that have proven successful in involving nurses in accomplishing this include decentralization to the unit level, committee systems, and governance systems.[23]

Nurses who pursue holistic nursing practice encourage clients to make decisions about health and health-care issues. Decisions about health-care policy are not controlled by health-care professionals. They are made by the business sector and according to sociopolitical and economic variables.

Nurses need to become policy analysts, since analysts use communication networks or structures as strategy to action. Communication with decision makers is crucial to effecting decision making. Nurses use networking and professional relationships to influence decision makers. They arrive at positions on health-care policy through interest groups. Membership in professional associations, committees, and interest groups, plus communication with or as analysts, leads to participation in policy decision making and changes in the primary health-care system.[24]

Shared governance is an organizational administrative model that has been used as a vehicle for increasing staff-nurse participation in decision making and problem solving. It often involves multidisciplinary groups. Shared governance has as its object the provision of a trusting and nonjudgmental environment in which nurses, along with others, use the decision-making and problem-solving processes to make productive changes in organizations. Improved communication is a product of the shared governance process.[25]

Exercise 12–1

The following exercise may be done individually or as a group. You may want to work with a group of your peers.

Case Study: You are Ms. Carrie Platt. You have been director of nursing of Mason General Hospital for 1½ years. Mason General is a 500-bed general hospital in a metropolitan area serving a population of 700,000. The city has four other hospitals and a University Medical Center. A local ADN nursing program affiliates with your hospital. Today is Monday, March 20. During the past week, on Thursday, March 16, and Friday, March 17, you were away from the hospital to conduct a two-day workshop. You have just arrived at 8:00 a.m. and must leave the hospital at 8:50 a.m. to be at the airport at 9:10 a.m. There has been an unexpected death in the family, and you will be gone the entire week. You notice that the in-basket contains several items. You should make decisions about these things before leaving.

INSTRUCTIONS: Three decision-making exercises appear on the following pages. Each exercise is composed of a memorandum or other message-carrying device and a decision worksheet format. Use the worksheet format to list ideas for action and arrive at a decision. If the information given lacks essential detail, make any assumptions necessary. The following are some examples of possible decisions:

- Take immediate action and state what the action is.
- Delegate the action to another person and state who the person is.

(continued)

- Postpone the action, stating when you will take action.
- Other course; please specify.

MEMORANDUM #1

TO: Ms. Platt
FROM: Kay Campbell, Nurse Manager-5 N
SUBJECT: Poor charting of I & O
Date: March 17

The I & O record on Mrs. East in 517 is incomplete for evening and night shifts for her postoperative period. Mrs. East went into shock in the recovery room and is in renal failure. Dr. Blake is *extremely* upset about the lack of thorough charting of I & O. One of the evening aides heard Mr. East call his lawyer about the possibility of a lawsuit. We thought you needed to be aware of this situation.

Decision Worksheet

Subject	Decision Alternatives	Decision Analysis	Decision Selected

MEMORANDUM #2

IMPORTANT MESSAGE

FOR _Ms. Platt_

DATE _March 17_   TIME _10¹⁵_   A.M. / P.M.

M _s_ _Tonia Cole, MSN_

OF _____Chicago_____

PHONE _____

AREA CODE   NUMBER   EXTENSION

TELEPHONED	X	PLEASE CALL	
CAME TO SEE YOU		WILL CALL AGAIN	
WANTS TO SEE YOU	X	RUSH	
RETURNED YOUR CALL		SPECIAL ATTENTION	

MESSAGE ___Called in reference to ad for clinical specialist. Will be in area Wed. and Thurs next week and would like appt.___

SIGNED _____

Exercise 12–1
(continued)

Decision Worksheet

Subject	*Decision Alternatives*	*Decision Analysis*	*Decision Selected*

MEMORANDUM #3
TO: Ms. Platt
FROM: Mrs. Back, In-Service Instructor
SUBJECT: Uniform Regulations
DATE: March 17

The meeting with the nursing assistants regarding uniform regulations has been scheduled for March 21 at 10:00 a.m. in In-Service Room 406. We appreciate your offer to discuss this matter with the nursing assistants.

Decision Worksheet

Subject	*Decision Alternatives*	*Decision Analysis*	*Decision Selected*

PROBLEM-SOLVING PROCESS

At this point, one may be wondering about the relationship between decision making and problem solving. The first step in decision making was to identify the problem. But problem solving can involve the making of several decisions. The best way to define the relationship between the two is to define the steps of problem solving.

Steps in the Process

In reality, the steps of the problem-solving process are the same as the steps of the decision-making process: assess and analyze, plan, implement, and evaluate. Assessment includes systematic collection, organization, and analysis of data related to a specific problem or need. It involves logical fact-finding, questioning all sources, and differentiating between objective facts and subjective feelings, opinions, and assumptions. Knowledge and experience guide the data collection and analysis of data. Before the process goes any further, assessment should also determine whether a commitment exists to implement a decision or an action.[26] Making certain that there is no readily apparent solution also saves the time of all the people who may become involved in problem solving. Once the problem is identified, it must be determined whether it requires other than routine handling—that is, whether it is a rare or unique situation rather than a recurrent one. This leads to the second step of problem solving: planning.

Planning involves several phases. In nursing terms, we determine priorities, set goals and measurable objectives, and plan interventions. Management literature essentially says the same thing: break the problem down into components and establish priorities; develop alternative courses of action; determine probable outcomes for each alternative; decide which course is best in relation to resources, goals, risks, and the like; and decide on and make a plan of action with a timetable for implementation.[27]

When determining priorities, nurses should relate the problem to the corporate mission. Decisions involve choosing among alternative courses of action. They must have an acceptable effect on those directly involved, other areas affected, and the entire organization. Plans should include when and how to alter a course of action when undesired results occur.

The third step is implementation of the plan. The nurse should keep informed of the status of the process because it is unlikely that she or he will be directly involved. This is the one step in the process most likely to be delegated to subordinates. Implementation requires knowledge and skills appropriate to the specific alternatives selected.

Evaluation, the final step in problem solving, includes determining how closely goals and objectives were met, the success or failure of actions taken in resolving the problem, and whether the plan should be terminated because the problem has been resolved or whether it should be continued, with or without modification.

Effective problem solving requires that the practitioner be frequently at a high cognitive level: the level of abstract thinking. The essential difference between problem solving and decision making is that in the former, the thinking process works to solve a problem whereas in the latter, it serves to reach a goal or condition. Students used to learn to do problem solving by actually solving clients' problems. In doing so, student and client collaborate. Computer simulations are available for problem solving. Students progress through several levels of cognitive problem solving and practice: novice, advanced beginner, competent, and proficient. A few interactive video discs are available for practice in solving clinical problems.[28]

Group Problem Solving

While each step of the problem-solving process can be approached by an individual, input from all affected individuals or areas promotes more complete data collection, creative planning, successful implementation, and evaluation indicating problem resolution. Managerial problem-solving groups are often formed in organizations, with the expectation that the group's effect will prove to be greater than the sum of its parts. Brightman and Verhoeven state that

> a team of problem-solvers has greater potential resources than an individual, can have a higher motivation to complete the job, can force members to examine their own beliefs more carefully and can develop creative solutions.[29]

WEB ACTIVITIES

- Visit www.jbpub.com/swansburg, this text's companion website on the Internet, for further information on Decision Making and Problem Solving.
- What resources are available on the Internet to help guide you to new methods of decision making?
- Using the Internet, what further information can you find regarding the place of intuition in the decision making process?

SUMMARY

Decision making and problem solving occur concurrently with all major functions of nursing. A model of the cognitive thinking skills involved in decision making is presented: the descriptive model.

Decision making involves having an objective, gathering data pertaining to the objective, analyzing the data, identifying and evaluating alternative courses of action to achieve the objective, selecting an alternative (the decision), implementing it, and evaluating the results. Nurses make the best decisions through knowledge and use of the theory of decision making combined with intuitive ability developed over years of experience.

Although problem solving is not the exact equivalent of decision making, it employs a similar thinking process. Decision making is different from problem solving in that the objective does not have to pertain to a problem. It can be an objective that relates to change, to progress, to research, and to implementation of any operational or management plan.

NOTES

1. W. Lancaster and J. Lancaster, "Rational Decision Making: Managing Uncertainty," *Journal of Nursing Administration,* September 1982, 23–28.
2. T. Peters, "This Is CNN: Chaos Is the Future of Business," *San Antonio Light,* 3 March 1992, B9.
3. H. A. Simon, *Administrative Behavior,* 3d ed. (New York: The Free Press, 1976).
4. Ibid.
5. J. H. Reitz, *Behavior in Organizations* (Homewood, Ill.: Richard D. Irwin, 1977), 154–199.
6. A. Orton, "Leadership: New Thoughts on an Old Problem," *Training,* June 1984, 28, 31–33.
7. K. Harrison, "Cost Benefit Analysis: A Decision-Making Tool for Physiotherapy Managers," *Physiotherapy,* July 1991, 445–448.
8. D. Graham and D. Reese, "There's Power in Numbers," *Nursing Management,* September 1984, 48–51.

9. R. M. Kanter, *When Giants Learn to Dance* (New York: Simon & Schuster, 1989), 114, 153–155.

10. W. H. Agor, "The Logic of Intuition: How Top Executives Make Important Decisions," *Organizational Dynamics,* winter 1986, 5–18.

11. Ibid., 9.

12. Ibid., 5–18.

13. L. Rew, "Intuition: Concept Analysis of a Group Phenomenon," *Advances in Nursing Science,* January 1986, 21–28.

14. S. Blakeslee, "Seat of Morality Inside the Brain," *San Antonio Express-News,* 30 May 1994, 24A.

15. L. Casebeer, "Fostering Decision Making in Nursing," *Journal of Nursing Staff Development,* November/December 1991, 271–274.

16. M. L. Botter and S. B. Dickey, "Allocation of Resources: Nurses the Key Decision Makers, *Holistic Nursing Practice,* November 1989, 44–51.

17. C. Barnard and M. Beyers, "The Environment of Decision," *Journal of Nursing Administration,* March 1982, 25–29.

18. R. C. Swansburg, *Management of Patient Care Services* (St. Louis: C.V. Mosby, 1976), 149–170.

19. P. S. McKay, "Interdependent Decision Making: Redefining Professional Autonomy," *Nursing Administration Quarterly,* summer 1983, 21–30.

20. American Hospital Association, *Strategies: Nurse Involvement in Decision Making and Policy Development,* 1984, 1–10.

21. M. A. Blegen, C. Goode, M. Johnson, M. Maas, L. Chen, and S. Moorhead, "Preferences for Decision-Making Autonomy," *Image,* winter 1993, 339–344.

22. D. J. Dwyer, R. H. Schwartz, and M. L. Fox, "Decision-Making Autonomy in Nursing," *Journal of Nursing Administration,* February 1992, 17–23.

23. American Hospital Association, op. cit.

24. N. J. Murphy, "Nursing Leadership in Health Policy Decision Making," *Nursing Outlook,* July/August 1992, 158–161.

25. B. Anderson, "Voyage to Shared Governance," *Nursing Management,* November 1992, 65–67.

26. A. Scharf, "Secrets of Problem Solving," *Industrial Management,* September–October 1985, 7–11.

27. B. Blai, Jr., "Eight Steps to Successful Problem Solving," *Supervisory Management,* January 1986, 7–9.

28. E. Klaasens, "Strategies to Enhance Problem Solving," *Nurse Educator,* May/June 1992, 28–30.

29. H. J. Brightman and P. Verhoeven, "Why Managerial Problem Solving Groups Fail," *Business,* January–March 1986, 24–29; D. E. Shaddinger, "Digging for Solutions," *Nursing Management,* May 1992, 96f, 96h.

IMPLEMENTING PLANNED CHANGE

- Identify reasons or need for change in nursing practice and nursing management.
- Match examples of change to Reddin's seven techniques for accomplishing change.
- Match examples of change to Lewin's three stages of change theory.
- Match examples of change to Lippitt's seven stages of change theory.
- Match descriptions of change theory to the correct theorist. Identify the causes of resistance to change.
- Develop plans, including strategies for overcoming resistance to change.
- Define creativity.
- Develop plans for recognizing and increasing the creativity and innovation of clinical nurses.
- Describe the need for nursing research in a service setting.
- Make a plan for nursing research activity in the service setting.

KEY CONCEPTS

change theory
change agent
creativity
nursing research

Manager behavior: Considers change the domain of executive nursing and initiates all efforts for change accordingly.

Leader behavior: Encourages all nursing employees to recommend changes in the practice of nursing and the environment in which nursing is practiced. Involves nurses in implementing change. Encourages nurses to be creative and involved in research activities.

As a catalyst, the nurse causes or accelerates changes by using knowledge and skills that are *not* permanently affected by the reaction to the changes. In essence, the nurse may be considered a change agent. Let us first consider the philosophy embodied in theories of human resource management, theories based on adequate assumptions about human nature and human motivation. Has the nurse organized money, materials, equipment, and personnel in the interests of providing quality services to patients and thereby giving them their money's worth? Have nursing employees had experiences of supervision that have made them passive and resistant to organizational needs? Or do nursing employees work under conditions that inspire them to develop their potential, assume increased responsibility, and work to achieve their personal goals as well as those of the organization? Are clinical nurses able to direct their own efforts?

Machiavelli said, "There is nothing more difficult to take in hand, more perilous to conduct, or more uncertain in its success, than to take the lead in the introduction of a new order of things.[1] With a few notable exceptions, such as the weather, most of the change that takes place in our society is planned. This means that nurse managers can plan with clinical nurses to implement change. It must first be decided that a new skill or technique using a new apparatus or technology is needed to improve patient care and the ability to deliver that care. Then nurse managers and clinical nurses can plan and carry out the changes they want to make.

Spradley defines planned change as "a purposeful, designed effort to bring about improvements in a system, with the assistance of a change agent."[2] Peters writes that planned change is the exception rather than the rule.[3] Change occurs whether one wants it to or not. New technology is developed; new treatments result, causing personnel and organizational adjustments. These changes need to be controlled or managed. Hence, we refer to the process as planned change.

THE NEED FOR CHANGE

Four general reasons for designing orderly change have been defined by Williams:[4]

1. To improve the means of satisfying somebody's economic wants.
2. To increase profitability.
3. To promote human work for human beings.
4. To contribute to individual satisfaction and social well-being.

To these reasons one must add the climate of the 1990s that the structures of health-care organizations will continue to change as are the structures of other businesses and industries. These changes encompass higher standards and superior performance, constant innovation in technology and corporate structure, the accomplishment of more for less, teamwork, customer preference, employee loyalties, industry regulations, corporate ownership, increased opportunities, shrinking resources, increased competition, more transactions, more paperwork, and more complexity.[5] The need for organizational change may involve not only the whole system but also each of its units. This change will require management of the political dynamics and transition as well as motivation of constructive behavior.[6]

The basic motivation for change could be that orderly change needs to be designed to improve patient care while lowering costs and increasing nursing's economic status. It could be that the organization would profit by being able to do more for less or for the same cost or by improving its reputation for quality of care. Or, change could improve individual satisfaction and social well-being for both patients and staff members.

Implementing planned change will alter nursing's status quo. New programs of patient care will modify existing relationships among nursing personnel and between them and other members of the health-care team.

Change can help achieve organizational objectives as well as individual ones. Individual nurses and the institution of nursing will grow and prosper if they change with improved technology, especially if that technology will cure disease, save infant lives, prolong life without increasing suffering, and in general promote social improvement.

Other changes include personnel and organizational adjustments, such as constant turnover of personnel or changes in organizational structure. Nurses are certainly aware of changing relationships with those who hold authority and power, changes in responsibility and status, and changes in organizational, departmental, and unit objectives. Some employees resist change, but others welcome it as an opportunity to make adjustments in existing work situations, alter their relationships with their associates, and achieve personal goals.

Adaptation to change has always been a job requirement for nursing. Nursing personnel work for numerous bosses, including individual patients, physicians, the nurse manager, and a different charge nurse on each shift. Nurse practitioners find their roles changed many times in a day, sometimes as a manager, sometimes as a clinical nurse, sometimes as a consultant, and always in multiple roles.

Among the reasons for change is the evidence that something needs changing. The nurse manager needs to recognize the symptoms, which can be glaring or subtle. An example of the latter would be offhand comments by float personnel, such as, "I'd rather work anywhere than ward 3F" or "Could you send me someplace else?"

The health-care system is constantly changing. Changes include a labor force that wants wages comparable to those in other professions, hours of work that fit their personal needs, and the power to make their own professional decisions about patient care. Many times the change focuses on technology, without consideration for human relationships and political sensitivities. A case in point was the American Medical Association's 1988 failed push to solve the nursing shortage by proposing a new health-care technician. Professional nurses later introduced their own assistive personnel proposals.

Nurses require extensive knowledge of community affairs, government trends and constraints, world affairs, international practices and procedures, the changing nature of individual needs, and group motivation. Even the supply and demand for nurses relates to these many areas. Within nursing, needs change with new computer systems, planning, business, accounting, control, and marketing.[7]

Younger nurses, like other younger professionals, are mobile and have salable skills. They want to use all of their skills and to be collaborative and democratic.[8]

Change is the key to progress and to the future.

CHANGE THEORY

Some widely used change theories are those of Reddin, Lewin, Rogers, Havelock, Lippitt, and Spradley.

Reddin's Theory

Reddin has developed a planned change model that nurses can use.

He has suggested seven techniques by which change can be accomplished:

1. Diagnosis.
2. Mutual setting of objectives.
3. Group emphasis.
4. Maximum information.
5. Discussion of implementation.
6. Use of ceremony and ritual.
7. Resistance interpretation.

The first three techniques are designed to give those who will be affected by the change an opportunity to influence its direction, nature, rate, and method of introduction. These individuals are then able to have some control over the change, to become involved in it, to express their ideas more directly, and to propose useful modifications.

Diagnosis (the first technique) is scientific problem solving. Those affected by the change meet and identify problems and the probable outcomes. Mutual objective setting (technique number 2) ensures that the goals of both groups, those instituting the change and those affected by it, are brought into line. It may be necessary for groups to bargain and compromise. Group emphasis (number 3) is sometimes referred to as team emphasis. Change is more successful when supported by a team rather than by a single person. "Groups develop powerful standards for conformity and the means of enforcing them."[9]

Maximum information (number 4) is important to the success of change. Management should make at least four announcements with regard to a proposed change:[10]

1. That a change will be made.
2. What the decision is and why it was made.
3. How the decision will be implemented.
4. How implementation is progressing.

Lewin's Theory

One of the most widely used change theories is that of Kurt Lewin. Lewin's theory involves three stages:

1. *The unfreezing stage:* The nurse manager or other change agent is motivated by the need to create change. Affected nurses are made aware of this need. The problem is identified or diagnosed, and the best solution is selected. One of three possible mechanisms provides input to the

initial change: (a) individual expectations are not being met (lack of confirmation), (b) the individual feels uncomfortable about some action or lack of action (guilt-anxiety), or (c) a former obstacle to change no longer exists (psychologic safety). The unfreezing stage occurs when disequilibrium is introduced into the system, creating a need for change.[11]

2. *The moving stage:* The nurse manager gathers information. A knowledgeable, respected, or powerful person influences the change agent in solving the problems (identification). A variety of sources gives a variety of solutions (scanning), and a detailed plan is made. People examine, accept, and try out the innovation.[12]

3. *The refreezing stage:* Changes are integrated and stabilized as part of the value system. Forces are at work to facilitate the change (driving forces). Other forces are at work to impede change (restraining forces). The change agent identifies and deals with these forces, and change is established with homeostasis and equilibrium.[13]

Rogers's Theory

Everett Rogers modified Lewin's change theory. Antecedents included the background of the change agent and the change environment. Rogers's theory has five phases: phase 1, *awareness,* corresponds to Lewin's unfreezing phase; phase 2, *interest,* phase 3, *evaluation,* and phase 4, *trial,* correspond to Lewin's moving phase. Phase 5, *adoption,* corresponds to the refreezing phase. In the adoption phase, the change is accepted or rejected. If accepted, it requires interest and commitment.[14]

Rogers's theory depends upon five factors for success:[15]

1. The change must have the relative advantage of being better than existing methods.
2. It must be compatible with existing values.
3. It must have complexity—more complex ideas persist even though simple ones get implemented more easily.
4. It must have divisibility—change is introduced on a small scale.
5. It must have communicability—the easier the change is to describe, the more likely it is to spread.

Havelock's Theory

Havelock's theory is another modification of Lewin's, expanded to six elements. The first three correspond to unfreezing, the next two to moving, and the sixth to refreezing. Havelock's phases are as follows:[16]

1. Building a relationship.
2. Diagnosing the problem.
3. Acquiring the relevant resources.
4. Choosing the solution.
5. Gaining acceptance.
6. Stabilization and self-renewal.

Lippitt's Theory

Lippitt added a seventh phase to Lewin's original theory. The seven phases of his theory of the change process are as follows:[17]

Phase 1: Diagnosing the problem. The nurse as change agent looks at all possible ramifications and involves those who will be affected. Group meetings are held to win others' commitment. To ensure success, key people in top management and policymaking roles are involved.

Phase 2: Assessing the motivation and capacity for change. Possible solutions are determined, and the pros and cons of each are forecast. Consideration is given to implementation methods, roadblocks, factors motivating people, driving forces, and facility forces. Assessment considers financial aspects, organizational aspects, structure, rules and regulations, organizational culture, personalities, power, authority, and the nature of the organization. During this phase, the change agent coordinates activities among a number of small groups.

Phase 3: Assessing the change agent's motivation and resources. The change agent can be external or internal to the organization or division. An external change agent may have fewer biases but must have expert credentials. An internal change agent, on the other hand, knows the people. The process could involve both. The change agent needs a genuine desire to improve the situation, a knowledge of interpersonal and organizational approaches, experience, dedication, and a personality to suit the situation. The change agent should be objective, flexible, and accepted by all.

Phase 4: Selecting progressive change objectives. The change process is defined, a detailed plan is made, timetables and deadlines are set, and responsibility is assigned. The change is implemented for a trial period and evaluated.

Phase 5: Choosing the appropriate role of the change agent. The change agent will be active in the change process, particularly in handling personnel and facilitating the change. Conflict and confrontation will be dealt with by the change agent.

Phase 6: Maintaining the change. During this phase, emphasis is on communication, with feedback on progress. The change is extended in time. A large change may require a new power structure.

Phase 7: Terminating the helping relationship. The change agent withdraws at a specified date after setting a written procedure or policy to perpetuate the change. The agent remains available for advice and reinforcement.

Exhibit 13–1 compares these theories.

It should be noted that all five theories are similar to the problem-solving process itself, indicating that the latter could be used to implement planned change. The nurse manager should select the theory she or he feels most comfortable with after identifying the change to be made. A management plan is then made to cover the phases of making the change. The planning phase requires gathering data to support a decision for change. To set objectives, the nurse manager would work with the nursing staff who will be affected by the change. Thus, the entire group becomes aware of and interested in the need for change. A relationship is built between the nurse manager and nursing employees. The plan can then be made cooperatively, implemented by an enthusiastic

Exhibit 13–1   Comparison of Change Theories

Reddin	Lewin	Rogers	Havelock	Lippitt
1. Diagnosis 2. Mutual objective setting	1. Unfreezing	1. Awareness	1. Building a relationship 2. Diagnosing the problem 3. Acquiring the relevant resources	1. Diagnosing the problem 2. Assessing motivation and capacity for change 3. Assessing change agent's motivation and resources
3. Group emphasis 4. Maximum information 5. Discussion of implementation 6. Use of ceremony and ritual	2. Moving	2. Interest 3. Evaluation 4. Trial	4. Choosing the solution 5. Gaining acceptance	4. Selecting progressive change objective 5. Choosing the appropriate role of the change agent
7. Resistance interpretation	3. Refreezing	5. Adoption	6. Stabilization and self-renewal	6. Maintaining the change 7. Terminating the helping relationship

group, and evaluated and maintained by the group. Decision making is implemented by planned change.

Spradley's Model

Spradley has developed an eight-step model based on Lewin's theory. She indicates that planned change must be constantly monitored to develop a fruitful relationship between the change agent and the change system. The following are the eight basic steps of the Spradley model:[18]

1. *Recognize the symptoms.* There is evidence that something needs changing.
2. *Diagnose the problem.* Gather and analyze data to discuss the cause. Consult with the staff. Read appropriate materials.
3. *Analyze alternative solutions.* Brainstorm. Assess the risks and the benefits. Set a time, plan resources, and look for obstacles.
4. *Select the change.* Choose the option most likely to succeed that is affordable. Identify the driving and opposing forces, using challenges that include assimilation of the opposition.
5. *Plan the change.* Planning includes specific, measurable objectives, actions, a timetable, resources, budget, an evaluation method such as the Program Evaluation Review Technique (PERT), and a plan for resistance management and stabilization.

6. *Implement the change.* Plot the strategy. Prepare, involve, train, assist, and support those who will be affected by the change.
7. *Evaluate the change.* Analyze achievement of objectives and audit.
8. *Stabilize the change.* Refreeze; monitor until stable.

Exhibit 13–2 illustrates this model.

The Change Agent

As one studies change theory, one notes that its application tends to mimic the problem-solving process. Operating as a change agent, the nurse uses change theory to identify and solve problems. This nurse learns to anticipate impending

Exhibit 13–2   Planned Change Model

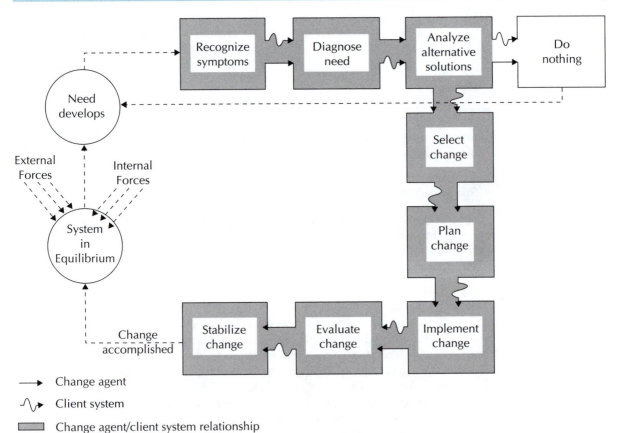

Change agent

Client system

Change agent/client system relationship

Source: B. W. Spradley, "Managing Change Creatively," *Journal of Nursing Administration,* May 1980. Reprinted with permission of J. B. Lippincott.

change, including that from interdependent systems, responds to change, and takes action to direct the change's course.

Nurses can compete successfully in the world of health care by doing things a new way. Professional nurses are expected to have the vision to change things and to be change agents.[19] Outsiders are resisted as change agents.

Examples of the Application of Change Theory

Retrenchments involving layoffs do not always use appropriate change theory. As a consequence, considerable unnecessary pressures, including unfavorable publicity, are placed on nurses. The organizational climate becomes tense and disruptive and gives personnel a sense of loss of security. Nurse managers feel tired and drained.

Causes of such problems include policies and plans that are developed after the fact, with few policies developed to deal with employees remaining with the organization. The media can be used to inform the public of changes in the health-care system that necessitated the layoff.

The following are among the positive responses that will minimize resistance to the change of retrenchment:[20]

1. Having a strong orientation toward reality, preparedness, knowledge of human behavior, stress management, and openness and honesty in dealing with employees.
2. Developing organizationwide retrenchment plans and policies with the advice of the personnel/human resource management department and legal counsel.
3. Considering the use of consultants.
4. Evaluating the criteria for layoffs: seniority, performance appraisal, and job categories. The principle of last hired, first fired should be weighed against the principle of keeping the best-qualified employees.
5. Having the public relations department (or a consultant) handle publicity.
6. Dealing positively with rumors through newsletters, informal discussions, and open meetings.
7. Reassuring remaining employees by being visible and available. Making frequent rounds.
8. Doing team building with chaplains, psychiatric specialists, and human resource specialists.
9. Forming a nurse manager support group that includes families, friends, colleagues, and nonnursing professional peers.
10. Being fair and honest and handling people with dignity and care.

Transformational change brings radical change to the mission, structure, and organizational culture of an organization. This change may be managed with consultation and employee participation. The nurse manager should keep training personnel abreast of organizational changes. Empowerment is a key factor in managing change, as empowered employees become change agents. Some coping strategies are problem-focused, some emotion-focused. Exhibit 13–3 lists individual coping strategies and organizational initiatives for coping with

Exhibit 13–3   Strategies for Coping with Organizational Change: Sources of the Strategy

Individual Coping Strategies	Organizational Initiatives
Use of coping efforts: problem-focused, emotion-focused Reliance on internal resources (personality traits, internal locus of control, hardiness, *sense* of mastery) Use of external resources and social supports (spouse, family, friends, managers, co-workers)	*Communication/Leadership* Empowering individuals to take control of change Provision of timely and accurate communication Training in communication The use of transformational leaders *Unlearning* Promotion of unlearning programs to deal with the removal of old elements of organizational culture; use of pre-merger diagnosis and integration workshops to determine elements of culture incompatibility *Job-Related Tasks* Classification of roles and relationships; establishment of support teams, improving person-job fit; job enrichment *Stress Programs* Provision of stress management interventions, including establishment of fitness and wellness programs

Source: V. J. Callan, "Individual and Organizational Strategies for Coping with Organizational Change," *Work & Stress,* March 1993, 68.

change. Change threatens a person's tenure, job role, career path, and status and power within the organization.[21]

Employees need time to adjust to change—sometimes a year or several years. They can use this time to learn new skills and become well trained. If they are to leave the organization, they need time to prepare resumes and do a job search. All employees should be treated with respect and concern. Whenever possible, change should give employees choices.[22]

RESISTANCE TO CHANGE

Resistance to change, or attempting to maintain the status quo when efforts are being made to alter it, is a common response. Change evokes stress that in turn evokes resistance.

Resistance is often based on a threat to the security of the individual, since change upsets an established pattern of behavior. If the problem-solving approach is used, answers should be provided to questions about the impact of the change, including the following: Will the change affect the work standard and subsequent employment, promotion, and raises? Will it mean an increased workload at an accelerated pace? Do employees visualize how they will fit into the picture if this change occurs? In-service and continuing education may help provide the answers.

Factors that stimulate resistance to change include habits, complacency, fear of disorganization, set patterns of response to change, conservatism, perceived loss of power, ego involvement, insecurity, perceived loss of current or meaningful personal relationships, and perceived lack of rewards.[23]

People are afraid of change because of lack of knowledge, prejudices resulting from a lifetime of personal experience and exposure to others, and fear of the need for greater effort or a higher degree of difficulty.

People have developed fears, biases, and social inhibitions from the cultural environment in which they live. Since they cannot be separated from these cultural factors, it is necessary to find ways of managing them within a system.

Barriers to change include a perception of implied criticism. "You are changing the system because you don't like the way I do it." Employees perceive that machines and systems are replacing them or making their jobs less interesting. As an example, a programmed system could be developed for patients to take their own nursing histories.

Change may demand the investment of a great deal of time and effort in relearning. If nurses are to be independent practitioners, what happens to those who are not prepared? "Probably the greatest single personal barrier is that individuals do not understand or refuse to accept the reasons for the change or the need for it. Unfortunately, it is not always easy to equate the reasons and the needs and to communicate them in meaningful and compelling language."[24]

People are members of a social system in a community and will resist change if it affects that social system. Social changes that threaten social customs, values, self-esteem, and security are resisted more than technical changes. One member of the social system may influence others even if unaffected by the change.

Other causes of resistance to change include time and pace; different generations of nurses have different rates of change.

Gillen claims that change stimulates increased levels of energy, which is called *hyper-energy* and is *not* stress. Hyper-energy is the heightened drive a person feels in response to a perceived challenge or threat. If not managed, hyper-energy is used by employees to think of surreptitious ways of preventing change. Hyper-energy can be pooled for collective resistance to change. It distracts employees, causing errors and accidents.[25] Skilled nurse leaders bring employees into the change process so that the employees do not view the change as a threat. Employees' hyper-energy is then channeled into involvement in the change process.

One reason for resistance to change is that hierarchical, bureaucratic frameworks with rules achieve stability. It should be kept in mind that both individuals and organizations need such stability through continuity in policies and procedures so that recurring needs can be dealt with routinely and problems do not have to be resolved anew each time they appear.

The major symptoms of resistance to change are confrontation; covert resistance such as nonpreparation for meetings or misunderstandings of the place or time; incomplete reports; refusal to accept responsibility; uncooperative employees; passive-aggressiveness; absenteeism; and tardiness.[26]

STRATEGIES FOR OVERCOMING OBSTACLES TO CHANGE

Managed Change

Change can be managed with nurse managers acting as change agents. One of the strategies a nurse manager can use is to hire a consultant who can make the diagnosis and recommend programs that will improve the productivity of nurse personnel while giving them job satisfaction. Such measures can include educational programs to improve the areas where problems exist.

Effective managed change leads to improvement of patient-care services, raised morale, increased productivity, and the meeting of patient and staff needs. Change is an art, the mastery of which can be exhilarating, refreshing, challenging, and exciting, because it represents opportunity. Change is facilitated when nurse employees are assigned to adapt to changing job requirements.

Preparation or Planning

Preplanning will help overcome many obstacles to change. Planning will keep interpersonal relationships from being disrupted if persons with common frames of reference are brought together. The planner can assist people to meet their goals while minimizing their fear and anxiety. Fear is stimulated by the external threat of change. Anxiety, which is self-induced dread, is internally stimulated. Planning will help people accept change without fear or anxiety.

In making changes, nurse managers should plan to help people unlearn the old (unfreeze) and use the new (refreeze). Implementation of nursing management information systems can refine much unfreezing and refreezing. Often, nurse managers help their staff learn the new without having them unlearn the old. This is a major problem in nursing today because of how the role of nurses is changing.

To prepare a plan carefully, the nurse manager should share information and decision making, work for common perception and understanding, and support and reinforce the nursing staff's effort to effect change. Clear statements of philosophy, goals, and objectives are needed in preparing for change.

Nursing in all areas, both clinical and managerial, must consider competition. The patient will go where there is high-quality nursing care, which results from effectively planned and managed change. Nurse educators should perform market surveys to determine the nursing products and services that consumers want.[27] This activity itself will constitute change and will result in changes.

Plans will list everyone on whom the change depends and their level of involvement. Who will oppose and who will support the change? The dominant coalition in the organization and the forces that will stimulate change should be identified and their support enlisted. Appropriate current events should be noted through reading and through meetings, highlighting those that will enhance the mission of the organization and for which the clinical nurses will claim or share ownership.[28] This activity brings new ideas and new knowledge to stimulate and justify the need for change.

Planning will also require thinking in multiple time frames: changes to be effected in six months, one year, and so on. The nurse manager should identify the trade-offs between nursing and other departments, between clinical and management staffs, and within the change process itself. List ways to enlist support.[29]

Nurse managers need to be careful not to overplan. They should leave some room for the people who will implement the change to exercise intelligent initiative. They need to be sure that the rewards or benefits to individuals and to the group are carefully communicated. If people want a change to work, they will make it happen.

Training and Education

The frequency of training and education should match the frequency of change. Nursing personnel will require constant staff development programs to keep from depreciating in knowledge and competence. From initial hiring and orientation, change should be portrayed as an integral part of the nurse's job.[30] Nurse managers should inform employees of the pressures that are making change necessary.

Rewards

Rewards for old behavior patterns should be removed after the individuals have been helped to see the reasons for the proposed change. Employees need to see the necessity for the new behaviors and should be given real incentives, financial or nonfinancial. Here is where job standards come in. The job standards should incorporate the new methods or skills and phase out the old ones. To provide an incentive, performance appraisal can be based on the new standards. Time must be allowed and opportunity provided for retraining. Nonfinancial rewards include enriching jobs and encouraging self-development. Such activities can satisfy individual needs.

Using Groups as Change Agents

Groups in themselves are often effective change agents. When the group appears to work in harmony and to have well-understood goals, it may be used to institute the change. If the idea can be planned in the group, it will be implemented more successfully. A group is more willing than most individuals to assume risks. Planning should make clear the need for change and provide an environment in which group members identify with such need. Objectives should be stated in clear, concise, and qualitative terms. Administrative policy should contain broad guidelines with understandable procedures for achieving the objectives, and the guidelines and procedures should be communicated to the group.

As agents of change, nurse managers need to utilize staff talents by using temporary work teams to solve specific problems and effect change. They need to participate on interdisciplinary task forces and prepare people for job mobility through experiences planned to facilitate it. Third-party critics may help diagnose and solve problems.

The informal group can promote and support change. It can be formed by enlisting the help of a strong leader and by forming a strong group that will communicate its perception of needed change to nurse managers and educators.[31]

Communications

Too often change is announced by rumor when it should be clearly introduced. Since changes split teams and kill friendships, causing productivity to drop, employees should be told about up coming changes before they become a rumor.[32] Announcements should be factual and comprehensive and should state objectives, nature, methods, benefits, and drawbacks of the change. An announcement that can be made face-to-face will be better received.

Discussion of implementation should give people maximum information. The discussion should cover the rate and method of implementation, including the first steps that will be taken and the rate, sequence, and people involved in each step.

Ceremonies may be effective in various aspects of the change. They are useful for retirements; promotion; introduction of a new co-worker, superior, or subordinate; a move to a new job; start of a new system; and reorganization. When used well, ceremonies focus on the importance of the ongoing institution and underline the importance of individual loyalty to that institution and its positions. They convey that the organization and the employees are both needed.

As change agent, the nurse manager discusses with people reasons for resisting change. When people understand the real reasons for the changes, they are not so resistant to it. They should be encouraged to sound off.

Planned change needs to be successfully communicated to all employees, even those who are not directly or immediately involved. Verbal announcements can be followed up with written ones and progress reports. Change occurs smoothly in direct proportion to the positive and democratic behavior that demonstrates management's philosophy and practice at all levels from the top down.

The Organizational Environment

Nurse managers could be more successful if they paid attention to the organizational environment into which change is introduced and the manner in which it is done. Managers need to be committed to a change and to support it by actions that express their attitudes. When the nurse leader attempts to impose change on people in an authoritarian manner, people often resist it.

Concern for employees is as important as concern for patients. Managers can establish an environment for change by doing the following:[33]

1. Emphasizing relationships with and between groups.
2. Bringing out mutual trust and confidence.
3. Emphasizing interdependence and shared responsibility.
4. Containing group membership and responsibility by limiting individuals from belonging to too many groups and ensuring that the same responsibilities are not given to several groups.

5. Having a wide sharing of control and responsibility.
6. Resolving conflict through bargaining and problem-solving discussions.

Other aspects of the organizational environment that support change include the following:

1. Permitting job movement to facilitate careers.
2. Anticipating and rewarding change, thus institutionalizing it.[34]
3. Modifying the nursing organizational structure to accommodate changes that provide growth and development.
4. Promoting a can-do attitude.
5. Providing predictability and stability by maintaining job security, sharing bad news early, and shifting concern to teamwork and process improvement.[35]

When the organizational climate changes, employees change behaviors. A desired organizational climate fosters high-quality patient care.[36]

Anticipating Potential Failures

Although preparation is the key to successful change, it should include anticipation of potential failure. Three questions need to be answered before actions for change begin. First, nurse leaders should determine the risks and how much they are willing to expend in terms of resources. Second, they should decide who will do the work. Third, they should have a flexible agenda and plan what will be done when it goes wrong.

Mistakes will happen. The importance of the change will determine how much risk the nurse leader is prepared to take. For example, one might risk a great deal and reorganize an entire unit to achieve the goal of having professional nurses perform as case managers. Changes can be introduced in one unit, evaluated, and modified before being extended to other units.

The positive aspect of resistance to change is that it pushes the change agent to plan more carefully, listen with sympathetic understanding, and reexamine goals, functions, priorities, and values. When properly addressed, resistance uses less of people's energy. Other effective responses to resistance are showing respect for honest questions and differences of opinion, altering of strategy and tactics, altering of composition of groups, and proceeding in an objective, firm, assertive, and nonjudgmental manner.[37]

Exercise 13–1   You may complete the following exercise as an individual or as a group.
Scenario: It was obvious to the entire nursing staff of a community hospital that the workload was decreasing. There were empty beds on every unit. Deliveries on the obstetrical unit were down to an average of one a day, and the daily census of the postpartum unit and newborn nursery was four to six patients. Workload and patient census on the pediatric unit were likewise low. Rumors were rampant. One was that the pediatric and obstetrical units would be combined. Another was that they would both be closed and their patients
(continued)

Exercise 13–1
(continued) would be combined with medical-surgical patients on other units. A third rumor was that the other community hospital was having similar problems and that negotiations were under way to combine several specialty services between the two institutions. It was even rumored that one hospital would become an extended-care facility and that the management of both hospitals would be combined. Worries of nursing staff gave way to gossip among various groups in corridors, at coffee breaks, in the dining room, and everywhere employees chanced to meet, including areas to which patients were transported, such as the x-ray lab, the physical therapy room, and the medical laboratory. Employees were concerned most about job security and institutional stability—whether there would be jobs for all of them and whether the job benefits would be the same if they worked at either hospital. At a clinical nurse managers' meeting, the director of nursing was asked whether any of the rumors were true. She stated that the administrator would make an announcement at the appropriate time and that until then the staff should continue with its work. That afternoon the local newspaper announced a merger of the two hospitals, describing in detail the missions and services each would provide to the community. No reference was made to the plans for employees.

Prepare a business plan (management plan) that embodies application of change theory that would be best under the preceding scenario.

CREATIVITY AND INNOVATION

Creativity Defined

Creativity is defined in *Webster's New Twentieth-Century Dictionary, Unabridged,* Second Edition, as "artistic or intellectual inventiveness." Innovation is defined as "the introduction of something new." These definitions suggest that the terms are interchangeable. A person could say that creativity is the mental work or action involved in bringing something new into existence, while innovation is the result of that effort.[38] If one wishes to differentiate the two, one might say that a nurse can create or invent a new nursing product, process, or procedure (creativity) or effect change by putting a new product, process, or procedure into use (innovation). Creativity is a way of using the mind.[39] Research indicates that creativity is *not* intelligence.[40]

Establishing a Climate for Creativity

For creativity to prosper, the organization should provide a warm, intellectual environment that gives employees recognition, prestige, and an opportunity to participate. Employees will gain a sense of ownership and commitment by being involved in planning their work and making decisions. Nurse managers promote creativity through sensitivity that gives people the attention they want and treats them as distinct individuals. Professionally competent managers inspire creativity by taking risks as well as by showing confidence, giving praise and support, being nourishing, using tact, and having patience.[41]

The External Environment

The external environment includes all aspects of the larger system, such as a hospital, that determines how conducive to creativity a group of clinical nurses perceives its climate to be.

The following task-related actions by nurse managers will help to develop and maintain a creative climate:[42]

1. Providing freedom to experiment without fear of reprimand.
2. Maintaining a moderate amount of work pressure.
3. Providing challenging yet realistic work goals.
4. Emphasizing a low level of supervision in performance tasks.
5. Delegating responsibilities.
6. Encouraging participation in decision making and goal setting.
7. Encouraging use of a creative problem-solving process to solve unstructured problems.
8. Providing immediate and timely feedback on task performance.
9. Providing the resources and support needed to get the job done.

Creative Problem Solving

Creative problem solving starts by using vague or ill-defined problems as challenges. Problems can be attacked intuitively to generate as many ideas as possible. Solutions may create new challenges and new cycles of creative problem solving.

There are several theories of creative problem solving. Lattimer and Winitsky suggest the following:[43]

1. *Thinking.* Identify the factors to be used in solving an issue or developing a strategic plan. The choice is between a risk-free alternative and one that involves risk.
2. *Decomposing.* Break down the situation into components—alternatives, uncertainties, outcomes, consequences; work with each and combine the results for a decision.
3. *Simplifying.* Determine the important components and concentrate on them. What are the most crucial factors and most essential relationships? Then make intuitive judgments.
4. *Specifying.* Establish the value of key factors, the probabilities for the uncertainties, and preferences for the outcomes.
5. *Rethinking.* Was the original analysis sensible regarding omissions, inclusions, order, and emphasis?

Creativity Training

Training can help people be creative. It can teach them to develop creative thinking skills and logic techniques that can lead to successful results. General Electric established creativity training for its engineers in 1937. Many other companies provide creativity training for employees. Before developing creativity training, nurse educators should establish some general concepts about the new products, techniques, markets, etc., they want employees to bring into existence.

Creativity training aims to increase the creative capacity or creative behavior of individuals or groups. The techniques of creativity training can include brainstorming, synectics, morphological analysis, forced fit, forced relationships, brainwriting, visualization, cueing, lateral thinking, and divergent thinking.[44] (See Exhibit 13–4).

Nurses will be motivated to be creative when nurse leaders encourage them to express their ideas openly and accept divergent ideas and points of view. Other motivators of creativity by nurses include providing assistance to develop new ideas, encouraging risk taking while buffering resisting forces, providing time for individual effort, providing opportunities for professional growth and development, encouraging interaction with others outside the group, promoting constructive intragroup and intergroup competition, recognizing the value of worthy ideas, and exhibiting confidence in workers.[45]

Research studies indicate that creative behavior is inherent in human nature and can be developed. Elements or pieces necessary for creating something new exist and must be arranged in new and useful combinations. Excessive motivation, caused by high rewards for performance or anxiety over possible failure, has been proven to inhibit creativity. It causes people to pursue ideas down blind alleys.

The following are actions for producing original, goal-oriented ideas:[46]

1. Assemble the separate elements that will be creatively combined to produce a product or a new procedure. The problem must be identified in terms of usefulness of this product or process. If a known element is missing, what is available to replace it?
2. Use the available and assembled elements in combinations that produce original ideas.
3. Remove inhibitions to creativity, such as excess motivation, anxiety, fear of taking risks, dependence upon authority, or habitual modes of thinking and talking about things. Creativity is not confined to a small, exclusive set of gifted people. Since language contains the potential for creative thought, everyone has the potential.
4. Study techniques of creativity so that the elements can be used.

Characteristics of a Creative Person

Creative people, including nurses, have a broad background of knowledge. They have the mental skills of curiosity, openness, sensitivity to problems, flexibility, ability to think in images, analysis, and synthesis.[47]

Creative nurses use their knowledge to stimulate their sensory perceptions. In addition to solving problems, they create new problems to solve by formulating questions about the whys and hows of established practices. To foster independence and creative talents, nurse managers will assume that creative nurses are not odd or eccentric. As a consequence, barriers will not be erected among peer groups. Nurse managers will communicate and cooperate with clinical nurses to set new goals or new practices for achieving goals.[48]

Exhibit 13–4   The Creativity Jargon Jungle

Here is a list of the ten techniques and terms we heard most often while researching the wonderful world of creativity training. Our thumbnail definitions are in no way USDA-approved. And remember that terms sometimes mean anything a particular speaker wants them to mean.

Creativity Training

According to the *Encyclopedia of Management* (Van Nostrand Reinhold, 1982), General Electric established in 1937 a two-year work/study program for engineers "showing creative promise during the first months of employment." This first recorded creativity training program focused on nurturing that promise through work assignments and educational experiences.

Today the term is used to cover a multitude of processes and means neither more nor less than the speaker wants it to mean. As used here, it refers to training that aims to increase the creative capacity or creative behavior of individuals or groups; it does not refer to efforts to foster a creative "climate" in an organization.

Brainstorming

A group-based idea-generating technique developed by Alex Osborn in 1938 and popularized in his book *Applied Imagination* (Scribner, 1953). Brainstorming is not a room full of people madly shouting out whatever comes into their heads. It is a structured, moderated process. The group is led by a chairman who controls time, presents the problem to be worked out, and controls the progress of the storm. Brainstorming usually starts with a warm-up wherein the participants review the rules ("no critiquing others' ideas, piggybacking is good, be far out, etc."), and loosen up with practice exercises ("How many uses can you think of for a sick cat?").

Then the real problem is presented and participants call out as many ideas as they can dream up. Someone records every idea. The idea-generation phase typically lasts an hour to 90 minutes. Participants then cluster and categorize the ideas, evaluate their potential, and recommend the most promising ones to the problem owner.

Brainstorming groups have been convened to find new uses for an old product, to name a new product, and to develop slogans for campaigns from sales to

safety. Proponents see the technique's uses as virtually unlimited. Brainstorming is the longest running act in the idea-generating business; there are probably as many variations as there are people who hold creativity sessions.

Synectics

A group-based problem-solving technique that stresses control over the creative environment and reasoning by analogy. In 1944, W. J. J. Gordon set out to study creativity through the psychoanalysis of inventors. George Price joined Gordon, popularized his findings, added to them and translated them into practical procedures. In 1960 they founded Synectics, Inc., which sells training in the method. The firm is credited with coining the expression, "making the familiar strange and the strange familiar." Synectics comes from the Greek *synetikos,* meaning "the joining together of apparently irrelevant elements." A short description of synectics is just about impossible. The major stages are: 1) problem as given, 2) short analysis of the problem as given, 3) purge (the problem as given is clarified and simplified), 4) problem as understood (the problem is reinterpreted in analogy or metaphor), 5) excursion (the group leaves the problem and "plays" with analogies), 6) fantasy force fit (a metaphor is forced onto the original problem), 7) viewpoint (the problem is redefined in a "new light").

Morphological Analysis

Developed in the late 1940s by a mathematician named Frank Zwicky, and refined later by Myron Allen, morphological analysis is a system of breaking an idea or problem into its components for study. It is seen as falling toward the logical end of the creative problem-solving spectrum.

You specify the attributes of the problem and then make a grid or cube of them. For instance, you're trying to come up with a new method of transportation. You choose "energy" as a minor dimension, and list under that heading all the ways that a thing can be powered (wind, gas, steam, etc.). That list forms one side of a morphological grid. Across the other axis you write "surfaces" and list ground, air, water, etc. This gives you a series of "boxes" where each factor listed under one of your major headings intersects with each factor listed under the other. Where "wind" and "water"

Exhibit 13–4   The Creativity Jargon Jungle *(Continued)*

intersect, we think of a sailboat. Ah, but what about "wind" and "ground"? Add a third major dimension and you can create a three-dimensional cube instead of a grid.

Force Fit/Forced Relationships

A basic idea in creative problem solving and in the creativity literature as a whole is that if you rub two old ideas together you sometimes come up with a new one. But ideas don't necessarily stick to one another easily: sometimes they have to be forced together and examined for fit. Force fitting refers to going back to a list of interesting, outrageous, preposterous—as well as sensible—ideas and twisting and squeezing them until they become a reasonable or at least a possible solution to the problem. Sometimes ideas are jammed together with objects, sights, sounds, etc. Smell, particularly, is considered a powerful sensory trigger.

The terms *direct force fit* and *get-fired technique* also show up in connection with this process. In get-fired the challenge to the group is to come up with solutions that would work, but that would lead to the sponsor getting fired. Once such a solution is determined, the task becomes to scale or tone it down so that the problem gets solved but the sponsor saves his or her job. Force-Fit Game is a team competition in idea-generating developed by Helmut Schlicksupp of the Battelle Institute in Frankfurt, Germany.

Brainwriting

This is an idea-generating technique for groups that aren't exactly groups, much like the Nominal Group Technique, Crawford Slip Method, and Collective Notebook. All are methods that encourage free association and the recording of ideas in writing, without verbal interaction with other people but with their "assistance." In brainwriting, originally developed by Bernd Rohrback, the technique is simple. Participants are given a set of forms, consisting mostly of lines and white space. They listen to an explanation of the problem and are asked to write four ideas (solutions, suggestions, thoughts, etc.) about the problem on the form. The teams are then exchanged. Reading others' ideas is supposed to stimulate more ideas, which are then written on the form. The process continues until no one can think of something else to write.

Visualization

Most of us have little movie projectors in our heads that we can use to review the past, speculate about the future or create "pictures" of impossibilities. For some time, psychologists have tapped into this ability to help people overcome phobias and fears in a process called *systematic desensitization.*

People like T. H. Carl Krueger of Encina Corp., Las Cruces, NM, have conducted several studies in high-technology settings that suggest that it is possible to control and harness this natural skill that 85% of us share (15% of the adult population cannot spontaneously visualize) and to fine-tune it for problem solving. A wide range of creativity consultants have been claiming that for years. Excursion, the generation of a fantasy scenario having no apparent relation to the problem being solved, is a form of visualization used in the Synectics process and in many other courses.

Lists

There are a lot of them: Osborn's list, Arnold's list, the Davis and Houtman list, Polya's checklist and more. They tend to be sets of specific questions to ask in specific problem-solving situations. For instance, if you are trying to make a change in a product, a checklist might ask, "Can you make it smaller? Larger? A different color?" The items on the checklists are intended to act as cues to new ways of considering the problem.

Attribute listing is a specific technique. The characteristics of a product or problem are spelled out. The group—or an individual—then speculates on ways of modifying the characteristics or obtaining the same characteristic in another way: "What can we substitute that has the same characteristics?" Walter Mettal uses the example of running out of packing material the evening before the moving trucks arrive. Packing material is "light, shock-absorbent, available, etc." These characteristics lead to a creative solution: "Go into the kitchen and pop a bushel or two of popcorn. Use the popcorn as packing material."

Lateral Thinking

A term coined by Edward de Bono to represent the need to escape from conventional ways of looking at problems to solve them. In his 1970 book, *Lateral Thinking* (Penguin Books), he divided problems into three types: those whose solutions require the processing of information,

Exhibit 13–4   The Creativity Jargon Jungle *(Continued)*

those where the "problem" is one of accepting what cannot be changed, and those that can be solved only by reorganizing information and assumptions about the problem. To solve the third type, you have to be illogical or "think laterally." Training in this area primarily involves learning to challenge assumptions and developing the awareness that methods other than straight logical reasoning can solve problems.

Divergent Thinking
A term that refers to expanding one's view of a problem. In divergent thinking, we roll the problem over in our minds and think about it in different ways without necessarily trying to solve it—just to "get a handle on it." Convergent thinking is just the opposite: the problem is cut into smaller and smaller pieces to obtain a manageable size and perspective. The key is to know when to do which. Predominantly, divergent thinkers are referred to as impractical, woolgatherers, perhaps scatterbrained. Insistently convergent thinkers are accused of jumping to solutions and being narrow-minded. Divergent thinking is most often stressed, but both skills are useful in creative problem solving.

Source: Reprinted with permission from the May 1976 issue of *TRAINING* Magazine. Copyright 1976, Lakewood Publications, Minneapolis, Minn. All rights reserved. Not for resale.

Creative people have been considered different from other people. This difference has been described by one writer:

> The public would have him nearsighted but farseeing, brilliantly innovative but absentminded, widely acclaimed but impervious to applause, capable of highly involved abstract thinking but naive and eccentric in his everyday reasoning. The truth of the matter is that the creative person *is* different but is *not* a monster strangely mysterious and incomprehensible.[49]

An individual may appear to have been gifted with a brilliant intellect. During childhood this individual may have been the curious type who searched for books to read and tasks to do that satisfied his or her curiosity. Searching for the approval and encouragement of parents, friends, or teachers but not receiving it, the person may have become somewhat of a loner.

Creative individuals value the work and association of other creative individuals. They stimulate each other to think and perhaps even to be competitively creative. Creative people can tolerate ambiguity; they have self-confidence, the ability to toy with ideas, and persistence.[50]

A clinical nursing coordinator had set up her own cancer clinic. She convinced the physicians of her ability to perform the functions and of the clinic's benefit to them and to the patients. Patients now make direct appointments with this clinic, which has expanded to become a health screening clinic for women. In addition to coming for a Pap test and breast examination, clients have a history taken by the nurse practitioner. They are referred to the physician only when there is evidence of pathology. Many patients now come for personal health counseling.

In another instance, an assistant to the director of nursing questioned the time-honored practice of nurses counting narcotics and controlled drugs three times a day. With the advice of legal counsel, it was determined that this was being done only because it had become common practice. Policy has been changed so that the narcotics and controlled drugs are inventoried by the pharmacist when the medications are ordered each morning and by the unit manager before leaving at the end of the shift. Discrepancies are reported to the nurse manager. Thus, nurses have lost another nonnursing function.

THE RELATIONSHIP OF NURSING RESEARCH TO CHANGE

The Need for Nursing Research

While there are many predictions of the future directions of health care, the future will probably differ from all of them. Nursing research is essential to preparing for the future and for competition within the health-care system. Nurse managers should have good information to keep nursing competitive with other caregivers in providing patient care. They should also have the knowledge to be competitive among employers and in a global economy. This requires the development and employment of nursing scientists who are researchers. Employment of these nursing researchers will commit nurses to developing research in managing humans beings to their full potential. It is an investment that keeps people, the future human capital, from depreciating.[51]

Nursing research improves nursing practice. A profession grounds practice in scholarly inquiry. Nurse educators will improve the quality of nursing practice when they promote nursing research and the application of the findings of nursing research. Nursing research will validate the discipline of nursing.[52]

Nurse managers, clinical nurses, instructors, and others are often eager to effect change. They like to try something new, to apply the latest technologies, and they can do so through the nursing research process. There are two kinds of research activities: those in which nurses are the subjects and those in which they develop their own nursing research program. Real research requires preparation and time.

Nursing Research in the Service Setting

It follows, then, that if there is to be research in nursing and if it is to be part of the organizational goals, there must be planning. Plans incorporate a budget, a staff, and defined problems for research. Staff nurses working in clinical jobs and management personnel usually do not have time for this kind of research. They can use the results of such research and apply them to their situation to build better health-care delivery systems.[53]

A nursing position filled by a scholar will enhance the chances that a nursing research program will be successful. A scholar will have the knowledge to increase nursing research of a high intellectual and professional caliber. A nurse researcher can promote the reunification model of nursing education and nursing service through joint appointments and joint nursing research endeavors, supporting cooperation between service and education.

Nursing faculty tend to disengage from practice because of the numerous demands of their teaching roles. One reason that faculty focus on wellness may be their disengagement from practice. Since nursing faculty are often well-prepared scientists, nursing managers should find ways to budget money for released time from faculty duties. Faculty may then do clinical practice and the service agency reimburses the school for their work. A coalition will benefit all nurses because faculty will be recognized for research activities that keep them up-to-date and managers will benefit from improved patient care.[54]

Nursing administration scholars will allow clinicians adequate time to develop their projects. They will provide a resource link to help clinicians find research partners with whom they can pursue relevant nursing research.[55]

A survey of nursing deans indicated increased demand for well-prepared nurse researchers. Researchers were most highly needed in the psychosocial and biophysical domains. Also needed would be those in health-care delivery systems and administration, education, and methodology and instrumentation. All areas of research are important to the profession and the development of its theory base.[56] The focus of the National Center for Nursing Research is upon funding for training in biological theory and measurements in nursing research.[57]

Nurse managers and administrators can improve the use of nursing research findings by encouraging replication of nursing studies, having research findings translated into understandable language, and rewarding nurses for implementing research findings. Otherwise, too much new nursing knowledge will continue to be lost.[58]

Nurse managers can facilitate the implementation of nursing research findings through specific continuing education programs and by providing sources of help in developing research activities, identifying available library services, and using computer networks. They should keep clinical nurses informed on institutional review policies. Seed money can often be found by institutional administrators. Research forums may be held once or twice a year. Research awards are excellent forms of recognition. They are even better when supported by funds for presentation when papers are accepted by professional organizations.[59]

Establishing a research program in a clinical institution requires administrative support, including funds for staffing, supplies, and equipment. The program coordinator may be established in the nursing division or the research and development department. Goals and priorities need to be established for the types of research to be done: education, administration, program evaluation, methodology, case study, and clinical nursing. A nursing research program requires a budget, funding, and strategies. One strategy may be to focus on research and not be distracted by other activities. Nursing research should focus on outcomes that will have values for clients and for nurses and nursing (see Exhibit 13–5).[60]

Efforts are being made to use research findings to change nursing practice. Laschinger and others designed a project to use the findings of research in nursing administration. Students chose the area of job satisfaction. They presented themselves as an external consultant team and chose the Conduct and Utilization of Research in Nursing (CURN) model as an approach. One project was to

Exhibit 13–5   Framework for Establishing a Clinical Nursing Research Program

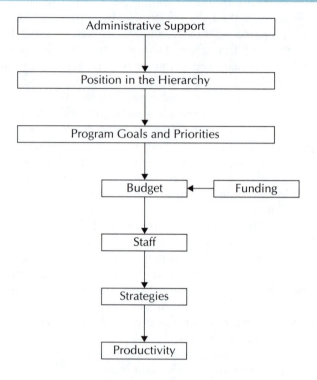

Source: L. Marchette, "Developing a Productive Nursing Research Program in a Clinical Institution," *Journal of Nursing Administration,* March 1985, 26. Reprinted with permission of J. B. Lippincott.

develop a program using research findings for nurse managers in an agency. The exercise represents a method for nurse managers and administrators to use research findings in nursing administration.[61]

To build a nursing research culture, nurse managers should create an environment that fosters it. This can be achieved by using the learning process. Resource individuals are academic nursing faculty and nurses prepared in research methodology at the graduate level. The nurse leaders provide continuing education to promote interest in nursing research. They support this interest with internal and external funding and pay for performance in productive research activities.[62]

The Nursing Research Process

The nursing research process includes both scientific and technical steps. The format for writing up research is a problem-solving one and includes the following sections:[63]

1. *Introduction.* Includes an overview of the problem and tells why the research is being done.
2. *Statement of the problem.* An explicit and precise expression of the research question.
3. *Purpose of the study.* Answers the question, What is the long-range goal of the research, the ultimate purpose that will be achieved by the findings? The statement also relates to current nursing concerns and the motivation for the study. If readers of a study cannot determine its purpose, they should read no further.
4. *Review of the literature.* A summary of the studies previously published and their results and a statement indicating what this study will add. The review should present a conceptual framework for the study, concepts and theories documented in previous studies, and evidence to support the approach. It should also indicate how the proposed study goes beyond what has already been achieved. The dependent variables to be measured and the independent variables to be manipulated should be identified.
5. *Hypothesis.* A formal statement of the research question, of what relationships are being tested and how they are to be measured. The variables are specifically defined.
6. *Methodology, or design.* Describes the setting, the subjects, how the subjects are chosen, procedures, analysis, and data collection. Measurement techniques used will be those appropriate to the hypothesis.
7. *Analysis.* A statistical test that measures the effect of the independent variable.
8. *Results.* Answers the research question objectively. The presentation of results stays within the parameters of the designed study.
9. *Discussion.* Includes any unexpected results as well as the conclusions reached.

This format can be used to evaluate research reports. Steps 1 through 5 indicate how to develop a research proposal; plans for steps 6 through 9 should be included in the proposal.

The Research Question   The research question comes from many intensive hours of thought, literature review, and reflection. It avoids value judgments and opinions. The research question needs more than one variable. It may be a question or a statement. The researcher begins by getting thoughts down on paper and by writing an annotated statement of the question without concern for grammar, which will be refined later. A literature search is undertaken to find out what facts are known about the subject, including relationships among facts and their level of confidence.

Written abstracts are made by the researcher, including types of studies and categories of variables. The researcher also defines the independent and dependent variables and has peers critique them. Questions answered include, Are these variables related so that change in one is apt to produce change in the other? and What variables other than the one to be tested could influence the variable(s) to be measured?[64] See Exhibit 13–6 for a sample research question.

Exhibit 13–6   Sample Research Question

Research Question
What is the difference in attendance between continuing education (CE) programs that are based on a needs survey and those that are not? (This question is researchable, while "Should a CE needs survey be done?" is not.)

Test	Other Factors	Measure
Independent variable: the variable being tested, examined, or manipulated. Provides measurement of the dependent variable.	Extraneous variables: conditions, behaviors, or characteristics known to exist but not considered of primary importance to the research. The research design may or may not control for these.	Dependent variables: the variables being measured, studied, or investigated to evaluate the impact of the first variable. The outcome or criterion: what will result from the study? *Attendance at CE programs*
Needs survey	*Cognitive mapping, rewards, threats, personal needs*	

Source: Adapted from C. A. Lindeman and D. Schantz, "The Research Question," *Journal of Nursing Administration,* January 1982, 6–10. Reprinted with permission of J. B. Lippincott.

According to Lindeman and Schantz, a good research question will meet the following criteria:[65]

1. It can be answered by collecting observable evidence or empirical data.
2. It contains reference to the relationship between two or more variables.
3. It follows logically and consistently from what is already known about the topic.

Lindeman and Schantz state that experimental studies should not be done if no descriptive ones exist.[66]

The Research Design.   The research design is the blueprint created to answer the research question. It follows development of the research question, the literature search, and statement of the hypothesis. The following are six elements of a good research design:[67]

1. *Setting.* This is the place where research will be done. There must be enough cases or variables specific to the intent of the research, thereby strengthening internal and external validity and the ability to generalize.
2. *Subjects.* Subjects should be profiled and limited to those most useful in answering the research question. Their human rights will be protected.
3. *Sampling.* This is the method for choosing the sample size or number of subjects. Increasing the size of a sample adds strength, power, and meaningfulness.
4. *Treatment.* Subjects of the sample are assigned to groups randomly: experimental versus control. They are manipulated to increase the difference between the groups.

5. *Measurement.* Statistical tests are selected to measure the differences between the groups. A reliable instrument produces consistent results. A valid instrument measures what it claims to measure.
6. *Communicating the results.* Data are analyzed and results reported to others. Findings related to the research question are given first, followed by surprise data.

Research Strategies

Nursing Research in a Health-Care Agency.   Utilization of nursing research findings is poor in all spheres of nursing. This is improving as nurse administrators establish nursing research programs within their organizations. Once the nurse administrator, with input from practicing nurses, defines the objectives of a nursing research program, a decision can be made regarding the organizational design for it. If resources are so scarce that additional budgeted personnel cannot be hired, a standing research committee can be established. A standing committee will promote stability by maintaining effective protocols and standards. The committee chair should have research expertise.

Since program resources are a determinant of the scope of the research program, the nurse administrator will need to establish a budget related to the objectives. This may include reallocation of money, generation of external funding, or revenue-generating activities by the professional nursing staff.

Budget permitting, the nurse administrator may hire a research specialist full- or part-time. Sometimes a budgeted position is shared by another nurse specialist. It could be a joint appointment with the college of nursing faculty.[68]

A research consortium can be established as a cooperative venture with other organizations within the community. It can include such organizations as hospitals, home-health-care agencies, and nursing homes.

Given a larger budget, the nurse executive can establish a research department as a separate cost center. Such a department will have direct accountability and clearly structured authority. It can even be self-supporting. Success will reflect strong commitment and will give increased visibility. Exhibit 13–7 shows examples of nursing research studies from one institution.

The ultimate purpose of service-based nursing research is to improve patient care. Nursing management research will answer questions related to the management of resources used in providing patient care. As practicing nurses become aware of the availability of competent nurse researchers, they will refer research questions to them.

Four phases occur in the application of research findings to practice:[69]

1. Evaluation of the strength of the research design.
2. Evaluation of the feasibility and desirability of making the change in practice.
3. Planning the introduction and implementation of the change.
4. Using a pretest and posttest to evaluate the effect of the proposed change on practice.

Exhibit 13–7   Nursing Research Studies Completed at Northeast Georgia Medical Center, 1986–1988

"A Comparison Study of Three Self-Monitoring Blood Glucose Meters," Shannon Garner, R.N., Debbie Cleland, R.N., and Susan Stone, R.N.

"The Recruitment and Retention of Registered Nurses in a Hospital Setting," Susan Stone, R.N., and Dan Walter, M.B.A.

"A Comparison Study of Heparinized Saline and Normal Saline in Maintaining INT Catheter Patency," Susan Stone, R.N., NGMC IV team.

"The Perceived Personal Needs of Families of Acute Brain-Injured and Spinal Cord–Injured Patients," Tracy Carlisle, R.N., and NGMC neuroscience nursing staff.

"ICU Mortality Prediction Model," Susan Stone, R.N., Ruth Kunkle, R.N., NGMC ICU Nursing Staff.

"Nurses' Attitudes Towards Alcohol-Dependent Clients," Joan Burnham, R.N., North Georgia College.

"The Effects of Music Therapy on Critically Ill Patients in an ICU Setting," Sonja Chaffin, R.N., Angela Chambers, R.N., Fran Rusk, R.N., and Susan Stone, R.N., NGMC ICU Nursing Staff.

"Nurse Retention: Staff Nurse Perspectives," D. Patricia Gray, R.N., Susan Stone, R.N., NGMC neuroscience nursing staff.

"The Effects of Nocturnal Bottle-Feeding Patterns on Infant Weight and Maternal Satisfaction," Gay Mortimer, R.N., and Susan Stone, R.N., NGMC newborn nursery staff.

Source: Reprinted with permission of Northeast Georgia Medical Center, 743 Spring Street, Gainesville, GA 30501-3899. The author visited this hospital and noted that while administration provided seed money, nursing research was expected to pay for itself through improved practice and cost savings.

Milieu.   A University of Michigan study of the Conduct and Utilization of Research in Nursing (CURN) model included participating hospitals with milieus that supported research. These milieus were found to include an active clinical faculty for such resources as undergraduate and graduate students, existing research programs, influential nurse administrators, and librarians. Each facility had experienced, degree-prepared nurses with flexible, autonomous roles who facilitated research. These nurses perceived nursing research to have increased the status and visibility of nursing in both education and practice.[70]

Organizational Considerations.   Once nurse administrators decide that nursing research will be a component of the nursing organization, they must plan the program design within the organizational structure. The mission, philosophy, and objectives will give direction to a nursing research program design. Input can be obtained from interested professional nurses at the planning stage. This can be done through an ad hoc committee that defines clear objectives for both clinical and administrative research activities. These objectives can include those for research conducted to satisfy departmental, personal, and interdisciplinary needs of the institution, graduate students, staff, faculty, and others. Other ad hoc committees can be formed to conduct research studies or to evaluate and implement research findings. Their composition will be determined by their objectives and by interest and expertise of participating nurses.

Research Strategies.   Protocols can be developed to benefit the entire institution. A hospital-wide research department or committee can include nurses. Such a committee can standardize procedures for approval, evaluation, and implementation of all research.

Staff development programs can support interest in the nursing research program. Instructors can communicate to the nursing staff the relevance of nursing research studies and teach nursing staff their roles. The nursing staff can be provided with rewards of nursing research in the form of money, improved care, and prestige. This will be supplemented with consistent communication in memoranda, study abstracts, literature, references, presentations, seminars, and conferences.[71] Exhibit 13–8 presents details of an actual research study.

Pressure is increasing to produce research that is congruent with societal need. This pressure reflects the public's view of costs versus benefits, of societal need versus scientific interest. Heads of U.S. corporations indicate that most innovation today is coming from industry rather than the research community. Americans tend to waste research money. Five major international research priorities are "human resources, cultural concerns (effect of socioeconomic status and culture on health practices, patterns of illness, and styles of intervention), health of women and children, models for delivery of nursing care, and models for education." Nursing research should result in a significant payoff to the public.[72]

Exercise 13–2   Scan the previous year's issues of ten different nursing journals and answer the following:
How many articles report *research* in management or administration? _____
Teaching? _____
Practice? _____

Exercise 13–3   Identify a published research study from one of the journals in Exercise #2. What was the research question? How does it meet the criteria of Lindeman and Schantz? Evaluate the study using the steps of the research process outlined in this chapter.

Exhibit 13–8   ICU Mortality Prediction Model

Purpose

As health care resources become limited and the cost of intensive care increases, reliable methods are needed to predict patient outcomes in the critical care setting. Determination of those patients who are most likely to benefit from the intensive care unit (ICU) could be useful to evaluate the need for admission and to estimate resources required for the ICU.

Northeast Georgia Medical Center (NGMC) was invited to participate in a national study funded by the National Center for Health Service Research Grant HS 04833. The purpose of this study was to describe the severity of illness of patients admitted to ICU and to predict the mortality of ICU patients based on clinical variables assessed on admission.

Study Design

A sample of 100 consecutive patient admissions was drawn from the ten-bed NGMC ICU. Each ICU nurse was instructed on the use of the ICU mortality prediction model (MPM) admission and discharge forms. Each MPM admission form was completed by an ICU nurse within four hours of the patient's admission to the ICU. Following patient discharge, the MPM discharge forms were completed and each was reviewed by the clinical nursing researcher. Confidentiality and anonymity were assured. Logistic regression and analysis were used to interpret the data.

Results

One hundred patients participated in the study. The mean patient age was 53 years. Fifty-eight percent were admitted to surgical service; 26 percent to medical service; 16 percent to neurological service. Average patient acuity according to the Medicus Patient Classification System was 3.91. Two of the patients were categorized as "do not resuscitate" by the physician.

The *actual* ICU mortality rate was 7 percent. The *predicted* ICU mortality rate, according to the ICU Mortality Prediction Model, was 16.5 percent. Among the other sixteen hospitals included in the study, the average predicted mortality rate was 17 percent. The predicted mortality range was 10 to 31 percent.

The average probability of dying among the living was 0.138 for NGMC. The average probability of dying among the dead was 0.519 for NGMC. Ninety-one of the 100 patients were correctly classified by the MPM. There were no patients who died who were predicted to live. For the ten highest calculated probabilities, 6.59 patients were expected to die and four actually died.

Source: Reprinted with permission Northeast Georgia Medical Center, 743 Spring Street, Gainesville, GA 30501-3899.

Exercise 13–4   Identify a published research study from one of the journals in Exercise #2 and apply the results. Use change theory to make a business or management plan for doing this.

Exercise 13–5   Form a group of your peers and have each identify something that can be improved in nursing. This may be a policy or a procedure; a change in a form to make the form's use more effective; an interdepartmental protocol, such as how tests are scheduled or patients transported or handled; or a change in clinical practice. Each person makes a plan for improvement and discusses it with the group. When the group decides that the plan merits implementation, present it to nursing administration where you work or are assigned as a student.

Exercise 13–6   Scan several nursing journals from the past year. Select research findings you would like to use in clinical nursing. Select a model for implementation such as the Conduct and Utilization of Research in Nursing (CURN) model. (See J. A. Horsley, J. Crane, and J. Bingle, "Research Utilization as an Organizational Process," *Journal of Nursing Administration* 8, no. 7 (1978): 4–6.) Prepare a plan and implement the findings.

WEB ACTIVITIES

- Visit www.jbpub.com/swansburg, this text's companion website on the Internet, for further information on Implementing Planned Change.
- Kurt Lewin developed three stages of change theory. Can you locate a website on his theory?
- What resources are available for planning strategies and increasing creativity to foster change?

SUMMARY

Ability to manage planned change is a necessary competency of all nurses, since it represents viability of the nursing organization. Since planned change is a necessity, nurse managers create the climate for its receptivity by nursing personnel. Change, the key to innovation and the future, has its basis in change theory.

Lewin's change theory is widely used by nurses and involves three stages: unfreezing, moving, and refreezing. In the unfreezing stage, employees are made aware of needed changes. A plan for change is made and tested in the moving stage. During the refreezing stage, the change becomes a part of the system, establishing homeostasis and equilibrium.

Rogers, Havelock, and Lippett each modified Lewin's original change theory. Reddin's theory has many similarities, and all these theories have common elements of problem solving and decision making.

Resistance to change is evoked by stress from threatened security of affected employees. It can be overcome by planning that involves those who will be affected, particularly if they can see a benefit. Established values and beliefs, imprinting, time perspectives, and hyper-energy all stiffen resistance to change.

The nurse as change agent is the manager of change and thus requires knowledge of the theory of change. Education and training are necessary for nursing personnel who will be affected. Intrinsic and extrinsic rewards are another management tool. Using groups to effect change will help absorb the risks of change, since risks are part of the process.

Creativity and innovation are important aspects of nursing that lead to better practice as new knowledge and skills are applied. The result is change that leads to maintenance of a competitive share of the health-care market, thus assuring the position of nursing.

Nursing educators can promote change through nursing research, thus committing nursing to a clinical practice based on scholarly inquiry. Promotion of nursing research effects change through application of research findings. Nursing research can be income-enhancing when it produces more effective and efficient nursing prescriptions.

Change involves nursing managers in many functions of nursing. It requires planning. The organization is adapted to accommodate the changes. The nurse manager uses communication, leadership, and motivation theory to overcome resistance and gain support in making the change work. The implemented change is continually evaluated to keep it working and effective.

NOTES

1. W. J. Reddin, "How to Change Things," *Executive,* June 1969, 22–26.
2. B. W. Spradley, "Managing Change Creatively," *Journal of Nursing Administration,* May 1980, 32–37.
3. T. Peters, "Vote for Change but Follow Through," *San Antonio Light,* 7 May 1991, B2.
4. E. G. Williams, "Changing Systems and Behavior," *Business Horizons,* August 1969, 53–58.
5. R. M. Kanter, *When Giants Learn to Dance* (New York: Simon & Schuster, 1989), 9–26.
6. D. A. Nadler and M. L. Tushman, "Organizational Frame Bending: Principles for Managing/Reorganization," *Executive,* March 1989, 194–204.
7. R. D. Brynildsen and T. A. Wickes, "Agents of Changes," *Automation,* October 1970.
8. Ibid.
9. W. J. Reddin, op. cit.
10. Ibid.
11. B. W. Spradley, op. cit.; L. B. Welch, "Planned Change in Nursing: The Theory," *Nursing Clinics of North America,* June 1979, 307–321.
12. Ibid.
13. Ibid.
14. L. B. Welch, op. cit.
15. Ibid.
16. Ibid.
17. Ibid.
18. B. W. Spradley, op. cit.
28. Ibid.
19. J. V. Roach, "U.S. Business: Time to Seize the Day," *Newsweek,* April 4, 1988, 10; M. Beyers, "Getting on Top of Organizational Change: Part 1, Process and Development," *Journal of Nursing Administration,* October 1984, 32–39.
20. J. Feldman and D. Daly-Gawenda, "Retrenchment: How Nurse Executives Cope," *Journal of Nursing Administration,* June 1985, 31–37.
21. V. J. Callan, "Individual and Organizational Strategies for Coping with Organizational Change," *Work & Stress,* March 1993, 63–75.

22. D. Rosenberg, "Eliminating Resistance to Change," *Security Management,* January 1993, 20–21.
23. E. G. Williams, op. cit.
24. M. J. Ward and S. G. Moran, "Resistance to Change: Recognize, Respond, Overcome, *Nursing Management,* January 1984, 30–33.
25. D. J. Gillen, "Harvesting the Energy from Change Anxiety," *Supervisory Management,* March 1986, 40–43.
26. M. J. Ward and S. G. Moran, op. cit.
27. M. Beyers, op. cit.
28. Ibid., D. J. Gillen, op. cit.
29. D. J. Gillen, op. cit.
30. R. E. Hunt and M. K. Rigby, "Easing the Pain of Change," *Management Review,* September 1984, 41–45.
31. M. J. Ward and S. G. Moran, op. cit,
32. Report on Victor E. Dowling's Change Theory, "How to Wage the War on Change," *Electrical World,* October 1990, 38–39.
33. R. E. Endres, "Successful Management of Change," *Notes & Quotes,* November 1972, 3.
34. R. E. Hunt and M. K. Rigby, op. cit.
35. Report on Victor E. Dowling's Change Theory.
36. M. Beyers, op. cit.
37. W. J. Ward and S. G. Moran, op. cit.
38. D. P. Newcomb and R. C. Swansburg, *The Team Plan: A Manual for Nursing Service Administrators,* 2d ed. (New York: Putnam, 1971), 136–172.
39. R. L. Lattimer and M. L. Winitsky, "Unleashing Creativity," *Management World,* April 1984, 22–24.
40. J. Gordon and R. Zemke, "Making Them More Creative," *Training,* May 1986, 30ff.
41. R. R. Godfrey, "Tapping Employees' Creativity," *Supervisory Management,* February 1986, 16–20.
42. A. G. Van Gundy, "How to Establish a Creative Climate in the Work Group," *Management Review,* August 1984, 24–25, 28, 37–38.
43. R. L. Lattimer and M. L. Winitsky, op. cit.
44. J. Gordon and R. Zemke, op. cit.
45. A. G. Van Gundy, op. cit.
46. S. Glucksberg, "Some Ways to Turn on New Ideas," *Think* (IBM) March–April 1968, 24–28.
47. R. R. Godfrey, op. cit.
48. D. P. Newcomb and R. C. Swansburg, op. cit.
49. H. Levinson, "What an Executive Should Know About Scientists," *Notes & Quotes,* (Hartford: Connecticut General Life Insurance Company, November 1965), 1.
50. R. R. Godfrey, op. cit.
51. T. R. Horton, "Poised for Tomorrow," *Newsweek,* 5 October 1987, S-4.
52. M. L. McClure, "Promoting Practice-Based Research: A Critical Need," *Journal of Nursing Administration,* November–December 1981, 66–70; American Hospital Association, *Strategies: Integration of Nursing Research into the Practice Setting* (Chicago: AHA Nurse Executive Management Strategies, 1985).
53. R. C. Swansburg, *Management of Patient Care Services* (St. Louis, Mo.: C. V. Mosby, 1968), 334.
54. M. L. McClure, op. cit.
55. K. P. Krone and M. E. Loomis, "Developing Practice-Relevant Research: A Model That Worked," *Journal of Nursing Administration,* April 1982, 38–41.

56. L. N. Sherwen, C. A. Bevil, D. Adler, and P. G. Watson. "Educating for the Future: A National Survey of Nursing Deans About Need and Demand for Nurse Researchers," *Journal of Professional Nursing,* July–August 1993, 195–203.

57. M. J. Cowan, J. Heinrich, M. Lucas, H. Sigmon, and A. S. Hinshaw, "Integration of Biological and Nursing Sciences: A 10-Year Plan to Enhance Research and Training," *Research in Nursing and Health* 16 (1993): 3–9.

58. L. R. Bock, "From Research to Utilization: Bridging the Gap," *Nursing Management,* March 1990, 50–51.

59. H. J. Krouse and S. D. Holloran, "Nurse Managers and Clinical Nursing Research," *Nursing Management,* July 1992, 62–64.

60. L. Marchette, "Developing a Productive Nursing Research Program in a Clinical Institution," *Journal of Nursing Administration,* March 1985, 25–30.

61. H.K.S. Laschinger, S. Foran, B. Jones, K. Perkin, and P. Boran, "Research Utilization in Nursing Administration," *Journal of Nursing Administration,* February 1944, 32–35.

62. G. C. Polk, "Building a Nursing Research Culture," *Journal of Psychosocial Nursing* 27, no. 4 (1989): 24–27.

63. C. A. Lindeman and D. Schantz, "The Research Question," *Journal of Nursing Administration,* January 1982, 6–10; D. Schantz and C. A. Lindeman, "Reading a Research Article," *Journal of Nursing Administration,* March 1982, 30–33.

64. C. A. Lindeman and D. Schantz, op. cit.

65. Ibid.

66. Ibid.

67. D. Schantz and C. A. Lindeman, "The Research Design," *Journal of Nursing Administration,* February 1982, 35–38.

68. American Hospital Association, op. cit.

69. E. A. Hefferin, J. A. Horsley, and M. R. Ventura, "Promoting Research-Based Nursing: The Nurse Administrator's Role," *Journal of Nursing Administration,* May 1982, 34–41.

70. K. P. Krone and M. E. Loomis, op. cit.

71. American Hospital Association, op. cit.

72. E. Larson, "Nursing Research and Societal Needs: Political, Corporate, and International Perspectives," *Journal of Professional Nursing,* March–April 1993, 73–78.

14

THE ORGANIZING PROCESS

OBJECTIVES

- Define "organizing."
- Apply or illustrate selected principles of organizing.
- Describe a bureaucracy.
- Identify the components of a nursing-care delivery system.
- Analyze an organizational structure.
- Use a set of standards to evaluate line and staff relationships of a nursing organization.
- Distinguish among various forms of organizational structures.
- Describe an informal organization.
- Use a set of standards to evaluate an organizational chart.

KEY CONCEPTS

organizing
chain of command
unity of command
span of control
specialization
bureaucracy
role theory
organizational development
autonomy
accountability
culture
climate
team building
organizational structure
restructuring
nursing-care delivery system
departmentation
organization chart
informal organization

Manager behavior: Maintains the nursing organization to support a bureaucratic structure through adherence to basic principles of organizing.

Leader behavior: Works with nursing employees to develop a modified organizational structure that supports autonomy, accountability, and a culture and climate conducive to satisfied patients, families, and physicians, nurses, and other staff.

ORGANIZATIONAL THEORY

Once plans are made, the mission, purpose, or business for which the organization exists has been established, the philosophy and vision statements have been developed and adopted, and the objectives have been formulated, resources are organized to sustain the philosophy, achieve the vision, and accomplish the mission and objectives. Organizations develop as goals become too complex for the individual and have to be divided into units that individuals can manage.[1]

Fayol referred to the organizing element of management as the form of the body corporate and stated that the organization takes on form when the number of workers rises to the level requiring a supervisor. It is necessary to group people, distribute duties, and adapt the organic whole to requirements by putting essential employees where they will be most useful. An intermediate executive is the generator of power and ideas.[2] The body corporate of the nursing organization includes executive management and staff, departmental managers (middle managers), operational managers (first-line managers), and practicing professional and technical nursing personnel. Reformed organizations eliminate middle management, with operational managers becoming the department heads. Professional nursing personnel manage the performances of technical nursing personnel. In a theory of nursing management, nurse managers have as their object the development of a nursing organization that facilitates the work of clinical nurses.

Definition of Organizing

Urwick referred to organizing as the process of designing the machine. The process should allow for personal adjustments, but these will be minimal if a design is followed. It should show the part each person will play in the general social pattern, as well as the responsibilities, relationships, and standards of performance. Jobs should be put together along the lines of functional specializations to facilitate the training of replacements. The organizational structure must be based on sound principles, including that of continuity to provide for the future.[3]

Organizing is the grouping of activities for the purpose of achieving objectives, the assignment of each grouping to a manager with authority for supervising the group, and the defined means of coordinating appropriate activities with other units, horizontally and vertically, that are responsible for accomplishing organizational objectives. Organizing involves the process of deciding the levels of organization necessary to accomplish the objectives of a nursing division, department or service, or unit. For the unit, it would involve the type of work to be accomplished in terms of direct patient care, the kinds of nursing personnel needed to accomplish this work, and the span of management or supervision needed.

Principles of Organizing

The following paragraphs discuss the established principles of organizing.

Chain of Command.   The chain of command principle states that to be satisfying to members, economically effective, and successful in achieving goals, organizations are established with hierarchical relationships within which authority flows from top to bottom. This principle supports a mechanistic structure, with a centralized authority that aligns authority and responsibility. Communication flows through the chain of command and tends to be one-way—downward. In a modern nursing organization, the chain of command is flat, with line managers and a technical and clerical staff that support the clinical nursing staff. Communication flows freely in all directions, with authority and responsibility delegated to the lowest operational level.

Unity of Command.   The unity of command principle states that an employee has one supervisor and there is one leader and one plan for a group of activities with the same objective. This principle is still followed in many nursing organizations but increasingly is modified by emerging organizational theory. Primary nursing modality and case management support the principle of unity of command, as does joint practice. Professional nurses and others frequently are in matrix organizations, where they answer to more than one supervisor.

Span of Control.   The span of control principle states that a person should be a supervisor of a group that he or she can effectively supervise in terms of numbers, functions, and geography. This original principle has become an elastic one—the more highly trained the employee, the less supervision is needed. Employees in training need more supervision to prevent blunders. When different levels of nursing employees are used, the nurse manager has more to coordinate. Some management experts recommend hiring up to seventy-five employees answering to one supervisor.[4]

Specialization.   The principle of specialization is that each person should perform a single leading function. Thus, there is a division of labor—a differentiation among kinds of duties. Specialization is thought by many to be the best way to use individuals and groups. The chain of command joins groups by specialty, leading to functional departmentalization.

The hierarchy or scalar chain is a natural result of these principles of organizing. It is the order of rank from top to bottom in an organization. These principles of organizing are interdependent and dynamic when used by nurse managers to create a stimulating environment in which to practice clinical nursing.

Bureaucracy

Bureaucracy evolved from the early principles of administration, including those of organizing. The term was coined by Max Weber. Bureaucracy is highly structured and usually includes no participation by the governed. The principles of chain of command, unity of command, span of control, and specialization support bureaucratic structures. These structures do not work in their pure form and have been greatly adapted in today's organizations.

Among the historical strong points of bureaucratic organizations is their ability to produce competent and responsible employees who perform by uniform rules and conventions, are accountable to one manager who is an authority, maintain social distance with supervisors and clients, thereby reducing favoritism and promoting impersonality, and receive rewards based on technical qualifications, seniority, and achievement.

The characteristics of bureaucracy include formality, low autonomy, a climate of rules and conventionality, division of labor, specialization, standardized procedures, written specifications, memos, and minutes, centralization, controls, and emphasis on a high level of efficiency and production. These characteristics frequently lead to complaints about red tape and to procedural delays and general frustration.[5]

Professionalism and Bureaucracy.   Hall studied the relationship between professionalization and bureaucratization. In a study using both structural aspects and attitudinal attributes of a profession, his findings were as follows:[6]

1. Attitudes are strongly associated with such behavior as participation in professional organizations and pursuit of certification.
2. Nurses are high in professionalism in terms of belief in service to the public, belief in self-regulation, and sense of calling to the field but are low in feeling of autonomy and using the professional organization as a reference point.
3. Nurses are high in bureaucratization, except in the area of technical competence.
4. Autonomous organizations have less hierarchy of authority. (Autonomous organizations are those that promote autonomy of professional practitioners.)
5. An organization's size does not affect hierarchy.
6. Autonomous organizations have less division of labor.
7. Autonomous organizations have fewer procedures.
8. Autonomous and heteronomous organizations emphasize technical competence. (These organizations promote differences in practice patterns among autonomous practitioners of nursing.)
9. Professionalism increases with decreased division of labor, decreased procedures, decreased impersonality, and increased autonomy. Hierarchy is accepted if it serves coordination and communication functions.
10. Bureaucracy inhibits professionalism.

The conclusion would be that the less bureaucratic the organization, the more nurses perceive themselves as professionals.

Role Theory

Role theory indicates that when employees receive inconsistent signals of what is expected and lack information, they will experience role conflict, leading to stress, dissatisfaction, and ineffective performance. Role theory supports the chain of command and unity of command principles. Multiple lines of authority are disruptive; they divide authority between profession and organization and create stress. They force employees to make choices between formal authority and professional colleagues. The result is role conflict and dissatisfaction for employees and reduced efficiency and effectiveness for the organization. Role conflict reduces trust of and personal liking and esteem for the person in authority, reduces communication, and decreases employee effectiveness. Role conflict and ambiguity can be reduced by management that provides for the following:[7]

1. Certainty about duties, authority, allocation of time, and relationship with others.
2. Guides, directives, policies, and the ability to predict sanctions as outcomes of behavior.
3. Increased need fulfillment.
4. Structure and standards.
5. Facilitation of teamwork.
6. Toleration of freedom.
7. Upward influence.
8. Consistency.
9. Prompt decisions.
10. Good, prompt communication and information.
11. Using the chain of command.
12. Personal development.
13. Formalization.
14. Planning.
15. Receptiveness to ideas by top management.
16. Coordinating work plans.
17. Adapting to change.
18. Adequacy of authority.

In a changing work environment, nurses are required to perform in new roles under new circumstances. Managers provide the education and support necessary for nurses coping with their role changes. Management support addresses the potential and real needs deficits that nurses will confront. The goal is to prevent role insufficiency by thoroughly preparing nurses to function in new roles. Managers may opt to do this through role modeling. Clear understanding of role changes and planned programs to support them will reduce role stress and prevent role strain.[8]

Effective use of role theory has a positive impact when changes have to be made in a nursing care delivery system. Role ambiguity, role stress, and role strain are minimized through educational programs aimed at socializing nurses into their new roles. Effective communication improves role changes.[9]

ORGANIZATIONAL DEVELOPMENT

Organizational development deals with changing the work environment to make it more conducive to worker satisfaction and productivity. An underlining premise is that "people planning" is as important as technical and financial planning. Organizational development allows managers to attend to the psychological as well as the physical aspects of organizations. Change is the terrain by which organizational development applies.

Organizational development can sustain the favorable or desirable aspects of bureaucracy, and change can modify the undesirable aspects. There is room for directive as well as nondirective leadership within organizations. Nurse managers have to be strong and tough in supporting the values of clinical nurses. They have to be proactive in planning, designing, and implementing new organizational structures and work environments. The object is to develop people, not to exploit them. Organizational development emphasizes personal growth and interpersonal competence.[10]

Autonomy and Accountability

Among the psychological and personality attributes of organizational development are autonomy and accountability, crucial elements of nursing professionalism. A professional nurse is obliged to answer for decisions and actions. Characteristics of professional autonomy include self-definition, self-regulation, and self-governance. Professional nurses respond to demographic changes in society to defining and reshaping the content of nursing practice. They address society's needs, including the needs for increased care for the elderly and the need to control resources. Autonomy will be strengthened by unbundling the hospital bill and by direct reimbursement for nursing services by third-party payers.

Self-governance for nursing includes a nursing administrator hired or elected with input from nurses, self-employment of nurses, approval of nursing staff privileges by peer review with privileges revoked by the nursing staff organization, and case management.[11]

Argyris describes people as complex beings who work for an organization for their own needs or gains. These needs exist in varying degrees or at varying depths that must be understood by organizations. People seek out jobs to meet their needs. They develop and live on a continuum from infant to adult that is reflected throughout life at work and at leisure.[12] Exhibit 14–1 shows the developmental continuum. Employees begin at the infant level of behavior in the organization and progress gradually to adult behaviors. This progress is helped or hindered by the organizational environment, which is, in turn, affected by employee behavior.

Culture

Organizational culture is the sum total of an organization's beliefs, norms, values, philosophies, traditions, and sacred cows. It is a social system that is a subsystem of the total organization. Organizational cultures have artifacts, perspectives, values, assumptions, symbols, language, and behaviors that have been effective in the past.

Organizational cultures include communication networks, both formal and informal. They include a status/role structure that relates to characteristics of employees and customers or clients. Such structures also relate to management styles—whether authoritative or participatory. Management style greatly impacts individual behavior. In a health-care setting, these structures promote either individuality or teamwork. The status/role structure relates to classes of people and could be identified through demographic surveys of both employees and patients.

The basic mission of the organization is part of its culture: employment, service, learning, and research. There is a technical or *operating* arm for getting the work done. Also, there is an *administrative* arm that covers wages and salaries, hiring, firing, and promoting; report making and quality control; fringe benefits; and budgeting.

The artifacts of an organizational culture may be physical, behavioral (rituals), or verbal (language, stories, myths). Verbal artifacts result from shared values and beliefs. They include traditions, heroes, and the party line and result in ceremonies that embody rituals. Such ceremonies include rewards for years of service, the annual picnic, the Christmas party, and the wearing of badges and insignia.[13]

Metaphors are used to characterize personalities and work styles:[14]

1. Military. Language includes such terms as battle zone, tight ship, captain, troops, battles, campaigns, enemies, and stars. Award ceremonies also contain military metaphors.
2. Sports. Terms such as teams, stars, and quarterback are used. Award ceremonies may also reflect the sports metaphor.
3. Anthropology. Terms include family, novice, big daddy, big momma, elder, and prodigal son.
4. Television. Terms include sitcom, soap opera, country club, playground, nursery, and jungle.
5. Mechanistic. Terms such as factory, assembly line, and well-oiled machine are used.
6. The "zoo." Terms such as sly fox, chicken, and top dog appear.

Dress, personal appearance, social decorum, and physical environment are all part of the organizational culture. They will require strict compliance through written or implied rules.

Values are the general principles, ideals, standards, and sins of the organization. Basic assumptions are the core of the culture. They include the beliefs that groups have about themselves, others, and the world.

Corporate culture is a concept that is created in people's minds. It originates as a vision of the leader and spreads throughout the company and sets the tone of the organization. Culture is termed *climate* or *feel* by some people. What does the leader do to nurture the feeling desired in his or her department? Culture is created by such rites and rituals as[15]

- Casual days, where workers wear jeans and sport shirts to create an atmosphere of creativity and friendship.
- Birthing rooms and sibling birth participation programs to promote family health.
- Focus on quality, service, and reliability.
- A strong communication network.
- Face-to-face contacts.
- Name tags with only first names.
- Open parking.
- Open dining.

Exhibit 14–1 Developmental Continuum

Infant	Adult
Dependent	Independent
Submissive	Autonomous
Few abilities	Many abilities
Shallow abilities	Deep abilities
Short time perspective	Long time perspective
Frustrated by	Motivated or inspired by
Lack of self-control	Self-control
Being controlled	Self-direction
Directive (authoritarian) leadership	Job involvement
	Participative (democratic) leadership (electing own leaders)
Lack of self-actualization	Self-actualization
Lack of opportunity to learn	Opportunity to learn
Lack of opportunity to advance	Opportunity to advance
Repetitive work	Variety in work
Dull work	Interesting work
Lack of equipment	Resources to do job
Lack of information	Feedback
Low pay	High pay
Powerlessness	Autonomy and responsibility
Fractionalized jobs	Job enlargement
Lack of education restricting job opportunity to lower levels	Education that increases job opportunity at higher levels
Structured jobs that inhibit individual growth	Opportunity for independent thought, action, growth, and feelings of accomplishment
Overstaffing	Understaffing (perform multiple roles)
Specialization of tasks	Generalization and wholeness of jobs
	Rewards for learning
	Self-governance
Routine work	Complex work
Responds by	Responds by
Fighting for redesign or control (union)	Allocating own tasks
Leaving (turnover)	Staying
Psychological apathy or indifference	Seeking out intrinsic rewards
Becoming oriented to payoffs of being market-oriented or instrumentally oriented	Increasing productivity
	Focusing on job content
Absenteeism	Attendance
Daydreaming	Being industrious and attentive
Aggression toward supervisors	Being innovative
	Cooperating
Aggression toward coworkers	Participation
Restricting output	
Making mistakes or errors	
Postponing difficult tasks or decisions	Accepting responsibility
Focusing on pay, fringe benefits, hours of work	Focusing on self-direction, self-expression, individual accomplishment, opportunity to use abilities or help people
Lack of interest in work	
Alienation	

Exhibit 14–1   Developmental Continuum *(Continued)*

Infant	Adult
Decreased job rating associated with	Increased job rating associated with
Reduced community participation	Increased community participation
Decreased leisure involvement	Increased leisure involvement
Decreased political activity	Increased political activity
Decreased participation in voluntary activities, culture, cerebral skills, group activities	Increased participation in voluntary activities
Being solitary	
Being withdrawn	

Source: Reprinted from "Personality and Organization Theory Revisited" by Chris Argyris, published in *Administrative Science Quarterly,* 18, 2 (June 1973): 141–167 by permission of *Administrative Science Quarterly.* © 1973 by *Administrative Science Quarterly.*

Culture is evident in the way workers relate to time, trust for each other, and authority relationships. It is evident in the dress and personal appearance of workers, promotion policies from within or outside, and where workers take meal breaks. Every organization has heroes to model after and antiheroes to be avoided. Artifacts of an organization include its written materials, such as the organizational chart. A project team could evaluate an organization's culture and recommend changes. A Clinical Nurse Specialist (CNS) could act as team leader.[16] Exhibit 14–2 lists suggested questions for organizational assessment.

Research indicates that a strong culture that encourages participation and involvement of employees in shared decision making that emphasizes customers, shareholders, and employees, and of leadership from managers at all levels positively affects an organization's performance. Such organizations outperform competitors two to one in return on investments and sales.[17] (See Exhibit 14–3.)

Exhibit 14–2   Suggested Questions for Organizational Assessment

- What were your first impressions when you initially came to this unit/institution?
- From this first impression, what factors were most pleasing for you to encounter?
- What factors were most anxiety-provoking?
- What do "they" say about the nurses who work on this unit/at this hospital?
- How can *you* tell that a nurse works on this unit/at this hospital?
- What is the most interesting story you ever heard about this unit/hospital?
- What do you think this story tells you?
- What is most helpful in contributing to excellent nursing care on this unit/at this hospital? Why?
- What is the most significant barrier to the delivery of excellent nursing care at this institution?
- Who, in this environment, is a hero? Why?
- What does it mean to be "the best"?
- What is the most important lesson, good or bad, that you've learned here? How did you learn it?

Source: Reprinted from "Assessment of Organizational Culture: A Tool for Professional Success" by C. Caroselli, with permission of *Orthopedic Nursing,* © May/June 1992:60.

Exhibit 14–3   The Effects of Management Style on Five Aspects of Corporate Life

Authoritarian Style	Participative-Management Style	Authoritarian Style	Participative-Management Style

Leadership Processes

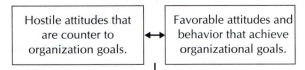

The degree of delegation.
The amount of initiative permitted.
The level of people's work load.
The usefulness of appraisal and feedback.

Communication Processes

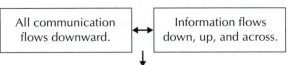

The realism of individual goals.
The retention of key executives.
The "buying into" or circumventing of the system.
The accuracy of business forecasts.
The art of gamesmanship at budget time.

Motivational Forces

Hostile attitudes that are counter to organization goals.	←→	Favorable attitudes and behavior that achieve organizational goals.

The effectiveness of management system.
The degree to which managers play it safe.
The determination of how well business decisions
   are implemented.

Interaction and Influence Process

Little interaction, characterized by fear and distrust.	←→	Extensive interaction with a high degree of trust and confidence.

The degree of cooperation and teamwork among
   individuals, functions, and departments.
The amount of information given or withheld.
The level of success or failure of project management.
The type of rules played on committees or task
   forces.

Authoritarian Style	Participative-Management Style

Decision-Making Process

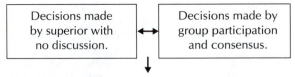

The quality of decisions.
The level of sales, profits, costs, and market position.
The degree to which potentially harmful problems surface.
The level of individual productivity and output.

Source: R. Desatnick, "Management Climate Surveys: A Way to Uncover an Organization's Culture," *Personnel*, May 1986.

Successful organizations have leaders and staff who share clear strategic visions, perform identifiable activities with confidence and within achievable time frames, and attain specific goals by department.

Research and Organizational Culture.   Through qualitative research, Ray discovered the theory of differential caring, which has multiple meanings, including the following:

■ Humanistic—empathy, love, and concern.
■ Political-legal—decision making, liability, and malpractice.
■ Ethical religious—trust, respect, acts of brotherly love, and ideals of doing unto others.
■ Economic—budget management and economic well-being.
■ Technological/physiological—use of machinery.
■ Educational—information, teaching, education programs.
■ Social—communication, social interaction and support, interrelationships, involvement, intimacy, knowing clients and families, humanistic potential for compassion and concern, love and empathy.

A formal theory of bureaucratic caring emerged from the substantive theory of differential caring (see Exhibit 14–4). The challenge for nurses is to create an organizational culture that supports the theory of bureaucratic caring.[18]

Fleeger studied organizational culture to arrive at the characteristics of consonant and dissonant cultures (see Exhibit 14–5). She recommends that managers promote a consonant culture through the following:[19]

■ Strategic planning sessions promoting employees involvement.
■ Identifying conflict situations as opportunities for creative change.

Exhibit 14–4   Differential Caring in an Organizational Culture: Caring Categories of Administrators

Role	Dominant Caring Descriptors	Structural Caring Categories
Nonnurse administrators	Empathy	Social
	Communication	Political
	Economic management	Economic
	Effective competition	Spiritual
	Responsibility/attitude	Ethical
Nurse administrators	Empathy	Social
	Communication	Political
	Time management	Economic
	Rapport	Spiritual
	Budget decisions	
	Spiritual concern	

Source: M. A. Ray, "The Theory of Bureaucratic Caring for Nursing Practice in the Organizational Culture," *Nursing Administration Quarterly,* Winter 1989, 37. © 1989 Aspen Publishers. Reprinted with permission.

Exhibit 14–5 Characteristics of Consonant and Dissonant Cultures

Consonant Cultures	Dissonant Cultures
• Collective spirit	• Mismatch between professional and organizational goals
• Golden rule norm	
• One superordinate goal	• Stronger union affiliations than organizational
• Frequent management/staff interactions	• Little staff representation on committees
• Clinical expertise valued	• Low staff participation in decision making
• Professional and organizational goals similar	• Do not have primary care models
• Goals same across work units	• Competitive spirit
• High cooperation between units	• Them versus us norm
• Primary care model promoting autonomy and independence	• Low staff/management interactions
• Formal and informal systems to address conflicts	• Staff feel undervalued
• Match between values and outcomes	• Mismatch between values and outcomes
• All nurses seen as members of same occupational group	• Nurse managers seen as outside occupational
• All members seen as working toward same goal	• Double standards exist for behaviors
• Behavior norms same for everyone	• Groups feel others not working toward common goal
	• Myths, stories, symbols not caring or positive

Source: M. E. Fleeger, "Assessing Organizational Culture: A Planning Strategy," *Nursing Management* 24, no. 2 (February 1993): 40.

- Planning job redesign and job enrichment activities in stagnant departments where personnel demonstrate signs of stagnation.
- Increasing both formal and informal staff interactions.
- Adapting a nursing care model that promotes autonomy and responsibility.

It takes a well-planned and executed unit orientation to integrate new employees into the corporate culture and subculture. The object is to achieve a fit between employee and organization. The organizational culture inventory is an instrument that can be used to measure culture as perceived by employees. It was used to profile the "ideal" nursing culture as described by a small group of nurses representing several hospitals (see Exhibit 14–6). Such instruments can be used to measure organizational culture to define what needs preservation versus what needs changing.[20]

Climate

The organizational climate is the personality of an organization, the perceptions and feelings shared by members of the system. It can be formal, relaxed, defensive, cautious, accepting, trusting, and so on. It is employees' subjective impressions or perceptions of their organization. Practicing nurses create, or at the very least, contribute to the creation of, the climate perceived by patients.

Managers create the climate in which practicing nurses work. If managers trust them, practicing nurses will provide their managers with good information

Exhibit 14–6   Ideal Culture Profile (n = 26 registered nurses)

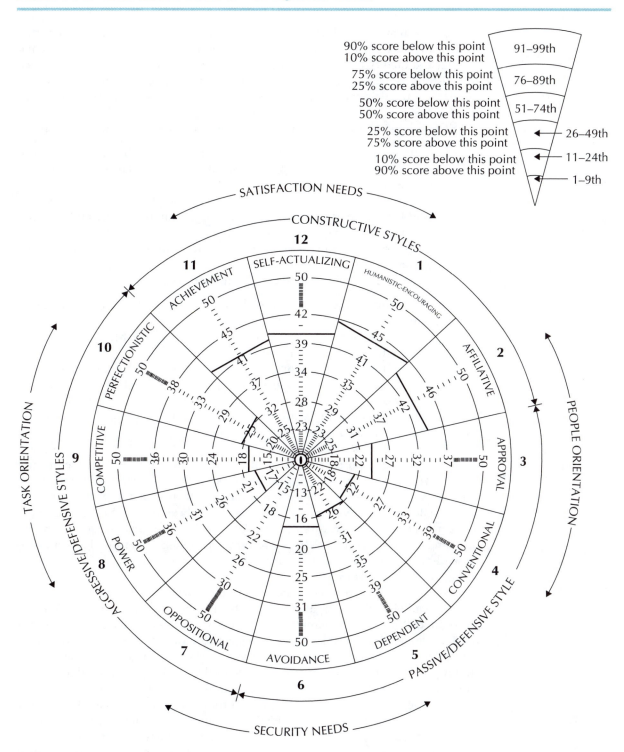

to keep their managers informed. This kind of climate promotes the concept that most hands-on employees can perform routine management, accounting, engineering, and quality tasks. Ninety percent of expert staff work can be performed by well-trained, well-equipped, self-managed work teams, the members of which are also good salespersons. The object of expert staff is to spread knowledge fast.[21]

The following are six sociological dimensions of organizational climate:

1. Clarity in specifying certification of the organization's goals and policies. This is facilitated by a smooth flow of information and management support of employees.
2. Commitment to goal achievement through employee involvement.
3. Standards of performance that challenge, promote pride, and improve individual performance.
4. Responsibility for one's own work, fostered and supported by managers.
5. Recognition for doing good work.
6. Teamwork—a sense of belonging, mutual trust, and respect.

The environmental dimensions of climate include room attractiveness, illumination, and the shape of the furniture.

The foregoing facets of organizational climate can be measured using the supervisory climate survey in Exhibit 14–7.[22]

Practicing nurses want a climate that will give them job satisfaction. They achieve job satisfaction when they are challenged and their achievements are recognized and appreciated by managers and patients. They achieve satisfaction from a climate of collegiality with managers and other health-care providers, a climate in which they have input into decision making.

Practicing nurses want a climate that provides good working conditions, high salaries, and opportunities for professional growth through counseling and career development experiences that will enable them to determine and direct their professional futures. They want a climate of administrative support that includes adequate staffing and shift options. It has been known for years that the personnel shortages, frustration, failure, and conflict in nursing required sweeping changes in intrinsic and extrinsic rewards, including career development programs that increase the ability of professional nurses to develop their self-esteem through self-actualization.

Many studies have been done to determine work climate within business, industry, and health-care organizations. Climate and philosophy result from the corporate culture, and changing the culture leads to climate change. One nurse manager designed and implemented a project to motivate the nursing staff of a medical unit to better service and greater self-satisfaction. She designed an employee-of-the-month motivational strategy that included measurable performance criteria. Although the staff were initially uninterested, they eventually increased their interest and participation. Productivity also increased, and new talents emerged. The strategy included a recognition ceremony, a free lunch or dinner, and the employee's picture on the bulletin board. By the end of six months, 25 of 144 employees had earned the title of employee of the month, their voluntary participation indicating that the strategy met some of their needs.[23]

Exhibit 14–7 Supervisory Climate Survey

Instructions

For each of the statements below draw a circle around one of the following: A—Always; F—Frequently; O—Occasionally; S—Seldom; N—Never.

For example, if you feel that you are frequently encouraged to come up with new and original ideas, you would circle the F in the following question:

A   F   O   S   N   1. We are encouraged to come up with new and original ideas.

Use only one evaluative letter code for each answer.

A   F   O   S   N   1. I have the opportunity to review my overall performance and effectiveness with my supervisor.

A   F   O   S   N   2. There is much respect between management and other personnel in this group.

A   F   O   S   N   3. In this organization, the rewards and encouragements you receive for effective performance outweigh the threats and criticisms.

A   F   O   S   N   4. Our people are encouraged to make decisions when the situation demands an immediate decision.

A   F   O   S   N   5. In this group I am given a chance to participate in setting the performance goals for my job.

A   F   O   S   N   6. The rooms in which we hold meetings for decision making are conducive to good interpersonal communication.

A   F   O   S   N   7. I feel that I am a member of a well-functioning team.

A   F   O   S   N   8. My supervisor is easily accessible to all of his or her employees.

A   F   O   S   N   9. We are encouraged to come up with new and original ideas.

A   F   O   S   N   10. In this group we are rewarded in proportion to how well we do.

A   F   O   S   N   11. As a group we can disagree without becoming disagreeable.

A   F   O   S   N   12. People are proud to belong to this group.

A   F   O   S   N   13. In this group what constitutes good performance has been identified.

A   F   O   S   N   14. Most of our meetings are held in attractive rooms.

A   F   O   S   N   15. The results I am supposed to achieve in my job are realistic.

A   F   O   S   N   16. In meetings we may sit wherever we wish.

A   F   O   S   N   17. In this group people demonstrate strong commitment to achieving group performance.

A   F   O   S   N   18. Things seem to be well organized in my group.

A   F   O   S   N   19. There is good communicative balance in my group.

A   F   O   S   N   20. People in this group help each other in solving job-related problems.

A   F   O   S   N   21. In this group people come to meetings well prepared.

A   F   O   S   N   22. We can disagree with our boss and not fear any form of reprisal.

A   F   O   S   N   23. I am involved in setting my own performance goals and in understanding how they relate to the overall goals of my group.

A   F   O   S   N   24. My supervisor does a good job in recognizing good performance.

A   F   O   S   N   25. Our overall organizational climate is a positive one.

Score the Supervisory Climate Survey in the following manner: Always, 4 points; Frequently, 3 points; Occasionally, 2 points; Seldom, 1 point; Never, 0 points.

Your organizational climate is excellent if you scored 90 to 100 points, good if you scored 80 to 89 points, average if you scored 70 to 79 points, fair if you scored 60 to 69 points, and poor if you scored less than 60 points.

Source: H. E. Munn, Jr., "Organizational Climate in the Health Care Setting," *The Health Care Supervisor,* October 1984, 27.
Reprinted with permission. Copyright © 1984 Aspen Publishers.

Other studies indicate the following:

1. Practicing clinical nurses obtain satisfaction from patient and family care and education; a variety of work experiences; interaction with staff members; their paycheck; mental challenges; being needed; friendly staff and physicians; observed patient improvement; patients' compliments; knowledge of a job well done; exciting and unpredictable work; the ability to contribute, learn, and achieve; the availability of senior professionals to assist and teach; developing new staff; and having predictable work schedules.[24]

2. The behaviors of professional nurses is positively affected by charge nurses who give honest pep talks, key in on feelings, make fair and equitable assignments, handle orders efficiently, help when the workload is great, listen to complaints and ideas, promote cooperation, treat their staff as resource persons for clinical expertise, value staffs' opinions, are up to date in knowledge and skills, and teach others.

3. Behavior was negatively affected by charge nurses who were two-faced, were phony, gossiped, took advantage, favored friends in making assignments, ignored questions, refused advice or help, did not help with patients when the need arose, did not communicate orders, did not follow suggestions they asked for, were disorganized, and did not know policies and procedures.

4. Staff nurses put high value on self-esteem and self-fulfillment, achievement, recognition, tasks assigned, advancement, and responsibility.[25]

5. Senior students indicate that practicing nursing meets their self-esteem needs. Job satisfiers include personal satisfaction (77.5 percent), collegial relationships (43.75 percent), security (12.5 percent), choice of work area (12.5 percent), and hours (11.25 percent).[26]

6. Medical-surgical and psychiatry practice areas have the greatest potential for problems with job satisfaction and require the greatest attention to organizational climate by nurse managers.[27]

7. Humor is motivating, stimulates creativity, and improves job performance. A positive work climate is created by steering conversations to the positive; brainstorming negative statements to make them humorous; keeping humorous things around you; encouraging laughter, which boosts the heart rate, blood circulation, and energy exchange; and never using put-down humor.[28]

The following activities promote a positive organizational climate:

1. Developing statements of the organization's mission, philosophy, vision, goals, and objectives, with input from practicing nurses, including their personal goals.

2. Establishing trust and openness through communication that includes prompt and frequent feedback and stimulates motivation.

3. Providing opportunities for growth and development, including career development and continuing education programs.

4. Promoting teamwork.

5. Asking practicing nurses to state their satisfactions and dissatisfactions during meetings and conferences and through surveys.
6. Marketing the nursing organization to the practicing nurses, other employees, and the public.
7. Following through on all activities involving practicing nurses.
8. Analyzing the compensation system for the entire nursing organization and structuring it to reward competence, productivity, and longevity.
9. Promoting self-esteem, autonomy, and self-fulfillment for practicing nurses, including feelings that their work experiences are of high quality.
10. Emphasizing programs to recognize practicing nurses' contributions to the organization.
11. Assessing unneeded threats and punishments and eliminating them.
12. Providing job security and an environment that enables free expression of ideas and exchange of opinions. Threats and recriminations, which may occur as downscaled performance reports, negative counseling, confrontation, conflict, or job loss, are not part of a positive organizational climate.
13. Being inclusive in all relationships with practicing nurses.
14. Helping practicing nurses overcome their shortcomings and develop their strengths.
15. Encouraging and supporting loyalty, friendliness, and civic consciousness.
16. Developing strategic plans that include decentralization of decision making and participation by practicing nurses.
17. Being a role model of performance desired for practicing nurses.

Exercise 14–1   Use the list of activities that promote a positive organizational climate in this chapter as a point of discussion for a group of your peers. Assess the organizational climate in the organization at which you are a student or an employee.

Team Building

The commonly used terms to describe the state of feeling of an organizational climate are *high morale* and *low morale*. Morale is a state of mind that reflects the zeal or enthusiasm with which someone works. A person who works courageously and confidently, with the discipline and willingness to endure hardship, would be manifesting high morale. Low morale is evident in the person who is timid, cowardly, devious, fearful, diffident, disorderly, unruly, rebellious, turbulent, or indifferent as a result of job dissatisfaction and the organizational milieu. Morale is a motivation factor related to productivity and quality of product or service outcomes. Firms want high morale among employees and use activities to promote it.

A team is a group of two or more workers interdependently striving for a common purpose or mission. The team members depend upon one another. The leader will emerge (if not appointed) as the person sustaining the confidence of the group. The leader will sustain the team's confidence through his or her expertise in the team's purpose or mission and by the enthusiasm expressed by his or her verbal and nonverbal behavior. High enthusiasm by the leader will spark high enthusiasm within the group, thereby boosting group morale and stimulating the group's esprit de corps, a spirit and sense of pride and honor.

Among the leader roles are those of guide, marketer, teacher, visionary, team player, entrepreneur, and idea broker.[29] The conditions for team building are collaboration, commitment, motivation, willingness, and timely feedback. Team building permits risk taking, encourages trust, and builds confidence. A strong team will have knowledge, be receptive and flexible, and promote freedom and openness. Team building is not needed when communications are working well for group and organizational needs.[30]

One continually hears such remarks as "This organization does not care about the employees!" or "This organization really cares about its employees!" It goes without saying that nurse managers want to hear the positive statement. People who have low morale are not satisfied with their work. Dissatisfied workers will not contribute positively to esprit de corps.

The objective of team building is to establish an environment of cohesiveness among shift personnel and among different shifts of a unit. The first step in team building is to find out why nursing employees are unhappy or dissatisfied. This can be accomplished through a questionnaire, although an open meeting is probably better. The meeting will be more productive if it is held away from the unit to eliminate interruptions and the shadow of the organization.

The nurse manager can assume the leadership or allow the group to select a leader. In any event, the nurse manager will have to explain what the effort is all about and what the group is supposed to accomplish. To set a positive note, the nurse manager should, if possible, begin identifying group satisfactions.

Next, the leader focuses on identifying problems and setting their priorities for action. If the nurse manager can assume the role of facilitator rather than leader, the group will probably proceed at a faster pace. The meeting style is a participatory management one with group ownership of activities and outcomes. The leader guides the members in defining each member's role on the team.

Problems or dissatisfactions are identified, and a calendar is established for addressing them. It is important to make a schedule of meetings and keep a list of attendees for all phases of team-building activities. Meetings should be held at times when most of the staff can be there. They should be short and focused on the problems and followed in priority sequence. It is best for the team to make a brief management plan that includes the problem, objectives, actions the team can accomplish on its own authority, actions needing management support, persons assigned specific responsibilities, target dates, and a list of accomplishments.

As the plan is put into effect it should be communicated to the entire staff of the unit, department, or division. Evaluation should occur on a continuous basis to keep the momentum going. Each person can be encouraged to fulfill commitments, and everyone's accomplishments should be recognized. While each shift can work on its own plans, an occasional open forum of personnel on all three shifts is essential for intershift problems.

Once the team is functioning, team building focuses on work production. Some meeting time should always be dedicated to morale, motivation, team skills, and discussion of team direction.[31]

Team building is a part of the self-directed work team organizational concept. Developing teams to their top potential is a tough job. The team leader identifies training needs of the team and of individual members. He or she also runs interference for the team, acts as liaison in negotiating for scarce resources, arranges publicity for accomplishments, and keeps abreast of information on outside events affecting the team. When conflicts arise as a result of misperceptions that some team members are doing more than their share of work or that the wrong members are getting promoted, the team leader deals with them. The dream team collaborates with enthusiasm to get a job done well. Self-directed work teams and team building will continue to increase.[32]

Though people participate in team building, they still want to retain their individuality. Nurse managers provide leadership that is flexible, fair, and mindful of tasks and people; inspires; and models the role of professional nurse.[33] Team building and self-managed work teams require continuous efforts by team leaders to maintain effective functioning.

Nave and Thomas suggest fifty specific techniques to boost employee morale (see Exhibit 14–8).[34]

| Exercise 14–2 | Refer to Exhibit 14–8, "Fifty Specific Techniques to Boost Employee Morale." Make a list of similar activities found in the organization at which you work as a student or as an employee. |

DEVELOPING AN ORGANIZATIONAL STRUCTURE

An organizational structure for a division of nursing must meet the needs of that division as written in the statements of mission, philosophy, vision, values, and objectives. Most existing institutions already have an organizational structure. Before the structure is changed, the nurse managers should engage in a systematic analysis as well as some sound thinking about altering the organization's design and structure, starting with objectives and strategy.

Work Activities and Functions

Work activities and functions to be analyzed and encompassed in identifying the building blocks of an organization include the following:

1. The operating work at the unit level includes primary nursing care (the basic mission, not the method or modality of nursing); operational nursing management, commonly referred to as nurse manager activities; and support activities essential to the application of primary nursing care, such as training and clerical work. Management at the unit level includes management of the clinical component of direct nursing care and management of nonnursing or indirect activities.

2. In any health-care institution, top management functions will need to be performed. In a small division, the nurse manager will be top manager of the department and a member of top management of the institution. In a large division with multiple missions and objectives, there will likely be enough functions and activities for a top management

Exhibit 14–8 Fifty Specific Techniques to Boost Employee Morale

The following are 50 of the techniques identified to boost employee morale. In reviewing them, keep in mind that there is no best answer for anyone. The best techniques are those that best suit your organization.

1. Supervisors greet employees with a handshake as the employees begin their shifts.
2. Supervisors write personal notes such as Thank You or Happy Birthday on payroll checks.
3. Members of employee groups meet regularly with management representatives to promote understanding and carry out activities of mutual interest.
4. Employees and management work side by side once a year on a community help project.
5. Employers are personally congratulated by supervisors when they exceed their goals.
6. Supervisors personally introduce new hires to each employee.
7. An employee's years of service are noted each year on the anniversary date of employment on a plaque or poster in the lobby.
8. When department supervisors enter the employee lounge, they treat all employees who happen to be there to a cup of coffee.
9. Supervisors personally hand employees in their department a silver dollar at Christmas as a "little something extra."
10. Relations with retired employees are maintained by means of an annual breakfast and personal delivery by the supervisors of a box of Christmas candy each year.
11. A cash reward is given each month to the employee with the "best idea" for the firm.
12. Part-time employees are invited to all social events.
13. The chief executive officer periodically has "brown bag" luncheon discussions with employees at which their concerns are addressed.
14. Employees are allowed to accept telephone calls at any time.
15. Letters of commendation are sent to employees for performance above and beyond normal expectations. Copies of the letter are included in the employees' personnel files.
16. The plant manager cooks at the supervisors' picnic. At another firm, supervisors serve the food at a company picnic.
17. Birthday cards are signed by the president of the firm or immediate supervisor and are sent to the employees' homes.
18. Free popcorn is always available for employees and customers.

19. Employee birthdays are celebrated with cake and by singing "Happy Birthday."
20. The safety department issues a monthly "safety for the family" newsletter that is mailed directly to the employees' homes.
21. Free meals are provided in the company cafeteria for employees working on special days such as Christmas and Thanksgiving.
22. At irregular intervals managers provide food for employees to munch in the break area.
23. Soft drinks, coffee, and/or snacks are provided for staff at departmental meetings.
24. Flexible working hours are permitted during slow work times.
25. Morale-building meetings are held at which management informs employees of the firm's successes.
26. Brief meetings are scheduled for all new employees with staff from the business office, security, facilities management, and the like to familiarize new hires with policies and procedures.
27. A worker is recognized by being named Employee of the Week or Employee of the Month. The recognition takes many forms, including presentation of a plaque, lunch with the president or supervisor, gifts, and mention in the company newsletter.
28. An activities committee has been established to plan social events, and new employees are introduced to a member of this committee so they become aware of company activities.
29. Snacks are available during employees' first break each day.
30. Employees missing one day or less due to illness or injury during the year receive a gift.
31. Factory eating areas are decorated on special occasions.
32. Free coffee is provided on special days.
33. Once a quarter, 10 to 12 employees selected by random drawing are taken on a guided tour of all plant facilities and have lunch on the house in the plant cafeteria.
34. A Halloween costume contest is held each year, employees wear their costumes the work day, and the winner receives one day off with pay.
35. Receptions are given for every employee who retires.

Exhibit 14–8   Fifty Specific Techniques to Boost Employee Morale *(Continued)*

36. In each month that new accounts exceed an established figure, all employees are taken out for dinner.
37. An annual awards banquet is held for employees on the last working day before a holiday.
38. Annual parties for occasions such as Christmas are given by the company.
39. An appropriate gift is distributed to all employees daily, weekly, or monthly, when a production record is established.
40. A cash drawing is held each month that there is no employee time lost due to accident. Variation: A drawing is held each month for employees who have not missed time due to injury or illness.
41. An annual employee appreciation dinner is given by the company.
42. Lunch and entertainment are provided "on the grounds" for all employees two or three times each year.

43. Some food for snacking is supplied by the company on a daily basis.
44. Positive comments on an employee by a customer result in the employee receiving a silver pin. Three such compliments during the year earn a gold pin.
45. Special food items are given to all employees on occasions such as Thanksgiving or Christmas.
46. Occasional boat rides on a cruiser are made available to all employees.
47. Company-wide potluck luncheons are held.
48. One firm sponsors a daily 15-minute radio program on which one of the employees is recognized/spotlighted.
49. When a new safety record is reached, employees receive a small memento and attend a cook-out hosted by management.
50. Lunch is provided for all employees on the last working day before a holiday.

Source: J. L. Nave and B. Thomas, "How Companies Boost Morale," *Supervisory Management,* October 1983, 29–33 © 1983, American Management Association, New York. Reprinted by permission. All rights reserved.

team in the division of nursing. The chair will still be a member of top management of the institution, functioning at the strategic planning level in both instances.

3. A technostructure of staff of varying size, depending upon the size of the institution, will support the management and clinical components of the nursing organization. These staff members will include experts in such areas as infection control, staff development, oncology nursing, and quality improvement. In some organizations, they are labeled consultants.

Context

Certain contextual variables relate to an organization's structure, such as organizational charter or social function, size, technology, environment, interdependence with other organizations, structuring of activities, concentration of authority, and line of control of work flow.[35]

Forms of Organizational Structure

A mixture of two common forms of organizational structure—hierarchical and free-form—is needed in nursing.

Hierarchical Structure. A hierarchical structure is commonly called a line structure (see Exhibit 14–9). It is the oldest and simplest form and is associated with the principle of chain of command, bureaucracy and a multitiered hierarchy, vertical control and coordination, levels differentiated by function and authority, and downward communications. These structures have all of the advantages and disadvantages of a bureaucracy. Most line structures have added a staff component. In nursing organizations, both line and staff personnel will usually be professional nurses.

Line functions are those that have direct responsibility for accomplishing the objectives of a unit. For the most part, they are filled by registered nurses, licensed practical nurses, and nursing technicians. Staff functions are those that assist the line in accomplishing the primary objectives of nursing. They include clerical, personnel, budgeting and finance, staff development, research, and specialized clinical consulting. The relationships between line and staff are a matter of authority. Line has authority for direct supervision of employees, while staff provides advice and counsel. There may be line authority within a staff section.

To make staff effective, top management assures that line and staff authority relationships are clearly defined. Personnel of both should work to make their relationships effective; they attempt to minimize friction by increasing mutual trust and respect.

Functional authority takes place when an individual or department is delegated authority over functions in one or more other departments. This has occurred in the development of infection control and quality improvement systems, where professional nurses have line authority to hospital management and staff authority to nursing management, or line authority to nursing management and staff authority to other divisions. The functional staff does this through delegated authority to consult and prescribe procedures and sometimes policies for the function as it is to be carried out in the other departments. These delegated authority functions are clearly defined and carefully restricted. They are usually limited to procedures and time frames and do not include personnel or context. They should not weaken or destroy the authority and thus the effectiveness of line managers. For example, staff personnel might be assigned authority to recruit nurses, with line managers retaining final authority over hiring. Exhibit 14–10 shows a set of standards for evaluating the effectiveness of line and staff relationships within nursing in a hierarchical organization. Exhibit 14–11 depicts several common organizational patterns.

Free-Form Structures. Free-form organizational structures are called *matrix* organizations (see Exhibit 14–12 on p. 380). The matrix design enables timely response to external competition and internally facilitates efficiency and effectiveness through cooperation among disciplines.

A matrix organization has the following characteristics:

1. Maintenance of old-line authority structures.
2. Specialist resources obtained from functional areas.
3. Promotion of formation of new organizational units.

Exhibit 14–9   A Hierarchical Organizational Structure

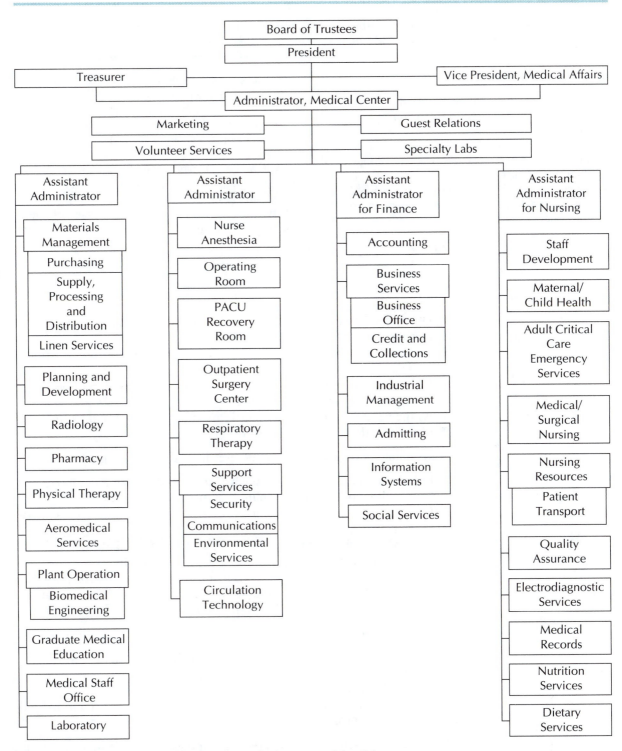

Source: Courtesy University of South Alabama Medical Center, Mobile, Alabama.

Exhibit 14–10 Standards for Evaluating the Effectiveness of Line and Staff Relationships in a Hierarchical Organization

Standards

1. Line authority relationships are clearly delineated and defined by the organizational and/or functional charts and policies.
2. Staff authority relationships are clearly delineated and defined by the organizational and/or functional charts and policies.
3. Functional authority relationships are clearly delineated and defined by the organizational and/or functional charts and policies.

4. Staff personnel consult with, advise, and provide counsel to line personnel.
5. Service personnel functions are clearly understood by line and staff personnel.
6. Line personnel seek and effectively use staff services.
7. Appropriate staff services are being provided by line nursing personnel and other organizational departments or services.
8. Services are not being duplicated because of line and staff authority relationships.

4. Decision making done at the organizational level, at a group consensus, first-line management level.
5. The exercising of authority by the matrix manager over the functional manager.
6. Cooperative planning program development and allocation of resources to accomplish program objectives.
7. Assignment of functional managers to teams that respond to the chief of the functional discipline and matrix manager.

Matrix nursing organizational structures have the following advantages:[37]

1. Improved communication through vertical and horizontal control and by coordination of interdisciplinary patient-care teams.
2. Increased organizational adaptability and fluidity to respond to environmental changes.
3. Increased efficiency of resource use, with fewer organizational levels and decision making closer to primary care operations.
4. Improved human resource management because of increased job satisfaction with achievement and fulfillment, improved communication, improved interpersonal skills, and improved collegial relationships.

Matrix nursing organizational structures have the following disadvantages:[38]

1. Potential conflict because of dual or multiple lines of authority, responsibility, and accountability relationships.
2. Role ambiguity.
3. Loss of control over functional discipline as a result of a multidisciplinary team approach.

A matrix management structure superimposes a horizontal program management over the traditional vertical hierarchy. Personnel from various

Exhibit 14–11   Several Common Organizational Patterns

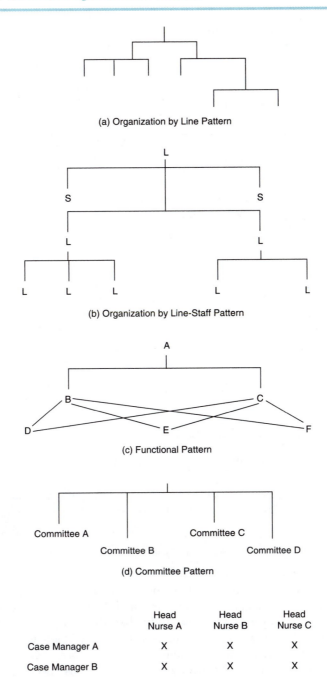

(a) Organization by Line Pattern

(b) Organization by Line-Staff Pattern

(c) Functional Pattern

(d) Committee Pattern

	Head Nurse A	Head Nurse B	Head Nurse C
Case Manager A	X	X	X
Case Manager B	X	X	X
Case Manager C	X	X	X

(e) Matrix Organization

Source: B. S. Barnum and K. M. Kerfoot, *The Nurse As Executive,* 4th ed. (Gaithersburg, Md.: Aspen, 1994), 66. Reprinted with permission. Copyright © Aspen Publishers.

Exhibit 14–12 Fully Evolved Matrix Organization

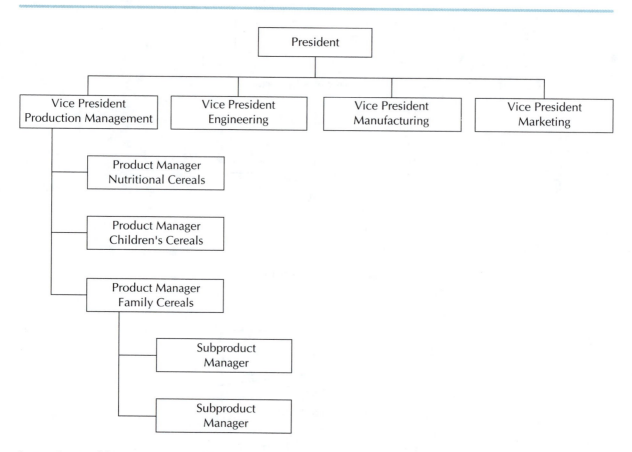

Source: Reprinted from *Organizations: Behavior, Structure, Processes,* 8th ed. by J. Gibson, J. Ivancevich, and J. Donnelly, with permission of Richard D. Irwin Inc., © 1994. (Burr Ridge, Il: Irwin, 1994): 487.

functional departments are assigned to a specific program or project and become responsible to two bosses—a program manager and their functional department head. Thus, an interdisciplinary team of core and extended team members is created. A longitudinal study of a geriatrics matrix team program showed that while costs increased initially, they were offset after a year by decreased acute-care readmission rates, emergency room use, and nursing-home placement. Mortality was significantly decreased, and the functional ability of patients increased.[39]

Adhocracy. "Adhocracy" models of organization are like matrix models. Simple teams or task forces exist on an ad hoc basis. They are formed, complete their goals, and are disbanded; and new groups are then formed to meet changing and dynamic missions and objectives.[40]

Matrix and adhocracy models employ participatory management. Xerox is an example of a company that has successfully used self-managing work teams. The teams once exceeded cost reduction targets of $3.7 million by one million dollars.

The expert is the authority that leads the team. Companies that use work teams are consultative organizations that delegate rather than tell; they encourage maverick behavior and reward results. Of 360 manufacturing companies studied, the forty-one that were most successful had fewer employees per sales dollar, encouraged risk taking, had smaller headquarters staff, had decentralized decision making, and had self-contained units or cost centers.[41]

Exercise 14–3   Use Exhibit 14–10, "Standards for Evaluating the Effectiveness of Line and Staff Relationships in a Hierarchical Organization," to evaluate the nursing division, department, service, or unit in which you work as a student or an employee. Involve your colleagues.

RESTRUCTURING NURSING ORGANIZATIONS

Survival of many hospitals is threatened as they compete for growth and a competitive edge in the marketplace. For this reason, Florey indicates that the governing boards may need to be reconstituted, with members focusing on patient care. Many hospitals include the chief nurse executives in governing board meetings as active participants.[42]

Kanter defines synergies as "interactions of businesses that would provide benefits above and beyond what the units could do separately."[43] Synergies are both a good and a bad consequence of restructuring in which organizations are downsized (employees cut), demassed (middle management cut), and decentralized. The aim of restructuring is to achieve synergies from the value of adding up the parts to create a whole.[44] One of the elements of restructuring would be to build a synergistic model for a governing body. Exhibit 14–13 depicts a synergistic model for the governing body as suggested by Florey.

Old organizational forms do not work in today's health-care environment. Sovie recommends development of special project teams to design the required structure and system change. She gives the following as the first five steps of restructuring:[45]

1. Create an organizational culture marked by commitment to high-quality care and superior, responsive service to all users, including patients and their families and physicians, nurses, and other staff.
2. Redesign the organizational structure to flatten it and eliminate or reduce barriers among departments, disciplines, and services.
3. Empower the staff, invest in employee education and training, and create mechanisms to ensure information flow.
4. Develop special project teams to design the required system changes; nurture and promote innovation and pilots of new approaches.
5. Celebrate accomplishments, innovators, and champions; care for the caregivers; support, recognition, and reward.

Exhibit 14–13 A Synergistic Model for a Governing Body

Governing Body Function	Contribution of Nurse Executive
1. Defining mission	• Patient and community advocate: provides focus of consumer needs and views. • Incorporates nursing philosophy and mission. • Educates nursing staff on agency's mission.
2. Quality of care	• Quality-of-care expert. • Presents evaluations and quality issues to the board. • Influences hospital-wide decision making regarding quality and health services.
3. Strategic planning	• Shares in responsibility of executive management in developing and implementing the strategic plan. • Meshes goals of the nursing department with organization's plan. • Presents nursing strategic plan.
4. Financial viability	• Participates on finance committee. • Oversees largest department operating budget. • Obtains resources for patient care. • Introduces productivity measures to create synergies.
5. Reduce risk and liability	• Acts as a guardian of the institution's welfare. • Presents policy and procedures focusing on potential liability. • Presents nursing risk-management plan and program. • Interprets standards and legislation affecting nursing service delivery.
6. Community relations	• Represents the agency in community-service programs and relations. • Presents community perspectives and needs regarding the agency's role in health-services delivery.
7. Organizational growth	• Interprets and communicates needs and visions of the nursing department and community in planning for growth. • Supports and assists the chief executive officer in implementing strategic vision and plan.
8. Policy development	• Educates trustees in issues regarding the delivery of care. • Represents nursing in overall policy development.
9. Service development	• Presents proposals for the enhancement of care services. • Provides a clinical focus to planning. • Acts as consultant to planning needs and operational needs.
10. Decision making	• Represents the voice of nursing in overall governance and decision making. • Provides insights from a nurse- and client-centered focus.

Source: D. L. Flarey, "The Nurse Executive and the Governing Body: Synergy for a New Era," *Journal of Nursing Administration* 21, no. 12 (December 1991): 13. Reprinted with permission of J. B. Lippincott.

The goals are improvement of patient care, organizational success, and staff satisfaction.

Restructuring of organizations includes downsizing and elimination of middle managers (see Exhibit 14–14). As a consequence of this, the hands-on workers are empowered to provide clients (customers, patients) with what they need and want. Before they can be empowered, hands-on nursing workers need to have management training for their new roles. The span of control is greater when hands-on workers are educated, trained, motivated, stable, and empowered. Such workers neither want nor need micromanagement. The manager with a widened or expanded span of control now becomes mentor, guide, facilitator, and coach.

Small departments can be consolidated under one department head through empowerment. One example would be physical therapy, occupational therapy, endoscopy, neurodiagnostics, sleep disorders, social services, and respiratory therapy into one department. Issues of loss of power and authority arise and must be resolved so that job shrinking and empowerment can occur. Managers who spend time protecting their turf decrease productivity of their workers.

Nurse managers of their units can do all hiring, resolve patient complaints, be given budget authority associated with staffing and patient loss, and do orientation of new managers. Middle managers can be incorporated into the structure as nurse managers of units or in staff functions, such as case managers. Clearly, the span of control for top managers can increase as first-line managers are empowered.

Empowerment increases responsiveness. It is better to eliminate jobs with attrition than to fire personnel. Excess managers should be turned back into service performers.[46]

Downsizing is common in today's corporate world, including health-care organizations and institutions. The goals of downsizing are to decrease costs and increase profits. Although decentralization and participatory management are sometimes identified with downsizing, the goals are not always the same. The former have as primary goals increasing job satisfaction and increased productivity.

Winning companies have three to nine fewer levels of management than losing companies. Winning companies have workers doing their own maintenance, self-inspection, direct costing, and just-in-time inventory management. Winning companies have few people at headquarters level. They decentralize database management, eliminate approval signatures, retrain middle managers, and increase spending authority at the unit level.[47]

An organizational analysis should be done to gain the theory and skills needed to intervene in complex organizational systems[48] (see Exhibit 14–15).

The Organization of Work

Work is organized according to the stages in the process. In some areas, the work moves to the skills and tools, good examples being coronary care nursing and operating room nursing. Sometimes a team moves different skills and

Exhibit 14–14 Restructured Nursing Department

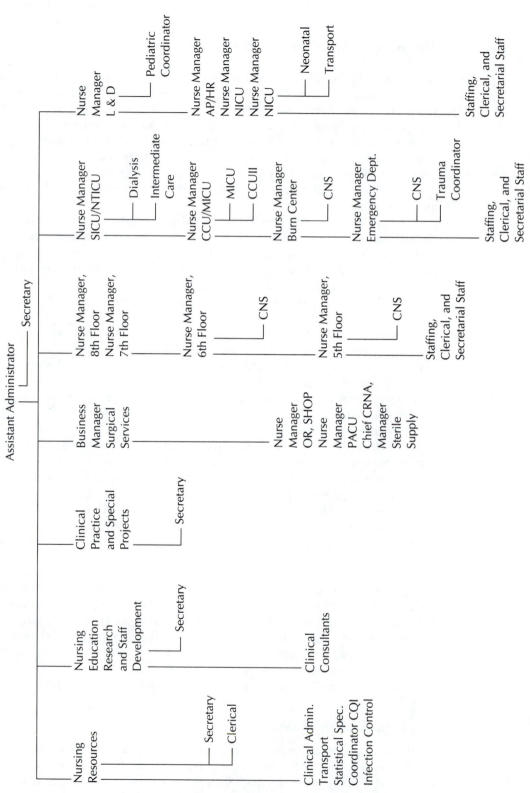

Source: Courtesy University of South Alabama Medical Center, Mobile, Alabama.

Exhibit 14–15   Organizational Analysis

Areas to be Assessed	Data Collection Strategies		Analysis Criteria

A. Formal organizational structure	A. Obtain a copy of the following:
	Philosophy and objectives—hospital and nursing
	Organization charts (table of organization (TO))
	Hospital, nursing, job descriptions—nursing
		(5%)	A. 1. Provides philosophies and objectives of hospital and nursing
			   a. Discusses compatibility of the two re formal mission
			   b. Discusses congruence between own philosophy of nursing and nursing department's philosophy
			2. Includes nursing job descriptions
			   a. Relates how CNS job description compares to New York State Nurses Association's position statement
			   b. Comments on appropriateness of other relevant nursing job descriptions
			3. Provides organizational charts

B. Power bases	B. Refer to
	   TO
	   Documents
	   Observations
	   Interviews
		(2%)	B. 1. States where power bases lie—formal and informal
			2. Names and describes sources of power identified

C. Decision-making and policy-making bases	C. Refer to
	   TO—Superimpose informal decision-making network on TO
	   Documents
	   Observations
	   Interviews
		(5%)	C. 1. States where formal bases lie
			2. Identifies informal networks
			3. Describes extent to which nursing is represented on major decision-making bodies in hospital and influences major decisions
			4. Discusses extent of nursing staff's participation at unit level; in what issues?
			5. Describes methods used in decision and policy making

D. Leadership	D. Documents
	   Observations
	   Interviews
		(2%)	D. 1. Relates predominant leadership styles of unit head nurse and CNS
			2. Describes nursing staff's response to styles used

E. Communication system	E. Refer to
	   TO
	   Staff communication books and all other communication methods
	   Documents
	   Observations
	   Interviews
		(4%)	E. 1. Discusses
			   a. Direction of flow
			   b. Openness of communication; clarity; distortions; omissions; overload
			   c. Primary sources of and participants in communication re task accomplishment (sociogram may be used)
			2. Identifies formal and informal methods of communication

Exhibit 14–15 Organizational Analysis *(Continued)*

Areas to be Assessed	Data Collection Strategies		Analysis Criteria
F. Organizational climate	F. Refer to Clark and Shea, pp. 29–30, for Walton's guidelines for analyzing the organizational climate Census and patient reports Analysis of staffing and assignments Professional development Activities Interviews Documents Observations	(3%)	F. 1. Discusses degree of individual autonomy 2. Describes compensation, working conditions, assignments 3. Relates opportunities for continued professional and personal growth
G. See criteria		(8%)	G. For each area A–E, based upon your clinical work as a CNS and the analysis, identifies and discusses the organizational-environmental factors that facilitate and inhibit nursing management and the functioning of the CNS
H. See criteria		(3%)	H. Based on G, identifies at least one potential, realistic project for planned change to be implemented in the spring semester

Source: M. Reddecliff, E. C. Smith, and M. Ryan-Merritt, "Organizational Analysis: Tool for the Clinical Nurse Specialist," *Clinical Nurse Specialist,* Fall 1989, 135. With permission of Williams & Wilkins.

different tools to the work, for example, when an operating room team moves to a delivery room to perform a caesarian section. We certainly can find other combinations in nursing.

Much of the work in nursing is accomplished by a functionally structured organization. Clarity is an advantage of the functional structure, since the individuals know where they stand and they understand their tasks. Functional structures are usually stable. A disadvantage is that sometimes the task neither relates to the whole structure nor contributes to the common purpose. Functional structures are rigid, and frequently they neither prepare nurses for the future nor train and test them.

Team organization has been tried in nursing for the past half century. It has been used mainly at the operating or primary-care level rather than at top or middle-management levels. "A team is a number of people—usually fairly small—with different backgrounds, skills, and knowledge, and drawn from various areas of the organization (their home) who work together on a specific and defined task. There is usually a team leader or team captain."[49]

A team must have a continuing mission, which nursing has. The team should be highly flexible, without a rigid chain of command. Like all organizational structures in business, industry, or health care, the team organization needs clear and sharply defined objectives. Leadership delegates on decision and command authority, and the team is responsible for accomplishing the tasks or mission. Team members know each other's functions, but leadership must first establish clear objectives and everybody's role. Everyone on the team should know the whole scope of work and be adaptable and receptive to innovation. The team leader gives continuing attention to clear communications and decision making. A team should be kept small for top management work and for innovative work. Otherwise, the team design complements the functional design. A combination may consist of employees who work in teams but produce work organized on the functional principle. This approach seems to work best in nursing and is probably better than either organizational structure in its pure form.

Nursing-Care Delivery Systems

Managed care and case management are leading innovations in health-care delivery. Benefits are controlled costs, improved outcome monitoring, reduced bureaucracy, less travel time for patients, and fewer people to sort out or confront. Patient-care needs and outcomes should be assessed and evaluated by nurses. Priority of patient-care tasks should be determined by nurses who refer needs to others. This is the essence of work redesign that will retain nursing autonomy and influence.[50]

Example 1—Nursing Practice Model.   Valley Baptist Medical Center in Harlingen, Texas, built a nursing practice model that included unit action committees on each nursing unit; a comprehensive integrated tool called the restorative-care path; variance analysis; permanent care teams with clinical managers, assistant clinical managers, licensed vocational nurses, and nursing assistants; and collaborative nurse-physician practice with a physician-nurse liaison committee. Since credentialing and recredentialing of physicians is considered the ultimate form of peer review, it should be considered for peer review of nurses.[51]

Example 2—Group Practice.   Nursing group practice at Catherine McAuley Health System "is a formal membership of professional nurses who contract to provide nursing care for a specific patient population." Nurses may contract privately or as employees of an organization. They provide 24-hour coverage 365 days a year. The group's staffing for cardiothoracic surgery includes sixteen nurses, two certified surgical technologists, and one clinical nurse manager, who reports to the clinical director of OR services. The group eliminated the first-line manager, making the clinical nurse manager a resource facilitator, liaison person, and mentor. A supportive climate emphasizes trust, accountability, and responsibility. The criteria for group practice membership includes clinical competence and leadership ability. Evaluating peers use a clinical ladder with described behaviors. The practice model is shared governance: practice, education, and quality assurance councils.

Staff satisfaction, cost, and quality all improved. Turnover rate decreased. Problems such as surgical complications and poor communication were prevented. Products and techniques were changed to reduce costs. Turnaround times were faster. Financial recognition was made quarterly. Incorrect sponge and instrument counts were reduced 25 percent.[52]

The following are suggested activities to implement such a group practice:

- Define roles and organization structure.
- Determine program costs.
- Decide on membership criteria and staffing mix.
- Set salary guidelines (e.g., hourly or salaried status).
- Work with the hospital administration in writing policies and planning for implementation.
- Plan to evaluate the success of the program using specific, predetermined instruments.

Example 3—Helper Model.   The Helper Model of health-care delivery is widespread. It matches RNs with nurse aides. To work efficiently, the Helper Model requires the following:[53]

1. Experienced RNs at the competent or proficient levels of practice.
2. Permanent RN/nurse aide pairs.
3. Enhanced primary nursing.
4. Support for agency and float nurses.
5. Policy for attendance that targets incentive and reward programs.
6. Thoroughly prepared RNs and nurse aides.
7. Support systems.
8. Follow-up in-services.

Example 4—Differentiated Practice.   Role theory underlies the concept of differentiated practice, which defines the levels of competence within which two categories of RNs will practice: nurses with bachelor's degrees and those with associate degrees.

The BSN (bachelor of science in nursing) level is the professional practice level; the ADN (associate degree in nursing) is the associate or technical practice level. These practice levels can function within a variety of different delivery systems, including team and primary systems. The premise for differentiated practice is that professional practice exercises the nurse's autonomous decisions, including personal acceptance of risks and responsibilities in making professional judgments. Extended education at a BSN level or higher is required preparation for this role at the professional practice level.[54]

The differentiated group professional practice model has three major components: (1) group governance, (2) differentiated care delivery, and (3) shared values.[55] The differentiated practice system or delivery model has the following components:

1. Differentiated registered nurse (RN) practice.
2. Use of nurse extenders.
3. Primary case management.

"Differentiated care delivery is designed so that nurses with varying educational preparation and work experience can most efficiently use their knowledge and skills while delegating nonnursing tasks to assistive personnel. Nurse extenders are delegated tasks rather than patient assignments."[56]

The differentiated practice role has three basic components:

1. Provision of direct care.
2. Communication with and on behalf of patients.
3. Management of patient care.

A differentiated practice maximizes available registered nurse resources for efficiency and effectiveness. "Differentiated practice is a strategy that calls for licensed and practicing nurses to be used in accord with their respective experience, ability, and formal and continuing education. Further, differentiated practice is defined as both a human resource deployment model and an alternative to primary nursing and case management."[57] It is role differentiation. More education and experience is needed for cognitive skills.

To use the differentiated practice model, the nurse's knowledge and skills are assessed (see Exhibit 14–16).

Exhibit 14–16 Differentiated Practice Assessment

RN Professional

BSN prepared
Makes complex decisions and interactions
Cost management of supplies, clinical alternatives, flexible scheduling of personnel, and caseloads
Structures the unstructured
Cognitive role and highly skilled tasks
Care manager
Independent judgments, initiative, problem solving
Coaches self-managed work team
Manages all resources, fiscal and material
Consults with other disciplines
Discharges patients

RN Associate or Technician

Non-BSN RN
Assists the professional nurse
Performs high-skill tasks such as chemotherapy
Special tests and procedures
May lead self-managed work team coached by professional nurse
Direct care provider
Uses common, well-defined diagnoses
Works in structured settings and situations

Tall Versus Flat Organizations

Line organizations are considered to be *tall,* or vertical, organizations, while matrix and adhocracy models are considered to be *flat,* or horizontal, organizations. In a study of the effects of tall versus flat organizational structures on job satisfaction of managers, flat organization were found to decrease need deficiencies in selected indicators of self-esteem and self-actualization. Tall organizations decrease need deficiencies for selected indicators of security, social needs, and self-esteem. Overall there was "no difference between tall and flat organizations in terms of perceived need deficiencies." Flat organizations are not superior to tall organizations for managers.[58] Research is needed along these lines for practicing nurses.

Future organizations will be unstructured, flat, flexible, and decentralized; authority will come from competence; leaders will change with goals. There will be no formal job descriptions. Employees will be salaried, collegial groups of equals who will respond quickly to change. Vertical integration will diminish with microprocessor communication technology and through artificial intelligence and robotization. People will go from manufacturing to the service, transportation, communication, and recreation industries. Employees will telecommute from home. Telecommuting programs already exist in 450 companies. Parents will be able to stay at home and have an improved quality of work life.[59]

The following does work: horizontal structures; temperance; leaders who treat key managers and employees alike; elevating human resources; clear tasks and goals; agreed-upon tasks, goals, and objectives; few reports; no rank; no boss; no seniority. The result is committed employees participating in decision making and accepting responsibility.[60]

ANALYZING ORGANIZATIONAL STRUCTURES IN A DIVISION OF NURSING

Analyzing the organizational structure of a division of nursing entails the following six main steps:

Step 1. Compile a list of the key activities as determined by the mission and objectives of patient care. The written philosophy and vision statements will help by indicating important values to be considered. Once this list is completed, it must be analyzed. Group similar activities together. What are the central load-carrying elements? Most will be related to primary care, and philosophy will usually dictate that excellence of patient care is a requirement for the accomplishment of objectives. The analysis of key activities can be done according to the kinds of contributions made. These will include (1) results-producing activities, (2) support activities, (3) hygiene and housekeeping activities, and (4) top-management activities.

Step 2. Based on the work functions to be performed, decide on the units of the organization. Decision analysis will be important here, since it must be decided which kinds of decisions will be required and who will make them. Decisions involving future commitments may have to be a top-management function, depending on the degree of futurity and the speed with which the decision can be reversed. It will be necessary to analyze the impact of decisions on other functions, the number of functions involved being an important factor. Qualitative factors, such as decisions involving ethical values, principles of conduct, and social and political beliefs, will have to be analyzed. The frequency of the decision will influence its placement: Is it recurrent, or is it rare? In principle, all decisions should be placed at the lowest level and as close to the operational scene as possible.

Step 3. Decide which units or components will be joined and which separated. Join activities that make the same kind of contribution. This will require relations analysis and will be related to the sequence of key activities or functions.

Step 4. Decide on the size and shape of the units or components.

Step 5. Decide on appropriate placement and relationships of different units or components. This will result from the relations analysis (step 3). There should be the smallest possible number of relationships, and each should be made to count.

Step 6. Draw or diagram the design and put it into operation. This will result in an organizational chart or schema.

These steps should be used when major organizational problems occur, such as friction among department heads over authority and staffing problems. They also apply to organizing a new corporation, division, or unit and to reorganizing an established entity.

Exhibit 14–17   Standards for Evaluation of Departmentation

1. Nursing activities have been grouped to attain goals and sustain the enterprise.
2. Nursing activities have been grouped for intradepartmental and interdepartmental coordination.
3. Personnel roles have been designed to fit the capabilities and motivation of persons available to fill them.
4. Personnel roles have been designed to help employees contribute to departmental or unit objectives.
5. Personnel roles provide optimum and economic job enlargement.
6. Nursing activities have been grouped for full use of resources, people, and material.
7. Nursing activities have been grouped for optimum cost benefits.
8. Nursing activities have been grouped to match special skills to special needs.
9. Nursing activities have been grouped to achieve an optimum management span.
10. Nursing activities and personnel have been grouped for optimum correlation for decision making and problem solving.
11. Nursing activities have been grouped to achieve minimal levels of management by providing for delegation of responsibility and authority to the lowest competent operational level.
12. Nursing activities and personnel have been grouped to eliminate duplication of staff services and centralized services of specialists.
13. Nursing activities and personnel have been grouped to facilitate production of products and services that will promote health of individuals and groups.
14. Nursing activities and personnel have been grouped to promote soundness of industrial relations programs and fiscal policies and procedures.
15. Nursing activities have been grouped to fulfill time demands of shifts.
16. Nursing activities have been grouped to achieve priorities and allow for change and flexibility in achievement of objectives.
17. Nursing activities have been grouped to facilitate training of employees.
18. Nursing activities have been grouped to facilitate communication.

Departmentation

Steps 3, 4, and 5 involve departmentation, the grouping of personnel according to some characteristic. Departmentation is an organizing process done by functional specialty, time, territory, and product.

At the present, nursing services are usually organized using a mix of departmentations. So long as the system is based on logic, it will provide a viable and efficient organization. Use Exhibit 14–17 on the previous page to evaluate departmentation of nursing service activities and personnel.

ORGANIZATION CHARTS

Most nursing organizations use a graphic representation called an organization chart to depict reporting relationships and communication channels. Charts of line organizations show supervisor and supervisee relationships from top to bottom of the nursing organization. Hierarchical relationships exist on which communication channels follow the line of authority to and through the chief nurse executive. (Refer to Exhibits 14–9, 14–11, 14–12, and 14–14.)

Staff charts show the advisory relationship of specialists, or experts, to the nurse administrators. This type of chart usually shows the title or rank of each line and staff position in the authority relationship structure. Staff charts denote how authority and responsibility are delegated as well as the direction of accountability for the goals of the nursing division.

Organization charts show how nursing responsibilities are distributed. These responsibilities may be divided according to one function or a combination of functions: contiguous geography, similar techniques, similar objectives, or like clientele. Exhibit 14–18 shows how to evaluate an organization chart of a nursing division, department, or unit.

THE INFORMAL ORGANIZATION

Every formal organization has a parallel informal one. The informal organization meets the needs of individuals with similar backgrounds, values, hobbies, interests, and physical proximity. It meets their needs for sharing experiences and feelings. The informal organization can help to serve the goals of the formal organization if it is not made the servant of administration. It should not be controlled. A major shortcoming in its use is that not all employees are part of the informal organization.

MINIMUM REQUIREMENTS OF AN ORGANIZATIONAL STRUCTURE

Minimum requirements of an organizational structure are clarity, economy, direction of vision, decision making, stability and accountability, and perception and self-renewal.

To apply design principles that are appropriate, the nurse manager uses a mixture of all that are productive.

Principle: Organizational needs derive from the statements of mission and objectives and from observation of work performed.

Exhibit 14–18 Evaluating Organizational Function

Answer the following questions as a final evaluation of your organizing function within a department or unit. For those checked No, plan changes so that they will result in effective organizing. Then implement the management plan.

	Yes	No
1. Is there evidence that organizing is an intentional and ongoing function of the division, department, service, or unit?	___	___
2. Is there evidence that organizing changes as plans, goals, or objectives change?	___	___
3. Is there evidence that managers are developed or replaced to fit organizational changes emerging from changed plans and objectives?	___	___
4. Are organizational managerial relationships clearly structured to give security to individual managers?	___	___
5. Has authority been delegated to appropriate levels of managers?	___	___
6. Is there evidence that delegation of authority has been balanced to retain control of appropriate administrative functions by the chief nurse executive?	___	___
7. Is information dissemination clearly separated from decision making?	___	___
8. Is the authority delegated commensurate with the responsibility?	___	___
9. Is there evidence of acceptance of responsibility and authority by subordinate managers?	___	___
10. Is there evidence that subordinate managers have the power to accomplish the results expected of them?	___	___
11. Is there evidence that authority and responsibility have been confined within divisional, departmental, service, or unit boundaries?	___	___
12. Is there evidence of balance in support and use of staff functions?	___	___
13. Is there evidence of balance in support and use of functional authority?	___	___
14. Is there evidence of maintenance of the principle of unity of command?	___	___
15. Is there evidence of efficient and effective use of service departments?	___	___
16. Is there evidence of too many levels of managers (overorganization)?	___	___
17. Is there evidence of unneeded line assistants to managers (overorganization)?	___	___
18. Is there evidence that the nursing division, department, service, or unit is organized to facilitate accomplishment of its specified objectives by its personnel?	___	___
19. Is there evidence that the nursing division, department, service, or unit structure has been modified to fit human factors after being organized to accomplish its specified objectives?	___	___
20. Is there evidence that the nursing division, department, service, or unit is organized to accomplish planning for recruiting and training to meet present and future personnel needs?	___	___
21. Is there evidence that the organizational process is flexible enough to adapt to changes in its external and internal environment?	___	___
22. Are changes in organization justified, based on deficiencies, experience, objectives, purpose, and plans?	___	___
23. Is there evidence that the organizing process is balanced between inertia and continual change?	___	___
24. Is there evidence that all nursing personnel know the organizational structure and understand their assignments and those of their co-workers?	___	___
25. Is there evidence that the nursing organizational charts are widely used?	___	___
26. Is there evidence that nursing organizational charts provide comprehensive information to all workers?	___	___
27. Is there evidence that there are job descriptions and job standards for every job and that they are widely used by nursing managers?	___	___

Exhibit 14–18   Evaluating Organizational Function *(Continued)*

	Yes	No
28. Is there evidence that nursing employees are all oriented to the nature of the nursing organizing process?	____	____
29. Is there evidence that the organizing process within the nursing division, department, service, or unit prevents waste or unplanned costs?	____	____
30. Is there evidence that the nursing organization has an effective span of control by managers?	____	____
31. Are the lines of authority within the nursing organization clear?	____	____
32. Is there evidence that the management information system is effective?	____	____
33. Is there evidence that each employee has only one supervisor?	____	____
34. Is there evidence that the CNE has absolute responsibility for subordinate nursing managers?	____	____
35. Is there evidence that all nursing managers are able to effect their leadership abilities?	____	____

Principle: Organizational design and structure develop to fit organizational needs so that people perform and contribute to achieving the work of the division of nursing.

Principle: A formal organization should be flexible and based on policy that promotes individual contributions to the achievement of organizational objectives.

Principle: A formal organization is efficient when it promotes achievement of objectives with a minimum of unplanned costs or outcomes. Most results should be planned for, should give satisfaction to supervisors and employees, and should not occasion waste and carelessness. When grouping activities for organizing purposes, the supervisor or administrator should examine the benefits and disadvantages of alternative groupings.

Principle: A formal organization should build the least possible number of management levels and forge the shortest possible chain of command. This eliminates stress and levels of friction, slack, and inertia.

Exercise 14–4   Describe the form of the organizational structure of the nursing division or unit in which you work as a student or an employee. Discuss the changes that could be made to make it more functional.

Exercise 14–5   Use Exhibit 14–18, "Evaluating Organizational Function," Exhibit 14–2, "Suggested Questions for Organizational Assessment," Exhibit 14–5, "Characteristics of Consonant and Dissonant Cultures," and Exhibit 14–17, "Standards for Evaluation of Departmentation," to evaluate the nursing organization chart of the organization at which you work as a student or an employee. Summarize your findings.

WEB ACTIVITIES

■ Visit www.jbpub.com/swansburg, this text's companion website on the Internet, for further information on The Organizing Process.
■ Explore different websites that help you to define and analyze organizational structure.
■ Use the Internet to distinguish between a manager's and a leader's behavior.

SUMMARY

No best design exists for a nursing organization, nor do universal design principles exist. Nurse managers need to work for an ideal organizational structure, and they need to be pragmatic. They should build, test, concede, compromise, and accept. They should design the simplest organization for getting the job done. They should focus on key activities to produce key results. The organization is productive when employees are delivering care that meets clients' needs and for which employees have a sense of accomplishment.

The nursing management function of organizing is evolving as nurse managers learn and apply the knowledge gained from research and experience in business and industry. Nurse managers further develop the organizing function through nursing research and experience in nursing management.

NOTES

1. C. Argyris, "Personality and Organization Theory Revisited," *Administrative Science Quarterly* 18 (1973): 141–167.
2. H. Fayol, *General and Industrial Management,* translated by C. Storrs (London: Sir Isaac Pittman & Sons, 1949), 53–61.
3. L. Urwick, *The Elements of Administration* (New York: Harper & Row, 1944), 37–39.
4. T. Peters, *Thriving On Chaos* (New York: Harper & Row, 1987).
5. J. L. Gibson, J. M. Ivancevich, and J. H. Donnelly, Jr., *Organizations: Behavior, Structures, Processes,* 8th ed. (Burr Ridge, Ill.: Richard D. Irwin, 1994), 539–541.
6. R. H. Hall, "Professionalization and Bureaucratization," *American Sociological Review,* February 1968, 92–104.
7. J. R. Rizzo, R. J. House, and S. I. Lirtzman, "Role Conflict and Ambiguity in Complex Organizations," *Administrative Science Quarterly* 15 (1970): 150–162.
8. M. Warda, "The Family and Chronic Sorrow: Role Theory Approach," *Journal of Pediatric Nursing,* June 1992, 205–210.
9. J. A. MacLeod and S. Sella, "One Year Later: Using Role Theory to Evaluate a New Delivery System," *Nursing Forum* April–June 1992, 20–28.
10. D. Dunphy, "Personal and Organizational Change—Status and Future Direction," *Work and People,* February 1983, 3–6.
11. E. C. Dayani, "Professional and Economic Self-Governance in Nursing," *Nursing Economics,* July–August 1983, 20–23.

12. C. Argyris, op. cit.

13. D. J. del Bueno and P. M. Vincent, "Organizational Culture: How Important Is It?" *Journal of Nursing Administration,* October 1986, 15–20.

14. Ibid.

15. W. W. Moore, "Corporate Culture: Modern Day Rites & Rituals," *Healthcare Trends and Transitions,* March 1991, 8–13, 32–33.

16. C. Caroselli, "Assessment of Organization Culture: A Tool for Professional Success," *Orthopedic Nursing,* May–June 1992, 57–63.

17. R. L. Desatnick, "Management Climate Surveys: A Way to Uncover an Organization's Culture," *Personnel,* May 1986, 49–54, 14–22.

18. M. A. Ray, "The Theory of Bureaucratic Caring for Nursing Practice in the Organizational Culture," *Nursing Administration Quarterly,* winter 1989, 31–42.

19. M. E. Fleeger, "Assessing Organizational Culture: A Planning Strategy," *Nursing Management,* February 1993, 39–41.

20. C. Thomas, M. Ward, C. Chorba, and A. Kumiega, "Measuring and Interpreting Organizational Culture," *Journal of Nursing Administration,* June 1990, 17–24.

21. T. Peters, "Experts' Strengths Can Be a Weakness," *San Antonio Light,* 24 September 1991, B3.

22. H. E. Munn, Jr., "Organizational Climate in the Health Care Setting," *The Health Care Supervisor,* October 1984, 19–29.

23. M. Holt Ashley, "Motivation: Getting the Medical Units Going Again," *Nursing Management,* June 1985, 28–30.

24. L. R. Campbell, "What Satisfies . . . and Doesn't?" *Nursing Management,* August 1986, 78.

25. R. L. Jenkins and R. L. Henderson, "Motivating the Staff: What Nurses Expect from Their Supervisors," *Nursing Management,* February 1984, 13–14.

26. T. K. Crout and J. C. Crout, "Care Plan for Retaining the New Nurse," *Nursing Management,* December 1984, 30–33.

27. C. Joiner, V. Johnson, J. B. Chapman, and M. Corkrean, "The Motivating Potential in Nursing Specialties," *Journal of Nursing Administration,* February 1982, 26–30.

28. S. Felgelson, "Mixing Mirth and Management," *Supervision,* November 1989, 6–8.

29. K. Russell-Babin, "Team Building for the Staff Development Department," *Journal of Nursing Staff Development,* September/October 1992, 231–234.

30. D. Heming, "The Titanic Triumvirate: Teams, Teamwork and Team Building," *CJOT,* February 1988, 15–20.

31. K. Russell-Babin, op. cit.

32. "Managing a Dream Team," *Modern Materials Handling,* January 1993, 23.

33. J. W. Frederickson, "The Strategic Decision Process and Organizational Structure," *Academy of Management Review,* April 1986, 280–297.

34. J. L. Nave and B. Thomas, "How Companies Boost Morale," *Supervisory Management,* October 1983, 29–33.

35. D. S. Pugh, D. J. Hickson, C. R. Hinings, and C. Turner, "The Context of Organizational Structures," *Administrative Science Quarterly,"* March 1969, 91–114.

36. M. L. McClure, "Managing the Professional Nurse: Part I. The Organizational Theories," *Journal of Nursing Administration,* February 1984, 15–21; M. M. Timm and M. G. Wavetik, "Matrix Organization: Design and Development for a Hospital Organization," *Hospital & Health Services Administration,* November/December 1983, 46–58; American Organization of Nurse Executives, *Organizational Models for Nursing Practice* (Chicago: American Hospital Association, 1984).

37. Ibid.

38. Ibid.

39. J. G. Newman and R. Boissoneau, "Team Care and Matrix Organization in Geriatrics," *Hospital Topics,* November/December 1987, 10–15.
40. B. Fuszard, "'Adhocracy' in Health Care Institutions," *Journal of Nursing Administration,* January 1983, 14–19; R. H. Waterman, Jr., *Adhocracy—the Power to Change* (New York: Norton, 1990).
41. R. H. Guest, "Management Imperatives for the Year 2000," *California Management Review,* summer 1986, 62–70.
42. D. L. Florey, "The Nurse Executive and the Governing Body," *Journal of Nursing Administration,* December 1991, 11–17.
43. R. Kanter, *When Giants Learn to Dance* (New York: Simon & Schuster, 1989, 36.
44. Ibid., 57–67.
45. M. D. Sovie, "Redesigning Our Future: Whose Responsibility Is It?" *Nursing Economic$,* January–February 1990, 21–26.
46. A. Lewis, "Too Many Managers: Major Threat to CQI in Hospitals," *Quality Review Bulletin,* March 1993, 95–101.
47. T. Peters, *Thriving on Chaos* (New York: Harper & Row, 1987), 424–438.
48. M. Reddecliff, E. L. Smith, and M. Ryan-Merritt, "Organizational Analysis: Tool for the Clinical Nurse Specialist," *Clinical Nurse Specialist,* fall 1989, 133–136.
49. P. F. Drucker, *Management: Tasks, Responsibilities, Practice* (New York: Harper & Row, 1973), 564.
50. D. L. del Bueno, "Paradigm Shifts—What's Good and Not So Good for Health Care," *Nursing & Health Care,* February 1993, 100–101.
51. R. A. Adams and A. R. Rentfro, "Strengthening Hospital Nursing: An Approach to Restructuring Care Delivery," *Journal of Nursing Administration,* June 1988, 12–19.
52. C. E. Schmekel, "Nursing/Group Practice," *AORN Journal,* May 1991, 1223–1226, 1228.
53. K. M. Metcalf, "The Helper Model: Nine Ways to Make It Work," *Nursing Management,* December 1992, 40–43.
54. M. Manthey, "Delivery Systems and Practice Models: A Dynamic Balance," *Nursing Management,* January 1991, 28–30.
55. D. Milton, J. Verren, C. Murdaugh, and R. Gerber, "Differentiated Group Professional Practice in Nursing: A Demonstration Model," *Nursing Clinics of North America,* March 1992, 23–29.
56. Ibid.
57. K. S. Erhat, "The Value of Differentiated Practice," *Journal of Nursing Administration,* April 1991, 9–10.
58. L. W. Porter and E. E. Lawler III, "The Effects of 'Tall' Versus 'Flat' Organization Structure on Managerial Job Satisfaction," *Personnel Psychology,* summer 1964, 135–148.
59. R. H. Guest, op. cit.
60. G. Klaus, "Horizontal Organization," *Executive Excellence,* November 1989, 3–5.

COMMITTEES AND OTHER GROUPS

- Define "committee."
- Distinguish between standing and ad hoc committees.
- Use a set of standards to evaluate nursing committees.
- Discuss group dynamics and the roles played by group members.
- Analyze the phases of groups.
- Analyze committee effectiveness.
- Define "groupthink" and give examples.
- Describe the characteristics of various group techniques.
- Describe the characteristics of self-directed work teams.

KEY CONCEPTS

committee
synergy
group dynamics
Delphi technique
brainstorming
focus group
groupthink
quality circle
self-managed work team

Manager behavior: Assigns managerial personnel to all agency committees.

Leader behavior: Organizes the nursing staff to have clinical nurses represented on major agency committees. Uses self-managed work teams to increase autonomy and productivity of nursing staff.

A committee is a group form that evolves out of a formal organizational structure. Committees are formed to make collective use of knowledge, skills, and ideas. They are a blend of the good characteristics of several or many individuals—a reason for making careful appointments or selections. The principle of synergy underlies committee activity; it puts the thinking power of a selected group together for the most effective outcome. What is the optimum number of people to produce the desired outcome of synergy? The answer is difficult because it depends upon the goals to be addressed, the characteristics of the committee members, and the environment within which these members function. The goal is to aim for the best combination of skills and energies.[1]

COMMITTEES AS GROUPS

Because the work of organizations is accomplished by groups, many persons have studied the dynamics of group function. While not all groups are committees, the management of a group of employees whose goal is to accomplish the objectives of the enterprise is similar to the leadership and management of a committee whose goal is to accomplish selective objectives. In the 1920s, researchers at Harvard Business School found that worker morale and productivity were positively influenced by small, informal work groups.[2]

Committees are formal groups that can serve useful functions in the organizational process of nursing and administration. In addition to being organizational entities, committees are a part of managerial planning, and in turn, they make plans. They are directed by leaders who are appointed by management or elected by constituents determined by management. Since professional nurses want autonomy but are mostly employed by organizations, formal groups, including committees, are a medium for promoting autonomy by giving them a voice in managing the organization. A committee's effectiveness can be controlled internally and externally. A committee that does not serve a useful function should be evaluated and restructured. When no longer needed, it should be selectively abandoned.

There are two common types of committee: *standing* and *ad hoc,* or *special.* Standing committees are advisory in authority, although some may have collective authority to make and implement decisions. They have continuity as organizational entities. Ad hoc committees are formed to fulfill a specific purpose and are disbanded upon achievement of the purpose.

Fuszard and Bishop use the term *adhocracy* to refer to the use of ad hoc committees in nursing organizations. They credit Toffler with originating the term. Applying adhocracy to nursing, a group would be formed to accomplish a specified mission, after which it would be dissolved. It could be called a task force, a project team, or an ad hoc committee. Team members would be those nurses with the special qualifications needed to accomplish the task.[3]

BENEFITS OF COMMITTEES

Committees can transmit useful information in two directions—toward administrators or managers and toward employees. They encourage and involve participation of interested or affected employees in the management of the nursing enterprise. Their advice can be helpful, and they can promote understanding of objectives and programs by other employees. They can promote loyalty. Some of the new ideas that keep nursing an open sociotechnical system come from committees. Committees provide face-to-face meeting of individuals for the purposes of gathering information, seeking advice, making decisions, negotiating, coordinating, and thinking creatively to resolve operational problems and improve the quality of services rendered by the organization.

Committees provide a pool of people with specific skills and knowledge that can be assimilated into plans of action. They can bridge gaps between departments or units. They can use the pooled expertise of specialists and people with special talents and leadership abilities. They give people an opportunity to participate in the social process of group dynamics. They can help reduce resistance to change. Supervision, control, and discipline can be reduced through committee activities. Care quality can be improved, personnel turnover reduced, and harmony promoted through committee work.

All of the positive or beneficial outcomes of committees can be achieved if the committees are appropriately organized and led. Otherwise, committees become liabilities to the organizing process by wasting time and money, deferring decisions or providing wrong information for the making of decisions, promoting too many compromises and stagnation, or being used by administrators to avoid decision making.

ORGANIZATION OF COMMITTEES

Every committee should have a purpose and short-range objectives, and every standing committee should have long-range objectives. Objectives need to be translated into plans of action with time frames and precise responsibility. Assignments should be given well in advance of the meeting so that presentations are ready by the time of the meeting. Committee chairs are accountable to a specific administrator who provides guidance to them through consultation. Committee members should be chosen according to their expertise and their capability of representing the larger group. Committees should be of manageable size for discussion and disagreement. They should have prepared agendas and effective chairs. Exhibit 15–1 lists standards for evaluating nursing committees.

Nursing should be represented on most health-care institution committees and always on those whose activities will affect nursing. It should have representation that will be effective in determining the outcomes of a health-team approach to patient-care services. In effect, nurses should determine how they will practice nursing. The organizational entity presented in Appendix 15–1 on p. 416 meets the goals of shared governance.

Exhibit 15–1   Standards for Evaluating Nursing Committees

1. The committee has been established by appropriate authority: by law, executive appointment, or other.
2. Each committee has a stated purpose, objectives, and operational procedures.
3. There is a mechanism for consultation between chairs and persons to whom they report.
4. Each committee meeting has a published agenda.
5. Committee members are surveyed beforehand to obtain agenda items, including problems, plans, and sharing of news.
6. Each committee has an effective chair.
7. Recorded minutes of each committee's meetings are used to evaluate the committee's effectiveness in meeting stated objectives.
8. Committee membership is manageable and representative of the expertise needed and the people affected.
9. Nurses are adequately represented on all appropriate institutional committees.

GROUP DYNAMICS

Each member of a group plays a role in achieving the work of the group. Since each member has a unique personality and individual abilities, to facilitate the group's effectiveness, the group leader needs a knowledge of how groups function. Original studies of group dynamics were done through observations of informal groups. The Hawthorne studies of 1924–1932 were conducted in four phases designed to discover what would make workers increase their output. The results of the studies indicate that employees respond to identification with their groups and to the interpersonal relationships with members of their small group by increasing their output.

Through interpersonal relationships, group members perform task roles, group-building and maintenance roles, and individual roles. In the performance of these roles, the group members share the power of the organization and its management.

Group Task Roles

Each member of a group performs a role related to the task of the group or committee to arrive cooperatively with the other group members at a definition of and solution to a common problem. Benne and Sheats identify twelve group task roles, each of which may be performed by a group member or by the leader; one person may perform several roles. These roles are as follows:[4]

1. Initiator-contributor, a group member who proposes or suggests new group goals or redefines the problem. (This may take the form of new procedures or group restructuring. There may be more than one initiator-contributor functioning at different times within the group's lifetime.)
2. Information seeker, a group member who seeks a factual basis for the group's work.
3. Opinion seeker, a group member who seeks opinions that reflect or clarify the values of other members' suggestions.
4. Information giver, a group member who gives an opinion indicating what the group's view of pertinent values should be.
5. Elaborator, a group member who suggests by example or extended meanings the reason for suggestions and how they could work.
6. Opinion giver, a group member who states personal beliefs pertinent to the group discussion.
7. Coordinator, a group member who clarifies and coordinates ideas, suggestions, and activities of the group members or subgroups.
8. Orienter, a group member who summarizes decisions or actions and identifies and questions differences from agreed-upon goals.
9. Evaluator-critic, a group member who compares and questions group accomplishments and compares them to a standard.
10. Energizer, a group member who stimulates and prods the group to act and to raise the level of their actions.

11. Procedural technician, a group member who facilitates the group's actions by arranging the environment.

12. Recorder, a group member who records the group's activities and accomplishments.

Group-Building and Maintenance Roles

Individual members of the group work to build and maintain group functioning. Again, each role may be performed by a group member or by the leader, and one person may perform several roles. The following are the seven group-building roles:[5]

1. Encourager, a group member who accepts and praises the contributions, viewpoints, ideas, and suggestions of all group members with warmth and solidarity.

2. Harmonizer, a group member who mediates, harmonizes, and resolves conflicts.

3. Compromiser, a group member who yields his or her position within a conflict.

4. Gate-keeper and expediter, a group member who promotes open communication and facilitates participation to involve all group members.

5. Standard setter or ego ideal, a group member who expresses or applies standards to evaluate group processes.

6. Group-observer and commentator, a group member who records the group process and uses it to provide feedback to the group.

7. Follower, a group member who accepts the other group members' ideas and listens to their discussion and decisions.

Individual Roles

Group members also play roles to serve their individual needs. To keep individual roles from disrupting the group's activities in meeting its objectives, selected group members are frequently trained in group dynamics. This training is particularly important for the group leader. Individual roles are not suppressed but are managed by the leader and the other trained leaders. The following are the eight individual roles:[6]

1. Aggressor, a group member who expresses disapproval or vetoes the values or feelings of other members through attacks, jokes, or envy.

2. Blocker, a group member who persists in expressing negative points of view and resurrects dead issues.

3. Recognition-seeker, a group member who works to focus positive attention on himself or herself.

4. Self-confessor, a group member who uses the group setting as a forum for personal expression.

5. Playboy, a group member who remains uninvolved and demonstrates cynicism, nonchalance, or horseplay.

6. Dominator, a group member who attempts to dominate and manipulate the group.
7. Help-seeker, a group member who manipulates members by sympathizing with expressions of personal insecurity, confusion, or self-depreciation.
8. Special interest pleader, a group member who cloaks personal prejudices or biases by ostensibly speaking for others.

Exercise 15–1   Attend meetings of several committees or groups for the purpose of identifying behavior of individual members in group roles. Identify the role each member is playing. Write a brief summary of your observations.

Phases of Groups

Groups have a natural history of development. The following are five generally accepted phases of a group:[7]

1. *Forming or orientation phase.* This is the phase during which group members are discovering themselves. They want uniqueness; they want to belong while maintaining personal identity. They test each other for appropriate and acceptable behavior. This is the time to exchange information, discover ground rules, size up each other, and determine fit.
2. *Conflict or storming phase.* During this phase, group members jockey for position, control, and influence. Leadership struggle and increased competition take place. The leader helps members through this phase, assisting with roles and assignments.
3. *Cohesion or norming phase.* Roles and norms are established, with a move toward consensus and objectives. Members reach a common understanding of the true nature of the opportunity to reach the group's goals. They will diagnose the root cause of the problem, the deviation from expected performance. They will be open to alternative definitions with multiple views. Morale and trust improve, and the negative is suppressed. The leader guides and directs as needed.
4. *Working or performing phase.* Members work with deeper involvement, greater disclosure, and unity. They complete the work. The leader may intervene as needed.
5. *Termination phase.* Once goals are fulfilled, the group terminates. The leader guides the members to summarize discussions, express feelings, and make closing statements. The group is reluctant to break up. A celebration can help.

Exercise 15–2   Examine the collective minutes of an ad hoc committee. Identify the phases of the committee and link each phase with recorded behaviors. Summarize your findings.

Selected Group Techniques

A number of group techniques have been developed to make groups effective and productive. Among them are the Delphi technique, brainstorming, the nominal group technique, and focus groups.

Delphi Technique.   The Delphi technique pools the opinion of experts. This technique can be used in nursing to pool the opinions of a group of leaders in the field. Each round of questioning has three phases. For example, the group is polled for input, which is analyzed, clarified, and codified by the investigator and given as feedback to the experts; the experts are polled for further commentary on the composite of the first round. This process can continue for three to five rounds. Exhibit 15–2 presents an example of a format for round one of a Delphi technique.[8]

Members of the group using the Delphi technique may never have the opportunity to meet personally, since most of the activities are done through correspondence or electronically.

Brainstorming.   As a group technique, brainstorming seeks to develop creativity by free initiation of ideas. The object is to elicit as many ideas as possible. The following are the steps in the brainstorming technique:[9]

1. The leader instructs the group, giving them the topic or problem and telling them to respond positively with any ideas or suggestions they have relative to it. No critical responses are allowed.

Exhibit 15–2   Delphi Technique, Round One

	Desirability			Feasibility			Timing probability (year by which probable event will have occurred)		
	High	Average	Low	High	Likely	Unlikely	10%	50%	90%
1. Case management will become dominant in nursing in a majority of hospitals.									
2. A majority of hospitals will have unbundled the hospital bill to cost and charge nursing services.									

Source: Adapted from R. M. Hodgetts, *Management: Theory, Process and Practice,* 5th ed. (Orlando, Fla.: Harcourt Brace, 1990), 286. Reprinted with permission.

2. The leader lists on a poster or chalkboard all ideas and suggestions as they are given and encourages their generation.
3. Ideas and suggestions are evaluated only after every group member has contributed all possible ideas and suggestions.

The Nominal Group Technique.   In this technique, the problem or task is defined. Members independently write down ideas about it, trying to make them problem-centered and of higher quality. Each member presents ideas to the group without discussion. The ideas are summarized and listed. Next the members discuss each recorded idea to clarify, evaluate, and assign a priority to each decision. The process takes about one and one-half to two hours and results in a sense of accomplishment and closure.[10]

Focus Groups.   Focus group methods stem from consumer market research. They do not provide quantitative research but provide a phenomenologic approach to qualitative research. Focus groups offer descriptions of the vicarious experiences of the participants. Groups of eight to twelve participants meet with a moderator who facilitates focused discussion on a topic. The focus process has three phases:[11]

Phase 1: Gathering data of internal and external conditions related to the group's objectives.
Phase 2: Designing the study—type and size of sample, group discussion method, and focus group format. Identify three to four focus groups of eight to twelve participants. During this phase, the role of the moderator is defined, and the script is developed.
Phase 3: Implementing the plan and providing participant confidentiality.

Group Leaders

Group leaders may be formal, informal, or specialized. Formal leaders are appointed by management or elected by management directive; they carry line authority or power to discipline and control group members. Informal leaders emerge from the group. Their influence inspires cooperation and mediation, and group members reach consensus about their contributions to effective functioning of the group in their quest of goals. Specialized leaders are often temporary leaders who have a special skill or ability that is needed by the group at a particular point in time.

To influence people, one must be viewed as having power. Power to influence groups includes the following attributes:[12]

1. Preparing prior to the meeting.
2. Dressing to influence, to be included, and to attain the next level position.
3. Being aware of body language, such as posture, facial expression, arm position, and eye contact. Noting attention, messages being received, and agreement.

4. Touching people on the forearm or the back of the hand to transmit confidence, reassurance, praise, and security. Saying the person's name.
5. Using space expansion—greater height, raised head, a standing position.
6. Holding meetings in one's own office or seating oneself at the one-o'clock position in relation to the leader.
7. Being attentive. Listening for information, concerns, and emotional overtones. Clarifying and repeating to verify.
8. Overcoming resistance to new ideas by giving others ownership. Proposing new ideas in a "what would happen if?" framework. Developing a yes pattern. Being an initiator.
9. Speaking clearly and with enthusiasm. Using declarative sentences. Tape recording and then evaluating one's own speech within a group.
10. Learning how to negotiate. Going for win-win results, giving deadlines for completing tasks, and getting concession even after the final negotiation.

MAKING COMMITTEES EFFECTIVE

Purposes of Committees

Organizations, through their meetings, which fulfill deep personal and individual needs, promote communication. The effective use of meetings by groups improves productivity. Committees can be effectively used to implement major policy changes, accomplish a job, and plan strategically. Problems requiring research and planning are better assigned to individuals. Day-to-day decisions should be handled by line managers.[13]

A major purpose of using groups or committees is to involve personnel in participatory management that gives representatives of employees at all levels a share in the decision-making process. According to Dixon, this goal can be accomplished by having the following:[14]

1. Enough groups to ensure representation at all levels.
2. Standing committees, ad hoc committees, town hall meetings, and small meetings so that all levels feel represented.
3. Representation by visible managers to ensure support.
4. Control of employees.
5. Planned absence of managers at selective meetings to encourage discussion.
6. Stimuli to employee participation with tangible results.
7. Members solicited as volunteers, appointed by managers, or selected by employees.
8. Technical assistance to identify problems, promote communication and solve problems.
9. A focus on the power of the group to act on its own recommendations, have its own budget, or access company resources.

Advantages of Committees

In addition to allowing for participation in decision making, committees allow for group deliberations and coordination. Research comparing two groups of interviewees in a public employment agency has shown that the more competitive the group, the less productive it is. On the other hand, in the more competitive group, the more competitive the individuals, the more productive they are. A cohesive group reduces anxiety, curbs competitive tendencies, fosters friendly personal relationships, and makes the group more productive. Personnel ratings that focus on production records increase anxiety and decrease cohesiveness and productivity. Supervisors who decrease employee anxiety and increase employee cohesiveness will increase efficiency and productivity.[15]

Another advantage of committees is their use as a medium of communication. Committees should not, however, supplant such communication techniques as personal executive action, written communications, individual and conference telephone calls, audiotapes, and closed-circuit television.

Meetings also provide an opportunity for managers to relate to employees. They provide a variety of input and a collective depth of knowledge upon which to make quality decisions. Meetings bring together people who advance more approaches to a problem. They blend concrete experiences, reflective observations, active experiments, and abstract conceptualization. Through group dynamics, committees increase acceptance of solutions and commitment to implementation of their decisions. Also, groups take risks.[16]

Disadvantages of Committees

Committees can waste time. Attendees become cynical, often benefiting more from the recreational than the educational aspects of a meeting. Committees do not always use the organization's own experience in a meaningful way. This can be remedied by using organizational personnel and events as part of the program.[17]

Participants complain that committee meetings and conferences do not allow enough individual input, lead to compromise, are expensive, sometimes have weak leaders who are dominated by other members, and act as substitutes for weak executives who cannot make decisions. If not trained, committee participants may arrive at premature decisions, especially those that are popular with a majority of members, and they may not change decisions when better approaches are found. Without trained leadership, committees can be dominated by one person, suffer disruptive conflicts, and be tormented by individuals who must win at all costs.[18]

Improving Committee Effectiveness

Nurse managers can improve the effectiveness of standing and ad hoc committees by establishing minimal ground rules, including the following:[19]

1. Establish clearly stated objectives. For ad hoc or specialized meetings, discuss the goals before planning the meetings. Base the goals on advancing the clinical and business goals of nursing. See Appendix 15–1.

2. Establish a committee structure to support the clearly stated objectives (see Exhibit 15–3).
3. Plan all meetings and events to meet the group's goals and objectives.
   a. Keep the committee or event at a manageable size. Define membership. *Assemblies* begin at one hundred and increase in size. They observe and listen but may have little participation. *Councils* may comprise forty to fifty persons who listen or comment. *Committees* should include around ten to twelve persons who all participate on an equal footing.
   b. Draw up a point-by-point agenda and send it to the attendees. Include the purpose of the meeting. Since the sequence of the agenda is important, the following points are helpful:
   (1) Put dull items early and "star" items last.
   (2) Decide whether to place divisive items early or late.
   (3) Plan a time for starting important items.
   (4) Limit committee meetings to two hours or less.
   (5) Schedule meetings to begin one hour before lunch or one hour before the end of the workday.
   (6) Avoid extraneous business on the agenda.
   (7) Read the agenda and write in comments before the meeting.
   c. Tailor the meeting room to the group and prepare it beforehand.
   d. Prepare for the meeting by learning the subject matter and preparing audiovisual materials to support it. Bring input via videotaped interviews from people who do not attend. Make events memorable.
   e. Time the agenda items. New or controversial subjects usually take more time. Attention spans diminish after the first hour. Use time efficiently, including mealtimes.
   f. Referee and set the pace of the meeting. Summarize and clarify as needed.
   g. Promote lively participation by involving attendees in the program with a warm-up, get-acquainted phase, a conflict phase, and a total collaboration phase. Bring out the personal goals of the individuals.
   h. Listen to what others say so there will be a sharing of knowledge, experience, judgments, and folklore.
   i. Bring the meeting to a definite conclusion by obtaining decisions and obtaining commitments.
   j. Follow up as necessary to eliminate loose ends. Evaluate whether the meeting's purpose was achieved.
   k. Circulate useful information with the minutes. Keep them brief, listing time, date, place, chair, attendance, agenda items and action, time ended, and the time, date, and place of the next meeting.

GROUPTHINK

Groupthink is inappropriate conformity to group norms. It occurs when group members avoid risk and fear to disagree, to challenge, or to carefully assess the points under discussion. The following are the symptoms of groupthink:[20]

Exhibit 15–3   Committee Structure

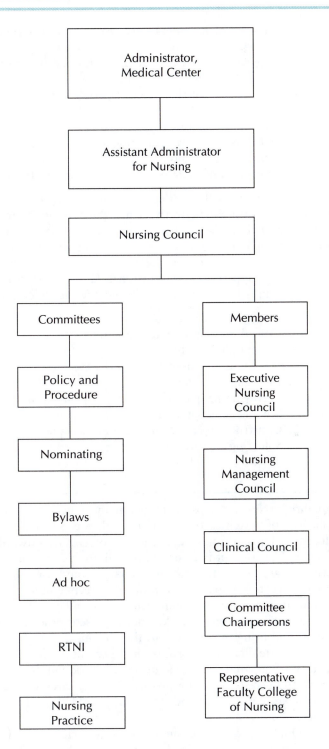

Source: Courtesy University of South Alabama Medical Center, Mobile, Alabama.

1. Illusions of invulnerability, leading to overconfidence and reckless risk taking.
2. Negative feedback ignored and rationalized to prevent reconsideration.
3. A belief of inherent morality.
4. Stereotyping of the views of people who disagree as wrong or weak or badly informed.
5. Pressure on members to suppress doubts.
6. Self-censorship by remaining silent about misgivings.
7. Unanimous decisions.
8. Protection of members from negative reactions.

Groupthink will not occur when members are aware of the potential for it. Groups are considered effective when their resources are well used; their time is well used; their decisions are appropriate, reasonable, and error-free; their decisions are implemented and supported by group members; problem-solving ability is enhanced; and group cohesion is built by promoting group norms and structuring cooperative relationships. The group's leader should teach group members cures for groupthink that include the following:[21]

1. Acting as devil's advocate.
2. Considering unlimited alternatives.
3. Thinking critically.
4. Providing increased time for discussion.
5. Changing directions.
6. Surveying people affected by the problem under discussion.
7. Seeking other opinions.
8. Constructing challenging group measures.
9. Soliciting input from people in the group who do not agree with you.

QUALITY CIRCLES

Quality circles are a participatory management technique that uses statistical analyses of activities to maintain quality products. The technique was introduced in Japan through the teaching of Dr. W. Edwards Deming after World War II. The concept is to use statistical analysis to make quality improvements. Workers are taught the statistical concepts and use them through trained, organized, structured groups of four to fifteen employees called quality circles. Group members share common interests and problems and meet on a regular basis, usually an hour a week. They represent other employees from whom they gather and bring information to the meetings.[22]

The quality circle process has become widespread in Japan, raising the quality of Japanese manufacturing to worldwide eminence. It involves workers in the decision-making process. Quality circles have spread to major manufacturing companies and to some health-care institutions in the United States.

Quality circles are similar to other elements of participatory management. Employees are trained to identify, analyze, and solve problems. Involved in the process, they make solutions work because they identify with ownership. As a result of being recognized, they develop goodwill towards their employers.

SELF-MANAGED WORK TEAMS

Self-managed teams tend to give workers a high degree of autonomy and control over their immediate behavior. Workers are organized into teams on the basis of relatively complete task functions. Workers make such decisions as who will work on what machine or work operation, how to address their interpersonal difficulties within the group, and how to resolve quality problems.

The change to self-managed work teams requires training of management personnel who are uncomfortable with the process and find their status and power threatened. Managers have to unlearn traditional autocratic approaches with punitive emphasis and tight controls on the workforce. Managers are trained to overcome feelings of threat and resentment to change; to perceive workers as mature and responsible; to believe that workers can train each other, that peer pressure can overcome absenteeism, and that a self-managed team gives them time to develop key people; and to be a resource to team members and a support group among themselves. They will be facilitators who work with the group. Managers transition to new roles with modified behavior and attitudes.[23]

One of the activities that self-managed work teams can do effectively is problem solving, a powerful service strategy that gets everyone working toward top performance. Employees feel that their ideas and efforts are valued. Once the self-managed work teams are formed, problem solving may be introduced in five steps, as follows:[24]

1. Brainstorm to identify problems. Team members are asked to describe problems they have observed or experienced.
2. Once all problems are listed, team members are asked to vote for the three problems they believe are most significant. The votes are tallied and the most important problem presented.
3. Brainstorm possible solutions to the problem. The most promising solution is selected. Team members are assigned to investigate the solution and gather further information to report on later. The meeting is then closed.

Exercise 15–3

1. Use Exhibit 15–4, "Checklist for Evaluating Meeting Effectiveness," and Exhibit 15–1, "Standards for Evaluating Nursing Committees," to evaluate a meeting in the organization in which you work as a student or as an employee.
2. When the minutes of the meeting have been distributed, use Exhibit 15–4 to evaluate them. Is there a difference between the actual meeting and the minutes? What is it? How can the meeting process be

(continued)

**Exercise 15–3
(continued)**

improved? Make a management plan (using the following format) to improve the committee's meetings and/or the minutes. Be tactful and use a positive approach in your planning.

Management Plan

Objective:

| Actions | Target Dates | Assigned To | Accomplishments |

Exhibit 15–4   Checklist for Evaluating Meeting Effectiveness

Standards	Yes	No
1. The meeting started on time.	____	____
2. A quorum existed.	____	____
3. The meeting agenda is on a schedule.	____	____
4. The agenda for the meeting reflects the purpose of the committee.	____	____
5. The chair acts as an equal member of the group, taking no special considerations.	____	____
6. The chair follows the agenda.	____	____
a. Dull items are scheduled early, star items last.	____	____
b. Divisive items are strategically placed.	____	____
c. Important items have a starting time.	____	____
d. The agenda avoids any business not on the agenda.	____	____
e. Meetings are scheduled for one hour before lunch or one hour before end of workday.	____	____
f. The chair is well-prepared for the meeting.	____	____
g. The chair referees, paces, summarizes, and clarifies discussion.	____	____
h. The meeting concludes with definite decisions and a commitment to them.	____	____
i. The chair follows up on necessary items.	____	____
j. Useful information is circulated with the minutes.	____	____
7. The chair allows adequate time for discussion.	____	____
8. The chair facilitates participation by all members.	____	____
9. Items requiring further study are referred to smaller groups as projects. Timetables for results are established.	____	____
10. Managers attend meetings when needed to assure support.	____	____
11. Managers plan absences from selected meetings to encourage discussion.	____	____
12. Technical assistance is provided to facilitate meeting success.	____	____

4. At the next meeting, the team reports its findings, which are discussed, including the positive and negative aspects.
5. The team chooses a solution through discussion and general agreement. Team members share the responsibility for putting the solution to work.

SUMMARY

Synergy, putting the thinking power of a selected group together for the most effective outcome, defines a committee's primary function. Committees provide employees with a representative voice in the management of organizations.

A standing committee has continuity as an organizational entity, while an ad hoc committee is formed for a specific purpose and disbanded when that purpose is fulfilled.

Adhocracy represents a system in which a project team exists for a single patient and disbands when its patient is discharged.

Committees can facilitate communication, promote loyalty, pool special human resources, reduce resistance to change, and give people opportunities to work together. They should have purposes, objectives, and operational procedures.

Chairs of committees need knowledge and skills of group dynamics, which can be provided through staff development programs for all nurses desiring it.

Group techniques include the Delphi technique, brainstorming, the nominal group technique, and focus groups, among others. Group leaders either are appointed or elected (formal leaders) or emerge from the group (informal leaders).

Groupthink, in which the entire committee conforms to group norms, should be prevented by training in group processes.

Quality circles have emerged as a participatory management technique that uses statistical analysis of activities to maintain quality products. Quality circles have the characteristics of groups and use group dynamics but are a regular part of the organization whose members are established work groups.

Self-managed work teams increase participatory management by broadening jobs and increasing employee cohesiveness.

NOTES

1. D. C. Mosley, P. H. Pietric, and L. C. Megginson, *Management: Leadership in Action* (New York: HarperCollins, 1996), 456.

2. E. Mayo, *The Human Problems of Industrial Civilization* (Boston: Harvard Business School, 1946).

3. B. Fuszard and J. K. Bishop, "'Adhocracy' in Health Care Institutions," in *Self-Actualization for Nurses,* ed. B. Fuszard (Rockville, Md.: Aspen, 1984), 90–99.

4. K. D. Benne and P. Sheats, "Functional Roles of Group Members," *Journal of Social Studies,* winter 1948, 41–49.

5. Ibid.

6. Ibid.

7. L. L. Northouse and P. G. Northouse, *Health Communication: A Handbook for Health Professionals* (Englewood Cliffs, N.J.: Prentice-Hall, 1985); H. J. Brightman and P. Verhowen, "Running Successful Problem Solving Groups," *Business,* April–June 1986, 15–23.

8. R. M. Hodgetts, *Management: Theory, Process and Practice,* 5th ed. (Orlando, Fla.: Harcourt Brace, 1990), 286.

9. D. C. Mosley et al., op. cit., 197.

10. L. L. Northouse and P. G. Northouse, op. cit., 240–241.

11. M. B. DesRosier and K. C. Zellers, "Focus Groups: A Program Planning Technique," *Journal of Nursing Administration,* March 1989, 20–25.

12. T. A. Kippenbrock, "Power at Meetings: Strategies to Move People," *Nursing Economics,* July–August 1992, 282–286.

13. B. J. Stevens, "Use of Groups for Management," *Journal of Nursing Administration,* January 1975, 14–22.

14. N. Dixon, "Participative Management: It's Not as Simple as It Seems," *Supervisory Management,* December 1984, 2–8.

15. P. M. Blau, "Cooperation and Competition in a Bureaucracy," *American Journal of Sociology,* May 1984, 530–535.

16. R. L. Veninga, "Benefits and Costs of Group Meetings," *Journal of Nursing Administration,* June 1984, 42–46.

17. R. M. Kanter, "Toward the World's Best Corporate Conference," *Management Review,* May 1986, 7–9.

18. R. L. Veninga, op. cit.

19. A. Jay, "How to Run a Meeting," *Journal of Nursing Administration,* January 1982, 22–28; B. Y. Auger, "How to Run an Effective Meeting," *Commerce,* October 1967, R. C. Swansberg, *Management of Patient Care Services* (St. Louis: C.V. Mosby, 1976); R. M. Kanter, op. cit; B. J. Stevens, op. cit; B. S. Barnum and R. M. Kerfoot, *The Nurse as Executive,* 4th ed. (Gaithersburg, Md.: Aspen, 1994); H. S. Rowland and B. L. Rowland, eds. *Nursing Administration Handbook,* 4th ed. (Rockville, Md.: Aspen, 1997).

20. E. H. Rosenblum, "Groupthink: The Peril of Group Cohesiveness," *Journal of Nursing Administration,* April 1982, 27–31; H. S. Rowland and B. L. Rowland, op. cit.; M. Leo, "Avoiding the Pitfalls of Management Think," *Business Horizons,* May–June 1984, 44–47.

21. B. S. Barnum and R. M. Kerfoot, op. cit.

22. The theory for quality circles was actually developed by Frederick Hertzberg and W. Edwards Deming of the United States approximately fifty years ago. S. Johnson, "Quality Control Circles: Negotiating an Efficient Work Environment," *Nursing Management,* July 1985, 35A–34B, 34D–34G; A. M. Goldberg and C. C. Pegels, *Quality Circles in Health Care Facilities* (Rockville, Md.: Aspen, 1984).

23. C. C. Manz, D. E. Keating, and A. Donellon, "Preparing for an Organizational Change to Employee Self-Management: The Managerial Transition," *Organizational Dynamics,* autumn 1990, 15–26.

24. K. L. Seelhoff, "Six Steps to Team Problem Solving," *Hotels,* August 1992, 26.

Appendix 15–1   Nursing Council By-Laws

ARTICLE I
Name

1.1 The name of this Committee shall be the Nursing Council.

ARTICLE II

The purpose of this Council shall be:

2.1 To ensure excellence in nursing care which will return patients to their best possible state of health or will enable them to die with dignity.
2.2 To provide a climate which will promote and support the practice of professional nursing.
2.3 To provide a forum for the discussion of management and patient care concerns.

The function of the Council shall be:

2.4 To ensure excellence in nursing care.
   a. Through the development and support of ad hoc committees.
   b. Through the support of USA Standards of Care.
2.5 To develop nursing service employees to their fullest potential.
   a. Through the development and support of ad hoc committees.
   b. Through the support of USA Standards of Care.

ARTICLE III
Member

The members of this Council shall be:

3.1 All members of Nurse Manager Council Group, Clinical Council, Executive Council, committee chairs, and representatives from the USA College of Nursing.

ARTICLE IV
Officers

The officers shall consist of:

4.1 Chair, Vice-Chair, and Parliamentarian
   a. All officers shall be elected by secret ballot.
   b. A majority of votes cast will be required to be elected.
   c. In the event a majority of votes is not achieved by the first ballot, a run-off between two candidates having the most votes shall be required.
   d. Ballots shall be counted by the Administrative Secretary and RTN I.
   e. Officers shall serve for one year and are eligible for reelection for one consecutive term.
4.2 Officers, together with the Assistant Administrator of Nursing, shall constitute a governing board.
4.3 In the event of a vacancy:
   a. The Vice-Chair replaces the Chair.
   b. The Parliamentarian shall replace Vice-Chair.
   c. The new Parliamentarian will be appointed by the governing body.
4.4 Duties of the officers:
   a. The Chair shall work closely with the other officers of the council. The Chair and other officers shall meet one week prior to each regular meeting for the purpose of developing and distributing the agenda and establishing time limits for discussion. The Chair is responsible to the Council for the smooth and effective functioning of its committees. The Chair is a voting member of the Executive Council and is responsible to the Council for communicating recommendations to the Executive Council. The Chair shall function according to the guidelines established in *Robert's Rules of Order*.
   b. The Vice-Chair shall assume the duties of the Chair in his or her absence and shall serve as Chair of the nominating committee.
   c. The Parliamentarian shall oversee that the Business of Nursing Council is conducted according to *Robert's Rules of Order*.
4.5 Qualifications for office-Must be members of Nursing Council.

ARTICLE V
Meetings

5.1 Regular meetings shall be held quarterly.
5.2 The annual meeting shall be held in November, at which time annual reports of officers and Chair shall be read and officers elected.
5.3 Special meetings shall be called by the Chair. The purpose of the meeting shall be stated in the call and at least two days notice will be given.

ARTICLE VI
Quorum

A quorum of the Council shall be one-third of the membership. The presence of a quorum shall be documented in the minutes.

Appendix 15–1   Nursing Council By-Laws *(Continued)*

ARTICLE VII
Committees

7.1 Policy and Procedures Committee
  a. Purpose
    1. To establish guidelines, policies, and instructions for performance of procedures in accordance with the current standards of nursing practice for personnel of the Department of Nursing. The guidelines are specific and prescribe the precise action to be taken under a set of circumstances.
    2. To annually appraise policies and procedures followed by nurses, and to develop new policies to meet present and future needs.
    3. To assure compliance between nursing policy and hospital policy.
  b. Membership
    1. Members shall be appointed from each of the divisions within the Department of Nursing and from the USA College of Nursing. One member shall be appointed from each of the following: Executive Council, Staff Development, and Nursing Resources. Two members shall be appointed from the USA College of Nursing. Three members (one Nurse Manager or Clinical Specialist, one staff RN, and one LPN) shall be appointed from each of the following divisions: Medical Surgical, Maternal Child, Critical Care, and Special Services.
    2. Each member shall have an alternate appointed to attend in the member's absence.
    3. Members are to be appointed to serve a two-year term, beginning January 1 of each year.
    4. Each representative may be reappointed for one consecutive term. Only one-half of the membership shall turn over annually.
  c. Meetings
    1. The policy and procedures committee shall meet at least six times annually.
    2. The time, date, and place of meetings shall be determined by the Chair.
    3. Minutes of the meeting shall be recorded and kept on file in Nursing Service.
    4. The Chair of this committee shall be elected by its membership.
  d. Duties

    1. To accept written recommendations from an individual or committee regarding the need for a policy or procedure.
    2. Identify independently the need for a policy or procedure.
    3. To research the literature and other resources to determine common, accepted nursing practice.
    4. To develop policy and procedures statements.
    5. To annually review and revise as necessary all current policies and procedures.
    6. To report to Nursing Council at each regular meeting.
    7. To prepare a written annual report outlining the accomplishments of the committee. The report shall be prepared by the Chair of the committee and submitted to the Chair of the Nursing Council.

7.2 Nominating Committee will meet during the last quarter prior to the annual meeting as called by the Chair. The slate of nominees shall be presented to Council for consideration one month prior to the annual meeting.

7.3 By-Laws
  a. Purpose—To review the by-laws of the Nursing Council and make recommendations to the Council for by-laws revision.
  b. Membership
    1. A Chair shall be elected from Nursing Council following the annual meeting.
    2. Members shall be volunteers from Nursing Council.
  c. Meetings
    1. The Chair shall determine the frequency, time, date, and place of meetings.
    2. Minutes of the meeting shall be recorded and kept on file in Nursing Service.

7.4 Ad Hoc Committees
  a. Purpose—To provide a vehicle by which specific tasks or programs can be assumed by a committee.
  b. Membership
    1. Membership shall follow the same format as for standing committees, unless the council decides that a smaller, more specific group, will be more appropriate.

(continued)

Appendix 15–1 Nursing Council By-Laws *(Continued)*

2. Members can be appointed by Nursing Council or the committee may elect its Chair during its first meeting.

c. Meetings

1. During the first meeting, the committee shall:
   a. Define its purpose.
   b. Outline the necessary steps to achieve the purpose.
   c. Establish a tentative timetable.
2. Minutes of the meetings shall be recorded and kept on file in Nursing Service.

d. Duties

1. The committee Chair shall report to Nursing Council during regular meetings.
2. When the committee has completed its task, a final recommendation is made to Nursing Council for approval. Upon acceptance of this final recommendation, the Ad Hoc Committee is dissolved.

7.5 RTN-I

a. Purpose—To provide a forum for the discussion of topics relating to the practice of professional nursing at USAMC.

b. Membership

1. RTN from each unit or area and float pool for term of one year.
2. Any RTN may attend as an observer.
3. Adviser chosen by the committee and approved by administration. The adviser is a non-voting member.
4. Officers are chosen by the committee.

c. Duties

1. To identify problems related to professional nursing and recommend solutions to Nursing Council.
2. To disseminate information to coworkers.
3. To review at monthly meetings all approved new and/or revised policies and procedures.
4. To accept and assume responsibility for projects delegated by Nursing Council.
5. To report to Nursing Council at each regular meeting. The report shall include:
   a. Problems identified concerning professional nursing.
   b. Recommendations for the solution of the identified problems.
   c. Progress on delegated projects.
   d. Summary of monthly committee activities.

6. To prepare an annual written report outlining the accomplishments of the committee. This report shall be prepared by the committee Chair and submitted to the Chair of Nursing Council.

7.6 Nurse Practice Committee

a. Purpose

1. To assist in identifying potential or actual problems related to quality of care, recommend corrective action, develop and plan for corrective action, and review effectiveness of corrective actions until an acceptable level of compliance is obtained. An additional charge of the committee is to develop and/or revise Nursing Standards of Care and Practice.

b. Membership

1. The Clinical Administrator for Nursing Practice shall assume position of Chair.
2. The Nurse Practice Committee is comprised of a Registered Nurse from each nursing unit within the hospital.

c. Duties

1. To review and evaluate Quality Assurance monitoring.
2. To evaluate the effectiveness of previous actions taken to improve care based on follow-up and tracking.
3. To plan appropriate actions that will improve the delivery of nursing care and affect patient outcomes.
4. To communicate and implement the planned action and follow-up at the unit level.
5. To identify trends for potential monitoring and evaluation.
6. To report Quality Assurance analysis to Nursing Council at each regular meeting.

d. Meetings

1. The committee will meet at least monthly or as called by the Chair.
2. Each committee member will receive written notice prior to meetings for attendance.
3. An annual written report summarizing the accomplishments of the committee shall be prepared by the Chair and shall be presented to Nursing and Executive Council.

Appendix 15–1   Nursing Council By-Laws *(Continued)*

ARTICLE VIII
Parliamentary Authority

The business of this group shall be conducted according to the *Robert's Rules of Order.*

ARTICLE IX
Amendments

The by-laws may be amended at any regular meeting by a majority vote. Any member of council may present an amendment for vote.

The proposed amendment must be presented to the Committee in writing one month prior to voting.

Source: Courtesy University of South Alabama Medical Center, Mobile, Alabama.

DECENTRALIZATION AND PARTICIPATORY MANAGEMENT

OBJECTIVES

- Describe decentralization.
- Give examples of the reasons for decentralization.
- Define participatory management.
- Give examples of the reasons for participatory management.
- Describe activities that promote participatory management.
- Illustrate the advantages and disadvantages of decentralization and participatory management.

KEY CONCEPTS

decentralization
participatory management
autonomy
vertical integration
horizontal integration
job enrichment
personalization
primary nursing
self-directed work team
shared governance
entrepreneurship
gain sharing
pay equity

Manager behavior: Delegates limited authority to selected professional nurses.
Leader behavior: Uses all possible vehicles over which the leader has authority for decentralizing decision making and involving nursing personnel in participatory management.

DECENTRALIZATION

Description

Decentralization refers to the degree to which authority is shifted downward within an organization to its divisions, branches, services, and units. Decentralization involves the management components of planning, organizing, leading, and controlling or evaluating. It includes the delegation of decision-making power, authority, responsibility, and accountability. Decentralization of these functions represents a management philosophy and reflects the management style of the chief executive officer and the chief nurse executive. Decentralization within organizations varies in degree but is never total. Top management bears ultimate responsibility for the success of an organization and the achievement of goals, objectives, outcomes, and profit or loss.[1]

The United States Compared with Japan and Europe

In Japan, when workers are asked, Who is in charge? they respond, I am! The Japanese style of management is a fad of the present era. Japan has an entirely different culture from the United States. The Japanese studied U.S. management and modified it to fit their culture. They have learned to manage complex organizations by applying the concepts of Theory Z, which Dr. William Ouchi developed after studying Japanese systems and similar management approaches in the United States. The following are the basic management principles of Theory Z:[2]

> Long-term employment.
> Relatively slow process of evaluation and promotion.
> Broad career paths.
> Consensus decision making.
> Implicit controls with explicit measurements.
> High levels of trust and egalitarianism.
> Holistic concern for people.

Decentralization is a U.S. business strategy that was instituted in the 1960s to aid in the penetration of European markets. It is considered necessary for the successful management of large firms. Both Europe and Japan have more family-held firms. Japanese firms retain collective, centralized, and strongly hierarchical organizational structures. Managerial reward systems in the United States usually emphasize individual rather than group performance, although this is changing with implementation of self-managed work teams.[3]

The United States has more formal business education schools than Europe and Japan have. European firms tend to provide management education and training in-house. While U.S. colleges and universities graduate over 78,000 MBAs annually, Great Britain graduates approximately 1,500, and Japan and Germany very few.[4]

Reasons for Decentralization

Health-care organizations are among the most complex in the world. Since their complexity increases with size, decisions are better managed at the specific site from which they originate. Communication does not have to travel up and down an organizational hierarchy. Sound decisions can be made and action taken more promptly when decision making is decentralized.

The variety and depth of nursing management problems have increased. Patient care must keep moving; delay in a diagnostic procedure or treatment can delay progress toward recovery and discharge, thereby increasing expense. Staffing is a complicated process that must account for many variables, a few of which are physician absences due to education, vacation, or illness; seasonal fluctuations resulting from such factors as school vacations; the random nature of tertiary care for such conditions as heart attacks, strokes, trauma, and cancer; third-party payer requirements; government rules and regulations related to patients and employees; coordination of multiple activities; increased technology with increased specialization; environmental and human stress; the complexity of managing human beings, including those with dual careers as nurses and homemakers; complaints; quality improvement; and staff development.

The object of decentralizing nursing is to manage decisions in their specific area of origin, thereby facilitating communication and effectiveness. Decentralization also supports role clarification to prevent overlapping and duplication of individual work.[5]

Studies have shown that decentralized decision making increases productivity, improves morale, increases favorable attitudes, and decreases absenteeism. One could conclude that decentralized decision making is good for health-care institutions because it is good for nursing personnel. Research on the decentralization of decision making confirms the hypothesis that it enhances job enrichment and job enlargement.[6]

To decentralize is to empower. Tom Peters suggests the following actions to empower employees:[7]

1. Give production people wide latitude to act when confronting a problem.
2. Take all employees seriously—listen to them and talk and act as if you hear them.
3. Delegate—give ownership.
4. Give high spending authority.
5. Require relatively infrequent formal reporting.
6. Have high standards, live them, transmit them to employees, demand them.
7. Have a crystal-clear vision.
8. Believe in people wholeheartedly.
9. Let the employee bite off more than he or she can chew.
10. Really let go. Do not take back. Give psychological ownership.
11. Love and respect your people.
12. Provide effective leadership and horizontal management to all employees.
13. Act to destroy bureaucracy.

Decentralization embodies the concept of participatory management, including shared governance.

PARTICIPATORY MANAGEMENT

When top management implements a philosophy of decentralized decision making, the stage is set for involving more people—perhaps even the entire staff—in making decisions at the level at which an action occurs. Both decentralized management and participatory management delegate authority from top managers downward to the people who report to them. In doing so, objectives or duties are assigned, authority is granted, and an obligation or responsibility is created by acceptance. The employee is accountable for results.[8]

In nursing, as in other organizations, delegation fosters participation. A professional nurse with delegated authority will contact another department to solve a problem in providing a service. The professional nurse does not need to go to his or her department head, who in turn would contact the department head of the other service, creating a communication bottleneck. The people closest to the problem solve it. This is efficient and cost-effective management.

The following sections detail some of the characteristics of participatory management.

Trust

Participatory management is based upon a philosophy of trust. The employee is trusted to complete the task, with periodic progress reports and a final review with management. The time and rate of participation should be managed to control stress. The entire task or decision should be delegated as much as possible. More and more professional nurses want to control their nursing practice. The manager can facilitate this by teaching them to make complete operational plans, including structuring priorities and setting deadlines. Such plans provide a documented standard for joint review. Managers who empower and facilitate employee performance communicate trust. This process will demonstrate the employee's capabilities and reveal shortcomings.

Motorola has had a participatory management program in effect since 1968, with almost all of its thousands of U.S. employees involved in it at some stage. The three basic ideas of their program embody trust:[9]

- Every worker knows his or her job better than anybody else.
- People can and will accept responsibility for managing their own work if that responsibility is given to them in the proper way.
- Intelligence, perspective, and creativity exist among people at all levels of the organization.

Commitment

Personal involvement in managing a nursing service requires commitment from the chief nurse and other nurse managers. Managers should be highly visible to the staff, supporting and nurturing them in the process. In turn, the staff should also be committed, a characteristic they will develop from association with the committed managers. They gain this commitment from seeing their bosses out at the production level where patients are being treated, from cooperating with their colleagues and managers in a spirit of teamwork, and from acquiring feelings of accomplishment. Nursing commitment comes from knowing that the purpose of the organization is patient care and that the managers are working with the nurses to produce that care. Staff share in making decisions and in coming to consensus with the bosses. This experience in participation turns them on and tunes them in so that they do not want to be lazy or mediocre or to featherbed. Commitment inspires staff to be industrious, outstanding, and productive. Under participatory management, commitment is elicited, not imposed.

Goals and Objectives

A key goal for a nursing organization is to keep itself healthy, and participatory management encourages a healthy work environment. Participation will make maximum use of employees' abilities without relinquishing the ultimate authority and responsibility of management. Professional nurses want to have input into decisions but do not want to perform the job of managers. They want the support of managers, to be able to talk with them and to be informed. Without this, they develop anger and hostility, which results in absenteeism and lower productivity.

Goal-setting activities can occur with reasonably frequent performance review and feedback. Nursing personnel bring their goals and objectives to conferences with management. The process is reciprocal, with the manager and employee together developing goals and objectives that are challenging, clear, consistent, and specific. Nurse managers and nurses will both be motivated. Healthy stress will be increased and undesirable stress reduced. (Conflict resolution is a major objective or goal of participatory management and is discussed in chapter 23.)

Autonomy

Autonomy is the state of being independent, of having responsibility, authority, and accountability for one's work as well as one's personal time. Professional employees indicate they want autonomy for practicing their profession and in making decisions about their work. They do not want their decisions made for them by hospital administrators, physicians, or others. They want to be treated as equal partners and colleagues in the health-care delivery system. This desire for autonomy has increased as nurses have developed increasingly sophisticated knowledge and skills and have used them with effective results.

Professional nurses want autonomous control over conditions under which they work, including pace and content. Such decisions are often in conflict with management's coordination role, a conflict that can be mitigated by involving professional nurses in delegating coordination of activities.[10]

Professional nurses are willing to assume and accept responsibility and to be held accountable for a charge. They want the authority, the rightful and legitimate power, to fulfill the charge. This authority comes from their expert knowledge and skill, their license, their position, and their peers.[11]

The autonomy of professional nurses is evident in an organization in which management trusts the nurses by giving them freedom to make decisions and take actions within the scope of their knowledge. Nurses are thus free to exercise their authority. This freedom is legitimized in the bylaws of their departments and in job descriptions, performance appraisals, and management support of their decisions. Nurses' independent behavior includes acknowledging mistakes, taking action to correct them, and preventing them from happening again.

The professional nurse is accountable for the consequences of his or her actions. Accountability is the "fulfillment of the formal obligation to disclose to referent others the purposes, principles, procedures, relationships, results,

Exhibit 16–1   Interlocking Major Concepts

Concept	Key Aspects
Responsibility	The charge
Authority	The rightful power to act on the charge
Autonomy	Freedom to decide and to act
Accountability	Disclosure regarding the charge

Source: F. M. Lewis and M. V. Batey, "Clarifying Autonomy and Accountability in Nursing Service: Part 2," *Journal of Nursing Administration,* October 1982. Reprinted with permission of J. B. Lippincott.

income, and expenditures for which one has authority."[12] The relationship between responsibility, authority, autonomy, and accountability is depicted in Exhibit 16–1.

To have autonomy, nursing employees should be involved in setting their own goals and be allowed to determine how to accomplish their goals. This principle applies to all nursing employees. When professional nurses work with other nursing employees, they should facilitate participation and input from these groups. This approach promotes these persons' interest, trust, and commitment.[13]

A study of nurse autonomy found variations in perceptions of whether the nurses were expected to exhibit autonomy and of whether they were supported in exhibiting it. The typical nurse exhibiting the highest level of autonomy was a female with a master's degree practicing in a clinical administrative role in the emergency room who perceived an expectation to function autonomously to a high degree. The typical nurse exhibiting the lowest level of autonomy was a male staff nurse in the operating room or post-anesthesia with less than a master's degree who perceived an expectation to practice autonomously to a low extent or was unsure of the expectation for autonomy. No change was found in the perceived levels of autonomy from studies done fifteen years ago. Highest scores were found among nurses practicing in the emergency room, psychiatry, and critical care, areas where institutions and physicians grant the greatest autonomy. Nurses at the master's level exhibited the highest scores in autonomy. Below that level, poor role definition, role confusion, and poor role modeling contribute to a socialization process that encourages all nurses to act the same. Conversely, nurses in administrative roles have clearer role expectations and correspondingly higher scores on autonomy. Apparently, they are not empowering their practice staff to have the same level of autonomy. The authors state that their findings may indicate that "hospitals do not expect or support autonomy in registered nurses."[14]

To foster greater autonomy, nurses need to be included in decision making, policy setting, and financial decisions. They need role clarity and to be educated at a higher level for autonomous practice. Greater attention needs to be paid to role modeling to facilitate understanding of nursing's independent, dependent, and interdependent aspects. When elements are identified within one area of practice that promote autonomy, they need to be incorporated into other areas as well.

A study of graduating students in one university indicated that the students ranked high on individual autonomy. It would appear that lack of professional status is not due to lack of autonomy in individual nurses. Therefore, consideration must be given to the denial of autonomy by employing institutions as the root cause. Nurses probably arrive at their first job with more autonomous attitudes than women in other industries. Serious consideration should be given to the role that institutions are playing in blocking nurses' efforts at achieving professional autonomy. Nursing education should address this issue by looking critically at existing programs and working to educate nurses who will be able to claim their rightful professional status.[15]

STRUCTURE OF DECENTRALIZED AND PARTICIPATORY ORGANIZATIONS

Flat organizational structures are characteristic of decentralized management. Traditional hierarchical structures with increasingly authoritative levels of management frighten employees, threaten their need for security, and make them uncomfortable. Economic events of the past decade favor horizontal organizational structures with no rank, no boss, and no seniority. Flat organizational structures are flourishing, increasing management/employee association and commitment, and deemphasizing the number of managers and manuals, titles, and executive suites.[16]

In nursing, there are reports of the elimination of head nurse positions, with committees of professional nurses elected by unit staff to manage unit activities. These nurses' efforts are facilitated by the new breed of leaders, who are democratic, participative, and laissez-faire, or free-rein, and who involve their followers in making decisions, setting objectives, establishing strategies, and determining job assignments. These nurse leaders place emphasis on people, employees, and followers and their participation in the management process. They are employee-centered and relationship-centered.

Decentralized organizational structures are compatible with primary nursing. Decisions are made, goals are set, peer review and evaluation take place, schedules are made, and conflicts are resolved by primary nurses. Levels of practice are built into staffing.[17]

Decentralized organizations call for increased involvement by the staff development department, which can also be decentralized. Each department (unit/specialty) is autonomous, with its own specific goals. Cooperation and sharing of ideas are increased, and goals and output are evaluated. Continuity of care is improved with a single department head and elimination of float personnel from other units. The department head is responsible for the hiring, training, performance, evaluation, and termination of personnel.

In one research study, eighteen of twenty hospitals had some decentralization; 77 percent had some decentralization down to the unit level. The overriding purpose was to increase worker satisfaction. Decentralization resulted in increased morale and job satisfaction and greater motivation among managers and workers. Personnel development, flexibility, and effective decision making all increased; conflict decreased, along with operational costs, negative attitudes, and underutilization of managers. The workforce stabilized and became more effective and efficient.[18]

Vertical Versus Horizontal Integration

Vertical integration combines decentralization with integration. When businesses and industries decentralize their operations into product lines and subsidiaries, each unit maintains its partnership and identity with the corporate structure. Prior to the advent of the prospective payment system and competition among hospitals, the industry was largely characterized by horizontal integration of departments within divisions. Some examples are nursing; operations related to patient-care services, such as pharmacy, physical therapy, and occupational therapy; operations related to plant management, including housekeeping; and finance.

As competition increased, hospitals began the quest to diversify into new markets. New corporate structures that included umbrella corporate management with subsidiary companies were formed. Among the objectives of vertical integration are (1) conversion of internal cost centers, such as medical supply and durable medical equipment, into revenue producers and (2) development of new and expanding markets for hospitals, including home health care.

The hospital is struggling for survival and has chosen vertical integration as a means of capturing lost revenues. Whether all efforts at vertical integration will be successful depends upon the market share of products and services captured.

Horizontal integration is also important to the success of participatory management. Integration of the decentralized decision-making process horizontally or laterally links traditionally separate functional hierarchies. The object here is to improve communication across functions, with mutually influential inputs from different interest groups whose individual values, objectives, and loyalties have previously been compartmentalized into obstructions to lateral integration. Horizontal integration is important to the success of participation. The organizational structure and functions require adaptation to models that will support participatory processes.[19]

THE PROCESS OF PARTICIPATORY MANAGEMENT

In the process of participatory management, professional nurses are involved in making decisions that affect them and in setting their own work standards. This process involves training, changed roles for supervisors, changed roles for unions, and communication. It also involves preparing managers for changed organizational structures. Participation requires the understanding and support of many levels of people in the organization.

As organizations grow, they are frequently geographically dispersed. In hospitals, this can occur as new services or products are added. Home health care is an example. When the mission is established, it is frequently housed in another building and sometimes in another part of the community. Geographic dispersion tends to result from vertical integration and to increase decentralization.

Health-care organizations grow as as they establish new missions for wellness, sports medicine, outpatient surgery, freestanding emergency and surgical centers, birthing centers, and auxiliary services and clinics of many kinds. Both diversity of specialization and the geographic distribution encourage decentralization and delegation of decision-making authority, responsibility, and accountability. Decentralization tends to increase if organizational growth is internal rather than external. As these products and services grow, it is more difficult to manage them effectively from a central office. It is important to have well-qualified product managers and unit managers, particularly when there is a great diversity of products and services.

Within a hierarchy, participation based on interaction and influence will succeed to the extent that it can operate independent of other parts of the organization. Product management will be done across organizational functions, so managers must attend to the quality of lateral arrangements. This includes integration of line and staff functions, such as production and marketing or production and education.

Even small companies are enlisting front-line workers as active participants in rethinking the business, organizing the work, and hiring new employees. Front-line workers are given such information as monthly sales figures and quarterly financial reports. Decentralization and employee participation and empowerment create turmoil. Managers respond with training and coaching. Some companies hire new employees only after worker interview and approval (along with the prospective manager and personnel professional). When teams hire members, they need training to be sure hiring laws are not violated.[20]

Training

Managers at all levels of nursing should subscribe to the philosophy of participatory management if it is to be successful. All managers and employees must unfreeze the present system of attitudes and values. This unfreezing process will require a comprehensive, well-planned training program. Training will promote a sense of job security by preparing everyone for changed roles. Staff at every level learn the reasons for participatory management, the advantages and disadvantages, and the roles they will play.

Managers may be threatened by the concept of participatory management if they perceive that their authority is being diminished. Their training program will require that their competencies be assessed. This will include developing their abilities to be frank with employees and willing to admit past failures, and to encourage contributions from their workers and be influenced by them. Managers need to learn to deal with justifying the existence of their jobs.[21]

More than one thousand businesses in the United States are involved in some form of participatory management. Many nursing organizations subscribe to the notion to some degree. Centralized management and authority is becoming history in the development of the science of human behavior.[22]

Because they have been subjected to centralized, authoritarian management for so long, nursing personnel will need to be schooled in the process of participatory management. This will include training to make input into collaborative decision making.

Changed Roles of Supervisors

Decentralization with participative management means that roles have to be redefined and coordinated to prevent conflict. Nurse managers and primary nurses have increased management responsibility. For some, this will mean decreased hands-on clinical responsibility. These nurses become mentors, role models, and facilitators. With a flattened organizational structure, some may lose jobs while others have the overall scope of their responsibility increased.[23]

In one experiment in decentralized patient education, all clinical nurses caring for patients became the teachers. The assistant head nurse became the facilitator—the person responsible for planning and developing objectives for patient education programs and for promoting staff interest and participation in all phases. The education department became the resource available to coordinate teaching programs in support of the primary nurse. The advantages of decentralized versus centralized patient education are summarized in Exhibit 16–2.[24]

In participatory management, the supervisor facilitates rather than directs the workforce. Traditional supervising functions are delegated downward. There must be clear delineation of managers' basic responsibilities, distinct from their behavioral or management style. Managers can gain satisfaction from their ability to make clinical nurses successful and satisfied. The interpersonal skills and conceptual abilities demanded of supervisors will increase. Supervisors should be challenged and should have a future. They should promote implementation of committee decisions, listen, and offer assistance.[25]

Exhibit 16–2 Decentralized Versus Centralized Teaching

Decentralized	Centralized
1. Utilizes all nursing and health personnel for education.	1. Specified individuals responsible for teaching patients and/or coordinating patient teaching activities.
2. Each nurse assumes professional responsibility education.	2. Concentrates responsibilities and accountability on individuals whose specific function is patient education.
3. Provides education to maximum number of patients and families.	3. Number of patients reached may be limited.
4. Educator(s) currently practicing in the clinical area. Possess up-to-date clinical skills and knowledge. Usually less formal training in education.	4. Educator(s) have more formal training in educational approaches. Clinical skills may or may not be in current use.

Source: S. Malkin and P. Luteri, "A Community Hospital's Approach—Decentralized Patient Education," *Nursing Administration Quarterly* 4, no. 2 (1980): 103–104. Reprinted with permission of Aspen Publishers. © 1980.

Changed Roles of Unions

Decentralized decision making and participatory management are not processes that give comfort to unions. Unions may view them as threats to their survival and to membership and as a prelude to efforts to decertify. Decentralization plans should include participation by union membership that emphasizes the common interests of union and management. Both entities want mutual trust, quality of work life, and employee involvement. Both want job security for their employees and members; successful participatory management programs give job security a high priority.

Some employers will promote decertification of unions while working to bond employees to them through involvement. Others will cooperate with their unions, promoting their active support. In the latter instance, traditional prerogatives of management are sometimes subjected to union influence. The risk/benefit ratio of mutual union-management involvement will have to be weighed by both sides.

The union's role will have to be defined. The goal is good labor-management relations. If they are to play a role, union shop stewards will be trained with company supervisors. There will need to be a memorandum of understanding for keeping grievance and contractual issues outside the employee involvement program.[26]

Communication

Good communication within the nursing organization is essential to an effective employee participation program. Good communication is effective communication; it is evident in employees who are informed about the business of nursing. Such employees know what management is saying and what management's intentions are. Management knows what employees are saying and how it squares with the perceptions management is working to develop. Broken communication contributes to stress and leads to direct economic losses through low productivity, grievances, absenteeism, high turnover, and work slowdowns or strikes. Flat organizational structures promote effective communication. Participation enhances commitment and interdepartmental and intradepartmental communication.

Decentralization requires a movement away from mainframe information processing toward distributed systems of smaller computers. This increases flexibility and control at lower organization levels, giving users heightened feelings of ownership of the system. Packaged software then offers fast relief for specific application needs. End-user involvement with computer application increases.[27]

ADVANTAGES OF PARTICIPATORY MANAGEMENT

The following is a list of the advantages of participatory management as cited by writers in business, industry, and health care, including nursing:[28]

1. High trust and mutual support.
2. Eliminated full-time-equivalent positions; fewer levels of management; fewer specialized departments.

3. Increased accountability of managers and employees.
4. Reduced ambiguity in work requirements for practitioners and employees as a result of improved communication.
5. Enhanced role for clinical nurse; self-supervision; active involvement of employees in identifying and solving problems; encouragement of employee contributions; career development.
6. Increased independence of the nursing division.
7. Legal clarity.
8. Increased efficiency resulting from higher nurse/patient ratio.
9. Teamwork (people become cooperative and independent as a result of increased motivation and initiative).
10. Improved organizational communication, with nurses being briefed on all phases of the nursing business, including revenues, costs, and strategic plans, thereby increasing employees' understanding of the organization.
11. Decreased absenteeism.
12. Increased effectiveness and productivity. Improved quality of work; higher level of mastery.
13. Uplifted morale and motivation at work. Increased excitement from fluctuating participation (participation makes work and values visible).
14. Fresh ideas for management decision making and problem solving.
15. Identification of potential leaders.
16. Fostering within professionals of a strong sense of identification with employer's goals and objectives.
17. Decreased turnover and increased stability of workforce.
18. Increased commitment as attitudes become positive.
19. Less overtime.
20. Lower cost.
21. Better utilization of professional nurses as participants' skills and talents are discovered and enhanced.
22. Increased job satisfaction.
23. Recognition of contributions because participation increases individual and organizational capacities to learn, adapt, and develop toward higher levels of excellence.

Exhibit 16–3 is a model of how participatory management works.

Practice and Research

In the Motorola participatory management program, factory-level employees in Plan I belong to groups of 50 to 250 people who set targets and valid standards that measure current cost, in-process quality, product deliveries, inventory levels, and housekeeping and safety. Representatives belong to working committees that review ideas, recommendations, and issues of waste and quality. The committees solve problems and send recommendations to a representative steering committee for review. Committee involvement of workers improves communication. Improved product quality or customer satisfaction is evident in increased sales and profits and results in financial bonuses to employees. In this process, each employee can see the effect of his or her contribution on the group and feel

Exhibit 16–3   A Model of How Participatory Management Works

Through the Types of Participation	Workers' Experience	Leading to Feelings of	Which Ultimately Result in

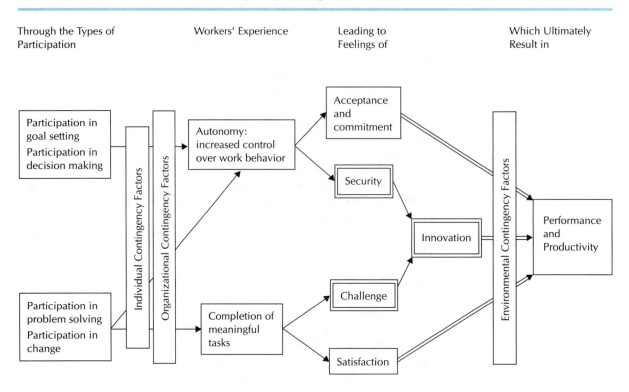

Source: M. Sashkin, "Participative Management Remains an Ethical Imperative," *Organizational Dynamics,* Spring 1986, 64. Reprinted by permission of American Management Association, New York. All rights reserved.

a sense of accomplishment. In one instance, as a result of the participatory management process at Motorola, a 4 percent loss of gold went to zero in two months. Production volume at one plant went up 33 percent with fewer employees. Team spirit and a sense of cooperation existed between management and employees, who worked with less supervision.[29]

Research studies have reported greater motivation and satisfaction when subordinates participate in performance appraisal. Research also indicates that mutual goal setting improves performances, increases productivity, satisfies employees' needs for fulfillment and self-actualization, and thus contributes to the well-being of the organization. Participatory management develops mature, healthy, self-directed personalities among employees.[30]

DISADVANTAGES OF PARTICIPATORY MANAGEMENT

Some of the disadvantages of participatory management are as follows:[31]

1. Occasional failures will occur.
2. Initiation of programs takes time and money.
3. Policies and procedures have to be changed.

4. It is sometimes difficult to determine which responsibilities are whose, even though other ambiguities are reduced.
5. The budget office and other offices or departments have to deal with several units in nursing service rather than a single department.
6. Lacking knowledge of the process, employers do not want it imposed upon them.
7. It is difficult to change management style to true participation.
8. Employees who view management as being autocratic perceive participatory performance appraisal as being insincere, patronizing, and manipulative. The person who initiates it has gone "soft."
9. Self-evaluation is threatening because the employee feels exposed to the view of others.

All of these disadvantages will be overcome by a committed chief nurse executive who prepares and implements a plan with supervisors and educators who are prepared psychologically, politically, and technically. The chief nurse executive selects and develops key people (the human beings developing human beings), works at a long-range future, and is accessible.

ACTIVITIES TO INVOLVE NURSES IN PARTICIPATORY MANAGEMENT

Some of the activities that can be used to involve nurses in participatory management are job enrichment, personalization, participation, primary nursing, self-directed work teams, shared governance, entrepreneurship, gain-sharing, pay equity, and response to identified factors causing job dissatisfaction. Most of these activities are discussed in the following subsections.

Job Enrichment

Job enrichment satisfies the motivation to fulfill higher-order needs, including variety within and among jobs and a strategy that challenges by emphasizing performance output over job processes. Job enrichment creates jobs with greater responsibility and more flexibility and promotes personal development. There are several approaches to job enrichment.

Herzberg's two-factor theory is one approach to job enrichment: growth and motivation factors are achievement, recognition, work, responsibility, and advancement. Reducing hygiene factors reduces dissatisfaction among employees but does not motivate them.

A job characteristics model structures work for effective performance, personal rewards, and job satisfaction. Job characteristics are variety, task entity, task significance, autonomy, and job-based feedback.

The Japanese style of management practices teamwork, group consciousness, harmony, training, and lateral transfers.

Quality-of-work-life approaches consider tasks, physical work environment, social environment within the organization, the administrative system, and the relationship between life on and off the job.

Job enrichment is affected by the workers' expressed interest (see Exhibit 16–4).

Exhibit 16—4 Job Characteristics Model for Job Redesign

	Job Enrichment	Job Characteristics	Japanese-Style Management	Quality of Work-Life Approaches (Sociotechnical Model)
Description	Based on motivation-hygiene theory. Focuses on changes in job content.	Based on job characteristics research. Focuses on job content.	Based on Japanese experience. Deals with organizational, job, and managerial factors.	Based on a variety of experiences in many countries and many types of organizations.
Motivational Assumptions	Two different needs are involved: increasing motivation and reducing dissatisfaction. Factors involved in increasing motivation relate to human characteristics; factors involved in reducing dissatisfaction relate to pain avoidance.	Work motivation is based on three psychological states: the knowledge of results, experienced responsibility, and experienced meaningfulness. These are achieved through five core job characteristics: task significance, skill variety, autonomy, task identity, and job feedback.	Motivation is based on "wa" (teamwork) or family-like norms and the organizational culture.	Motivation is based on jobs designed according to sociotechnical criteria and the capacity of individuals to make choices in designing their work.
Critical Techniques	• Direct feedback. • A client relationship. • A learning function. • The opportunity for each person to schedule his or her own work. • Unique expertise. • Control over resources. • Direct communications. • Personal accountability.	• Combining tasks. • Forming natural unity of work. • Establishing client relationships. • Using vertical loading. • Opening feedback channels.	• Intensive socialization. • Lifetime employment. • Competitive education. • Rotation and slow promotion. • Behavior evaluation. • Work-group task assignments. • Nonspecialized career paths. • Open communication. • Consultational decision making. • Concern for employees. • Compensation.	• Technical systems changes. • Job changes. • Participation/consultation. • Structural changes. • Pay/reward systems. • Compressed shift schedules. • Training and recruitment. • The operating philosophy statement. • Collective agreement modifications. • Group management.
Implementation Procedures	• Interview to identify critical changes in the person's feelings. • Group results into general motivation/hygiene categories.	• Diagnose the need for change. • Assess motivation and satisfaction. • Assess the motivational potential of the job.	• Audit the organizational philosophy. • Define the desired philosophy. • Implement the change. • Develop interpersonal skills.	• Define the need for change. • Obtain agreement. • Hold search conference. • Form action group. • Analyze the technical system.

Implementation Procedures	• Brainstorm changes. • Screen for generalities, vagueness, and horizontal and vertical suggestions. • Avoid participation. • Set up a controlled experiment.	• Assess particular job problems. • Assess readiness for change. • Implement changes, conduct training, and assess the impact.	• Test. • Involve the union. • Stabilize employment. • Install systems for slow promotion and career development. • Implement.	• Analyze the social system. • Develop design hypotheses. • Implement and evaluate. • Adjust to normal operations. • Implement in other settings.
Implementation Requirements	Worker participation or consultation is appropriate.	Worker participation or consultation is appropriate.	Emphasis on diagnosis or consultation is appropriate. Quality circles require involvement.	Broad-based participation. Emphasis is on "philosophy" of organization with corresponding job involvement. Emphasis is on the development of a "philosophy" of organization with corresponding changes in the job-classification plan emphasizing teamwork. Focus is on changing the management approach based on sociotechnical needs.
Job Classification Changes	Many supervisory tasks should become workers' responsibilities. Emphasis is on doing tasks at higher classification levels.	Emphasis is on enlarging the job and doing tasks at the same classification level. Some higher-level tasks may be appropriate.	Requires major changes in job-classification structure, although quality circles may not affect the classification plan.	
Types of Settings or Occupations	Probably more successful with operational/production jobs in which tasks can be defined and broken down.	Probably more successful with operational/production jobs in which tasks can be defined and broken down.	Focus is on changing the management approach based on concepts of Japanese management.	
Issues	• Criteria of motivation may be questioned. • No role for union. • Relatively easy to implement because of limited scope, although it suggests workers should perform higher-level tasks.	• Criteria of motivation may be questioned. • Undefined union role. • Relatively easy to implement because of limited scope. • Consultational in nature.	• Criteria of motivation may be cultural. • Undefined union role. • May be culturally bound and require value changes. • Attempts to shift decisions to workers.	• Criteria of motivation are based on the situation. • Requires union role. • Implementation requires value changes.
Key Employee Questions	Do workers need more responsibility, variety, growth?		Do workers need more responsibility, variety, growth?	Do workers need more responsibility, variety, growth? Do workers desire to work in teams in making decisions? Do workers see the organization as part of their identity?
Key Classification Questions	What job design ideas can be implemented without changing the job-classification plan? What job-classification plan adjustments should be made, and when would they be appropriate?		What job design ideas can be implemented without changing the job-classification plan? What job-classification plan adjustments should be made?	What job design ideas can be implemented without changing the job classification plan? What structural adjustments should be made? How should the job-classification plan be altered to respond to structural changes?

Source: J. B. Cunningham and T. Eberle, "A Guide to Job Enrichment and Redesign," *Personnel*, February 1990, 59. Reprinted by permission of American Management Association, New York. All rights reserved.

Personalization

Personalization is a strategy that focuses on people and knowledge, not numbers and politics. Its users stress empathy and involve professionals in making critical decisions that affect them. Career development opportunities are facilitated by advertising jobs, allowing transfers, giving feedback to job applicants, allowing and providing liberal training and development, and promoting workers based on objective measures.[32]

Primary Nursing

Primary nursing as a modality of nursing-care delivery makes nursing worthwhile work, enhances nurses' self-esteem through performing a complete function, produces results of personal endeavor, and realizes collegial and collaborative relationships.[33] Other nursing modalities compatible with participatory management are modular nursing, team nursing, case management, and collaborative practice models.

Self-Directed Work Teams

A self-directed work team is a functional group of employees (typically eight to fifteen). The team shares responsibility for a particular unit of production (including units of service or information). Members are cross-trained in all the technical skills necessary to complete the tasks assigned. They have the authority to plan, implement, and control all work processes. Members are responsible for scheduling, quality, and costs—responsibilities that have been clearly defined in advance. Exhibit 16–5 compares a self-directed team management model with a traditional management model. The nine characteristics of a self-directed work team are compared with those of a traditional work group in Exhibit 16–6. Employers indicate that self-directed work teams improve quality, increase productivity, decrease operating costs, and foster greater commitment from workers. Employees state that they feel "in on things," involved in decisions, challenged, and empowered and have increased job satisfaction.

Self-directed work teams have leaders. During early phases, the leader is appointed by upper management. As the team grows and changes, it selects its leader. Eventually, the role rotates. The team leader is an internal facilitator. Middle managers are trained to become external facilitators.[34]

Self-managed work teams are empowered to make all decisions about the work they do. Federal Express and IDS claim productivity up 40 percent with self-managed work teams. A survey of Fortune 1000 companies indicates that 68 percent use self-managed work teams, although only 10 percent of workers are in them.

To make self-managed teams successful, employers should do the following:

1. Empower the teams with decision making.

2. Provide them with with electronic mail communication systems so the teams can talk with each other.

Exhibit 16–5   Team Models

TRADITIONAL MANAGEMENT MODEL

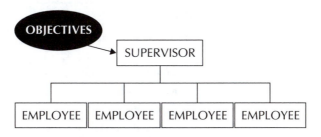

SELF-DIRECTED TEAM MANAGEMENT MODEL

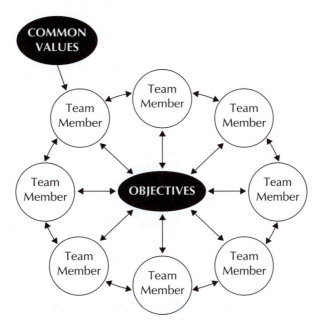

Source: L. Ankarlo, *Implementing Self-Directed Work Teams* (Boulder, Colo.: Career Track Publications, 1992), 5. Reprinted with permission.

3. Create teams only for work that can be done by teams.

4. Make teamwork the centerpiece of a pay-for-performance system.

5. Inspire the teams to increase morale, productivity, and innovation.

6. Use the right team for the right job. Form a problem-solving team to solve a problem; then disband it. Use work teams to do the day-to-day work. Work teams should be self-managed, have power to change the order of things, and have budgets.

Exhibit 16–6 Nine Characteristics of a Self-Directed Work Team vs. a Traditional Work Group

Traditional	Self-Directed
Top-down	Bottom-up
Unilateral	Consensus
Narrow focus	Big picture
Narrow training	Ongoing diverse training
Move up	Move around
Helplessness	Empowerment
Stuck/complacent	Challenged/innovative
Internal competition	External competition
Work together	Work and celebrate

Source: L. Ankarlo, *Implementing Self-Directed Work Teams* (Boulder, Colo.: Career Track Publications, 1992). Reprinted with permission.

7. Create a hierarchy of teams that make decisions on the spot. To build the 777, Boeing used three layers of teams: a top-management team to see that the plane was built correctly and on time; leader teams from engineering and operations to oversee the work teams; and cross-functional work teams. A fourth layer of airplane integration teams with access to everyone in the organization was added later. Problems were identified and solved early.

8. Maintain trust and morale. When restructuring, bring employees into the process. Plan for job loss by retraining, reassigning, retiring, and attrition.

9. Tackle people problems head-on by spending time to get people to work together.

Virtual teams are work teams whose members talk by computer, fly in and out as needed, and take turns as leader.[35]

Shared Governance

Shared governance is defined as the allocation of control, power, or authority among mutually interested parties. Data supporting reduction in turnover and increases in levels of nursing satisfaction are evidence of successful outcomes of shared-governance processes. The principles of shared governance are more consistent with the principles of professionalism than are the principles of participatory management. The following are the main principles of shared governance:

1. Shared governance is not a form of participatory management. Participatory management means allowing others to participate in decisions over which a line manager has control.

2. Shared governance is not management-driven. All activities that are neither direct caregiving nor related to that process are in support of it.
3. Shared governance has no locus of control. Accountabilities of a role are attributed to the role from within the role; they can never be assigned, nor can they be given away.
4. Models should be based on a clinical rather than an administrative organization.
5. Governance should be representative in nature, not democratic.
6. Representatives should be elected, not selected.
7. Bylaws should provide a system of checks and balances, and they should be passed by a majority vote of the entire nursing staff.

Under collaborative governance, managers become integrators, facilitators, and coordinators. Clinical managers are educated in decision making, team building, group dynamics, goals and objectives development, interviewing skills, budgeting, and disciplining and rewarding. Unit personnel develop policy. Structure is kept informal except for areas governed by law, regulations, and efficiency, where representative central committees operate. Unit personnel decide whether their unit will be "open," where personnel float in and out, or "closed." For the system to work, all unit employees must buy into it. It takes years to build a successful collaborative governance. A successful system is in constant state of flux and chaos. This system is based upon twelve shared beliefs (see Exhibit 16–7).[37]

Entrepreneurship

As decentralization and vertical integration strategies are implemented in healthcare organizations, a great opportunity exists for professional nurses to be involved in entrepreneurship. Nurses can form small companies with the sup-

Exhibit 16–7   Twelve Shared Beliefs

1. Knowledge is power.
2. Given adequate information, people will make appropriate decisions.
3. Individuals are unique in their contributions.
4. A sense of purpose results when organizational and personal values are congruent.
5. Maximum productivity results when organizational and personal values are congruent.
6. Risk-taking, with or without success, is growth.
7. People are honest and trustworthy and will work hard to achieve their full potential.
8. Individuals are accountable and responsible for their practice.
9. All problems identified are mutually owned and responsibility for resolution begins with problem identification.
10. Weaknesses and strengths are the same characteristics used differently. (Weaknesses are strengths in excess.)
11. Our decisions will acknowledge federal and state regulations and reasonable economic restraints.
12. Full cooperation with other divisions must be maintained to fulfill the hospital's mission.

Source: J. Jacoby and M. Terpstra, "Collaborative Governance: Model for Professional Autonomy," *Nursing Management,* February 1990, 42. Reprinted with permission.

port of government agencies and private businesses. Such companies require venture capital, which can, with sufficient preparation, be obtained from government and the private health-care industry. As an example, in the face of professional nurse shortages, health-care agencies could find it advantageous to contract with corporate nurse personnel agencies or vertical integration spin-offs that become, for example, nurse staffing subsidiaries, durable medical goods subsidiaries, and clinical nursing-care subsidiaries.

Gain-Sharing

Gain-sharing is a group incentive program in which employees share in the financial rewards of improved performance. It has many of the same advantages and disadvantages as other methods of participatory management. Top management are sensitive to the employees' goals, and employees identify with the organization through greater involvement.

The results of gain-sharing are measurable: savings, improved labor-management relations, fewer grievances, less absenteeism, and reduced turnover. Gain-sharing adds money to intrinsic rewards. Stock ownership and profit sharing are economic rewards similar to gain-sharing.

Pay Equity

Pay equity between management and employees is an issue of participatory management. Employees resent announcements of huge salary increases, fringe benefits, and perquisites for top management. Incentive programs for employees are a part of participatory management programs. While employees receive intrinsic satisfaction from public recognition and praise, they also obtain extrinsic rewards from financial bonuses, stock options, and profit sharing.[38]

Exercise 16–1

1. Form groups of six to eight persons each.
2. Select group leaders and recorders.
3. List characteristics of decentralization and participatory management evident in your organization. (15 minutes)
4. List characteristics of centralized management evident in your organization. (15 minutes)
5. List changes you would like to see implemented to increase decentralization of decision making in your organization. (20 minutes)
6. Report. (20 minutes)

Exercise 16–2   Delegation from nurse managers to clinical nurses is a part of the participatory management process. Mature nurse managers accept the principle of delegation, which leads to a more productive and enjoyable relationship with clinical nurses.

(continued)

Exercise 16–2
(continued)

1. Use Exhibit 16–8, "Delegation Audit," to audit your ability to delegate duties to licensed practical nurses, nursing assistants, and other professional registered nurses when appropriate.
2. Review your delegation audit. Choose three areas you intend to refine, assign them priorities, and outline three steps to improve your performance in each area.
3. Narrate to your group from exercise #1 an experience in delegating that convinced you of the importance of exercising this basic responsibility and strengthened your confidence in your ability to delegate effectively.

Exercise 16–3   Use the standards in Exhibit 16–9 to evaluate decentralization of authority in the division, department, service, or unit in which you work.

Exhibit 16–8   Delegation Audit

How effective are you in

	Low					High
1. Establishing work priorities for your subordinates?	1	2	3	4	5	6
2. Giving subordinates the necessary freedom and authority to work effectively?	1	2	3	4	5	6
3. Building confidence through guidance and direction?	1	2	3	4	5	6
4. Defining requirements clearly but not rigidly when you delegate work?	1	2	3	4	5	6
5. Relinquishing work you would like to do to others who can do it as well?	1	2	3	4	5	6
6. Spelling out the purpose and importance of a task, as well as other related duties?	1	2	3	4	5	6
7. Assigning someone to coordinate your activities when you are away?	1	2	3	4	5	6
8. Taking advantage of others' specialized skills when delegating?	1	2	3	4	5	6
9. Injecting challenge and motivation into tasks that you delegate?	1	2	3	4	5	6

TOTAL = _____
AVERAGE (total divided by 9) = _____
INTERPRETATION: Average Score of: 5–6—Terrific; 3–4—So-So; 1–2—You're "Doing," not "Delegating"

Source: E. C. Murphy, "Delegation—From Denial to Acceptance," *Nursing Management*, January 1984, 56. Permission requested and granted.

Exhibit 16–9 Standards for Evaluating Decentralization of Authority in a Nursing Division, Department, Service, or Unit

Standards

1. Authority for decision making is delegated to the lowest operating level consistent with
   a. Competence of subordinate managers
   b. Responsibility and accountability
   c. Economic management of enterprise
   d. Costs involved
   e. Need for uniformity and innovation of policy
   f. Management philosophy
   g. Subordinate managers' desires for independence
   h. Development of subordinate managers
   i. Need for evaluation and control
   j. Physical location of subordinate managers
   k. Organizational dynamics
2. Delegated authority is clear, specific, certain, and written. It is known by each subordinate manager.
3. Delegated authority supports the organizational, departmental, service, and unit goals, policies, standards, and plans.
4. Delegated authority is consistent with requirements of regulatory agencies, private and governmental.

WEB ACTIVITIES

- Visit www.jbpub.com/swansburg, this text's companion website on the Internet, for further information on Decentralization and Participatory Management.
- Search the Internet for examples of decentralization.
- Using the Internet, what can you learn about the advantages and disadvantages of decentralization and participatory management?

SUMMARY

Decentralization disburses authority and power downward to the operational units of an organization. Japanese organizations practice decentralization by eliciting consensus decision making in management. Decentralization in nursing organizations facilitates communication and effective decisions and clarifies roles.

Increased productivity, improved morale, increased favorable attitudes, and decreased absenteeism are the products of decentralized decision making. Decentralization supports participatory management, the characteristics of which are trust, commitment, involvement of employees in setting goals and objectives, autonomy, inclusion of employees in decision making, change and growth, originality, and creativity.

Decentralized and participatory organizations are usually flat or horizontal, employee-centered, and relationship-centered. They are also vertically integrated to enhance revenue production by developing new markets for health-care organizations.

Training is essential to the success of participatory management because managers often feel threatened by loss of authority. Managers have to be prepared for their new roles. Practicing nurses need to be able to perform as collaborators in the management of the nursing organization and the health-care institution. With their new roles comes increased accountability for practicing nurses. Managers become facilitators.

Decentralization and participatory management are consistent with union participation. A memorandum of understanding is needed to keep grievance and contractual issues outside the employee involvement program. Some employers will opt to promote union decertification while bonding employees to the organization through participatory management.

Increased participation of nurses on organizational boards and committees will improve communication. Communication among units and departments becomes direct and, hence, faster and more accurate.

Despite the numerous benefits or advantages of participatory management, there are some disadvantages, among which are occasional failures, occasional difficulty in determining employee responsibilities, and difficulty in changing employee perceptions of previously authoritarian management.

Nurses can be involved in participatory management through such activities as job enrichment, personalization, primary nursing, entrepreneurship, gain-sharing, and pay equity.

NOTES

1. D. C. Moseley, P. H. Pietri, Jr., and L. C. Megginson, *Management: Leadership in Action,* 5th ed. (New York: Harper & Row, 1996), 274–277; H. Shoemaker and A. El-Ahraf, "Decentralization of Nursing Service Management and Its Impact on Job Satisfaction," *Nursing Administration Quarterly,* winter 1983, 69–76.
2. C. W. Joiner, Jr., "SMR Forum: Making the 'Z' Concept Work," *Sloan Management Review,* spring 1985, 57–63.
3. R. Edfelt, "A Look at American Management Styles," *Business,* January–March 1986, 51–54; B. O'Reilly, "Reengineering the MBA," *Fortune,* 24 January 1994, 38–40, 42.
4. Ibid.
5. B.J.A. Simons, "Decentralizing Nursing Service—Six Months Later," *Supervisor Nurse,* October 1980, 59–64; R. B. Fine, "Decentralization and Staffing," *Nursing Administration Quarterly,* summer 1977, 59–67.
6. H. Shoemaker and A. El-Ahraf, op. cit.
7. T. Peters, *Thriving on Chaos* (New York: Harper & Row, 1987), 2, 9, 230, 525, 545–550.
8. D. C. Moseley, P. H. Pietri, Jr., and L. C. Megginson, op. cit., 274–277, 349, 582.
9. W. J. Weisz, "Employee Involvement: How It Works at Motorola," *Personnel,* February 1985, 29–33; G. W. Poteet, "Delegation Strategies: A Must for the Nurse Executive," *Journal of Nursing Administration,* September 1984, 18–27.
10. J. A. Raelin, C. Sholl, and D. Leonard, "Why Professionals Turn Sour and What to Do," *Personnel,* October 1985, 28–41.
11. M. V. Batey and F. M. Lewis, "Clarifying Autonomy and Accountability in Nursing Services: Part 1," *Journal of Nursing Administration,* September 1982, 13–17.
12. F. M. Lewis and M. V. Batey, "Clarifying Autonomy and Accountability in Nursing Services: Part 2," *Journal of Nursing Administration,* October 1982, 10.
13. J. E. Bragg and I. R. Andrews, "Participative Decision Making: An Experimental Study in a Hospital," in *Self-Actualization for Nurses,* ed. B. Fuszard (Rockville, Md.: Aspen, 1984), 102–110.

14. S. S. Collins and M. C. Henderson, "Autonomy: Part of the Nursing Role?" *Nursing Forum* 26, no. 2 (1991): 23–29.

15. S. Boughn, "Nursing Students Rank High in Autonomy at the Exit Level," *Journal of Nursing Education,* February 1992, 58–64.

16. G. Klaus, "Corporate Pyramids Will Tumble When Horizontal Organizations Become the New Global Standard," *Personnel Administrator,* December 1983, 56–59.

17. E. A. Elpern, P. M. White, and A. F. Donahue, "Staff Governance: The Experience of the Nursing Unit," *Journal of Nursing Administration,* June 1984, 9–15.

18. H. Shoemaker and A. El-Ahraf, op. cit.

19. C. W. Clegg and T. D. Wall, "The Lateral Dimension to Employee Participation," *Journal of Management Studies,* October 1984, 429–442.

20. M. Levinson, "Playing with Fire," *Newsweek,* 21 June 1993, 46–48; M. Levinson, "When Workers Do the Hiring," *Newsweek,* 21 June 1993, 48.

21. W. J. Weisz, op. cit.

22. R. E. Walton, "From Control to Commitment in the Workplace," *Harvard Business Review,* March–April 1985, 77–84.

23. B.J.A. Simons, op. cit.

24. S. Malkin and P. Lauteri, "A Community Hospital's Approach—Decentralized Patient Education," *Nursing Administration Quarterly,* winter 1980, 101–106.

25. R. E. Walton, op. cit.

26. Ibid.; M. H. Schuster and C. S. Miller, "Employee Involvement: Making Supervisors Believers," *Personnel,* February 1985, 24–28.

27. M. A. Robinson, "Decentralize and Outsource: Dial's Approach to MIS Improvement," *Management Accounting,* September 1991, 27–31.

28. H. Shoemaker and A. El-Ahraf, op. cit.; M. P. Lovrich, "The Dangers of Participative Management: A Test of Unexamined Assumptions Concerning Employee Involvement," *Review of Public Personnel Administration,* summer 1985, 9–25; W. J. Bopp and W. P. Rosenthal, "Participatory Management," *American Journal of Nursing,* April 1979, 671–672; J. A. Fanning and R. B. Lovett, "Decentralization Reduces Nursing Administration Budget," *Journal of Nursing Administration,* May 1985, 19–24; G. W. Poteet, op. cit.; R. E. Walton, op. cit.; S. R. Hinkley, Jr., "A Closer Look at Participation," *Organizational Dynamics,* winter 1985, 57–67.

29. W. J. Weisz, op. cit.

30. M. P. Lovrich, op. cit.; M. H. Schuster and C. H. Miller, op. cit.

31. H. Shoemaker and A. El-Ahraf, op. cit.; M. P. Lovrich, op. cit.; W. J. Weisz, op. cit.; C. L. Cox, op. cit.

32. J. A. Raelin, C. Sholl, and D. Leonard, op. cit.

33. J. E. Bragg and I. R. Andrews, op. cit.

34. L. Ankarlo, *Implement Self-Directed Work Teams* (Boulder, Colo.: Career Track, 1992); *Implementing Self-Directed Work Teams,* workshop, San Antonio, Texas, 1993.

35. B. Dumaine, "The Trouble with Teams," *Fortune,* 5 September 1994, 86–88, 90, 92.

36. T. Porter-O'Grady, *Implementing Shared Governance* (St. Louis: C. V. Mosby, 1992).

37. J. Jacoby and M. Terpstra, "Collaborative Governance: Model of Professional Autonomy," *Nursing Management,* February 1990, 42–44.

38. R. E. Walton, op. cit.

17

THE DIRECTING (LEADING) PROCESS

"Directing or leading is best done with maximum attention to employee participation and employee self-management."

OBJECTIVES

- Define "directing."
- Identify the nature of the directing function of nursing management relative to the physical acts of directing.
- Make a plan for delegating duties, tasks, and responsibilities.
- Make a plan for using management by objectives (MBO).
- Use a set of standards for evaluation of the directing function.

KEY CONCEPTS

directing (leading)
delegating
MBO
organizational development (OD)
management by objectives (MBO)

Manager behavior: Directs the operation of a nursing unit or agency to achieve its plans and using its organizational structure.

Leader behavior: Applies up-to-date principles of leadership, motivation, and communication, coaching nursing personnel who have been delegated major responsibilities for achieving the mission of the organization.

INTRODUCTION

In describing the functions of management, Fayol stated that the manager must know how to handle people and be able to defend his or her point of view with confidence and enthusiasm. The manager learns continuously and educates people at all levels for success in their assigned tasks.[1]

Fayol stated that command occurs when the manager gets "the optimum return from all employees of his [sic] unit in the interest of the whole concern."[2] To do this, the manager must know the personnel, eliminate the incompetent, be well-versed in binding agreements with employees, set a good example, conduct periodic audits, confer with chief assistants to focus on unity of direction, not become mired in detail, and have as a goal unity, energy, initiative, and loyalty among employees.[3] Fayol defined "coordination" as creating harmony among all activities to facilitate the working and success of the unit.[4] In modern management, "command" and "coordination" are labeled "directing," or "leading."

According to Urwick, it is the purpose of command and the function of directing to see that individual interests do not interfere with the general interest.[5] Command (directing) protects the general interest and should ensure that each unit has a competent and energetic head. Command functions to promote esprit de corps and to carefully select a staff that can be of most service.[6] It was Urwick's premise that bringing in new blood rather than promoting from within may excite resentment. Urwick indicated the need for a grievance procedure, for common rules to be observed by all, and for regulation that allows for self-discipline. Managers should explain regulations and cut red tape. They should "decarbonize," clean out rules and regulations as needed.[7]

Leading has become a more acceptable term for the directing function. All of the effective principles of nursing management are to be applied by nurse leaders. They begin with accomplishing the mission, goals, and objectives of a division, department, or unit. Since statements of mission, goals, objectives, philosophy, and vision direct the work of all nursing personnel, it is important that they be functional. All leading or directing activities will be guided by them. The actions of nurse leaders should inspire nursing personnel to produce services and products that please customers and maintain the vitality of the organization. The following are activities related to the leading or directing function:[8]

1. Implementing the theory (knowledge) base of nursing.
2. Making and using strategic and tactical plans with input from nursing personnel. Facilitating operational planning.
3. Facilitating the achievement of organizational mission, vision, goals, and objectives.
4. Providing and maintaining resources: people, supplies, and equipment.
5. Maintaining morale.
6. Providing education and training programs to maintain competency.
7. Providing, interpreting, and maintaining standards in the form of policies, procedures, rules, and regulations.
8. Facilitating maximum communication.
9. Coordinating among disciplines.
10. Providing leadership.
11. Facilitating and maintaining intrapersonal relationships.
12. Counseling and coaching.
13. Acting to inspire trust, teamwork, and cooperation.
14. Resolving conflict.
15. Using controlling (evaluating) processes that increase and maintain quality and productivity.
16. Facilitating group dynamics.
17. Organizing human resources.
18. Maintaining the physical plant.

In the 9, 9-oriented Grid® style developed by Blake and Mouton, the directing function of management is described by the statement, "I keep informed of progress and influence subordinates by identifying problems and revising goals or action steps with them. I assist when needed by helping to remove barriers."[9]

DIRECTING AND NURSING MANAGEMENT

Directing is a physical act of nursing management, the interpersonal process by which nursing personnel accomplish the objectives of nursing. To understand fully what directing entails, the nurse manager examines the conceptual functions of nursing management, that is, planning and organizing.[10] From the statement of mission or purpose, the statement of beliefs or philosophy, the vision statement, and the written objectives of the organization, the nurse manager develops management plans, the process by which methods and techniques are selected and used to accomplish the work of the nursing unit. Directing is the process of applying the management plans to accomplish nursing objectives. It is the process by which nursing personnel are inspired or motivated to accomplish work. Three of the major elements of directing are embodied in supervision of nursing personnel: motivation, leadership, and communication[11] (discussed in succeeding chapters).

Effective directing increases subordinates' contributions to achievement of nursing management goals and creates harmony between nursing management goals and nursing workers' goals. Effective directing is the management function wherein the nurse manager acts as facilitator and coach. The effective facilitator and coach provides the education needed for primary nurses and case managers to become first-line managers. Nurse managers teach nursing personnel to manage themselves in self-managed teams. Nursing personnel learn to do planning, self-scheduling, personnel management, and budgeting; effect change; make decisions and solve problems; and build teams for doing research. Nurse managers encourage and inspire their workers every step of the way.[12]

DELEGATING

Delegating is a major element of the directing function of nursing management. It is an effective management competency by which nurse managers get the work done through their employees. One of the criticisms of new nurse managers is that they emerge from clinical nurse roles and fail to identify with their management roles. These nurses have been rewarded for their nursing, not for their skill in leading other nurses. Delegation is a part of management; it requires professional management training and development to accept the hierarchical responsibilities of delegation. Nurse managers need to be able to delegate some of their own duties, tasks, and responsibilities as a solution to overwork, which leads to stress, anger, and aggression.

The following list suggests ways for nurse leaders to successfully delegate:[13]

1. Train and develop subordinates. It is an investment. Give them reasons for the task, authority, details, opportunity for growth, and written instructions, if needed.

2. Plan ahead. It prevents problems.
3. Control and coordinate the work of subordinates. Do not peer over their shoulders. To prevent errors, develop ways of measuring the accomplishment of objectives with communication, standards, measurements, and feedback. Nursing employees want to know the nurse leader's expectations of them. They understand expectations where clear, consistent messages and behavior exist that prevent confusion. They understand expectations from clearly defined jobs, work relationships, and expected results.
4. Visit subordinates frequently. Spot potential problems of morale, disagreement, and grievance.
5. Coordinate to prevent duplication of effort.
6. Solve problems and think about new ideas. Emphasize employees solving their own problems.
7. Accept delegation as desirable.
8. Specify goals and objectives.
9. Know subordinates' capabilities and match the task or duty to the employee. Be sure the employee considers the task or duty important.
10. Agree on performance standards. Relate managerial references to employee performance.
11. Take an interest.
12. Assess results. Expect what is clearly and directly asked for as the deadline for completing and reporting arrives. The nurse manager should accept the fact that employees will perform delegated tasks in their own style.
13. Give appropriate rewards.
14. Do not take back delegated tasks.

Build professional nurses' self-esteem by delegating as much of the authority for nursing practice as possible. Professional nurses want authority over their practice and can be educated to perform management tasks related to it. Nurse managers will determine what authority to delegate through communication with clinical nurses. Authority should be commensurate with assigned responsibility. As professional nurses gain individual self-esteem, organizational self-esteem follows. Employees respond to participation in decision making and gain satisfaction with their jobs and the organization.

The nurse manager should be careful not to misuse the clinical nurse by delegating tasks that can be done by nonnurses or nonlicensed personnel. This error can be avoided by consulting with clinical nurses to determine what authority they want.

Techniques for Delegating

Nurse managers at all levels can prepare lists of duties that can be delegated, from nurse executive to department or unit head and from department or unit head to clinical nurse. Delegation includes authority to approve, recommend, or implement. The list of duties should be ranked by time required to perform them and their importance to the institution. One duty should be delegated at a time.

When Not to Delegate

Do not delegate the power to discipline, responsibility for maintaining morale, overall control, a "hot potato," jobs that are too technical, or duties involving a trust or confidence. These are complicated areas of nursing management requiring specialized knowledge and skills. Nurse managers who handle them should be well-educated in the sciences of management and behavioral technology. Delegating these duties and responsibilities will cause clinical nurses to assume that managers are incompetent to handle these areas of nursing leadership and management.

Barriers to Delegating

Barriers to delegating can exist in the delegator, the delegatee, or the situation. Exhibit 17–1 lists a number of such barriers to delegating.

MANAGEMENT BY OBJECTIVES

Management by objectives (MBO) as a directing element was first advocated by Peter Drucker and made famous by George Odiorne, who defined it as

> a process whereby the superior and subordinate managers of an organization jointly identify its common goals, define each individual's major areas of responsibility in terms of the results expected of him [sic], and use these measures as guides for operating the unit and assessing the contribution of each of its members.[14]

Exhibit 17–1   Barriers to Delegating

Barriers in the Delegator
1. Preference for operating by oneself.
2. Demand that everyone "know all the details."
3. "I can do it better myself" fallacy.
4. Lack of experience in the job or in delegating.
5. Insecurity.
6. Fear of being disliked.
7. Refusal to allow mistakes.
8. Lack of confidence in subordinates.
9. Perfectionism, leading to excessive control.
10. Lack of organizational skill in balancing workloads.
11. Failure to delegate authority commensurate with responsibility.
12. Uncertainty over tasks and inability to explain.
13. Disinclination to develop subordinates.
14. Failure to establish effective controls and to follow up.

Barriers in the Delegatee
1. Lack of experience.
2. Lack of competence.
3. Avoidance of responsibility.
4. Overdependence on the boss.
5. Disorganization.
6. Overload of work.
7. Immersion in trivia.

Barriers in the Situation
1. One-person-show policy.
2. No toleration of mistakes.
3. Criticality of decisions.
4. Urgency, leaving no time to explain (crisis management).
5. Confusion in responsibilities and authority.
6. Understaffing.

Source: Reprinted, with permission of the publisher, from *The Time Trap* by Alec Mackenzie, © 1972 AMACOM, a division of American Management Association. All rights reserved.

MBO spells out the results expected of the clinical nursing unit and of the unit in relation to other units. It emphasizes teamwork and team results. It will include short-range and long-range objectives, as well as tangible and intangible objectives. Intangible objectives include development of the individual, performance and attitude of workers, and public responsibilities. Objectives should include those that indicate the contributions to higher levels of the enterprise.

MBO allows people to control their own performance, measure themselves, and exercise self-control. Through MBO, clinical nurses make demands upon themselves. Nurse managers will assume that clinical nurses want to be responsible, want to contribute, want to achieve, and have the strength and desire to do so. According to Drucker:

> What the business enterprise needs is a principle of management that will give full scope to individual strength and responsibility, as well as common direction to vision and effort, establish team work, and harmonize the goals of the individual with the commonweal. Management by objectives and self-control make the commonweal the aim of every manager. It substitutes for control from outside the stricter, more exacting, and more effective control from inside. It motivates the manager to action, not because somebody tells him [sic] to do something or talks him into doing it, but because the objective task demands it. [The manager] acts not because somebody wants him to but because he himself decides that he has to—he acts, in other words, as a free man.
>
> I do not use the word "philosophy" lightly; indeed I prefer not to use it at all; it's much too big a word. But management by objectives and self-control may properly be called a philosophy of management. It rests on a concept of the job of management. It rests on an analysis of the specific needs of the management group and the obstacles it faces. It rests on a concept of human action, behavior, and motivation. Finally it applies to every manager, whatever his [sic] level and function, and to any organization whether large or small. It ensures performance by converting objective needs into personal goals. And this is genuine freedom.[15]

Procedure and Process

Training.   The training for the MBO process should begin with the nurse managers of the enterprise. Managers will learn the characteristics of the process, the objectives of initiating an MBO program, the procedures to be used, and the methods for evaluating the program's effectiveness. During this training program, nurse managers can simulate the procedures to be used.

Once nurse managers are trained, all nursing employees are given similar training. Employees will be made aware of the necessity for writing and working towards their personal objectives as they seek to achieve those of the organization. They will be taught the value of synergism of personal and organizational objectives and will be asked to bring their written lists of objectives to the first meeting with their superior (see Exhibit 17–2).

First Meeting.   The first MBO meeting should be held in quiet surroundings, with sufficient time for discussion. The nurse manager should put the employee at ease. Most survival and safety needs of nurses are reasonably satisfied. Nurses' social, ego, and self-fulfillment needs are predominant at this time. As

Exhibit 17–2   Summary of MBO Cycle

Phase	Key Activities	Participants
Planning	Identify and define key organizational goals.	Manager
	Identify and define key departmental goals that stem from overall goals.	
	Identify and define performance measures (operational goals) for employees.	
	Formulate and propose goals for specific job.	Subordinate
	Formulate and propose measures for specific jobs.	
	Participate in management conferences.	Manager and subordinates
	Achieve joint agreement on individual objectives and individual performance.	
	Set up timetable for periodic meetings for performance review.	
Performance review	Continue to participate in management conferences.	Manager and subordinates
	Adjust and refine objectives based on feedback, new constraints, and new inputs.	
	Eliminate inappropriate goals.	
	Readjust timetable as needed.	
	Maintain ongoing comparison of proposed timetable and actual performance through use of control monitoring devices, such as visible control charts.	
Feedback to new planning stage	Review overall organizational and departmental goals for the next planning period, such as the next fiscal year.	Manager

Source: J. G. Liebler, R. E. Levine, and H. L. Dervitz, *Management Principles for Health Professionals,* p. 253. Copyright © 1984 Aspen Publishers.

the nurse presents each personal objective, the nurse manager relates it to an objective of the enterprise. Thus, the manager creates the conditions for fulfilling the nurse's needs. This includes the removal of obstacles, encouragement of growth, and provision of guidance.

During this first meeting, the nurse manager and clinical nurse set goals that are specific, promote teamwork, are measurable (in the sense that they can be quantified or described qualitatively), and are attainable. Goals should involve enough risk to challenge but not defeat. They should include objectives that are routine, problem-solving, creative or innovative, and for personal development.[16]

At the end of the first meeting, both nurse manager and clinical nurse should be satisfied with the written objectives. Each party will have a copy of these objectives. The nurse manager and clinical nurse will part with an understanding of how future meetings will progress and mutual expectations and will have set a time for the next meeting.

Actions   Between meetings, employees perform work that meets their agreed-upon objectives. They should periodically review these objectives and summarize their accomplishments.

Second Meeting.   Conditions for the second MBO meeting will be as for the first meeting. This meeting will provide a time for evaluation of results, review, appraisal, and the setting of further goals.

The employee should be encouraged to spell out gratifying and exhilarating experiences, do self-examination, and relate his or her thoughts about work. The nurse manager should listen and make the employee feel safe while helping him or her to have a person-to-organization fit.

The nurse manager examines his or her own reactions without criticizing the employee. This helps to build trust and confidence as well as an ethical relationship. In doing so, the manager and subordinate establish an organizational climate for personal and organizational achievement.[17]

Both nurse manager and employee should exit this meeting with a sense of accomplishment. This does not mean they will not be made aware of deficiencies or shortcomings. The latter will be recognized in the form of needed additions or changes, increased progress, and even deletions. All will be tied to patient care and organizational development. The feedback process tells employees what is expected and when they make errors.

This process will be repeated at intervals, with dates and times agreed upon at each meeting. At the end of an appraisal period, a performance results contract will be signed by both the employee and the supervisor and sent to the personnel department to be included in the employee's record. The performance appraisal can be used to identify promotion potential and to determine merit pay increases.

Problems with MBO

MBO must be viewed as genuine and fair by all employees. It must allow for errors and for adjustments resulting from work constraints and individual capabilities. The following are some specific problems of MBO:

1. Top management not supportive.
2. Inconsistency among managers.
3. Goals too easy or unattainable.
4. Conflict of goals and policies.
5. Accountability beyond control of subordinates.
6. Lack of commitment of subordinates.

MBO is a superb tool if the objectives are "(1) simple, (2) focused on what's important, (3) genuinely created from the bottom up (the objectives are drafted by the person who must live up to them, with no constraining guides), and (4) a 'living' contract, not a form-driven exercise."[18] MBO should promote flexibility.

Organizational Development

MBO is needed for organizational development, and vice versa. It allows the organization to be managed against goals and for results. Organizational development occurs as management skills and organizational processes are applied to shape and develop the conditions for human effectiveness. These conditions are (1) interpersonal competence, (2) meaningful goals, (3) helpful systems, and (4) achievement/self-actualization.[19]

The management philosophy should permit these conditions for human effectiveness to occur. In addition, it should emphasize meaningful work in which the doers are involved in all aspects of the job. Managers should delegate decisions and ensure that the decisions are made, that limits are known, that support is provided, and that accountability is met by evaluating results. MBO is a total management process that includes planning, organizing, directing (leading), and controlling (evaluating).

Exhibit 17–2 summarizes the MBO process, and Exhibit 17–3 lists the standards for evaluating the directing function of nursing management.

A theory of nursing management explores the cause-and-effect relationship between clinical nurses and their performance. It has as its object the removal of controls that create distrust, fear, and resentment, and the promotion of conditions (climate) that provide opportunities for clinical nurses to achieve their goals.

Exercise 17–1 Look at the statements of mission, philosophy, vision, and objectives of a nursing agency in which you work as a student or an employee.

1. What is the work of the unit or division?
2. What is the inference for the directing function of the unit or division?

Exhibit 17–3 Standards for Evaluating the Directing Function

1. Managers have established a medium by which nursing workers feel free to ask for advice, counsel, and consultation.
2. Needed written directions are available in the form of policies, procedures, standards of care, job analyses, job descriptions, job standards, and nursing care plans. They are clearly stated and current and are kept to a minimal number.
3. A training program is in effect that meets nursing employees' needs as they perceive them. They participate.
4. Supervisors are competent in needed knowledge and skills of administration and clinical specialization.
5. Nurse managers periodically work evening, night, weekend, and holiday shifts to keep abreast of clinical and administrative behaviors peculiar to these shifts.
6. The nurse administrator has operationalized the ANA Scope and Standards for Nurse Administrators.
7. The nurse managers have operationalized the ANA *Standards of Clinical Nursing Practice.*
8. Nurse managers are knowledgeable about and apply the appropriate standards of the Joint Commission on Accreditation of Healthcare Organizations, National League for Nursing, Medicare, and Medicaid.
9. The nurse administrator uses techniques of operations analysis. (This service is available at no charge to member hospitals of the American Hospital Association and its state affiliates.)
10. Nurse managers use a system of management by objectives or results.
11. The nurse administrator works with the consent and knowledge of patients and solicits input from consumers regarding nursing services desired.
12. Nursing unit personnel are organized into and working as direct care personnel and clerical personnel.
13. Nurse managers use the physical plant to the best advantage for patients and personnel.

Exercise 17–2   *Scenario:* Jennie Lynd, RN, has been working in the newborn nursery for one year. Her performance in caring for babies, teaching parents, and supporting other unit personnel has been exemplary. She has been told this. Jennie Lynd tells her nurse manager she is interested in transferring to the pediatric intensive care unit. With a group of your peers, decide how the nurse manager should handle this request.

Exercise 17–3   *Scenario:* As a nurse manager, Ms. Pressley, RN, has studied career development theory because she believes that clinical nurses do not really have careers. This is particularly true when a clinical ladder is nonexistent. Ms. Pressley plans to counsel her clinical nurses regularly and to push for a clinical promotion ladder that recognizes advanced competence, education, and certification. This activity falls within the directing category of management. Compare Ms. Pressley's actions with those of several other nurse managers you know or have known. Summarize your findings.

Exercise 17–4   Select one or more goals you would like to accomplish in the unit in which you work as a student or an employee. Make a management plan to accomplish them. The process should

1. Cover *your* individual objectives.
2. Be discussed and adjusted with your boss.
3. Have a plan for achieving each objective.
4. Set a time to evaluate accomplishment with your boss.

Exercise 17–5   Use Exhibit 17–3, "Standards for Evaluating the Directing Function," to evaluate one of the entities in the organization where you work as a student or an employee. Identify one concrete example for each standard. Summarize your results. If the directing function does not meet the standards, use a problem-solving approach and implement a plan of improvement.

WEB ACTIVITIES

- Visit www.jbpub.com/swansburg, this text's companion website on the Internet, for further information on Directing or Leading Process.
- Find websites that discuss the difference between managing and leading.
- Using the Internet, explore the distinctions between a nurse's direction function versus the physical act of giving someone directions.

SUMMARY

Effective directing will result in greater harmony in the actions of supervisors and subordinates and in the achievement of the objectives of personnel as well as of the enterprise. Directing will be most effective when subordinates have superiors who provide direct personal contact. Directing that encourages leadership, motivation, and communication techniques and emphasizes the human aspects of managing individuals is most desirable. It can be fostered by nursing administrators who desire to improve their directing or leading activities.

NOTES

1. H. Fayol, *General and Industrial Management* translated by C. Storrs (London: Sir Isaac Pitman & Sons, 1949), 82–96.
2. Ibid., 97.
3. Ibid., 97–98.
4. Ibid., 103.
5. L. Urwick, *The Elements of Administration* (New York: Harper & Row, 1944), 77.
6. Ibid., 81–82.
7. Ibid., 90–96.
8. T. Kron and E. Durbin, *The Management of Patient Care: Putting Leadership Skills to Work,* 10th ed. (Philadelphia: W. B. Saunders, 1987), 155–176; L. M. Douglass, *The Effective Nurse: Leader and Manager,* 5th ed. (St. Louis: C. V. Mosby, 1996), 153–185.
9. R. R. Blake and J. S. Mouton, *The Managerial Grid III,* 3d ed. (Houston: Gulf Publishing, 1985), 94.
10. C. Arndt and L. M. D. Huckabay, *Nursing Administration: Theory for Practice with a Systems Approach,* 2d ed. (St. Louis: C. V. Mosby, 1980), 92–106.
11. H. Koontz, C. O'Donnell, and H. Weihrich, *Essentials of Management* 5th ed. (New York: McGraw-Hill, 1990), 300.
12. R. C. Swansburg, *The Directing Function of Nursing Service Administration* (Hattiesburg, Miss.: University of Southern Mississippi School of Nursing, 1977), 3–5.
13. B. B. Beegle, "Don't Do It—Delegate It!" *Supervisory Management,* April 1970, 2–6; J. K. Matejka and R. J. Dunsing, "Great Expectations," *Management World,* January 1987, 16–17.
14. G. S. Odiorne, *Management by Objectives* (New York: Pitman, 1965), 55–56.
15. P. F. Drucker, *Management: Tasks, Responsibilities, Practices* (New York: Harper & Row, 1973, 1974), 430–442.
16. M. L. Bell, "Management by Objectives," *Journal of Nursing Administration,* May 1980, 19–26.
17. H. Levinson, "Management by Whose Objectives?" *Harvard Business Review,* July–August 1970, 125–134.
18. T. Peters, *Thriving on Chaos* (New York: Harper & Row, 1987), 603–604.
19. A. C. Beck, Jr., and E. D. Hillman, "OD to MBO or MBO to OD: Does It Make a Difference?" in *Readings in Basic Management* ed. A. T. Hollingsworth and R. M. Hodgetts (Philadelphia: W. B. Saunders, 1975), 190–196.

18

LEADERSHIP

by Sharon Farley, Ph.D., RN

Fail to honor people
They fail to honor you
But of a good leader, who talks little
When his work is done, his aim fulfilled
They will all say
"We did this ourselves."

—Lao Tsu

OBJECTIVES

- Define leadership.
- Explain trait theories of leadership.
- Match examples to Gardner's nine tasks to be performed by leaders.
- Match examples to individual leadership behavioral theorists.
- Match examples to the theory of transformational leadership.
- Discuss similarities between leadership and management.

KEY CONCEPTS

Leadership
Trait theory
Behavioral theory
Leadership style
Transformational leadership

Manager behavior: Maintains position power and delegated authority while working to solve problems with focus on results, analysis of failures, and tasks. Emphasizes control and decision making while focusing inward.

Leader behavior: Leader/managers think longer term; look beyond their units; expand their jurisdiction; emphasize vision, values, and motivation; exhibit political skill; and think renewal.

Florence Nightingale was both leader and manager.

Florence Nightingale, after leaving the Crimea, exercised extraordinary leadership in health care for decades with no organization under her command.[1]

One of the purest examples of the leader as agenda-setter was Florence Nightingale. Her public image was and is that of the lady of mercy, but under her gentle, soft-spoken manner, she was a rugged spirit, a fighter, a tough-minded system changer. In mid-19th Century England a woman had no place in public life, least of all in the fiercely masculine world of the military establishment. But she took on the establishment and revolutionized health care in the British military services. Yet she never made public appearances or speeches, and except for her two years in the Crimea, held no public position. She was a formidable authority on the evils to be remedied, she knew exactly what to do about them, and she used public opinion to goad top officials to adopt her agenda.[2]

LEADERSHIP DEFINED

Researchers have studied leadership for decades, but experts still do not agree on exactly what it is. Many persons use the term *leadership* as if it were a magic quality, something one is born with or simply has a talent for. However, like talent for music and art, talent for leadership involves much knowledge and disciplined practice. Many definitions of leadership have been written, among them that of Stogdill, who defines it as "the process of influencing the activities of an organized group in its efforts toward goal-setting and goal achievement."[3] A difference in responsibilities exists among group members, and each member influences the group's activities. A leader is one others follow willingly and voluntarily.[4]

Stogdill's definition of leadership can be applied to nursing. In nursing practice, goals of patient care are set. Each patient has a nursing-care plan that lists the problems that interfere with achieving physical, emotional, and social needs. For each problem, a goal is set and an approach or nursing prescription is written. An interdisciplinary team may identify problems, set goals, and write prescriptions. The team is influenced by the most highly skilled nurse available, the registered nurse who coordinates the care. Each interdisciplinary team member assumes different responsibilities in performing the total team functions. This process holds true when team nursing is practiced with a mixed staff of RNs, LPNs, and nurse extenders.

The same principles may be applied to the entire division of nursing. Usually, the title of the head of the division is assistant administrator, vice president, chair, or director of nursing services. The division head is responsible for influencing all nursing employees toward achieving the stated purpose and objectives of the division of nursing. The nurse administrator is influenced by a stated philosophy or statement of beliefs about the kinds of services to be rendered by the personnel of the division of nursing. The total staff includes personnel in different job categories, including nurse managers, assistant nurse managers of shifts, and clinical nursing personnel, each with different responsibilities.

Gardner defines leadership as "the process of persuasion and example by which an individual (or leadership team) induces a group to take action that is in accord with the leader's purposes or the shared purposes of all."[5] Numerous other definitions of leadership exist. Embodied in these definitions are the terms *leader, follower* or *constituent, group, process,* and *goals.* One would conclude that leadership is a process in which a person inspires a group of constituents to work together using appropriate means to achieve common mission and common goals. Constituents are influenced to do this willingly and cooperatively, with zeal and confidence and to their greatest potential.[6]

Leadership is a social transaction in which one person influences others. People in authority do not necessarily exert leadership. Rather, effective people in authoritative positions combine authority and leadership to assist an organization to achieve its goals. Effective leadership satisfies four primary conditions: (1) a person receiving a communication understands it, (2) this person has the resources to do what is being asked of him or her, (3) the person believes the behavior being asked of her or him is consistent with personal interests and values, and (4) the person believes the request is consistent with the purposes and values of the organization.[7]

According to McGregor, "There are at least four major variables now known to be involved in leadership: (1) the characteristics of the leader; (2) the attitudes, needs, and other personal characteristics of the followers; (3) the characteristics of the organization, such as its purpose, its structure, the nature of the task to be performed; and (4) the social, economic, and political milieu."[8] Leadership is a highly complex relationship that changes with the times, such changes being brought about by management, unions, or outside forces. In nursing, changes in leadership are wrought by nursing management, nursing educators, nursing organizations, unions, and the expectations of the clientele—patients and their families.

In all of the definitions, leadership is viewed as a dynamic, interactive process that involves three dimensions: the leader, the followers, and the situation. Each dimension influences the others. For instance, the accomplishment of goals depends not only on the personal attributes of the leader but also on the follower's needs and the type of situation.[9]

LEADERSHIP THEORIES

Trait Theories

Much of the early work on leadership focused on the leader. This research was directed toward identifying intellectual, emotional, physical, and other personal traits of effective leaders. The underlying assumption was that leaders are born, not made.

After many years of research, no particular set of traits has been found that predicts leadership potential. There are several possible reasons for this failure. According to McGregor, "Research findings to date suggest that it is more fruitful to consider leadership as a relationship between the leader and the situation than as a universal pattern of characteristics possessed by certain people."[10] This statement implies that leadership is a human relations function and that different situations may require quite different characteristics from a leader. Is it not to a large degree universally accepted in nursing that authoritarian power is effective in times of crisis but that it otherwise promotes instability?

In spite of the shortcomings of the trait theory, some traits have been identified that are common to all good leaders. Exhibit 18–1 lists some of the most researched traits.

Gardners' Leadership Studies

Two major treatises of Gardner's that relate to the traits of leadership are *The Tasks of Leadership* and *Leader-Constituent Interaction.* A brief summary of Gardner's ideas on these topics follows.[11] Gardner identifies nine tasks to be performed by leaders:[12]

1. Envisioning goals. These include a vision of the best a group can be, solving problems, and unifying constituencies.
2. Affirming values. Communities have "shared assumptions, beliefs, customs, ideas that give meaning, ideas that motivate." Society celebrates its values in art, song, ritual, historic documents, and textbooks. People will strive to meet standards that affirm their values and motivate them. Values must be continually rebuilt or regenerated, with leaders assisting to rediscover and adapt traditions to the present. Leaders reaffirm values verbally, through policy decisions, and through their conduct.
3. Motivating. Leaders stimulate people to serve society and solve its problems. They balance positive attitudes and acts with reality. They look toward the future with confidence, hope, and energy.
4. Managing. Leadership and management overlap. Leaders set goals, plan, fix priorities, choose means, and formulate policy. They also build organizations and institutions that outlast them. Leaders keep the system functioning by setting agendas and making decisions. Leaders mold public opinion and exercise political judgments.
5. Achieving workable unity. Leaders function in a pluralistic society in which conflict is necessary if there are grievances to be settled. Conflict

---

Exhibit 18–1   Traits Associated with Leadership Effectiveness

Intelligence	Personality	Abilities
Judgment	Adaptability	Ability to enlist cooperation
Decisiveness	Alertness	Popularity and prestige
Knowledge	Creativity	Sociability (interpersonal skills)
Fluency of speech	Cooperativeness	Social participation
	Personal integrity	Tact, diplomacy
	Self-confidence	
	Emotional balance and control	
	Independence (nonconformity)	

Source: Adapted from B. M. Bass, *Stogdill's Handbook of Leadership* (New York: Free Press, 1982), 75–76, in *Organizations: Behavior Structure, Processes,* 8th ed., J. Gibson, J. Ivancevich, and J. Donnelly (Burr Ridge, Ill.: Richard D. Irwin, 1994), 406.

must be resolved to achieve cohesion and mutual tolerance, internally and externally. Conflict resolution requires political skills: brokering, coalition formation, mediating conflicting views, deescalation of rhetoric and posturing, saving face, and seeking common ground. People must trust each other most of the time to prevent or resolve conflict. Leaders raise the level of trust.

6. Explaining. Leaders must communicate effectively. They teach.
7. Serving as a symbol. Leaders speak for others. They represent unity, collective identity, and continuity.
8. Representing the group. All human systems are interdependent. Leaders view events affecting them broadly.
9. Renewing. Leaders blend continuity with change. They are innovators who awaken the potential of others. They visit the front lines and keep in touch. Leaders sustain diversity and dissent, and they change the social order.

Leader-Constituent Interaction

Charismatic Leaders.   Gardner defines "charisma" as the quality that sets one person apart from others: supernatural, superhuman, endowed with exceptional qualities or powers. Charismatic leadership can be good or evil. Charismatic leaders emerge in troubled times and in relation to the state of mind of constituents. They eventually run out of miracles and "white horses," even though these leaders are magnetic, persuasive, and spellbinding.

Masses of people will often follow the charismatic leader. Such masses have historically been labeled unstable. The worry about mob rule and instability still exists. Social disorder is embodied in the Constitution of the United States.

Influence of Constituents on Leader.   Constituents and leaders have an equal influence on each other. Constituents confer the leadership role. Good constituents select good leaders and make them better. Loyal constituents support leaders who help them meet their needs and solve their problems.

Influence of Leader on Constituents.   Leaders choose to be leaders. They must adapt their leadership style to the situation and to their constituents. In doing so, they weigh the following considerations: the degree of structure they want in relationships with constituents, the degree of hierarchy of authority, formality, discipline, constraint, control, and the amount of focus on task versus people.

Leaders influence their superiors and their subordinates and have the courage to defy their constituents. Sam Houston was a leader of this type. He opposed the secession of Texas from the United States, going contrary to his constituents. A leader may show different faces to pluralistic groups of constituents, including special interest groups.

Transforming Leaders.   Transforming leaders respond to people's basic needs, wants, hopes, and expectations. They may transcend the political system or even attempt to construct it to operate within it. Transforming leadership is innovative and evolutionary.

The best leadership may be that which focuses on self-development and self-actualization. Leaders should develop the strengths of constituents and make them independent.[13]

It should be noted that many of Gardner's leadership qualities embody concepts of management.

Behavioral Theories

Among the behavioral research and theories are those of Douglas McGregor's Theory X and Theory Y, Rensis Likert's Michigan Studies, Blake and Mouton's Managerial Grid®, and Kurt Lewin's studies. Each of these is described here in more detail.

McGregor's Theory X and Theory Y.   McGregor related his theories to the motivation theories of Maslow. Security is a condition of leadership. Constituents need security and will fight to protect themselves against real or imagined threats to this need in the work situation. Leaders must act to give subordinates security through avenues such as fair pay and fringe benefits. Unions act to solidify job security.

A leader provides a further condition for effective leadership by creating an atmosphere of approval for subordinates. Such an atmosphere is created through the leader's manner and attitudes. Given the genuine approval of their leader, constituents will be secure. Otherwise, they will feel threatened, fearful, and insecure.

Knowledge is another condition of effective leadership espoused by McGregor. A person has security when she or he knows what is expected of her or him.

Consistent discipline is another condition for effective leadership. People are met with approval when they do their job according to the rules. They should know what to expect in terms of disapproval when they break these rules. Leaders should be consistent in setting standards and expecting constituents to meet them. Even discipline must occur in an atmosphere of approval.

Security encourages independence, another condition for effective leadership. Insecurity causes a reactive fight for freedom. Security that stimulates independence is desired. Constituents need to be actively independent by becoming involved in contributing ideas and suggestions concerning activities that affect them. When workers are secure and are encouraged to participate in solving the problems of work, they provide new approaches to solutions. They work to achieve the goals of the organization and feel they are a part of it.

With security and independence, constituents develop a desire to accept responsibility. The level of responsibility can be increased at a pace commensurate with preservation of their security. Taking responsibility will give constituents pleasure and pride. Leaders need security before they can delegate responsibility to constituents.

All constituents need provision for appeal, for an adequate grievance procedure by which they can take their differences with their superiors to a higher level in the organization. Leaders who do the job expected of them, who treat constituents in ways that meet their needs and give them security, achieve self-realization and self-development.[14]

McGregor's Theory X and Theory Y are further discussed in chapter 19.

Likert's Michigan Studies. Likert and his associates at the Institute for Social Research at the University of Michigan did extensive leadership research. They identified four basic styles or systems of leadership: (I) exploitative-authoritative, (II) benevolent-authoritative, (III) consultative-democratic, and (IV) participative-democratic. These systems are summarized in Exhibit 18–2.

It is generally conceded that leadership behavior improves in effectiveness as it approaches system IV.[15]

Blake and Mouton's Managerial Grid®. The Managerial Grid® is a two-dimensional leadership model. Dimensions of this model are tasks or production and the employee or people orientations of managers. The following Grid® synopsis describes this model:

Exhibit 18–2 Likert's Leadership Systems

Authoritative		Democratic	
System I Exploitative-Authoritative	System II Benevolent-Authoritative	System III Consultative-Democratic	System IV Participative-Democratic
Top management makes all decisions	Top management makes most decisions	Some delegated decisions made at lower levels	Decision making dispersed throughout organization
Motivation by coercion	Motivation by economic and ego motives	Motivation by economic, ego, and other motives such as desire for new experiences	Motivation by economic rewards established by group participation
Communication downward	Communication mostly downward	Communication down and up	Communication down, up, and with peers
Review and control functions concentrated in top management	Review and control functions primarily at top	Review and control functions primarily at the top but ideas are solicited from lower levels	Review and control functions shared by superiors and subordinates

Source: Adapted from R. Likert, *The Human Organization* (New York: McGraw-Hill, 1967), 4–10. © 1967. Reproduced with permission of McGraw-Hill Book Co.

Two key dimensions of managerial thinking are depicted on the Grid®: *concern for production* on the horizontal axis, and *concern for people* on the vertical axis. They are shown as nine-point scales, where 1 represents low concern, 5 represents an average amount of concern, and 9 is high concern.

These two concerns are interdependent; that is, while concern for one or the other may be high or low, they are integrated in the manager's thinking. Thus, both concerns are present to some degree in any management style. Study of the Grid® enables one to sort out various possibilities and the attitudes, values, beliefs and assumptions that underlie each approach. When one is able to objectively see one's own behavior compared to the soundest approach, it provides motivation to change in order to more closely approximate the soundest management. When group members come to share 9,9 values, beliefs, attitudes, and assumptions, they develop personal commitment to achieving group goals as well as their individual goals. In doing so they develop standards of mutual trust and respect that cause them to elevate cooperation and communication.

Blake and Mouton contend that the 9,9 style is the one most likely to achieve highest quality results over an extended period of time. The 9,9 style, unlike the others, is based on the assumption that there is no inherent conflict between the needs of the organization for performance and the needs of people for job satisfaction.

Finally, as an orienting framework, the Grid® serves as a road map toward more effective ways of working with and through others. When group members have this common frame of reference for what constitutes effective and ineffective approaches to issues of mutual concern, they are enabled to take corrective action based on common understanding and agreement about the soundest approach and objectivity when actions taken are less than fully sound.[16]

Exhibit 18–3 illustrates general management application of the Grid®, while Exhibit 18–4 illustrates its application to the job of the nurse administrator.

Kurt Lewin's Studies.   Lewin's leadership studies were done in the 1930s. Lewin examined three leadership styles related to forces within the leader, within the group members, and within the situation. These three leadership styles are summarized in Exhibit 18–5.

Other behavioral studies include the Ohio State studies that use a quadrant structure that relates leadership effectiveness to initiating structure, with emphasis on the task or production, and to consideration, with emphasis on the employee. These studies identified four primary leadership styles, as illustrated in Exhibit 18–6 on p. 466.[17]

Exercise 18–1   Kurt Lewin suggests that there are three leadership styles: autocratic, democratic, and laissez-faire.

1. Which leadership style does your supervisor exhibit?
2. List three of your supervisor's activities or decisions that illustrate that style.
3. How does your supervisor's leadership style affect your work and attitude?

Exhibit 18–3   The Leadership Grid Figure

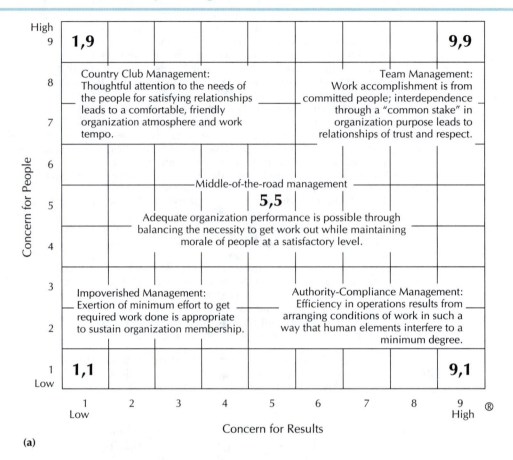

(a)

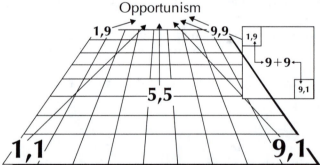

In Opportunistic Management, people adapt and shift to any Grid style needed to gain the maximum advantage. Performance occurs according to a system of selfish gain. Effort is given only for an advantage or personal gain.

(b)

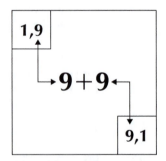

9+9 Paternalism/Maternalism
Reward and approval are bestowed to people in return for loyalty and obedienc failure to comply leads to punishment.

(c)

Source: The Leadership Grid® figure, Paternalism figure, and Opportunism Figure from *Leadership Dilemmas—Grid Solutions,* by Robert R. Blake and Anne Adams McCanse (Houston: Gulf Publishing Company). (Grid figure: p. 29, Paternalism figure: p. 30, Opportunism figure: p. 31). Copyright 1991 by Scientific Methods, Inc. Reproduced by permission of the owners.

Exhibit 18–4 The Nurse Administrator Grid®

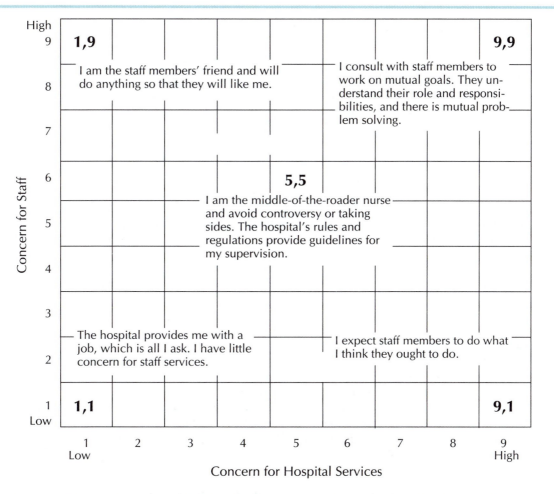

Source: Robert R. Blake, Jane S. Mouton, and Mildred Tapper, *Grid Approaches for Managerial Leadership in Nursing* (St. Louis: C. V. Mosby, 1981), 2. © 1984 by Robert R. Blake and Jane Srygley Mouton. Reproduced by permission of owners.

Exhibit 18–5 Kurt Lewin's Studies of Leadership Styles

Autocratic. Leaders make decisions alone. They tend to be more concerned with task accomplishment than with concern for people. Autocratic leadership tends to promote hostility and aggression or apathy and to decrease initiative.

Democratic. Leaders involve their followers in the decision-making process. They are people-oriented and focus on human relations and teamwork. Democratic leadership leads to increased productivity and job satisfaction.

Laissez-faire. Leaders are loose and permissive and abstain from leading their staff. They foster freedom for everyone and want everyone to feel good. Laissez-faire leadership results in low productivity and employee frustration.

Source: From *Management: Concepts and Applications,* 2d ed., by Leon Megginson et al. Copyright © 1986 by Harper & Row. Reprinted by permission of HarperCollins Publishers.

Exhibit 18–6   Ohio State Leadership Quadrant

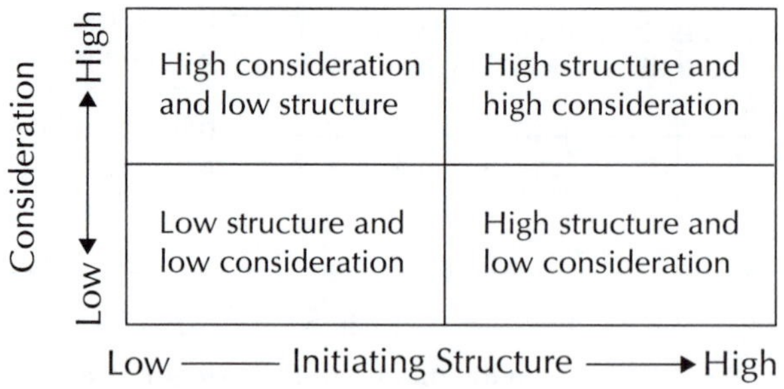

Source: From *Management: Concepts and Applications,* 2d ed., by Leon Megginson et al. Copyright © 1986 by Harper & Row. Reprinted by permission of HarperCollins Publishers.

LEADERSHIP STYLE

Other studies of leadership focus on style, including contingency-situational leadership models that focus upon a combination of factors, such as the people, the task, the situation, the organization, and a number of environmental factors. These models combine theories of Fred F. Fiedler, Paul Hersey, Kenneth H. Blanchard, D. E. Johnson, and William J. Reddin, whose contributions are discussed in the following sections.

Fiedler's Contingency Model of Leadership Effectiveness

There must be a group before there can be a leader. Fiedler indicates three classifications that measure the kind of power and influence the group gives its leader. The first and most important of these is the relationship between the leader and the group members. Personality is a factor, but its influence depends on the group's perception of the leader. Second is the task structure, the degree to which details of the group's assignment are programmed. If the assignment is highly structured, the leader will have less power. If the assignment requires planning and thinking, the leader will be in a position to exert greater power. Third is the positional power of the leader: It should be noted that great power does not yield better group performance. The best leader has been found to be one who has a task-oriented leadership style. This style works best when the leader has great influence or power over group members. When the leader has moderate influence over group members, a relationship-oriented style works best.

Fiedler's theory is one of situations. Leadership style will be effective or ineffective depending upon the situation.[18]

Theory of Hersey, Blanchard, and Johnson

Hersey, Blanchard, and Johnson follow a situational approach to leadership. A person's leadership style focuses on a combination of task behaviors and relationship behaviors. Focus on task behaviors is "characterized by endeavoring to establish well-defined patterns of organization, channels of communication, and ways of getting jobs accomplished." Focus on relationship behaviors relates to "opening up channels of communication, providing socio-emotional support, actively listening, 'psychological strokes', and facilitating behaviors."[19] These definitions evolve from the Ohio State Leadership Quadrant. Hersey, Blanchard, and Johnson add an effectiveness dimension to this Quadrant because leader effectiveness depends on how appropriate one's leadership style is to the situation in which one operates.

Reddin's Three-Dimensional Theory of Management

Reddin combined Blake and Mouton's Managerial Grid® with Fiedler's contingency leadership model. The outcome was a three-dimensional theory of management, the dimensions being adapted from (1) Managerial Grid® theory, (2) contingency leadership style theory, and (3) effectiveness theory. These possible combinations result in four basic leadership styles (see Exhibit 18–7).

1. Separated, in which both task orientation and relationship orientation are minimal.
2. Dedicated, in which task orientation is high and relationships orientation low. Dedicated leaders are dedicated only to the job.
3. Related, in which relationship orientation is high and task orientation is low. Related leaders relate primarily to their constituents.
4. Integrated, in which both task and orientation relationships are high. Integrated leaders focus on managerial behavior, combining task orientation and relationship orientation.

These management styles are graphically represented by the first two dimensions (height and width) of Exhibit 18–7.

- Executive leaders are integrated and more effective than compromiser leaders, who are less effective integrated leaders.
- Developer leaders are related and more effective than missionary leaders, who are less effective related leaders.
- Bureaucrat leaders are separated and more effective than deserter leaders, who are less effective separated leaders.
- Benevolent autocrat leaders are dedicated and more effective than autocrat leaders, who are less effective dedicated leaders.

The range of effectiveness is a continuum. As in other theories of leadership, the effective behavior of the leader is relative to the situation. Effective leaders apply leadership styles after assessing situations.[20]

Exhibit 18–7   Reddin's Three-Dimensional Management Styles

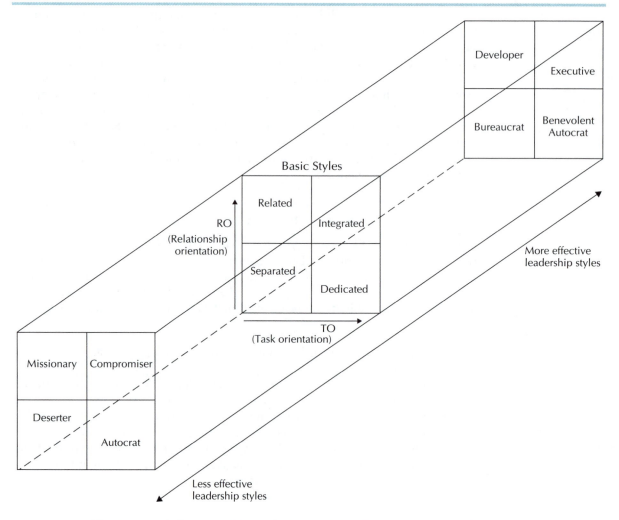

Source: W. J. Reddin, *Managerial Effectiveness* (New York: McGraw-Hill, 1970), 230. Reprinted with permission of W. J. Reddin.

TRANSFORMATIONAL LEADERSHIP: A NEW THEORY OF LEADERSHIP

The health-care system is experiencing change and chaos, and problems of the organization are increasingly complex. This change is causing uncertainty and anxiety among both health providers and consumers. Hospitals are downsizing and realigning in anticipation of health-care reform. Hospital nurses are being laid off and must be retrained for positions in community organizations. Health care is becoming prohibitively expensive for many Americans. Hospitals and emergency rooms are financially burdened by the uninsured who suffer from violence, drug overdose, and HIV infections. Many people, especially in rural areas and inner cities, do not have access to health care because hospitals are closing and there is a shortage of health-care personnel. Effective leaders in this atmosphere of rapid change will acknowledge uncertainty, be flexible, and consider the values and needs of constituents.[21]

Bennis and Nanus describe a new theory of leadership called *transformational leadership*. They describe a transformational leader as one who "commits people to action, who converts followers into leaders, and who may convert leaders into agents of change."[22] They believe that the nucleus of leadership is power, which they define as the "basic energy to initiate and sustain action translating intention into reality."[23] Transformational leaders do not use power to control and repress but instead empower constituents to have a vision about the organization and trust the leaders so that they work for goals that benefit the organization and themselves.

Leadership is thus not so much the exercise of power itself as the empowerment of others. This does not mean that leaders must relinquish power, but rather, that reciprocity, an exchange between leaders and constituents, exists. The goal is change in which the purpose of the leader and that of the constituent become enmeshed, creating a collective purpose. Empowered staff become critical thinkers and are active in their roles within the organization. A creative and committed staff is the most important asset that an administrator can develop.[24]

Transformational leaders will mobilize their staff by focusing on the welfare of the individual and humanizing the high-tech work environment. For the future, experts favor a leadership style that empowers others and values collaboration instead of competition.[25] People are empowered when they share in decision making and when they are rewarded for quality and excellence rather than punished and manipulated. When the environment is humanized and people are empowered, the people feel part of the team and believe they are contributing to the success of the organization. Leaders who share power motivate people to excel by inspiring followers to be part of a vision rather than punishing them for mistakes.[26] In nursing, empowerment can result in improved patient care, fewer sick days for staff, and decreased attrition.

Nurse managers who like to feel in charge may feel threatened by the concept of sharing power with staff. So they need to be personally empowered to assist in the empowerment of others. They will have a sense of self-worth and self-respect and a confidence in their own ability. Bennis and Nanus believe the most important essential trait of successful leaders is having a positive self-regard.[27] Self-regard is not, however, self-centeredness or self-importance; rather, leaders with positive self-regard recognize their strengths and do not emphasize their weaknesses. Interestingly, a leader who has positive self-regard seems to create in others a sense of confidence and high expectations. Techniques used to increase self-worth include the use of visualization, affirmations, and letting go of the need to be perfect.[28]

Bennis, through his research and observations, defined four competencies for dynamic and effective transformational leadership: (1) management of attention, (2) management of meaning, (3) management of trust, and (4) management of self.[29] The first competency is the management of attention, achieved by having a vision or sense of outcomes or goals. Vision is the image of a realistic, attainable, credible, and attractive future state for an organization.[30] Vision statements are written to define where the health-care organization is headed and how it will serve society. They differ from mission and philosophy statements in that they are more futuristic and describe where energies are to be focused.[31] People are committed to visions that are mutually developed, are based on a sense of quality, appeal to their values and emotions, and are feasible yet challenging.

The second leadership competency is management of meaning. To inspire commitment, leaders have to communicate their vision and create a culture that sustains the vision. Creating a culture or social architecture as described by Bennis and Nanus is "intangible, but it governs the way people act, the values and norms that are subtly transmitted to groups and individuals, and the construct of binding and bonding within a company."[32] Barker believes that "social architecture provides meaning and shared experience of organizational events so that people know the expectations of how they are to act."[33]

Nursing leaders will transform the social architecture or culture of health-care organizations by using group discussion, agreement, and consensus building, and they will support individual creativity and innovation. To do this, Barker believes that the nurse transformational leader will pay attention to the internal consistency of the vision, goals, and objectives; the selection and placement of personnel; feedback; appraisals; rewards; support; and development.[34] For example, rewards and appraisals must relate to the goals, and the vision must be consistent with the goals and objectives. Most importantly, all the elements must enhance the self-worth of individuals, allow creativity, and appeal to the values of nurses. For many nurse leaders, these are new skills that will take time and support from mentors to develop.

Since vision statements are a new concept to many, nursing leaders should provide opportunities for staff to openly explore feelings, criticize, and articulate negative reactions. Face-to-face meetings between nursing leaders and staff are desirable because in reactions involving trust and clarity, memorandums and suggestion boxes are not substitutes for direct communication.[35]

The third competency is the management of trust, which is associated with reliability. Nurses respect leaders whose judgment is sound and consistent and whose decisions are based on fairness, equity, and honesty. Staff can be heard to comment about a leader they trust with a statement such as "I don't always agree with her decision, but I know she wants the best for the patients." Bennis believes that "people would much rather follow individuals they can count on, even when they disagree with their viewpoint, than people they agree with but who shift positions frequently."[36]

The fourth competency is management of self, which is knowing one's skills and using them effectively. It is critical that nurses in leadership positions recognize when they lack management skills and then take responsibility for their own continuing education. Incompetent leaders can demoralize a nursing unit and contribute to poor patient care. When leadership skills are mastered by nurse leaders, stress and burnout are reduced. Nurse leaders thus need to master the skills of leadership.[37]

Although effective leaders are supportive of shared power and decision making, they continue to accept responsibility for making decisions even when their decisions are not popular. Constituents like to have their wishes considered, but there are times when they want prompt and clear decisions from a leader, especially in times of crisis.[38] Transformational leaders are flexible and able to adapt leadership styles to situations.

Differences Between Leadership and Management

Managers come from the "headship" (power from position) category. They hold appointive or directive posts in formal organizations. They can be appointed for both technical and leadership competencies, usually needing both to be accepted. Managers are delegated authority, including the power to reward or punish. A manager is expected to perform such functions as planning, organizing, directing, and controlling. Informal leaders, by contrast, are not always managers performing functions required by the organization. Leaders often are not even part of the organization. Florence Nightingale, after leaving the Crimea, was not connected with an organization but was still a leader.

Zaleznik indicates that the manager is a problem solver who succeeds because of "persistence, tough-mindedness, hard work, intelligence, analytical ability, and, perhaps most important, tolerance and good will."[39]

Managers focus on results, analysis of failure, and tasks, management characteristics that are desirable for nurse managers. Effective managers also need to be good leaders. Managers who are leaders choose and limit goals. They focus on creating spirit, and in doing so, they develop committed constituents. Manager-leaders do this by seeking advice and solutions to problems. They ask for information and provide positive feedback. Leaders understand the power of groups. They empower their constituents, making their subordinates strong—the chosen ones, a team infused with purpose. Mistakes are tolerated by manager-leaders who challenge constituents to stretch their potential.

Managers emphasize control, decision making, and decision analysis. As manager-leaders, they are concerned with modeling appropriate behavior as symbols of values and norms. Effective manager-leaders are technically capable and provide assurance in crises.

Managers focus inward but add the leadership dimension of connecting their group to the outside world, focusing intense attention on important issues. They escalate issues and complaints up the organization to be handled quickly and appropriately rather than try to control them.[40]

While managers are sometimes described in less glowing terms than leaders, successful managers are usually successful leaders. Leadership is a desirable and prominent feature of the directing function of nursing management.

Similarities Between Leadership and Management

Gardner asserts that first-class managers are usually first-class leaders. Leaders and leader-managers distinguish themselves beyond the general run of managers in six respects:[41]

1. They think longer term—beyond the day's crises, beyond the quarterly report, beyond the horizon.
2. They look beyond the unit they are heading and grasp its relationship to larger realities—the larger organization of which they are a part, conditions external to the organization, global trends.

3. They reach and influence constituents beyond their jurisdiction, beyond boundaries. Thomas Jefferson influenced people all over Europe. Gandhi influenced people all over the world. In an organization, leaders overflow bureaucratic boundaries—often a distinct advantage in a world too complex and tumultuous to be handled "through channels." Their capacity to rise above jurisdictions may enable them to bind together the fragmented constituencies that must work together to solve a problem.
4. They put heavy emphasis on the intangibles of vision, values, and motivation, and understand intuitively the nonrational and unconscious elements in the leader-constituent interaction.
5. They have the political skill to cope with the conflicting requirements of multiple constituencies.
6. They think in terms of renewal. The routine manager tends to accept the structure and processes as they exist. The leader or leader/manager seeks the revisions of process and structure required by ever-changing reality.

Good leaders, like good managers, provide visionary inspiration, motivation, and direction. Good managers, like good leaders, attract and inspire. People want to be led rather than managed. They want to pursue goals and values they consider worthwhile. Therefore, they want leaders who respect the dignity, autonomy, and self-esteem of constituents.[42] Effective nurse managers combine leadership and management. Effective nurse leader-managers will work to achieve these same requisites.

That a relationship between leadership and management exists seems scarcely arguable. Leadership is a subsystem within the management system. It is included as an element of management science in management textbooks and other publications. In some publications, the term *leading* has replaced the term *directing* as a major function of management. In such a context, communication and motivation would be elements of leadership, a concept that could be debated according to management theorists' philosophical bent.

Management includes written plans, clear organizational charts, well-documented annual objectives, frequent reports, detailed and precise job descriptions, regular evaluations of performance against objectives, and the administrative ordering of theory.[43] Nurse managers who are leaders can use these tools of management without making them a bureaucratic roadblock to autonomy, participatory management, maximum performance, and productivity by employees.

Exercise 18–2   Gardner asserts that first-class managers are usually first-class leaders. He believes that leaders and leader-managers distinguish themselves beyond the general run of managers in six respects (refer to beginning of this subsection). Give brief examples of how nurses you know fit all or some of the six characteristics.

Preparation of Nursing Leaders

Gardner believes that 90 percent of leadership can be taught.[44] Education begins in basic nursing education programs. To develop risk-taking behaviors and self-confidence, students should be encouraged to create new solutions and to disagree and debate and should be allowed to make mistakes without fear of reprisal. Faculty should encourage and support students who exercise their leadership abilities in projects and organizations on campus and in the community.

When nurses graduate and enter the workforce, most are not ready to assume a leadership role. They require opportunities for self-discovery to understand their strengths and for skill building. This skill building occurs through on-the-job training, along with support from peers and mentorship from effective leaders. Mentors must be dynamic, not status-quo-seeking role models who teach nurses how to preserve sameness. Tack writes that to prepare leaders for the future, they must be mentored by "those who see the world differently and project a dramatically different future, those who tend to shake things up rather than follow established precedents."[45]

Organizational managers, including nurse executives, will teach managers the nature of leadership. They will train nurse managers in leadership skills and will put managers in the proper environment to learn leadership. This will include "starting up an operation, turning around a troubled division, moving from staff to line, working under a wise mentor, serving on a high-level task force and getting promoted to a more senior level of the organization."[46]

Nurse executives and managers should be trained to coach their constituents on leadership skills. Constituents can be trained to help managers in leadership. Leaders can listen and articulate, persuade and be persuaded, use collective wisdom to make decisions, and teach subordinates to relate or communicate upward.

GENDER ISSUES

Since the majority of nurses are women, it is essential to understand the gender issues in nursing. Research indicates that gender differences do exist in leadership styles and competencies.[47] Masculinity has been associated with being task-oriented and using the direct approach for solving problems. Femininity has been characterized as people-oriented and supportive, sharing feelings and caring for others. Desjardins and Brown conducted two-hour interviews of seventy-two college presidents that included leadership-related questions concerning, for example, power, conflict resolution, and learning style. The findings indicated that the majority of women practiced leadership in a care-connected style.[48] This orientation, first described by Gilligan, values intimacy and nurturing in interactions with others.[49] The majority of men made decisions in the justice and rights mode, as was first described by Kohlberg in his work on moral reasoning.[50] This style of decision making values autonomy, objectivity, and fairness.

Rosener's research seems to support the thesis that leadership style is connected to gender issues. Rosener describes four major areas of difference in the women leaders whom she studied. First, these women tend to encourage participation; second, they share power and information more readily; third, they attempt to enhance the self-worth of others; and fourth, they energize others.[51]

It is important to remember that the modes and traits described by both researchers are gender-related but not gender-specific. Women and men fall into both modes, but more men are found in the justice and rights mode.[52] Also,

Rosener's work seems to indicate that men operate more often out of what Rosener sees as management transactions, exchanging rewards for services rendered or punishments for poor performance. Men, she found, also work more out of the power of their positions.[53]

The authoritarianism of traditional, male-oriented leadership styles is uncomfortable for many women.[54] Because women approach leadership roles differently from men, many women lack self-confidence. Therefore, staff development programs to develop nursing leaders should provide opportunities for self-awareness and skill building in new areas. Working with a supportive mentor who provides coaching through the real-world administrative environment will allow nurses to be successful and gain self-confidence.

Gender differences in leadership style and competencies do not translate into one style being better than the other. However, if nurses are sensitized to such differences, they will accept and utilize individuals for their unique leadership strengths instead of resisting them. This accepting atmosphere will encourage nurses (both men and women) to develop self-confidence and become strong leaders. Research is needed on gender issues related to nursing leadership.

LEADERSHIP AND NURSING

Nursing is usually conspicuous by its absence from lists of national leaders. National consumers do not perceive nurse leaders as having power. The health-care system has failed to recognize nurses as professionals with knowledge useful in creating solutions to complex problems. Cutler's perspective of nursing educators and nursing service personnel is that they have been the product of directive and authoritarian leadership.[55]

Historically, nurses have avoided opportunities to obtain power and political muscle. The profession now understands that power and political savvy will assist in achieving its goals to improve health care and to increase nurses' autonomy. Also, if the health-care system is to be reformed, nurses must participate individually and collectively. Nurses need to find ways to influence health-care policymaking so their holistic voice is heard.[56] Milio believes that nurses have the capacity for power to influence public policy and recommends the following steps to prepare:

1. Organize.
2. Do homework: learn to understand the political process, interest groups, specific people, and events.
3. Frame arguments to suit the target audience by appealing to cost containment, political support, fairness and justice, and other data relevant to particular concerns.
4. Support and strengthen position of converted policymakers.
5. Concentrate energies.
6. Stimulate public debate.
7. Make the position of nurses visible in the mass media.
8. Choose as the main strategy the most effective one.
9. Act in a timely fashion.

10. Maintain activity.
11. Keep the organizational format decentralized.
12. Obtain and develop the best research data to support each position.
13. Learn from experience.
14. Never give up without trying.

Nurses in leadership positions are most influential.[57]

Exercise 18–3 The following questions pertain to your personal knowledge of a nurse leader.

1. Name a nurse you consider to be an outstanding leader.
2. State why you consider her or him to be outstanding.

Exercise 18–4 Brower describes the leader in politics as a person of stature who can rally the people, a person with outstanding ability and character. He says there is an emotional bond between the leader and the led, a "bond which must exist between a leader and his people if either is to confront greatness."[58] He thinks that the abrasive strains of television may have irreparably damaged the bond between leader and led. Television shows the weaknesses in leaders because it constantly focuses on them. Formerly it had been thought that talent such as Jefferson pictured in a natural aristocracy would freely rise to the top. American leaders would be people of ability and morality; they would be wise and virtuous. According to Brower:

> Leadership, a relationship, depends very much on the basis of current enthusiasm or negation. Indeed it cannot exist at all in this country without the consent of the governed. We may very well be short on leadership because we are short on ourselves.[59]

Assuming that the characteristics of leadership are universally applicable to occupations, to government, to business, to industry, and certainly to service institutions and professions, list three characteristics described by Brower and apply them to nursing by writing a summary of examples you have observed.

Exercise 18–5 From the theory of leadership described in this chapter, describe and discuss actual examples of leadership demonstrated by persons in your organization. Consider the following:

1. Gardner's nine tasks performed by leaders.
2. A charismatic leader.
3. A transforming leader.
4. McGregor's Theory X and Theory Y.
5. Likert's authoritative and democratic systems.
6. Leadership style.
7. The implications for staff development.

SUMMARY

The theory of nursing leadership is a part of the theory of nursing management.

Leadership is a process of influencing a group to set and achieve goals. There are several major theories of leadership. One of the earliest is the trait theory, which suggests that leaders have many intellectual, personality, and ability traits. Trait theory has been succeeded by other leadership theories, indicating that managers, including nurse managers, can learn the knowledge and skills requisite to leadership competencies.

Behavioral theories of leadership include McGregor's Theory X and Theory Y, Likert's Michigan studies, Blake and Mouton's Managerial Grid®, and Lewin's studies.

Other studies of leadership focus on contingency-situational leadership styles and factors such as people, tasks, situations, organizations, and environment. Theorists include Fiedler, Hersey, Blanchard and Johnson, and Reddin.

Bennis and Nanus define a new theory of leadership they call transformational. This leadership method involves change in which the purposes of the leader and constituent become intertwined. The effective leader creates a vision for the organization and then develops a commitment to the vision. Bennis and Nanus believe that the wise use of power is the energy needed to develop commitment and to sustain action.

John W. Gardner's study of leadership includes the nature of leadership, identification of leadership tasks, leader-constituent interaction, and the relationship between leadership and power.

NOTES

1. J. W. Gardner, *The Nature of Leadership: Introductory Considerations* (Washington, D.C.: Independent Sector, January 1986), 8.

2. J. W. Gardner, *The Tasks of Leadership* (Washington D.C.: Independent Sector, March 1986), 15; E. Huxley, *Florence Nightingale* (New York: Putnam, 1975).

3. C. R. Holloman, "Leadership or Headship: There Is a Difference." *Notes & Quotes* No. 365, January 1969, 4; C. R. Holloman, "'Headship' vs. Leadership," *Business and Economic Review,* January–March 1986, 35–37.

4. L. B. Lundborg, "What Is Leadership?" *Journal of Nursing Administration,* May 1982, 32–33.

5. J. W. Gardner, *The Nature of Leadership,* op. cit., 6.

6. C. R. Holloman, "'Headship' vs. Leadership," op. cit. A. Levenstein, "So You Want to Be a Leader?" *Nursing Management,* March 1985, 74–75; G. R. Jones, "Forms of Control and Leader Behavior," *Journal of Management,* fall 1983, 159–172; D. McGregor, *Leadership and Motivation* (Cambridge, Mass: MIT Press, 1966), 70–80.

7. R. K. Merton, "The Social Nature of Leadership," *American Journal of Nursing,* December 1969, 2614–2618.

8. D. McGregor, op. cit., 73.

9. J. Kilpatrick, "Conservative View," Biloxi, Miss., *Sun-Herald,* February 2, 1974, 4.

10. D. McGregor, op. cit., 75.

11. J. W. Gardner, *The Tasks of Leadership,* op. cit; J. W. Gardner, *The Heart of the Matter: Leader-Constituent Interaction:* and *Leadership and Power* (Washington, D.C.: Independent Sector, October 1986).

12. J. W. Gardner, *The Tasks of Leadership,* op. cit., 7.

13. J. W. Gardner, *The Heart of the Matter: Leader-Constituent Interaction,* op. cit.

14. D. McGregor, op. cit., 49–65.

15. R. Likert, *The Human Organization* (New York: McGraw-Hill, 1967), 4–10.

16. The Grid® synopsis was furnished courtesy Scientific Methods, Inc., Box 195, Austin, TX 78747.

17. L. Megginson, D. Mosley, and P. Pietri, Jr., *Management: Concepts and Applications,* 3d ed. (New York: Harper & Row, 1989), 346–347, 352–353.

18. F. E. Fiedler, "Style or Circumstance: The Leadership Enigma," *Notes & Quotes* No. 358, March 1969, 3; L. Megginson, D. Mosley, and P. Pietri, Jr., op. cit.

19. P. Hersey, K. H. Blanchard, and D. E. Johnson, *Management of Organizational Behavior: Utilizing Human Resources,* 7th ed. (Englewood Cliffs, N.J.: Prentice-Hall, 1996), 134–135.

20. W. J. Reddin, *Managerial Effectiveness* (New York: McGraw-Hill, 1970), 230; R. M. Hodgetts, *Management: Theory, Process and Practice,* 4th ed. (Orlando, Fla.: Academic Press, 1986), 319–320.

21. A. M. Barker, "An Emerging Leadership Paradigm," *Nursing and Health Care,* April 1991, 204–207.

22. W. Bennis and B. Nanus, *Leaders: The Strategies for Taking Charge* (New York: Harper & Row, 1985), 3.

23. Ibid., 15.

24. S. P. Lundeen, "Leadership Strategies for Organizational Change: Applications in Community Nursing Centers," *Nursing Administration Quarterly,* fall 1992, 60–68.

25. M. W. Tack, "Future Leaders in Higher Education: New Demands and New Responses," *Phi Kappa Phi Journal,* winter 1991, 29–31; C. Desjardins and C. O. Brown, "A New Look at Leadership Styles," *Phi Kappa Phi Journal,* winter 1991, 18–20.

26. W. Bennis and B. Nanus, op. cit.

27. Ibid., 57.

28. A. M. Barker, op. cit.

29. W. Bennis, "Learning Some Basic Truisms About Leadership," *Phi Kappa Phi Journal,* winter 1991.

30. W. Bennis and B. Nanus, op. cit.

31. A. M. Barker, *Transformational Nursing Leadership: A Vision for the Future* (Baltimore: Williams & Wilkins, 1990).
32. W. Bennis and B. Nanus, op. cit.
33. A. M. Barker, "An Emerging Leadership Paradigm," op. cit., 207.
34. Ibid.
35. J. W. Gardner, *The Heart of the Matter: Leader-Constituent Interaction,* op. cit.
36. W. Bennis, "Learning Some Basic Truisms About Leadership," op. cit., 24.
37. R. P. Campbell, "Does Management Style Affect Burnout?" *Nursing Management,* March 1986, 38A–38B, 38D, 38F, 38H.
38. J. W. Gardner, *The Heart of the Matter: Leader-Constituent Interaction,* op. cit.
39. A. Zaleznik, "Managers and Leaders: Are they Different?" *Harvard Business Review,* May–June 1977, 68.
40. J. H. Zenger, "Leadership: Management's Better Half," *Training,* December 1985, 44–53.
41. J. W. Gardner, *The Nature of Leadership,* op. cit., 12.
42. J. H. Zenger, op. cit.
43. Ibid.
44. J. W. Gardner, *The Nature of Leadership,* op. cit.
45. M. W. Tack, op. cit., 30.
46. J. H. Zenger, op. cit.
47. C. Desjardins and C. O. Brown, op. cit.
48. Ibid.
49. C. Gilligan, *In a Different Voice: Psychological Theory and Women's Development* (Cambridge, Mass.: Harvard University Press, 1982).
50. L. Kohlberg, *The Philosophy of Moral Development, Moral Stages and the Idea of Justice* (San Francisco: Harper & Row, 1981).
51. J. Rosener, "Ways Women Lead," *Harvard Business Review,* November–December 1990, 19–24.
52. C. Desjardins and C. O. Brown, op. cit.
53. J. Rosener, op. cit.
54. C. Desjardins and C. O. Brown, op. cit.
55. M. J. Cutler, "Nursing Leadership and Management: An Historical Perspective," *Nursing Administration Quarterly,* fall 1976, 7–19.
56. N. J. Murphy, "Nursing Leadership in Health Policy Decision Making," *Nursing Outlook,* July/August 1992, 158–161.
57. N. Milio, "The Realities of Policy Making: Can Nurses Have an Impact?" *Journal of Nursing Administration,* March 1984, 18–23.
58. B. Brower, "Where Have All the Leaders Gone?" *Life,* 8 October 1971, 70B.
59. Ibid.

MOTIVATION

OBJECTIVES

- Differentiate between content (exogenous) theories of motivation and process (endogenous) theories of motivation.
- Illustrate Maslow's hierarchy of needs.
- Describe nurse dissatisfactions associated with productivity and the nurse as knowledge worker.
- Describe nurse satisfactions associated with productivity and the nurse as knowledge worker.
- Describe nurse satisfactions associated with applications of the science of human behavior.
- Choose examples that indicate the value of career planning, communication, self-esteem, and self-actualization as management strategies.

KEY CONCEPTS

motivation
content theories
process theories
science of human behavior
theory X and Theory Y
self-esteem
self-actualization
self-concept

Manager behavior: Makes the goals of management known to the organization's employees.

Leader behavior: Applies motivation theory to the management of the organization's employees, using the philosophy that satisfied workers increase productivity.

THEORIES OF MOTIVATION

Motivation is a concept used to describe both the extrinsic conditions that stimulate certain behavior and the intrinsic responses that demonstrate that behavior in human beings. The intrinsic response is sustained by sources of energy, termed *motives,* often described as needs, wants, or drives. All living people have them. Motivation is measured by observable and recorded behaviors. Deficiencies in needs stimulate people to seek and achieve goals to satisfy those needs.

Why do some registered nurses pursue an area of nursing specialization to the extent of continuously acquiring new knowledge and skills that enable them to make rapid and accurate nursing diagnosis and prescription? Why does a pediatric nurse pursue development of a role that extends professional practice into areas such as teaching parents to enjoy their children, providing follow-up health observations of high-risk newborns, and teaching health practices to the parents of newborns after they have been discharged to their homes? Why does that nurse go a step further and teach others to extend themselves and then write articles to provide the information for everyone?

Why does a mental health nurse pursue a role in off-duty time as a co-therapist of a group in addition to rotating shifts as a staff nurse? Why does another work to sell the concept and then conduct a psychodrama therapy program and ask for the privilege of answering mental-health consultations for medical and surgical patients? Why does a professional nurse work many hours as a committee member for a district nurses' association?

What makes some nurses come on duty on time, work hard and without error, maintain a pleasant demeanor, and meet all standards of performance, appearance, and behavior, while others do just the opposite? Some persons do not do well in an organization. This does not mean that these persons are not useful; the organization may be lacking the means of making them productive, useful, satisfied employees.

The answer to the preceding questions is motivation. Some nurses are motivated to excel and be creative; others put forth just enough effort to do the job. To get goods and services to the customer, managers care about people and their motivation. Managers' beliefs about motivation are reflected in their personal management styles.

Theories of motivation have been classified into content theories and process theories.[1] Work motivation theories have also been classified as dealing either with exogenous causes or with endogenous causes.[2]

Exogenous theories focus on motivationally relevant independent variables that can be changed by external agents, such as organizational incentive and rewards, and social factors, such as leader and group behavior. There are seven exogenous theories: motive/need theory, incentive/reward theory, reinforcement theory, goal theory, personal and material resource theory, group and norm theory, and sociotechnical system theory. Exhibit 19–1 summarizes some approaches to improving work motivation using these theories.

Exogenous theories are content theories of which three are presented here.[3]

Content Theories of Motivation

Content theories of motivation focus on factors or needs within a person that energize, direct, sustain, and stop behavior. The most widely recognized work in motivation theory is that of Maslow. Although not universally accepted, because of its lack of scientific evidence or research base, it is universally known, and many managers attempt to use it as they turn to a human behavior approach to management.

Much has been said in support of Maslow's theories of motivation relative to human needs and goals. Like every science, nursing is a human creation stemming from human motives, having human goals, and being created, renewed, and maintained by human beings called nurses.

Like other scientists, nurses are motivated by physiological needs, including the need for food; needs for safety, protection, and care; social needs

Exhibit 19–1 Approaches to Improving Work Motivation

Exogenous Variables

Imperative and Programs	1. Personal Motives and Values	2. Incentives and Rewards	3. Reinforcement	4. Goal-Setting Techniques	5. Personal and Material Resources	6. Social and Group Factors	7. Sociotechnical Systems
Motivational imperative	Workers' motives and values must be appropriate for their jobs	Make jobs attractive, interesting, and satisfying	Effective performance must be positively reinforced but not ineffective performance	Work goals must be clear, challenging, attainable, attractive	Provide needed resources and eliminate constraints to performance	Interpersonal and group processes must support goal attainment	Personal, social, and technological parameters must be harmonious
Illustrative programs	Personnel selection Job previews Motive training Socialization	Financial compensation Promotion Participation Job security Career development Considerate supervision Job enrichment Benefits Flexible hours Recognition Cafeteria plans	Financial incentive plans Behavioral analysis Praise and criticism Self-management	Goal setting Management by objectives Modeling Quality circles Appraisal and feedback	Training and development Coaching and counseling Equipment Technology Supervision Methods improvement Problem-solving groups	Division of labor Group composition Team development Sensitivity training Leadership Norm building	Quality of work-life programs Sociotechnical systems designs Organizational development Scanlon plan

Source: R. A. Katzell and D. E. Thompson, "Work Motivation," *American Psychologist,* February 1990, 147. Copyright 1990 by the American Psychological Association. Reprinted by permission.

for gregariousness, affection, and love; ego needs for respect, standing, and status, leading to self-respect or self-esteem; and a need for self-fulfillment or self-actualization. Many, but not all, are also motivated by cognitive needs for sheer knowledge and understanding. They voraciously question others; read textbooks, journals, and patients' charts; and regularly pursue courses in their specialty and in the liberal arts, particularly the humanities. Others are motivated by aesthetic needs for beauty, symmetry, simplicity, completion, and order and by their need to express themselves. How many of these needs are related to a nurse's desire to keep learning and applying new knowledge and skills? What can the nurse manager do to spark in a nurse the motive of curiosity that sets in motion a desire to understand, explain, and systematize? These and many other human needs may serve as the primary motivations for a person pursuing a career in nursing who wants to update and expand knowledge and skills. The motivation may be a feeling of identification and belonging with people in general, love for human beings, a desire to help people, the need to earn a living or express oneself, or a combination of all these needs working together. Certainly an individual's needs are both diverse and unique.[4]

A second content theory of motivation was developed by Alderfer, who reduced Maslow's hierarchy of needs from five levels to three: existence (E), relatedness (R), and growth (G)—thus the term *ERG theory*. In comparing Alderfer's scheme with Maslow's, existence needs are equivalent to physiological and safety needs; relatedness needs to belongingness, social, and love needs; and growth needs to self-esteem and self-actualization.

Whereas Maslow's theory proposes that the next level of needs emerge when the predominant (satisfaction-progression) ones have been fulfilled, Alderfer's theory adds a frustration-regression process. When higher-level needs are frustrated, people will regress to the satisfaction of lower-level needs.[5]

Herzberg did research on a third content theory, which he called a two-factor theory of motivation. One set of factors—dissatisfiers—are extrinsic conditions or hygiene factors. They include salary, job security, working conditions, status, company procedures, quality of technical supervision, and quality of interpersonal relations among peers, with supervisors, and with subordinates. They must be maintained in quantity and quality to prevent dissatisfaction. They become dissatisfiers when not equitably administered, causing low performance and negative attitudes. The other set of factors—satisfiers—are intrinsic conditions or motivators. They include achievement, recognition, responsibility, advancement, the work itself, and the possibility of growth. They create opportunities for high satisfaction, high motivation, and high performance. The individual must be free to attain them. Herzberg's research was criticized for its limited sample of only accountants and engineers and for being simplistic.[6]

Exercise 19–1   With a group of your peers, identify how content theories of motivation affect your practices. How can they be used to improve your practices? Write a summary of your conclusions.

Process Theories of Motivation

Endogenous theories deal with process or mediating variables such as expectancies and attitudes "that are amenable to modification only indirectly in response to variation in one or more exogenous variables."[7] Four endogenous theories are operant (reinforcement) theory, expectancy theory, equity theory, and goal-setting theory.

Skinner advanced a process theory of motivation called *operant conditioning,* also called behavior modification. Learning occurs as a consequence of behavior. Behaviors are the operants; they are controlled by altering the consequences with reinforcers or punishments, as illustrated in Exhibit 19–2.

Positive or desired behaviors should be rewarded or reinforced. Reinforcement motivates, increasing the strength of a response or inducing its repetition. Continuous reinforcement speeds up early performance. Intermittent reinforcement at fixed or variable ratios sustains performance. Research indicates higher rates of response, with ratio rather than interval schedules. Reinforcers tend to weaken over time, and new ones have to be developed.

Undesirable organizational behavior should not be rewarded. Negative reinforcement occurs when desired behavior occurs to avoid negative consequences of punishment. Although frequently used, punishment creates negative attitudes and can increase costs. Behaviorists believe that people will repeat behavior when consequences are positive.

Behavior modification research uses a scientific approach. Application of behavior modification is occurring in large companies. Benefits or results claimed include improved attendance, productivity, and efficiency and cost savings. Reinforcers center on praise, recognition, and feedback. The problem-solving method is used to apply behavior modification. Critics of the behavior modification theory consider rewards to be bribes.[8]

A second process theory of motivation is Vroom's expectancy theory, which postulates that most behaviors are voluntarily controlled by a person and are therefore motivated. There is an effort-performance expectancy, or a person's belief that a chance exists for a certain effort to lead to a particular level

Exhibit 19–2 Reinforcement Theory

S_1	$\rightarrow$	R_1	$\rightarrow$	S_2	$\rightarrow$	R_2
A memo that instructs subordinate to prepare budget		Preparing weekly budgets		Receiving valued praise from the superior		A sense of satisfaction
Conditioned stimulus		Conditioned operant response		Reinforcing stimulus		Unconditioned response
(Antecedent)		(Behavior)		(Consequence)		

Source: J. Gibson, J. Ivanovich, and J. Donnelly, *Organizations: Behavior Structure Processes,* 8th ed. (Burr Ridge, Ill.: Richard D. Irwin, 1989), 4. Reprinted with permission.

of performance. The performance-outcome expectancy or belief of this person will have certain outcomes. Given choices, the individual selects the one with the best expected outcome.[9]

Equity theory is a third process theory. Persons believe they are being treated with equity when the ratio of their efforts to rewards equals that of others. Equity can be achieved or restored by changing outputs, attitudes, the reference person, inputs or outputs of the reference person, or the situation. Research on equity theory has focused on pay.[10]

A fourth process theory of motivation is the goal-setting theory of Locke. This theory is based on goals as determinants of behavior. The more specific the goals, the better the results produced. Research indicates that goals are a powerful force. Goals must be achievable; their difficulty level should be increased only to the ceiling to which the person will commit. Goal clarity and accurate feedback increase security.[11]

Exercise 19–2   With a group of your peers, identify how process theories of motivation affect your practices. How can they be used to improve your practices? Write a summary of your conclusions.

Maslow

Maslow's theory of motivation is a positive one and is based on a holistic-dynamic theory. At the base of a needs system are the physiological needs, based on homeostasis, a condition of constancy of body fluids, functions, and states. The constancy is maintained automatically by uniform interaction of counteracting processes. It should be noted that human beings do not just eat; they eat selectively to maintain homeostasis. The same is probably true of other physiological needs, although not all physiological needs are homeostatic. Some are relatively independent of each other while at the same time are interdependent. For example, smoking may satisfy the hunger need in some persons. Some needs are in opposition to each other, such as the tendency to be lazy and the desire to be industrious.

Maslow proposed that human needs are organized in a hierarchy of prepotency: Higher needs emerge as lower needs are satisfied. When the physiological needs are satisfied, the human being is no longer motivated by them. However, a person tolerates deprivation of a long-satisfied need better than one that has been long or previously deprived.

When unsatisfied, physiological needs are the most prepotent, the strongest, of human needs. A starving person will steal food and perform other acts that threaten a person's safety. The dominance of a physiological need changes the individual's philosophy for the future.

Safety needs are the second group in the hierarchy. Among these are security, protection, dependency, and stability; freedom from anxiety, chaos, and fear; need for order, limits, structure, and law; and strength in the protector. Satisfaction of these needs influences a person's values and philosophy of life. What threatens the safety of nursing? Are nurses threatened by increased consumer interest in their shortcomings, which may lead to consumer control of practice? What motivates people? Is it a fear of the high cost of extended illnesses and results of poor care? The average person likes law, order, predictability, and organization. This may be one reason why people resist change. Insurance programs, job tenure, and savings accounts are expressions of safety needs.

Once the physiological and safety needs have been satisfied, the needs for love, affection, and belongingness emerge. Most individuals in nursing today have had their physiological and safety needs satisfied. Now they want to be part of a group or family with love, acceptance, friendliness, and a feeling of belonging. Are these needs thwarted by frequent moves? How are the needs of the individual, as well as those of the organization, satisfied? A society that wants to survive and be healthy will work to satisfy these needs. Otherwise, people will be maladjusted and will exhibit severe emotional and behavioral pathology.

Two categories emerge under the fourth set of needs—the esteem needs. All people share these needs. First, they desire strength, achievement, adequacy, mastery and competence, confidence before the world, independence, and freedom. Second, they desire reputation or prestige, status, fame and glory, dominance, recognition, attention, importance, dignity, or appreciation. A person whose self-esteem is satisfied has feelings of self-confidence, worth, strength, capability, adequacy, usefulness, and being needed in society. For it to be stable and healthy, one's self-esteem must be based on known or deserved respect. The reason for it must be known and recognized by its recipient.

Finally, at the pinnacle of the hierarchy of needs is the emotional gold— the need for self-actualization, the effort of people to be what they can be. Nurses want to become everything they are capable of becoming, achieve their potential, be effective nurses, be creative, and meet personal standards of performance.

Certain conditions are prerequisites to satisfying basic needs. When basic needs are thwarted, the individual feels threatened. These conditions include

1. Freedom to speak—communication.
2. Freedom to do what one wishes to do without harming others—choice of jobs, friends, and entertainment.
3. Freedom to express oneself—creativity.
4. Freedom to investigate and seek for information.
5. Freedom to defend oneself—justice, fairness, honesty, and orderliness in the group.

Human beings want to gain new knowledge, to solve problems, to bring order, and to explore, and they will voluntarily face dangers to do so.

The hierarchy of needs is not a simple classification. Individuals order their needs differently, some placing self-esteem before love. Others place creativity before all else. Certain people have low levels of aspiration. Permanent loss of love needs results in a psychopathic personality.

A long-satisfied need may become undervalued. A person who has never been deprived of a particular need does not regard the need as important. If two needs emerge, a person will probably want the more basic one satisfied first. People who have loved and been well-loved and who have had many deep friendships can hold out against hatred, rejection, or persecution.

Most normal persons in our society have partially satisfied and partially dissatisfied basic needs at the same time. They may have more satisfied physiological needs and correspondingly fewer satisfied self-actualization needs. New needs emerge gradually and are more often unconscious than conscious. Basic needs are common throughout different cultures. Most behavior is multidetermined: All of the basic needs are involved. A single act of an individual could be analyzed to show how it addresses physiological needs, safety needs, love needs, esteem needs, and self-actualization needs. Not all behavior is internally motivated; some is stimulated externally. Some is highly motivated, some weakly, and some not at all. Some is expressive and some rote. A gratified or satisfied need is not a motivator of behavior. Healthy persons are primarily motivated by the need to develop and actualize their fullest potentialities and capacities.

Usefulness to Nurse Managers

Motivational theory has been used in a number of studies of behavior modification for smoking cessation, weight control, exercising, and general reduction of cardiovascular risk factors. To date, modifying risk-taking behavior of people has had limited positive results. For example, since nicotine has been touted as a highly addictive substance, motivational theory may have to be combined with other treatment regimens to sustain cessation of smoking. The same may be true of other risk-taking behaviors. This area presents an opportunity for nurses to expand motivational research.[12]

Although there are many theories and much has been written about motivation, there is no easy way to motivate employees. Human motivation is diverse, subtle, and complex. To use the available information on motivation effectively, the nurse will study it and select and use those elements that appear to be practical and workable.

Knowledge of motivation theories is essential to improving the job performance of employees. Individual employees have different needs and goals. Nurses will learn and use motivation theories selectively.

DISSATISFACTIONS

Dissatisfactions of nurses can be alleviated by nurse managers who apply learned approaches to change within nursing organizations.

Productivity

Nurses respond negatively and become dissatisfied when managers use force, control, threats, and repeated applications of institutional power. Productivity decreases or stagnates. The new breed of nurses questions authority and gives loyalty to those who earn it. An attitude of mutual respect between clinical nurses and managers is essential to productivity.

To promote mutual respect, free interaction and communication must take place in which expectations are clarified and feedback on performance is given through role modeling of expected and desired performance. In addition, promises that cannot be fulfilled must be avoided. In more than seven out of ten working relationships, the employee does not know what is expected of her or him. Expectations must be clear. In a productivity attitude test developed and administered to production workers by Pryor and Mondy over a two-year period, 75 percent of respondents said that their supervisors did not keep promises they made. Broken promises anger employees and decrease productivity.[13]

The Nurse as Knowledge Worker

Drucker indicates that knowledge workers are productive only with self-motivation, self-direction, and achievement. No one dominant dimension to working exists. People are motivated to work based on Maslow's hierarchy of needs. Even when satisfied, a human need remains important. Economic rewards that are not properly taken care of create dissatisfaction with work and become deterrents to job satisfaction and productivity.[14]

Nurses are knowledge workers. Their basic economic needs are related to other human needs or human values. Performing work of equal difficulty, they want economic rewards of equal value to those of other knowledge workers. Pay is part of the social or psychological dimension of nurses. Nurses also want increased rank, power, and status commensurate with other knowledge workers.

More formal education and skills translate into higher real incomes and increased living standards. Boosts in investment in education, research and development, and updated equipment result in increased productivity. Ideas rather than physical resources result in economic value added. Highly skilled workers can switch jobs more easily and therefore spend less time unemployed. Money invested in education is an investment in the economic health and future of the United States.[15]

The nurse as knowledge worker is self-directed and takes responsibility. Rewarding and reaffirming self-direction and responsibility produce learning; fear produces resistance. Psychological manipulation is only a replacement for the carrot-and-stick approach to management. It does not work.

SATISFACTIONS

The Science of Human Behavior

How do we apply the knowledge of the social sciences so that our human organizations will be truly effective? We have the knowledge, just as we have the knowledge of physical sciences to develop alternative sources of energy such as solar, tidal, atomic, and geothermal energy. Application of vast knowledge in both physical and social sciences is expensive and time-consuming.

Theory X and Theory Y.   Although Douglas McGregor died in 1964, his theories of leadership and motivation live on. Unfortunately, his Theory X has not been replaced by his Theory Y. Theory X, as he described it for the world of business, was summarized in the following points:[16]

1. Management is responsible for organizing the elements of productive enterprise—money, materials, equipment, people—in the interest of economic ends.
2. With respect to people, this is a process of directing their efforts, motivating them, controlling their actions, modifying their behavior to fit the needs of the organization.
3. Without this active intervention by management, people would be passive—even resistant—to organizational needs. They must therefore be persuaded, rewarded, punished, controlled—their activities must be directed. This is management's task—in managing subordinate managers or workers. We often sum it up by saying that management consists of getting things done through other people.
4. The average man is by nature indolent—he works as little as possible.
5. He lacks ambition, dislikes responsibility, prefers to be led.
6. He is inherently self-centered, indifferent to organizational needs.
7. He is by nature resistant to change.
8. He is gullible, not very bright, the ready dupe of the charlatan and the demagogue.

How many nurse managers demotivate practicing nurses by falling into the trap of voicing the very statements embodied in Theory X? How may nurse managers motivate practicing nurses by applying the following precepts of Theory Y?[17]

1. Management is responsible for organizing the elements of productive enterprise—money, materials, equipment, people—in the interest of economic ends.
2. People are not by nature passive or resistant to organizational needs. They have become so as a result of experience in organizations.
3. The motivation, the potential for development, the capacity for assuming responsibility, the readiness to direct behavior toward organizational goals are all present in people. Management does not put them there. It is the responsibility of management to make it possible for people to recognize and develop these human characteristics for themselves.
4. The essential task of management is to arrange organizational conditions and methods of operation so that people can achieve their own goals *best* by directing *their own* efforts toward organizational objectives.

McGregor's Theory Y was used to change personnel behavior in a skilled nursing facility. An "audit process created unit expectations which provided a sense of accomplishment, personal growth and motivation to seek more responsibility."[18] The staff was provided with extensive in-service education. "Noting," the leaving of notes for the responsible staff person to correct noncompliance, was accepted as peer review to foster responsibility and accountability. The goal was to manage personnel to meet their needs for self-respect and improvement.

Exercise 19–3   With a group of your peers, discuss McGregor's Theory X and Theory Y. Which factors of each are evident in your place of work? Which can be changed to improve productivity? Discuss how this can be achieved. Summarize your discussion.

Nurse Managers and Motivation

Motivation is an emotional process; it is psychological rather than logical. The nurse manager should first learn how a nurse wants to feel and then help that nurse use the tools that will encourage attainment of those feelings. These tools may derive from such areas as associations with people on the job that make the nurse feel accepted, performance of those acts for which the nurse is highly skilled, and recognition for a satisfactory performance.

As previously stated, motivation is basically an unconscious process. When asked why she or he did a certain thing, a nurse may not be able to give an answer. Even though people's basic motives are hidden and intangible, their actions or behavior make sense to them. Motivational patterns are learned early and followed for years. There is no conscious selection, judgment, or decision making involved in 95 percent of what people do.

Each person is unique, with the key to one's behavior lying within the self. A leader uses judgment to figure out why each person reacts in a given way to a certain situation. Within each individual, motivating needs differ from time to time. The key is to figure out which need is currently predominant.

Human beings, including nurses, motivate themselves. The nurse leader will provide practicing nurses or deprive them of the opportunity to satisfy their needs.

> The motivational theory under discussion asserts that man if he is freed to some extent, by his presence in an affluent society, from the necessity to use most of his energy to obtain the necessities of life and a degree of security from the major vicissitudes—will by nature begin to pursue goals associated with his higher-level needs. These include needs for a degree of control over his own fate, for self-respect, for using and increasing his talents, for responsibility, for achievement both in the sense of status and recognition and in the sense of personal development and effective problem solving. Thus freed, he will also seek in many ways to satisfy more fully his physical needs for recreation, relaxation, and play. Management has been well aware of the latter tendency; it has not often recognized the former, or at least it has not taken into account its implication for managerial strategy.[19]

Observation and the evidence of the social sciences indicate that employees' behavior shapes itself to management perceptions. This behavior results not from inherent nature but from the nature of organizations, management philosophy, policy, and practice. The nurse leader looks for simple, practical, immediate ideas to solve personnel problems. There are no magic wands, but that does not mean there are no solutions.

Solutions

Career Planning.   Career planning is a continuous process of self-assessment and goal setting. It is a cooperative venture between the organization and the employee, the career counselor (who could be a mentor or sponsor) and the individual nurse. Career planning is an organized system with short-term and long-term career goals fitted to those of the organization.

To build a career development program requires major effort. The following outline stresses the major activities:

1. Assess the future goals and labor power needs of the nursing organization relative to recruitment, promotion, hiring, placement, retention, and turnover.
2. Develop job structures with career paths and qualifications, including career opportunities within the nursing organization.
3. Recruit qualified applicants, including those already employed within the nursing organization.
4. Assess each applicant for personal expectations.
5. Develop an individual career development plan for each nurse.
6. Provide developmental opportunities for the individual nurse to achieve career goals.

Most nurses will benefit from participation in a career development program, even if it improves only the quality of their working lives.[20]

Communication.   To produce quality nursing products and services requires highly motivated practicing nurses. Nurse leaders can motivate nurses by sharing information about the organization. Consultative leaders consult with nurses on problems, solutions, and decisions and share information about results.

Teamwork.   Nurse leaders can motivate practicing nurses by encouraging teamwork. Teams can be built from work groups to discuss and resolve work-related issues. Teams should have identifiable output, inclusive membership, leaders with carefully circumscribed authority, agreement on purpose, rules of procedure, and measurable goals, resources, and feedback. Teams are successful because they pool interpersonal skills, knowledge, and the expertise needed to accomplish goals effectively and efficiently.

By using teams, Hewlett-Packard has cut labor costs, reduced defects, solved vendor problems, eliminated jobs, decreased inspections, cut scrap production, and reached targets ahead of schedule. Teamwork helps workers to achieve personal recognition, raise self-esteem, and increase motivation and commitment. It is stimulated by trust, support, completion, acknowledgement, communication, and agreement.[21]

Teamwork raises the spirits of nurses during a time of economic recession, cutbacks, and curtailment of capital expenditures. Teamwork is used to clarify the purpose or mission of a department or unit, to define a vision of the process and product of team effort, to identify blocks and barriers to team members' vision, to look at ways the work group members support each other, to make requests and agreements about how each can work better with others on the team, and to plan the team's work goals and activities and commit each member to accomplishing them. The result would be an effective team in which each member felt personal satisfaction.[22]

Team processes are developmental. A summary of the developmental stages for teams is shown in Exhibit 19–3.

Exhibit 19–3 Summary of Developmental Stages for Teams

Stage	Characteristics	Team Leader Tasks	Member Tasks	Ideal Outcomes
Orientation	Opinions expressed cautiously Long pauses Artificial politeness Few interruptions Efforts unfocused	Promote atmosphere of acceptance and trust Encourage discussion of personal expectations Recognition of member insecurities as new relationships emerge	Get acquainted Develop trust in others Learn what is expected of them	Members develop trust in each other Members begin to learn and accept those things expected of them
Adaptation	Team norms developing Members start to assume appropriate team roles Some open disagreements	Help members identify strengths and contributions Provide opportunities to enhance member's self-esteem Provide direction and goals Provide structure and climate conducive to accomplish tasks	Find appropriate role as team member Identify own strengths and contributions Begin to identify role in team	Team norms developed and accepted Members begin to assume appropriate task and maintenance team roles Team identity beginning
Emergence	Conflict, disagreement, defending of opinions Power struggles Alliances forming Appropriate roles assumed Emergence of "we" identity	Provide support for team to express opinions without negative repercussions Monitor and manage conflict and power struggles	Able to differ, confront, communicate, and collaborate Assume appropriate role in team Commit to team Acceptance of team leadership	All necessary team roles enacted Conflict is managed well "We" and "Our team" often expressed
Production	Open, honest communication Shared leadership, decision making, responsibility Bargaining and negotiation replace conflict Members achieve goals	Support team in planning, making decisions, and dealing with difficult problems Assess and evaluate progress toward team goals	Value other team members Accept positive and negative feedback Open to various points of views Support team efforts and team goals	Mutual support of each other Enthusiasm for team work Cohesiveness among members Collaboration of efforts Team goals supersede individual goals

Source: M. J. Farley, "Teamwork in Perioperative Nursing: Understanding Team Development, Effectiveness, Evaluation," *AORN Journal,* 53, no. 3 (March 1991): 732–733. Reprinted with permission.

Exhibit 19–4   Examples of Self-Esteem Through Strength

1. Educators have strength when they know that other employees want to hire them because of their demonstrated influence with nurses, physicians, and others. They have self-esteem when this gives them satisfaction.
2. Nurse administrators have strength when chosen by top management to expand their spheres of respon-

sibility to direct other departments and when recognized by other administrators for skills and knowledge—being consulted by legislators or leaders in nursing and health care. They have self-esteem when this gives them satisfaction.

Self-Esteem

Having self-esteem means having a stable, firmly based, usually high evaluation of oneself, having self-respect and self-confidence from the ability to act independently, the achievement of one's personal and professional goals, and competence in personal and professional skills and knowledge. Being held in esteem by others because of one's personal accomplishments and reputation gives a person status and recognition. It makes one feel appreciated and respected and increases one's self-esteem. It satisfies the desire to have strength among family, friends, colleagues, supervisors, patients, visitors, and others.[23] Exhibit 19–4 above presents examples of self-esteem based on strength.

Self-esteem entails satisfying the desire for achievement of personal, professional, and organizational goals, as illustrated in Exhibit 19–5.

Self-esteem comes from satisfaction of the desire for adequacy, feeling worthwhile as a person in society and as a worker, as illustrated in Exhibit 19–6.

Self-esteem involves satisfying the desire for mastery of and competence in the knowledge and skills needed to perform a role in clinical practice, management, education, or research, as a member of a family, and as a citizen, as shown in Exhibit 19–7.

Self-esteem comes from acquiring a feeling of confidence in the face of the world, as in Exhibit 19–8.

Exhibit 19–5   Examples of Self-Esteem Through Achievement of Goals

1. A professional nurse satisfies the need for self-esteem by running for and winning a government office or an office in some service or professional organization.
2. A professional nurse satisfies the need for self-esteem by achieving credentials such as certification, an advanced degree, or computer skills.

3. A professional nurse manager satisfies the need for self-esteem by lowering the absenteeism and turnover rates of personnel in the nursing division.

Exhibit 19–6   Examples of Self-Esteem Through Adequacy

1. A professional nurse feels that she is a good wife and mother because she can work a schedule compatible with her husband's, be involved in the activities of her family, and save money for her children's college education.

2. A staff nurse in the recovery room feels she has the time to assess, plan, and give good care and attend to good documentation of care. She even has an opportunity to obtain reading references needed to keep professional knowledge and skills updated.

Exhibit 19–7   Examples of Self-Esteem Through Mastery

1. A nurse educator involves clinical nurses in preparing strategic objectives for a unit. The plan is approved by the organization's administrators.

2. A clinical nurse is selected to implement a theory of nursing about which the nurse is considered an authority.

Exhibit 19–8   Examples of Self-Esteem Through Confidence

1. A professional nurse goes to work confident of being able to perform as well as any other nurse and better than some; confident of being able to learn whatever is needed to do a job well; confident that her or his abilities will be recognized and credit given, that full merit pay will be earned, that the employer's standards as well as those of the

ANA, the JCAHO, and other internal and external agencies can be met.

2. A professional nurse decides to win support and run as a candidate for president of the district nurses association and wages a successful campaign.

Self-esteem involves satisfying the desire for independence and freedom. A person must be free to speak, to act without hurting others, to express herself or himself, to investigate and seek information, and to defend herself or himself. Each person must be treated with justice, fairness, honesty, and orderliness (see Exhibit 19–9).

People meet their esteem needs in different ways. They are influenced by culture, including the culture of the organization in which they work. The ends or results of achieving self-esteem are more important than the roads taken to achieve those ends or results. All human beings want to be esteemed unless they are pathological. Persons lacking self-esteem feel inferior, weak, helpless, and discouraged. They become indolent, passive, resistant to change, irresponsible, and unwilling to follow a dialogue. In the workplace, they focus on salary and fringe benefits, making unreasonable demands for economic benefits. They can become neurotic or emotionally sick when they have a deficiency in self-esteem.[24]

Exhibit 19–9   Examples of Self-Esteem Through Independence

1. A supervisor decides to learn something about joint practice as a modality of nursing and obtains information and writes a position paper on it. The administrator suggests making a plan to practice it. The supervisor sets a specific schedule to orient and gain approval of first the clinical nurses and then the physicians who use the unit.

2. Clinical nurses are given complete freedom to manage the care of their patients, including coordination with personnel of x-ray, medical laboratory, nutrition and food service, physicians, and others.

Direction and control are useless in motivating professional nurses whose social, ego, and self-fulfillment needs are predominant. Intellectual creativity is a characteristic of professional nurses who do not get ego satisfaction from wages, pensions, vacations, or other benefits of work. The job itself must be satisfying and fun if professional nurses are to satisfy their self-esteem needs. Professional nurses get their ego needs met by having a voice in decision making. They will commit to organizational objectives when they are allowed to determine the steps to take to achieve them. They want to collaborate with other professionals, both internal and external to the environment in which they work.

Self-esteem involves the personhood of all professional nurses, be they managers, clinical nurses, researchers, or teachers. Each person should enrich the esteem of the other person and should be the peer pal, mentor, sponsor, and guardian of each person within the profession. Esteem results in leading and influencing. One can listen to other people, treat them as individuals, show earnest exhilaration in responding to their creativity, offer ideas for improvement, and share the excitement of their successes and their victories. Success gives one a positive self-image and builds self-esteem. It avoids the pain of failure.[25]

Exercise 19–4   With a group of your peers, discuss the examples of self-esteem listed in Exhibits 19–4 through 19–9, how do these apply to your group? Are changes needed? If so, list them.

Self-Actualization

Self-actualization was defined by Maslow as an ego need at the top of the needs hierarchy. It does not exist by itself, and in some persons it may be no stronger than the love and belonging need or the self-esteem need.

Self-actualized people are better able to distinguish the real world, seeing reality more clearly. Comfortable with the unknown, self-actualized people are attracted to it. All are creative in whatever they do and perceive.

Accepting and adjusting to their own shortcomings, self-actualized people are less defensive and less artificial. They feel guilty if they are not doing something to improve their shortcomings, prejudice, jealousy, envy, and the other faults of humanity. They have autonomous codes of ethics yet are the most ethical of people. They conform when no great issues are involved.

In the area of values, self-actualized people accept their own nature, human nature, the realities of social life, and the constraints of physical reality. Self-actualized people are problem-centered, not ego-centered. Their values are broad and universal. Being deeply democratic, as opposed to authoritarian by nature, they respect people and have a strong sense of right and wrong, of good and evil. Self-actualized people are not interested in hostile humor. Their humor is of a philosophical bent, stated only to produce a laugh.

Self-actualized people like solitude and privacy. They are detached and objective under conditions of turmoil. They are self-movers. While they generally want to help the human race and can sometimes feel like strangers in a strange land, their relationships with people are more profound and their circle of friends small. They love children and humanity but can be briefly hostile to others when it is deserved or for the others' good. In social terms, self-actualized people are godly but not religious. While they are not conventional, they conform to social graces with toleration. They can be radical.

Maslow indicates that living at the higher need level is good for growth and health, both physically and psychologically. Self-actualized persons live longer, have less disease, sleep and eat better, and enjoy their sexual lives without unnecessary inhibitions. For them, life continues to be fresh, thrilling, exciting, and ecstatic. They count their blessings.

Self-actualized people have mystic or peak experiences. These are natural experiences. Happiness can cause tears. It comes from transcendence of appreciation for poetry, music, philosophy, religion, interpersonal relationships, beauty, or politics. They can have the peak experience from doing or sensing.

Self-actualized people are "metamotivated." Their motivations are for character growth, character expression, maturation, and development. They place more dependence upon self-development and inner growth than the prestige and status of others' honors.

Pursuit and gratification of higher needs have desirable civic and social consequences: loyalty, friendliness, civic consciousness. People who are living at this level make better parents, spouses, teachers, public servants, and so on. They also create greater, stronger, and truer individualism. They are synergistic.

One possible conclusion is that the self-actualized person achieves a highly satisfactory quality of life, that this quality of life extends from the gratified self-actualized person into society. Gratification or satisfaction of the higher-level needs can be positively influenced by the social environment of work, family, community, government, and the like.

Applying these insights to nursing, the nurse leader would selectively apply knowledge and skills of the social and behavioral sciences to creating an environment or climate in which practicing nurses could become self-actualized. In doing so, nurse managers themselves become self-actualized, and the products and services of nursing increase in quantity and quality.

Although critics of Maslow's work say it is based on too narrow a population, the theory is widely accepted and used. Maslow analyzed the profiles of sixty subjects, including Lincoln, Jefferson, Einstein, and Frederick Douglas. He suggested that the self-determined population may be limited to being from 5 percent to 30 percent of the total, another forecast criticized by other scientists.[26]

Self-Concept

Self-concept has been analyzed as a nursing diagnosis. Its components include body image, self-esteem, and personal identity. The nursing diagnoses under Human Responses Pattern, Perceiving, include body image disturbance, personal identity disturbance, and chronic low or situational self-esteem disturbance. Self-concept results from experience and is a determinant of behavior. LeMone adapted Roy's definition of self-concept as follows: "Self-concept is a composite of thoughts, values, and feelings that one has for one's physical and personal self at any given time formed from interactions with the environment and with other people, and directing one's behavior."[27] Maslow emphasized self-actualization as the motivating force in developing one's unique self-concept.

Other Activities to Stimulate Motivation

Motivation is stimulated by activities such as job enrichment, praise, empowerment, employee stock ownership plans (ESOPs), lateral promotions, inclusion in organizational activities, and focus on vision, values, and strategy. (Some of these activities and strategies have been discussed in other chapters.)

All employees should be able to describe the values of their employer (see Exhibit 19–10). These values are identified, defined, prioritized, and communicated through such means as booklets and orientation programs. Values are critical in empowerment. Managers should emphasize the value of people by trusting, respecting, and encouraging them. They should tie rewards to values of teamwork, innovation, safety, growth, and profitability and provide employees with financial and nonfinancial rewards.

Managers should motivate employees by including them in the group's mission. Employees are motivated by detailed explanations, praise, tangible rewards, and constructive criticism. They need time to improve unsatisfactory performance, and when they cannot do so, they should be encouraged to seek another post within the organization.[28]

Firms are using flexible work plans (see Exhibit 19–11) to cut costs and keep the best people. These plans, which reduce forced layoffs, include the following:

1. Paternity leave or work-at-home policies. Of firms surveyed in 1987 by Hay/Haggins Company, none had such policies. By 1991, nearly half offered paternity leave, and 14 percent offered telecommuting options. Flexible hours policies increased from 35 percent in 1987 to 40 percent in 1991. These numbers have expanded greatly. Website http://search.yahoo.com lists dozens of new work-at-home jobs. There is even a work-at-home online magazine. Website http://sprint.snap.com

Exhibit 19–10   Value Focus

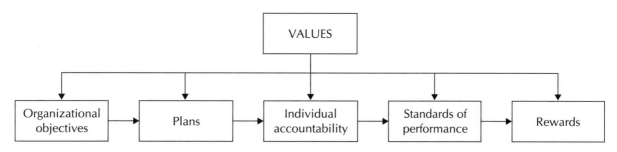

Source: Reprinted from L. Ginsburg and N. Miller, "Value-Driven Management," *Business Horizons,* May/June 1992, 24. Copyright 1992 by the Foundation for the School of Business at Indiana University. Used with permission.

has more than 232,000 pages on flexible hours and more than 168,000 pages on paternity leave policies.
2. Reduced workweek schedule, job sharing, unpaid leaves of absence, and early retirement.
3. Rearranged workdays to allow parents to attend child's school functions or meet other personal and family needs.
4. Childcare assistance.

The companies surveyed included DuPont, Philadelphia Newspapers, IBM, and Avon Products.[29]

Exercise 19–5   Small-Group Session

1. Each person will write a statement that provides a vision of what he or she wants to accomplish in stimulating the motivation of his or her peers or employees. (20 minutes)
2. Each person will outline a process for accomplishing this vision. (20 minutes)
3. Each person will report to the group. (20 minutes)

Exercise 19–6   Complete Exhibit 19–12, "Checklist for Assessing Job Satisfaction," and use it to develop goals that you can achieve. Keep in mind that all responsibility for personal satisfaction in life is ultimately your own. We have to take action to help ourselves, to be informed, to become better educated, to improve our interpersonal relationships, and to make our lives meaningful.

Exhibit 19–11   Flexible Work Plans

Favorite Arrangements

Percentage of companies on the Conference Board's Work-Family Research and Advisory Panel with these flexible work arrangements:

Reason	Percentage
Personal leave	97.0%
Part-time work	94.7
Flextime	92.4
Family/medical leave	89.4
Telecommuting	75.8
Compressed workweek	68.7
Job sharing	67.4
Sabbaticals	39.5
Phased retirement	30.8

Reasons for Flexible Plans

Top seven reasons companies initiate flexible work plans:

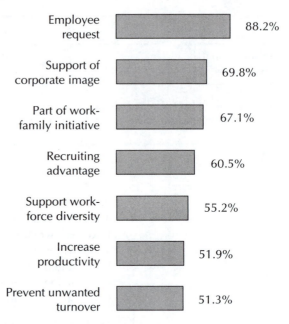

Employee request	88.2%
Support of corporate image	69.8%
Part of work-family initiative	67.1%
Recruiting advantage	60.5%
Support work-force diversity	55.2%
Increase productivity	51.9%
Prevent unwanted turnover	51.3%

Setting personal goals is a way of planning ahead. It gives people momentum because it means that they have decided to pursue what they want and obtain the necessary qualifications. It is important that they recognize their personal limitations and abilities and use that awareness to initiate the changes needed to achieve their goals. Social and leadership goals gained from such aspects of living as family, community, and church are often overlooked credentials for achieving self-improvement and self-fulfillment. Use Exhibit 19–13, "Future Goals Worksheet," to develop a list of goals. Once you have your goals written down, you can evaluate them using Exhibit 19–14, "Goal Evaluation Checklist."

Exhibit 19–12   Checklist for Assessing Job Satisfaction

In my current job I am	Yes	No or Insufficient
Happy with being able to help others.		
Intellectually stimulated and challenged.		
Given opportunity to progress educationally.		
Learning new skills.		
Sharpening old skills.		
Learning a new discipline.		
Qualifying for more responsibility.		
Qualifying for more respect.		
Given opportunities to attend staff meetings, patient-care conferences, and staff-development programs.		
Rewarded for doing my job well.		
Adequately paid.		
Given opportunity for advancement.		
Given opportunity to innovate and be creative.		
Given opportunity to choose shifts and hours of work.		
Given opportunity to be a leader.		
Given opportunity to grow as a bedside nurse.		
Able to trust my supervisors and peers.		
Supported by administration.		
Communicated with by administration.		
Being paid for my total knowledge and experience.		
Confident of job security.		
Working with adequate staffing.		
Feeling satisfied with my accomplishments.		
Supported by nursing management in resolving physician-nurse conflict.		
Able to resolve peer conflict.		
Adequately paid for overtime.		
Given opportunity to schedule extra time off above and beyond holidays and vacation.		
Given opportunity to schedule my working hours.		
Prepared to function as a team leader or charge nurse.		
Supported by competent professional nurses who assist and teach me.		

(continued)

Exhibit 19–12   Checklist for Assessing Job Satisfaction *(Continued)*

My job satisfaction could be increased by:

Identify specific steps to gather the information or make the changes that will help you reach your goal.

One of my job satisfaction goals is:

As a step toward reaching this goal I will talk to:

about:

and I will undertake the following activities myself:

Exhibit 19–13   Future Goals Worksheet

You will want to set goals in at least three areas:

1. **Personal Goals.** What would you really like to do with your life? Write down the personal goals you want to accomplish. Examples are "Become a role model for the profession," "Achieve as a writer in the field of staff development," or "Serve people who need but lack the means to buy health care."

   _____

   _____

2. **Family Goals.** Do you want to save money to travel? To put yourself and your family through school? To supplement a primary income? To buy something special? You may want to discuss these with your spouse and children.

   _____

   _____

3. **Professional goals.** Do you want to become a professor, a director of nursing, a consultant in nursing care of cancer patients, a clinical researcher, something outside of nursing altogether?

   _____

   _____

Exhibit 19–14   Goal Evaluation Checklist

Standards for Evaluating Goals	Yes	No
1. I have reviewed my short-range goals within the past three months.		
2. I have reviewed my long-range goals within the past year.		
3. My goals reflect my personal philosophy or beliefs and the purpose or reason I want to achieve them.		
4. My goals can be measured or verified as being achieved.		
5. I have set my goals in the priority or sequence in which I want to accomplish them.		
6. My goals are clear to me. They are specific and indicate actions to take to achieve them.		
7. My goals are flexible and realistic so that I will have as many opportunities as possible.		
8. I have the resources to accomplish my goals.		
9. My goals are stated for a specific job.		

WEB ACTIVITIES

■ Visit www.jbpub.com/swansburg, this text's companion website, for further information on Motivation.
■ Get motivated! Explore the many websites related to getting yourself motivated and how to motivate others.
■ Using the Internet, find examples of content theories of motivation and process theories of motivation.

SUMMARY

To summarize:

1. A person is motivated.
2. A person has goals.
3. Management has goals.
4. A condition or environment needs to be established whereby a person can achieve personal goals by achieving management's goals (and vice versa).
5. The person is rewarded by work achievements that are successful. Management practice provides the setting for success, perhaps by removing restraints or giving other intrinsic rewards. High-level ego needs are met on the job.

6. A cooperative interaction is fostered between manager and employee, since the latter participates in decisions that affect her or him.

7. Motivation occurs.

8. Personal and motivational goals are met as the nurse is motivated to be ambitious and responsible, to show initiative, to be proud of fellow nurses and the employing institution, to welcome change, and to demonstrate individual abilities.

The following law will apply to successful leadership in nursing: Find out where nurse persons want to go and what they want to accomplish, and bring these goals into line with those of the organization. Then nurses will accomplish organizational goals as they achieve their own.

NOTES

1. R. M. Hodgetts, *Management: Theory, Process, and Practice*, 5th ed. (Orlando, Fla.: Harcourt Brace Jovanovich, 1990), 460.

2. R. A. Katzell and D. E. Thompson, "Work Motivation," *American Psychologist*, February 1990, 144–153.

3. Ibid.

4. A. H. Maslow, *Motivation and Personality*, 2d ed. (New York: Harper & Row, 1970).

5. J. L. Gibson, J. M. Ivancevich, and J. M. Donnelly, Jr., *Organizations: Behavior, Structure, Processes*, 8th ed. (Burr Ridge, Ill.: Richard D. Irwin, 1994), 151–193.

6. R. M. Hodgetts, op. cit., 478–479; D. McGregor, *Leadership and Motivation* (Cambridge, Mass.: MIT Press, 1966).

7. R. A. Katzell and D. E. Thompson, op. cit.

8. J. L. Gibson, J. M. Ivancevich, and J. M. Donnelly, Jr., op. cit., 168–193; K. L. Roach, "Production Builds on Mutual Respect," *Nursing Management*, February 1984, 54–56; R. B. Youker, "Ten Benefits of Participant Action Planning," *Training*, June 1985, 52, 54–56.

9. J. L. Gibson, J. M. Ivancevich, and J. M. Donnelly, Jr., op. cit, 168–193.

10. Ibid.

11. Ibid.

12. J. Fleury, "The Application of Motivational Theory to Cardiovascular Risk Reduction," *Image*, fall 1992, 229–239.

13. K. L. Roach, op. cit.; M. G. Pryor and W. Mondy, "Mutual Respect Key to Productivity," *Supervisory Management*, July 1978, 10–17.

14. P. F. Drucker, *Management: Tasks, Responsibilities, Practices* (New York: Harper & Row, 1973–74), 176, 195–196.

15. P. Konstam, "Greenspan Joins Cry for Better Education," 12 February 1992, G1.

16. D. McGregor, op. cit., 5–6.

17. Ibid., 15.

18. M. Griffin, "Assumptions for Success," *Nursing Management*, January 1988, 32U–32X.

19. M. Miller, "Understanding Human Behavior and Employee Motivation," *Advanced Management Journal*, April 1968, 47–52; D. McGregor, op. cit., 211–212.

20. M. K. Kleinknecht and E. A. Hefferin, "Assisting Nurses Toward Professional Growth: A Career Development Model," *Journal of Nursing Administration*, July–August 1982, 30–36; J. C. Crout, "Care Plan for Retaining the New Nurse,"

Nursing Management, December 1984, 30–33; R. C. Swansburg and P. W. Swansburg, *Strategic Career Planning and Development for Nurses* (Rockville, Md.: Aspen, 1984).

21. M. C. Allender, "Productivity Enhancement: A New Teamwork Approach," *National Productivity Review,* spring 1984, 181–189.

22. P. Cornett-Cooke and K. Dias, "Teambuilding: Getting It All Together," *Nursing Management,* May 1984, 16–17.

23. A. H. Maslow, op. cit.

24. B. Fuszard, ed., *Self-Actualization for Nurses: Issues, Trends, and Strategies for Job Enrichment* (Rockville, Md.: Aspen, 1984), 140.

25. Ibid., 207.

26. A. H. Maslow, op. cit.

27. P. LeMone, "Analysis of a Human Phenomenon: Self-Concept," *Nursing Diagnosis,* July/September 1991, 126–130.

28. L. Hicks, "Motivation Key to Successful Employment," *San Antonio Express-News,* 17 March 1994, 1E–2E.

29. C. Trost, "To Cut Costs and Keep the Best People, More Concerns Offer Flexible Work Plans," *The Wall Street Journal,* 18 February 1992, B1.

20

COMMUNICATION

"Between two beings there is always the barrier of words. Man has so many ears and speaks so many languages. Should it nevertheless be possible to understand one another? Is real communication possible if word and language betray us every time? Shall, in the end, only the language of guns and tanks prevail and not human reason and understanding?"

Joost A. M. Meerloo[1]

OBJECTIVES

- Illustrate the components of communication.
- Interpret the elements of communication.
- Evaluate the climate for effective communication.
- Distinguish between communication as perception and communication as information.
- Compare communication with feedback to communication without feedback.
- Distinguish among causes of listening habits.
- Explain techniques that will improve listening.
- Distinguish among media of communication.
- Apply the Gunning Mueller Fog Index to an assigned reading.
- Contrast future impacts on communication.

KEY CONCEPTS

communication
perception
information
feedback
listening
media

Manager behavior: Provides information to employees through written and oral media.

Leader behavior: Solicits input from employees through several media of communication. Provides feedback that indicates communication has been effective.

COMPONENTS OF COMMUNICATION

In answering the question of who is involved in communication, one could simply answer, everyone! However, several aspects are to be considered. The first of these is that the person who wants to be heard is involved in communication. For example, the Bantam fried chicken facility wants to sell chicken and wants people to know that it has chicken to sell. Its manager will therefore advertise in an effort to communicate this desire to sell an appetizing product. The manager will do this through such media as newspapers, billboards, radio, television, and the internet. All kinds of tempting pictures will be portrayed in these advertisements. If the manager is successful and people buy lots of Bantam fried chicken as a result of the advertisements, then the people have received the message and the manager has communicated to them.

A second aspect of communication occurs when a person seeks out desired information. Suppose a working person is just plain tired of cooking and wants Bantam fried chicken to serve the family for Sunday dinner. That person knows where the nearest location is, having heard or seen it advertised. She or he may have driven past the facility and seen the sign and markings that identify the product. That person may have been reminded of the product while reading the Sunday paper that morning. And even if the person cannot remember the address, she or he can always refer to the Yellow Pages for an address and phone number or call directory assistance. When a person wants information, there are many sources from which to obtain it. All these sources are media of communication.

Elements of Communication

At least two people are involved in communication; a sender, or provider, and a receiver. A sender usually has something he or she wants to communicate, even if the information is distasteful. A receiver usually has need of some information, whether good or bad. Regardless of the medium, information is transmitted from sender to receiver, and a communication occurs.

Whether or not money is exchanged, communication always involves a buyer or a seller. The buying or selling is based on a need. Sometimes the receiver's need to hear is not as acute as the sender wants it to be. An example of this is the communication between a parent and a child, or vice versa. The parent can tell the child to be in by midnight on Saturday, but perhaps the parent has said the same thing before and when the child did not return by midnight, nothing happened. As a result, now the child does not even hear the parent, since she or he has no reason to listen. However, when the child returns after midnight and is then told the hour to get home will be 8:00 p.m. for four weeks, the child does have a reason to listen. Communication now takes place, since the child finds sufficient reason for listening.

Communication is a human process involving interpersonal relationships—and therein lies the problem. In the workplace, some managers view their knowledge of events as power; sharing knowledge through communication is sharing power, and these managers do not want to share. Other managers do not realize the importance of communication in an information age because they are not up-to-date on the advantages of decentralization and participatory management. These managers frequently fall into crisis management, treating the symptoms of poor communication and never identifying the root causes. A third group of managers recognizes that communication is like the central nervous system. It directs and controls the management process.

Over 80 percent of a higher-level manager's time is spent on communication: 16 percent of that time is spent reading, 9 percent writing, 30 percent speaking, and 45 percent listening. Is there any question that communication skills are absolutely essential to career advancement in nursing?[2] Effective communication has three basic principles:

1. Successful communication involves a sender, a receiver, and a medium.
2. Successful communication occurs when the message sent is received.
3. Successful nurse managers achieve successful communication.

Climate for Communication

Organizational climate and culture were discussed in Chapter 14, "The Organizing Process." The communication climate should be in harmony with the corporate culture and should be used to encourage positive values, such as quality, independence, objectivity, and client service, among nursing employees. Communication is used to support the mission (purpose or business) and vision of the nursing organization and to tell the consumers or clients that nursing is of high quality. The media used will include performance, nursing records, and marketing. Communication will be objective when it is accurately portrayed with descriptions of factual outcomes judged on the basis of objective outcome criteria.

Nursing literature abounds with evidence of nurses' desire for autonomy and knowledge they may use to communicate their support of autonomy. They may also provide a climate in which the nursing business remains as free of political constraints as possible. When political considerations are imperative, the imperative will be communicated to employees, who make decisions based on the institution's values and beliefs.

Cultural Agendas.   Cultural agendas publicize the mission or business of the organization. They tell what the organization stands for and what the nursing division, department, or individual unit places value on.

Cultural agendas are used to communicate promotions, new hires, marriages, deaths, and other personal news about personnel. Heroes are highlighted with features that illustrate support of desired values and beliefs: the nurse who presents a paper, authors a book, achieves prominence in the profession or in the community; the nurse who is a champion bowler, an elected officer in an organization, an appointed official in the health-care system; the nurse who is a volunteer in community activities. The cultural agendas are used also to publicize nursing units and special achievements, such as ongoing research in burn care or rehabilitation.

Various media, including newsletters, memoranda, awards ceremonies, and external communications—publications, radio, television, and organizational meetings—are used to publicize cultural agendas. Such communications will be most effective when they depict the people who are directly involved in the publicized events.

Cultural agendas can be effectively used to change the organizational climate and culture.[3] The nurse leader has to establish the climate for effective communication. Wlody recommends the following:[4]

Step I: Review your own communication technique.
Step II: Concentrate the staff's attention on communication as a needed skill that everyone can develop.
Step III: Lead the staff into more positive interaction within the unit.
Step IV: Make daily rounds with the whole team.
Step V: Form a group to reduce stress.

Nature of Communication Climate.   Important communication occurs between supervisor and employees at the work level where climate is set. A supportive climate encourages employees to ask questions and offer solutions to problems. Exhibit 20–1 compares the characteristics of supportive and defensive communication climates. Nurse leaders would strive for a supportive climate. A strong relationship exists between good communication skills and good leadership.

A supportive climate will produce clear communication to support productive nursing workers and effective teamwork. It will provide for identification of communication problems by designing instruments to collect data during specified periods of time. Real communication patterns and problems will be diagnosed from analysis of the data and can be related to communication climate and solved by using problem-solving techniques.

Communication problems have been listed as the source of job dissatisfaction. Organizational communication systems are powerful determinants of an organization's effectiveness. Communication rules are organization-specific and are either explicit or implicit. Explicit rules are codified. They govern formal activities, such as access to superiors. Their violation may result in sanctions. Implicit rules mimic norms of behavioral expectations and are not codified but are mutually shared. Conformation to rules reduces dissonance and maintains stability. A questionnaire may be used to assess communication in six areas: "(1) accessibility of information, (2) communication channels, (3) clarity of messages, (4) span of control, (5) flow control/communication load, and (6) the individual communicators"[5] (see Exhibit 20–2).

Negotiation.   When disagreements about the intent of a communication occur, negotiation is indicated to prevent conflict, resignation, or avoidance between supervisor and employee. When there is lack of confidence between supervisor and employee or among employees, nurse leaders can solve the communication

Exhibit 20–1 Supportive Versus Defensive
Communication Climate in the Workplace

Supportive Climate	Defensive Climate
1. The individual is free to talk to managers at any level of the organization without fear of retribution of any kind. Opportunities for this are planned and made known to the entire staff.	1. The individual works within traditional management principles of chain of command, line of authority, and span of control.
2. Equality: management by objectives supports equality by encouraging two-way communication in which both supervisor and employee evaluate progress and make future plans.	2. Superiority: pyramids, hierarchies, and chains of command support superiority.
3. Descriptive evaluation with management analysis and employee input. The employee gets information at specific intervals and when indicated.	3. Traditional evaluation with one-way communication done on an annual basis.
4. Spontaneity.	4. Strategy is kept at managerial planning level.
5. Problem orientation emphasizes joint view, bringing employee into the process.	5. Control emphasizes supervisor's view.
6. Provisionalism encourages adaptation and experimentation.	6. Certainty is dogmatic; it squelches.
7. Empathy indicates concern and respect. Managers should use it to counteract neutrality by using non-traditional management techniques.	7. Neutrality indicates nonconcern. It is fostered by orientation to numbers as in outcomes, profits, and even standardization of orientation procedures.

Source: Adapted from C. E. Beck and E. A. Beck, "The Manager's Open Door and the Communication Climate," *Business Horizons* (January/February 1986), 15–19. Copyright 1986 by the Foundation for the School of Business at Indiana University. Used with permission.

problem through a climate of openness that restores confidence through agreement and promotes individual autonomy as well as esprit de corps.[6] Communication and change require negotiation. Cooperation, or win/win negotiation, is best. The following are the steps of the negotiation process:[7]

1. Preparing for negotiation (e.g., introducing a topic at a meeting);
2. Communicating a general overview of what is to be accomplished during the process;
3. Relating the history of why negotiation is required;
4. Redefining the issue to be addressed;
5. Selecting when issues will be worked on;
6. Encouraging discussion during the conflict stage of the issue;
7. Addressing the fall-back or compromise for both parties on the issue;
8. Agreeing in principle during the settlement stage;
9. Recapping and summarizing the agreement; and
10. Monitoring subsequent compliance of the agreement (after settlement).

During the negotiation process, the nurse leader is always positive in explaining ideas, suggestions, and benefits. The nurse leader actively listens to employee responses, gaining perceptions, identifying concerns, and explaining

Exhibit 20–2   Communication Assessment Questionnaire

Please circle the number representing the extent to which you believe the statement is true for you in your work
  environment.

1 = the statement is not at all accurate
5 = the statement is completely accurate

1. I have the information I need in order to do my job in the most effective and efficient manner.	1	2	3	4	5
2. I know where I can get the information I need in order to do my job well.	1	2	3	4	5
3. I receive information about my job from					
a. my immediate supervisor	1	2	3	4	5
b. my co-workers	1	2	3	4	5
c. notices posted on bulletin boards	1	2	3	4	5
d. personnel from departments other than nursing	1	2	3	4	5
4. I receive the information about any changes that might affect my job in a timely manner.	1	2	3	4	5
5. The communications I receive are clear and understandable.	1	2	3	4	5
6. I am satisfied with the frequency of communications I have with my immediate superior.	1	2	3	4	5
7. I receive too little information about things that are happening in this organization.	1	2	3	4	5
8. I believe that nursing administration shares critical and pertinent information with nursing personnel.	1	2	3	4	5
9. People in administration effectively communicate with employees.	1	2	3	4	5

Source: M. J. Farley. "Assessing Communication in Organizations." *Journal of Nursing Administration,* 19, 12 (December
1989): 28. Reprinted with permission of J. B. Lippincott.

obstacles to these ideas, suggestions, and benefits. The nurse leader encourages
explanations and suggests ways of overcoming obstacles. Questions are
phrased to obtain discussion and answers. A supportive environment includes
a favorable location.

Successful negotiations have win/win outcomes that indicate progress,
maintain self-respect, leave positive feelings, are sensitive to each other's needs,
achieve a majority of each other's objectives, and facilitate future negotiation.
Change theory is involved in negotiation.[8]

Open-Door Policy.   Communication climate influences the success of an open-
door policy. An open-door policy of a nurse manager implies that an employee
can walk into the manager's office at any time. Usually, however, since the manager does follow a schedule, it is more convenient for both parties if the
employee makes an appointment.

A nurse manager who believes in the open-door policy will clearly state
the rules, including whether the employee needs anyone else's permission to
make an appointment with the manager. A democratic manager who believes

in setting a climate for open communication will encourage visits. Such a manager knows how to deal with confidential communication to protect employees and their supervisors.

Exercise 20–1 | Have a group of co-workers evaluate your current recognition program. Discard those activities that are not working if they cannot be fixed. Give an infusion of excitement to the other activities. Consider having an "attaboy" and "attagirl" award where customers can fill out a short form when they feel especially good about something an employee has done. Recognize the employee immediately, such as at change-of-shift report, breakfast, lunch, or dinner. Send out ten thank-you notes a month to employees, ten more to customers.

Exercise 20–2 | Make notes of calendar events, such as birthdays and work anniversaries, and serve doughnuts or cake to celebrate the events.

Exercise 20–3 | Be the first to make a contribution to the United Way or other community agency. Lead the charge when supporting a voluntary effort for a community activity. Recognize those who put forth community effort.

COMMUNICATION AS PERCEPTION

In nursing, as in other disciplines, communication is perception. Sound is created by the sensory perceptions people have associated with it. The sound aspect of communication is voice. Communication takes place only if the receiver hears and the person hears or perceives only that which he or she is capable of hearing. It is important that the communication be uttered in the receiver's language, and the sender must have knowledge of the receiver's experience or perception capacity.

Conceptualization conditions perception; a person must be able to conceive to perceive. In writing a communication, the writer must work out his or her own concepts first and ask whether the recipient can receive them. The range of perception is physiological, since perception is a product of the senses. However, the limitations to perception are cultural and emotional. Fanatics cannot receive a communication beyond their range of emotions.

Different people seldom see the same thing in a communication, since they have different perceptual dimensions. Drucker has said that to communicate, the sender must know what the recipient, *the true communicator,* is able to see and hear, and why. Perhaps if we focus on the recipient as the true communicator, we will improve communication. The unexpected is not usually received at all or is ignored or misunderstood. The human mind perceives what it expects to perceive. To communicate, the sender must also know what the recipient expects to see and hear. Otherwise, the recipient has to be shocked to receive the intended message.[9]

People selectively retain messages because of emotional associations and receive or reject them based on good or bad experiences or associations. Communication makes demands on people. It is often propaganda and so creates cynics. It demands that the recipient become somebody, do something, or believe something. It is powerful if it fits aspirations, values, and goals. It is most powerful if it converts, since conversion demands surrender.

Leveling with Employees

Leveling is being honest with employees. It makes all information, both the good and the bad, known to them. It gives employees a chance to improve. Managers can control the content of negative information, not by concealing it but by sharing ideas, feelings, and information with affected employees. Nurse managers address issues as they arise. They focus on employee needs, offering help as indicated. Communication is a major factor in performance evaluation.[10]

COMMUNICATION DIRECTION

For effective communication, the place to start is with the perceptions of the recipients. Listeners do not receive the communication if they do not understand the message. Nurse managers need to know what listeners are able to perceive, what they expect to perceive, and what they want to do. Then they need to formulate their message. Many nurse managers focus on what they want to say and then cannot understand why they are not understood by the recipients.

Feedback

Feedback completes or continues communication, making it two-way. Today's workers are better managed under a climate that promotes Theory Y and participation or involvement. Most are more affluent, are better educated, have increased leisure, and retire earlier, all indications of their changed values.

Feedback is one of the most important factors influencing behavior. People want to know what they have accomplished and where they stand. Feedback works best when specific goals are set to note the improvements sought, measurable targets, deadlines, and specific methods of attaining goals.

Effective communication includes giving and receiving suggestions, opinions, and information. If this two-way interaction does not occur, little or no communication takes place. Communication requires mutual respect and confidence.

Research shows that feedback increases productivity. One study showed an 83 percent increase in productivity as measured by staff treatment programs and client hours, using the technique of private group feedback. Using the technique of public group feedback, productivity increased 163 percent in thirty-eight weeks.

When suggestions were answered promptly in a mental health organization of eighty employees, the number of suggestions increased 222.7 percent over a thirty-two-week period. In other studies, feedback plus training has been found to be even more effective. A review of twenty-seven empirical studies indicated that objective feedback worked in virtually every case.[11]

A study was done to test the effect of feedback on process versus outcomes of reality orientation in a psychiatric hospital serving elderly patients. Subjects were psychiatric nurses. They were divided into three groups, two being given appropriate feedback, while the third group did not receive any feedback. The nurses in the process feedback group showed "substantial increases" in process behavior over the control group that did not receive feedback. They had increased patient contacts, but it was not determined that their patients had increased reality orientation.[12]

Successful synergies require leadership, cooperative management plans, joint incentives, information sharing, computer networks, face-to-face relationships, shared experiences, mutual need, and a shared future. Communication is involved in almost every one of these activities. Kanter states that the communication imperative is that "more challenging, more innovation, more partnership-oriented positions carry with them the requirement for more communication and interaction."[13]

INFORMATION

Although they are interdependent, communication and information are different. Communication is perception; information is logic. Information is formal and has no meaning. It is impersonal and not altered by emotions, values, expectations, and perceptions.

Computers allow us to handle information devoid of communication content, an example being personnel information. Information is specific and economical, based on need by a person and for a purpose. Information in large amounts beyond that which meets a person's needs is an overload.

Communication may not be dependent on information; it may be shared experience. Information should be passed to the person who needs to know it, and that person must be able to receive it and act on it. Perception and communication are primary to information, and as information increases, the communicator or receiver must be able to perceive its meaning.[14] In the interest of time management, nurse managers need skills that sort information according to its import. These skills require clear communication and acute perception.

Exercise 20–4   Provide employees with a list of all the information about the job and work environment that pertains to the previous week. Schedule meetings with all the employees. Give them the information and leave them with a printed version.

LISTENING

Communication takes place between employer and employee; herein lies the crux of the matter. To have satisfied, productive employees, an employer must hear what the employees are saying as well as what they are *not* saying. Additionally, to really hear someone requires concentration. Consider, for example, what happens at church on Sunday. The preacher speaks, but the congregation hears only by concentrating on what the preacher is saying. Otherwise, the people supposedly listening to the preacher are planning next week's work or the rest of the day's events. Many managers do not listen effectively to what people are saying to them and thus discourage the person who perhaps wants to point out a problem but knows that either he or she will not be heard or the suggestion will have no effect.

One reason nursing personnel find it difficult to listen to a change-of-shift report is that a person can listen four times faster than the 125 to 150 words per minute that are being spoken. The listener who is tuned out may not hear a message about an appointment or a directive regarding a patient. As a result, it is usually more efficient for the person to read the change-of-shift report or listen to it on a tape recorder.

Most working persons are engaged in some form of verbal communication 70 percent of the waking day, or approximately eleven hours and twenty minutes out of sixteen hours. Of that time, 45 percent is spent listening to what is 50 percent forgotten within twenty-four hours. Another 25 percent is forgotten in the next two weeks.[15] If this is true of nursing personnel, they will forget 75 percent of what they hear today within the next two weeks. Some claim that immediately after a ten-minute speech, we remember only 50 percent of what we heard. Twenty-five percent is considered a good retention level.[16]

By learning the art of listening and observing, managers better understand what people mean by what they say. They receive cues from employees' words and actions. Leaders learn that men and women communicate differently. Learning the art of listening creates a better organization with better relationships and better outcomes.[17]

Causes of Poor Listening Habits

The following can result in poor listening habits:

1. Calling a subject uninteresting or boring.
2. Criticizing the speaker's delivery.
3. Being overstimulated by the subject.
4. Avoiding the speaker's eye contact, since 60 percent of a message is nonverbal.
5. Being defensive about the speaker's message when it threatens the listener with blame or punishment for something; when it indicates the sender is trying to control the receiver; when it is regarded as deceitful; when the sender is perceived as being unconcerned about a group's welfare; when speech, verbal or nonverbal, indicates superiority; or when certainty indicates dogmatism.[18]
6. Thinking employees do not expect them to listen.
7. Thinking employees have nothing of value to say.
8. Thinking listening is not part of their job.
9. Thinking employees should listen to them.
10. Thinking employees will change their minds and will have to be reevaluated.[19]

Techniques to Improve Listening

Improving listening ability can be accomplished in many ways. One method is to summarize what is being said for better understanding and retention. The listener should give empathetic attention to the speaker and try to understand the substance of what is being said; seek to be objective and to apply creativity; go beyond the speaker's dialect, stance, gestures, and attire to understand the meaning of the speaker's words; and try to counter his or her own emotionality or prejudice even though the speaker and listener may have opposite convictions.

It is important to discriminate among those to whom one listens. People should listen to those who keep them informed and lighten their workload or save time, listen to those who argue constructively and use their arguments to sharpen the listener's judgment, know the kind of people who want to listen to them and the situation in which they will try to make the listener hear, learn to recognize when the listener is and is not prone to listen. Some people give good information, and people should listen to such people. These people are trusted troubleshooters, line managers in charge of the bread-and-butter functions of primary patient care, staff specialists who have been delegated special tasks, and reliable decision-makers. Nursing personnel should graciously avoid exaggerators, opportunists, office politicians, gossips, and chronic complainers.[20]

Things said by the speaker and the speaker's appearance, facial expression, posture, accent, skin color, or mannerisms can turn off the listener. A person who wants to hear must thus put aside all preconceived ideas or prejudices and give the speaker full attention so that the speaker will be motivated to do a better job of communicating while the person is talking, the listener analyzes what is being said for ideas and facts. The receiver must also listen for feelings—which are the background to the performance—in the tone of voice, gestures, and facial expressions.

Mnemonics.   A mnemonic is a device used to help one remember. The following are two examples of mnemonics:

1. AIDA: Capture *a*ttention, sustain *i*nterest, incite *d*esire, and get *a*ction.
2. PREP: *P*oint, *r*eason, *e*xample, *p*oint.

Such formulas are useful for preparing impromptu comments. The AIDA formula causes the speaker to focus on the listener's needs, interests, and problems. The PREP formula is ideal for spur-of-the-moment speaking. The first *point* reminds the speaker to clearly express a point of view on the subject. In giving the *reason,* the speaker explains why this is his or her point of view. The reasons should be illustrated with as specific *examples* as possible: statistics, personal experiences, authoritative quotes, examples, analogies, anecdotes, and concrete illustrations to clarify and substantiate the point. In the final *point,* the speaker brings the speech to a close with a restatement of the initial point of view. These formulas are intended to gain the attention of the listener and to elicit a positive response.

Other Practical Suggestions.   The following are some practical suggestions for encouraging people to listen:[21]

1. Be prepared by answering the questions who? and what?
2. Identify and evaluate the purpose of your remarks.
3. Organize and outline the report or speech to convey the facts.
4. Make efficient notes and use them.
5. Remember that you are part of the package.
6. Make your voice work for you with proper breathing and pitch.
7. Communicate with your eyes.

Since critical-thinking skills require interpretation of events based on present experience and factual data collection, they are also communication skills. Conceptualization, which is a part of both the communication and the critical-thinking processes, supports this conclusion. Also, the set of information and belief-generating and -processing skills and abilities and the habit, based on intellectual commitment, of using these skills and abilities to guide behavior support the integration of critical-thinking ability and communication skills. Leaders use their critical-thinking ability to identify feelings and become aware of beliefs, values, and attitudes of employees so as to communicate and respond to their needs. Active listening through use of all senses is required of managers who need to recognize and respond to verbal and nonverbal messages from employees.[22]

To become a good listener requires practice. Listening to the patient can prevent errors. During a patient's temporary stay in a skilled nursing facility, a medication error was made because the nurse refused to listen to the patients, a husband and wife admitted to the same room. The nurse communicated with a physician who did not know either patient. Unneeded laboratory tests were done and reported late. A further irony was that the wife was an RN, the husband a medical doctor, and both were mentally alert. Every nurse manager and practicing nurse should work at improving their listening skills.

Good listeners get out from behind the desk and circulate with their customers. Good listening turns people on. Listening to employees empowers them. A good listener is an engaged listener and take notes. It's okay to ask so-called dumb questions when one needs information. Knowledge will always be power and should never be hoarded. Since information is frequently leaked before it happens, managers should provide it to the first-line people who need it. Information motivates employees by giving them critical information and making them potent partners. Information facilitates continuous improvement. It discourages unneeded controls and delays. Information speeds up problem solving and decision making. It stirs the juices of competition by stimulating ideas. Useful information begets more of the same. Information abets the flattened organizational pyramid. To get information flowing requires an extensive training program in basic management skills.[23]

Results of Effective Listening

The results of effective listening are that (1) two people hear each other, (2) beneficial information is furnished on which to base right decisions, (3) a better relationship between people is established, and (4) it is easier to find solutions to problems.[24]

Exercise 20–5   Check your in-box. If you are not receiving communication from your customers (clinical nursing personnel, patients, and others), start a personal listening ritual. Call three customers a day and ask them how they are doing and what their problems are and listen to their responses.

Exercise 20–6   From your communications (calls, memos, etc.) follow up on complaints or problems. Help resolve them.

Exercise 20–7   Have a group of internal and external customers meet with you to discuss communication and information problems. Listen to them. Guide them to good solutions. Facilitate action.

COMMUNICATION MEDIA

Meetings

Meetings of all kinds are a medium for communication, often for purposes of dissemination of information as well as true communication.

To make his company successful, Robert Davies, founder and president of SBT Corporation, changed his management style. To keep his employees motivated, he decided to include two employees in all management meetings. The employees provide ideas from the production level of the organization. Davies encourages employees to risk telling what they really think through an e-mail suggestion system. This computer suggestion box is connected to all employees via more than 100 stations. It assures anonymity and in six months spawned over 100 suggestions—which must be read and answered. For example, employees kept requesting relaxation of the dress code, which was changed and became successful. Even Robert Davies dresses casually, and employees are more comfortable talking to him. Technology combined with good listening results in consensus, support for decisions, and a company in which employees do their best.[25]

Supervisors

Supervisors or managers at all levels are also a medium for communication. To be successful in today's complicated environment, the nurse manager should be out and about. Managers and supervisors should be visible. Peters recommends the following actions for increasing visible management:[26]

1. Put a note card in your pocket and write on it: "Remember, I'm out here to listen."
2. Take notes, promise feedback—and deliver. Fix things.
3. Cycle your actions through the chain of command and give managers the credit for fixing things.

4. Protect informants.
5. Be patient.
6. Listen, but preach a little, too, by killing unneeded red tape.
7. Give some, but not much, advance notice and travel alone. Take your own notes.
8. Work some night shifts; take a basic training course.
9. Watch out for the subtle demands you put on others that cut down on their practice of visible management.
10. Use rituals to help force yourself and your colleagues to get out and about.

We live in an information society. Communication is the necessary ingredient for accomplishing mission and objectives. An effective communicator is an effective leader. An effective communication creates meaning for people. It should be an act of persuasion.

The effective nurse manager should share information! She or he should share all the information possible. A person cannot have too much information about the company she or he works for. The only information a manager does not share is that protected by law and ethics and decency. A nurse manager who holds information as a source of power is not an effective manager or leader.

Recognition programs promote communication. Nurse managers should recognize fairly mundane actions, send short written notes for work well done, do special recognition, such as serving doughnuts or cake to celebrate an individual or a group achievement. They should be sure that all acts of special effort are heartfelt. They should not be a phony. They should do a few big rewards and many small ones, be systematic, and celebrate events they would like repeated.[27]

Exercise 20–8   Walk around your area of responsibility. Note at least one hassle that can be fixed each day (or week or month). Fix it!

Exercise 20–9   Identify and analyze your worst failure each month. How can it be fixed? Fix it!

Questions

Asking questions is an important method of communicating. Questions are asked to obtain information; the goal is mutual understanding. The tone of voice must encourage confidence and trust from the person being questioned. Facial expression is important, as is the physical conduct of the questioner. The nurse manager should always go beyond the answer to a primary question and not flatly agree or disagree when questioned.

The following types of questions should be used:[28]

1. Open questions that give the other person the opportunity to freely express thoughts and feelings, rather than closed questions that force a receiver to become the sender of information.

2. Leading questions that give direction to the reply, rather than loaded ones that restrict by putting the respondent into a hot spot.
3. Cool questions that appeal to reason, rather than heated ones reflecting the emotional state of asker and answerer.
4. Planned questions that are reflective and asked in logical sequence, rather than impulsive ones that just happen to occur to the asker.
5. Complimentary or "treat" questions that tell the respondent that he or she can make an important contribution to the asker's views, rather than trick ones that place the respondent on the spot.
6. Window questions that elicit the respondent's true thoughts and feelings, rather than mirror ones that reflect the point of view of the questioner.

Successful questioning consists of creating and maintaining a climate for communication, asking the right questions in the right way, and listening to the responses.

Exercise 20–10   Conduct a group session in which you construct questions following the six types described. Test the questions on each other. How did they work? Can they be improved? Discuss situations in which they would be useful.

Oral Communication

Oral communication is the most common form of communication used by executives, who spend 50 percent to 80 percent of their time communicating. Since oral communication takes so much time, a nurse manager should use the most effective words. Verbal messages are said to be 7 percent verbal (word choice), 38 percent vocal (oral presentation), and 55 percent facial expression.[29]

An advantage of face-to-face communication is that a person can respond directly to another or to others. The larger the group, the less effective is face-to-face communication. An effective message requires a knowledge of words and their meanings as well as of the contexts within which the words can be used. Thus, effective communication may depend on use of the dictionary for effective vocabulary.

When giving a speech, one needs to keep in mind that the members of the audience are usually informed and sophisticated and have access to information. The members of the audience want the speaker to talk things over with them, not talk at them. The speaker must be sincere and respect the listeners. To present an effective speech, the speaker needs to develop an outline and hold to four or five main ideas, put other ideas under the main topics as subordinate ideas, open with an introduction and close with a brief summary, type the speech for easy reading, practice reading the speech, maintain eye contact during the speech, and keep the voice and manner informal and conversational. After learning the speech, the speaker should practice it without notes. A speaker should know the audience and its members' knowledge of the subject, intellectual level, attitudes, and beliefs. Former Vice-President Hubert Humphrey said, "The necessary components to build a speech are full understanding of the facts of the subject, thorough understanding of the particular audience, and a deep and thorough belief in what you are saying."[30]

Exhibit 20–3 lists other techniques to use in preparing and giving an effective oral presentation.

Written Communication

Writing is a common medium of communication, not only in nursing but also in society in general. It comes in massive quantities: memos to be read and passed on, even if they go into someone else's wastebasket; letters that need to be answered; newspapers and magazines that collect in stacks; junk mail; posters and flyers and notices and newsletters. How should one go about handling all this material? First, one should make a mental decision to deal with each piece of paper. One should establish a system for assigning priorities to the mass of written communications, skim through everything, and then answer or delegate that which can be handled immediately. One should lay aside whatever can be taken care of at a future date but not put things where they will be forgotten. Papers can be placed in a folder according to priority.

The writer is writing to the receiver: a reader, viewer, listener, observer, or member of an audience. The receiver is not interested in the writer but is interested only in the message the writer is sending. One should therefore write everything to the reader or listener—the receiver, use good marketing techniques, and sell the product.[31] Exhibit 20–4 lists nine rules to follow when writing.

Words obviously are important to written communication. The writer should put the reader's interest first, begin with a provocative question or striking statement to jar the receiver, and get right to the point: the purpose of the written communication and, if needed, the request for action. When writing a letter, a personal letter is always better than a form letter. One should use a friendly tone, with first names and personal pronouns, which express an interest in the reader. The following are some simple suggestions for communicating effectively through the written word:[32]

- Use active voice verbs to give strength to written communication. About 10 percent of total words should be verbs.
- Use strong nouns.
- Use the subject and main verb early in a sentence.
- Avoid overuse of adjectives and adverbs and be specific when using adjectives. State the specific amount, such as 100, instead of "much," "any," or "a lot."
- Be as brief as possible.
- Use short rather than long words.
- Use sentences that contain one idea and are generally no longer than sixteen to twenty words, and vary the sentence length.
- Write naturally, using friendly, conversational language (although contractions such as "didn't" and "aren't" should be used with discretion).

Exhibit 20–3   Techniques for Effective Public Speaking

1. Prepare carefully. What is the goal of your presentation? Is it to inform? Persuade? Entertain? It can be a combination of these and, to be effective, should probably combine at least two, such as entertainment with information or persuasion.
2. Prepare the presentation carefully. Make an outline and develop the content to fit the outline. Start well in advance so that you can read and adjust the material for a smooth flow of ideas.
   a. What is the purpose of the presentation? Did you select the topic, or was it given to you? In either instance, clarify the purpose with the organizers of the event or whoever engaged you to do the presentation.
   b. Prepare an introduction that will gain the attention of the audience. Spark their interest. Humor often helps, but be careful of using cynicism or making derogatory remarks. References to religion, sex, and other controversial subjects should be carefully selected, if used at all. They are better avoided if you wish to persuade or inform, unless they are a part of your topic. Remember, words convey feelings, attitudes, opinions, and facts. Use them to turn the audience on, not off.
   c. Make the main points in the body of the presentation. Support them with appropriate and specific examples.
   d. Prepare or select visual aids to effectively support the key points of the presentation. They are an extension of your presentation designed to appeal to the senses and increase reception.
   e. Know who the audience will be and tailor the message to it. Provide useful material.
   f. Plan for audience participation with questions or appropriate exercises to involve listeners.
   g. Tie the message together with interval summaries and an effective conclusion. How do you want to leave the audience?
   h. If you plan to speak extemporaneously, make notes on cards or put outlines on a visual aid such as a poster, a chalkboard, an overhead transparency, or a slide projection screen.
3. Prepare the environment beforehand. Surroundings are important and should be as attractive as possible. Bear this in mind when you have input into selection.
   a. If you want to speak from a podium, make sure it is in place. If you want to sit, have a table and chair in place.
   b. Check lighting and sound equipment.
   c. Check audiovisual equipment.
   d. Remove unneeded barriers such as screens, furniture, and other movable objects. If pillars are in the way, rearrange your position or the audience seating, if this is possible. Arrange your proximity to the group to facilitate a feeling of closeness.
   e. Prepare your person for the presentation. Wear clothes that present you best. Conventional clothes are best, as the audience will focus on your words rather than your appearance. Be well-groomed.
   f. Good preparation will help you to be relaxed. Get a good night's sleep the night before the presentation. Plan your schedule so as not to be excited beforehand. Eat and drink moderately. Sit and do deep-breathing exercises immediately before.
4. Be on time and use time effectively.
5. Speak to be heard.
   a. Use your voice, varying pitch, volume, rate, and tone for planned effect.
   b. Practice pronouncing words with which you have trouble.
   c. Pause to enhance your delivery. Short silences emphasize points and allow the audience to think about them.
   d. Make your presentation sound natural even if you read it.
6. Use body language effectively.
   a. Slowly develop the audience's awareness of your nonverbal behavior. Be aware of it yourself.
   b. Maintain eye contact.
   c. Plan your movements: walking, standing. Your posture should convey energy, interest, approval, confidence, warmth, and openness.
   d. Keep the space between you and the audience open.
   e. Use positive gestures.
   f. Use head movements for effect.
   g. Use facial expression for effect.
   h. Know where your hands and feet are at all times.
   i. Be genuine! An audience can quickly identify a fake.
7. Adapt to audience feedback, being sensitive to listeners' interests and moods.
   a. Listen for unrest, shifting in seats, whispering, muttering.
   b. Watch for nonverbal responses. Pay attention to body language, facial expressions, gestures, body movements. Leaning backward or away is perceived as a negative response.
   c. Be prepared to answer questions if there are breaks in the presentation. You may want to plan for them. Repeat them before answering, regardless of whether they are oral or written. You are giving additional information.
   d. Treat your audience with respect in every way, and they will view you as genuine.

Exhibit 20–4   Nine Rules to Follow When Writing

1. Empathize. Be sensitive to the needs and desires of those who will read what you are writing. Arouse and maintain the reader's interest by appealing to the mind and emotions. For example, compose a message that will transmit respect for the nurse while offering a credible and unique inspiration to taking nursing histories or preparing nursing care plans. When giving orders, explain why you are asking for the task to be done. You-centered rather than I-centered communications are interesting to the reader or listener. Give people honest and deserved praise, the kind of flattery that makes them feel they are worth flattering. If you are addressing a particular person, a unique human personality, put that person's name in the salutation as well as in the body of the letter or memo. Make an effort to please the receiver by using tact, respect, good manners, and courtesy.
2. Attempt to avoid the COIK ("clear only if known" to the reader or listener already) fallacy. Think of the misunderstandings that could occur in a written message using abstract terms. Your aim should be to create mental pictures using language that is suitable to the experience and knowledge level of the receiver.
3. Do not repeat anecdotes frequently, or the reader will be insulted. Avoid overcommunication, overdetailing, and redundancy. Necessary repetition can be achieved by using pleasant and meaningful examples, illustrations, paraphrasing, and summaries. Repetition is essential to the mastery of a skill.
4. Express yourself in clear, simple language. Lincoln's Gettysburg Address contains 265 words, three-fourths of them of one syllable. Abstract, technical-sounding jargon, cliches, and trite platitudes may cover up insecurity in a writer afraid of committing herself or himself in writing. Avoid archaic commercial expressions, specialized in-house jargon, and fading journalese by writing clearly and concisely.
5. Make yourself accessible to the reader by positively and courteously requesting a response. You can ask a direct question and expect a reply by a certain date. You can also encourage response by giving a special return address, a private box or phone number, writing instructions, a postcard, or a return envelope. Make it easy, desirable, and pleasant for the reader to reply.
6. Use the format of the newspaper story: accuracy, brevity, clarity, digestibility, and empathy. Arouse the reader with a headline opener. Follow it with a summary that tells significant highlights in the opening paragraph. Then tell the details. Here is an example of a memo form that has worked for others.

> Date_____   Time_____
>
> To:_____   Subject:_____
>
> From:_____
>
> Objective:_____
>
> 1. _____
>   _____
> 2. _____
>   _____
> 3. _____
>   _____

7. Break up a solid page of print with a variety of forms: underline, space, italicize, capitalize, enumerate, indent, box, summarize, and illustrate. Make your reading attractive and digestible.
8. Back up what you write by what you do; build a reputation for integrity.
9. Organize your material.
   a. Outline key points.
   b. Compile data into groups according to commonality.
   c. Arrange materials in a logical sequential order:
      (1) Chronological.
      (2) Cause-effect relationship.
      (3) Increasing complexity.
   d. Tie the groups together using transitional devices:
      (1) Time-order words (first, later, finally).
      (2) Guide words (as a result, therefore, on the other hand).
   e. Link the communication with the previous message by referring to:
      (1) Date.
      (2) Subject.
      (3) Sender of correspondence.
   f. Furnish appropriate excerpts from past correspondence.

■ Reread and revise your written communication. Look at the nouns and verbs; study the simplicity or wordiness of your sentences. Determine that you have said what you mean and that you mean what you said. Eliminate unneeded words.

■ You may want to add a personal handwritten note at the bottom.

Exercise 20–11	Evaluate a sample of your writing using the Gunning Mueller Fog Index presented in Exhibit 20–5. Evaluate this chapter using the same instrument.

Written Reports

Written reports should indicate how the nursing objectives are being met. If a twenty-four-hour nursing report is made from the patient units to the director of nursing, the information provided should show progress in relation to the achievement of unit and department objectives. The information should be provided in a simple, functional or practical, and qualitative rather than complex and quantitative manner. In providing the information, the reporter should consider its relative value and purpose, eliminate any overlap or duplication, and put the report in perspective. The report should indicate the workload and state pertinent facts describing patients' status, why the patients are hospitalized, and the nursing diagnosis and prescription. The following are other factors to consider in writing useful reports:

1. Size and cost of reports should not exceed need or strength.
2. A strong report will not be contaminated with individual bias. For that reason, a computer printout has value over a hand-prepared report.
3. A strong report will be useful to many people, providing them with vital information to run the operation.
4. A strong report will have authentic and reliable sources of information—people with knowledge and skills required to judge what information needs to be transmitted. Some information can be given by clerks, some by technicians, and some, of necessity, by the nurse manager.
5. If the report is going to a group of people with limited time, such as a board of directors, the report writer should add an executive summary at the beginning of the report and highlight what she or he wants the readers to act on. This may speed up their response.

Sometimes managers have a tendency to eliminate reports. Although the busy nurse manager may hope that reports would all be eliminated, doing so without consensus sometimes drives them underground. Since reports and forms tend to proliferate, every report or form should have an elimination date, at which time it will be eliminated unless it is rejustified.

Interviews

Interviewing is a basic tool of communication. A prospective employee is interviewed. If good counseling and guidance techniques are practiced, interviews are used to apprise employees of their performance. An interview is essential to

Exhibit 20–5   The Fog Index

The Gunning Mueller Fog Index presents a way to measure the reading ease of a piece of writing. It produces a number that approximates the grade level at which a person must read to comprehend the material. Here is how to use it.

Take a 100-word sample of your writing and

1. Find the average number of words per sentence. (If the final sentence in the sample runs beyond the hundredth word, use more than 100 words for this step.)
2. In the first 100 words, count the number of words that contain three or more syllables. Do not count proper nouns, combinations of short words like bookkeeper or manpower, or verbs made into three syllables by adding -ed or -es.

3. Add the average number of words per sentence and the number of words containing three or more syllables. Multiply the sum by 0.4.

The result tells you the grade level of the writing sample. Remember, the average person reads at about a ninth-grade level, and anything above a seventeenth-grade level is difficult for college graduates.

Caution: Do not let the formula restrict your writing. Use it only to spot-check your writing periodically. Slavish devotion to the formula could result in choppy writing.

Source: Reprinted with permission from "How to Write to Be Understood," Communications Briefings, *Business,* January–March 1985, 39–40.

practicing management by objectives because this is done on an employer–employee process. In disciplining an employee, it is necessary to interview the individual. When an employee leaves, an exit interview is desirable to learn why the person is leaving and to gain ideas for strengthening the personnel management program. Interview questions should be worded to obtain the most beneficial information. The following are suggestions for conducting effective interviews:

1. Use plain and direct language rather than technical, professional, or slang terms.
2. Keep questions short.
3. Use familiar illustrations.
4. Don't assume the interviewee knows something. Check the extent of the interviewee's knowledge beforehand.
5. Avoid improper emphasis so as not to indicate the answer you hope to elicit.
6. Be sure the interviewee gives words the same meaning as you do.
7. Be precise in picking words. Use accurate synonyms.
8. Use words with one pronunciation.

Organizational Publications

Barnard stated that the first function of an executive is to develop and maintain a system of communication.[33] The bigger the organization, the more difficult it is for the director of nursing to communicate to the employees who give direct care to patients. This problem is further complicated by the requirement for twenty-four-hour-a-day, seven-day-a-week services. The medium for communication between nurse executives and employees is an organizational publication such as a newsletter or in-house magazine. This publication does not have to be confined to nursing but can be supported and used by nursing staff. Certainly the nurse executive will have input into the development and evaluation of such an organizational publication.

Electronic Media

Electronic linkages are a key to a successful management strategy. To increase productivity in the workplace, nurse managers need to be aware of development within the telecommunications industry. Fax machines provide quick and accurate transmission of orders from physicians to nurses. Will they improve the output of clinical nurses if the nurses can use them to get drugs from the pharmacy more quickly and accurately? Will they improve response times and accuracy of diagnostic testing with linkage to medical laboratories, radiology, and other departments? Will fax machines increase therapeutic response times among clinical nurses, physicians and physical therapists, respiratory therapists, and others?

Numerous other electronic linkages are available, including computer bulletin boards for fast memos and software programs that can be used to control supply inventories and provide just-in-time supplies. Electronic networks provide sources of fast, up-to-date information about diagnoses and treatments. Cellular phones, electronic memo pads, and all the latest in telecommunications technology should be evaluated by nurse managers for use within and among patient-care units. They should be a part of the strategic planning process. Their adoption should be evaluated on the basis of value added to individual and corporate performances and cost/benefit analysis.

The management information system or nursing information system should be transformed into a customer information system. Lack of electronic memos or faxes or other communications may indicate to personnel and patients that a nurse manager is not listening.

OBTAINING INFORMATION

Receivers have a responsibility for obtaining information. Professional employees feel some conflict between their personal needs and the demands of the organization. Communication, the giving and receiving of information, helps an employee to control or tolerate this conflict. Assume that management controls the information that will be given to the employees. A conservative manager will give employees as little information as possible, since that manager considers that too much information might be distorted or misunderstood.

A director of nursing stated that although the registered nurse in the recovery room was totally competent, she would not give her the title of nurse manager and bring her to nurse manager meetings because she would misinterpret the statements made there. The enlightened manager—a time leader—will be direct and honest, believing that employees need all the information they can get to do their job. Bad news usually leaks, and trying to keep it covered up only creates distrust and anxiety.

Communication of information is a joint responsibility of employer and employee. If you need to know something, ask. Find out how your organization is developing and what its future prospects are. Learn whether its requirements continue to be compatible with your personal goals.

THE FUTURE

Survival in the information age will depend upon a combination of technology and strategic insights. Service organizations will have to find people who need services and deliver these services to them. During the past 6,000 years, information has belonged to the power structure, which did not trade it, market it, or give it away. The service industries of the information age will market services that are heavily information-based.

Technology is always in arrears; both people and systems can quickly become obsolete. Managers should go after strategic, not technical, gains. They should not computerize what does not work or maintain obsolete technology in hiring people. The people have to be developed and updated, adjusted to the system, or they will career hop within and without the organization. Turnover is expensive, as it throws away assets. Human resource assets generate more value added when they are managed, enriched, and involved in the enterprise.[34]

Organizations

A successful organization has effective communication at all levels. A good communication system does the following:[35]

- Aids in cost savings, improves efficiency, and enhances productivity. People who know the system uncover and fix any problems.
- Keeps management better informed as it supports trust.
- Keeps employees informed of the company's plans, policies, goals, philosophies, and requirements. Informed employees act positively.
- Improves morale. Information means happy employees not swayed by outside influences.
- Makes employees feel they are part of a team. Again—spirit and trust support common goals.
- Maintains a work environment free of outside adversaries and unwanted third-party influences.
- Provides some confidentiality for mutual trust and respect.
- Responds promptly and completely.
- Provides a means for employees to ventilate.
- Provides sufficient information.
- Recognizes employees as individuals.

WEB ACTIVITIES

- ■ Visit www.jbpub.com/swansburg, this text's companion website on the Internet, for further information on Communications.
- ■ What resources are available through the Internet for discovering new listening methods?
- ■ What organizations or journals could you search for information on future impacts on communication?

SUMMARY

Communication occurs between numerous groups of people. It includes a sender, a receiver, and a message. Communication is a product of perception and is different from information. It can be improved by feedback. Communication occurs between people *only if they want it to*. The products of lack of communication—misinformation, misunderstanding, waste, fear, suspicion, insecurity, and low morale—are too costly to accept.

People have difficulty accepting the fact that communication is not the answer to all the problems of human relations and personnel management. A gap exists between senders and receivers that must be recognized before it can be bridged—a gap in background, experience, and motivation.

Good communication is frequently an illusion. It is not achieved with open doors, geniality, or jokes. It is helped by listening to what people are really saying and perceiving what they are projecting through their words, their facial expressions, their tone of voice, and their actions. To induce greater numbers of people to accept direction and not undermine it, these people must be encouraged to participate. They will listen for genuineness in the word of the boss as demonstrated by actions.

Communication is achieved through both the spoken and the written word in a number of arenas, such as meetings, interviews, speeches, and computers. Today, a great deal of communication is done through electronic media. Good communication requires both good sending and good listening (receiving) skills.

NOTES

1. J. Anderson, "What's Blocking Upward Communication?" *Personnel Administration,* January–February, 1968, 5+.
2. P. Morgan and H. K. Baker, "Building a Professional Image: Improving Listening Behavior," *Supervisory Management,* November 1985, 34–36; J. A. Griver, "Communication Skills for Getting Ahead," *AORN Journal,* August 1979, 242–249.
3. W. J. Corbett, "The Communication Tools Inherent in Corporate Culture," *Personnel Journal,* April 1986, 71–72, 74.
4. G. S. Wlody, "Communicating in the ICU: Do You Read Me Loud and Clear?" *Nursing Management,* September 1984, 24–27.
5. M. J. Farley, "Assessing Communication in Organizations," *Journal of Nursing Administration,* December 1989, 27–31.
6. P. S. O'Sullivan, "Detecting Communication Problems," *Nursing Management,* November 1985, 27–30.
7. C. H. Smeltzer, "The Art of Negotiation: An Everyday Experience," *Journal of Nursing Administration,* July/August 1991, 26–30.
8. Ibid.
9. P. F. Drucker, *Management: Tasks, Responsibilities, Practices* (New York: Harper & Row, 1973), 483.
10. W. D. St. John, "Leveling with Employees," *Personnel Journal,* August 1984, 52–57.
11. A. Levenstein, "Feedback Improves Performance, *Nursing Management,* February 1984, 64, 66.
12. A. Levenstein, "Back to Feedback," *Nursing Management,* October 1984, 60–61.
13. R. M. Kanter, *When Giants Learn to Dance* (New York: Simon & Schuster, 1989), 108–114.
14. P. F. Drucker, op. cit., 487–489.
15. R. Haakenson, "How to Be a Better Listener," *Notes & Quotes* No. 297, February 1964, 3.
16. P. Morgan and H. K. Baker, op. cit.
17. L. Sousa, "We Need to Teach Life 101," *San Antonio Express-News,* 1 May 1993, 6B.
18. J. R. Gibb, "Defensive Communication," *Journal of Nursing Administration,* April 1982, 14–17.
19. D. E. Shields, "Listening: A Small Investment, A Big Payoff," *Supervisory Management,* July 1984, 18–22.
20. N. Stewart, "Listen to the Right People," *Nation's Business,* January 1963, 60–63.
21. J. Guncheon, "To Make People Listen," *Nation's Business,* October 1967, 96–102.
22. J. H. Woods, "Affective Learning: The Door to Critical Thinking," *Holistic Nursing Practitioner,* April 1993, 64–70.
23. T. Peters, *Thriving on Chaos* (New York: Harper & Row, 1981), 524–532.
24. N. B. Sigband, "Listen to What You Can't Hear?" *Nation's Business,* June 1969, 70–72.
25. R. Davies, "Managing by Listening," *Nation's Business,* September 1992, 6.
26. T. Peters, op. cit., 608–613.
27. W. Bennis and B. Nanus, *Leaders: The Strategies for Taking Charge* (New York: Harper & Row, 1985), 14, 33–43, 106–108, 366–367.
28. E. D. Nathan, "The Art of Asking Questions," *Personnel,* July–August 1966, 63–71; M. A. Pulick, "How Well Do You Hear? *Supervisory Management,* November 1983, 27–31; P. Morgan and H. K. Baker, op. cit.
29. W. D. St. John, "You Are What You Communicate," *Personnel Journal,* October 1985, 40–43; D. Caruth, "Words: A Supervisor's Guide to Communication," *Management Solutions,* June 1986, 34–35.

30. H. P. Zelko, "How to Be a Better Speaker," *Notes & Quotes* No. 311, April 1965, 3.
31. R. Wilkinson, "Communication: Listening from the Market," *Nursing Management,* April 1986, 42J, 42L.
32. R. Dulik, "Making Personal Letters Personal," *Supervisory Management,* May 1984, 37–40.
33. C. I. Barnard, *The Functions of the Executive* (Cambridge, Mass.: Harvard University Press, 1938), 226.
34. P. A. Strassman and S. Zuboff, "Conversation with Paul A. Strassman," *Organizational Dynamics,* fall 1985, 19–34; A. J. Rutigliano, "Naisbitt and Aburdene on 'Re-Inventing' the Workplace," *Management Review,* October 1985, 33–35.
35. K. L. Gilberg, "Open Communication Provides Key to Good Employee Relations," *Supervision,* April 1993, 8–9.

21

NURSING INFORMATICS

OBJECTIVES

- Differentiate among elements of an NMIS.
- Illustrate uses of an NMIS.
- Discuss future uses of NMISs.

KEY CONCEPTS

artificial intelligence
data
database
expert system
hardware
information system
program
spreadsheet
word processing
(See also Appendix 21–1, "Glossary of Commonly Used Computer Terms.")

Manager behavior: Supports those computerized operations of other departments that impact nursing.

Leader behavior: Plans informatics that improve nursing operations, including management, education, research, and clinical practice. Does so with input from representative nurses.

As the year 2000 approaches, it is time we all face the fact that the technorevolution is firmly upon us. "The process of computerization is moving through our world with the power of its own momentum, transforming our experiences of life and culture."[1] Wherever we turn, we encounter products of the computer age: watches, automatic teller machines, credit and debit cards, televisions and VCRs, home appliances, FAX machines, home computers, and computers in the workplace are just a few. The realization is that we need to come to terms with the problems and opportunities computers in our society present.[2]

The challenge of embracing and utilizing computers will be critical for the management of health care in transition. Nurses will have to assimilate the knowledge and expertise required to understand and interact with this constantly changing technology, and then they must be capable of teaching this new knowledge and expertise to others. Any barriers to these assimilation and conveyance processes will need to be overcome.

Ethical and legal issues will need to be advanced in scope to address new and changing technology. Concepts of privacy, confidentiality, and security should be instilled in nursing personnel not only in terms of operational guidelines (data and physical security, policies, and procedures) but also in terms of professionalism and responsibility. Control of information needs to be taught as a management issue, not a technical one.

Computer interaction may be further complicated by exposure to multiple hardware and software platforms. There will be a new focus towards the integration of these distributed and often highly differentiated environments. The problems of computer phobia may be lessened with the implementation of graphical user interfaces (GUI, a visual system by which the user will interact with the computer) and pointing devices. The tools used by nurses should also be representative of these changes as interactive multimedia becomes commonplace.

As computers are brought into the home and are increasingly used in elementary, middle, and high school education, they are also being incorporated into our nursing curriculums at advanced levels. They are being merged into all facets of professional nursing. This explosive growth of computer use in health care, the complexity and cost of different computer systems, and rapid changes in health-care computer technologies place nurses in critical positions. Nurses must have knowledge of computers and information systems in general and an understanding of the key issues involved in automation in order to make computer tools useful to nursing practice.[3]

THE STATE OF THE ART

"State of the art" is one of those phrases that in the beginning meant a set of circumstances characterizing a craft or its principles, or a branch of learning.[4] Now it tends to be a cliché that salespeople and consultants commonly use to impress upon others the idea that something is as advanced as is technologically possible. Even nursing information systems specialists use the cliché. For example, Romano states, "To prepare nurses to practice in the increasingly technological environments of the future, and to direct and control the impact of technology on nursing are no small challenges. An awareness and involvement with the state of the art of computers and technology in health care can be that awesome first step."[5] In describing computing resources to support nursing informatics, Heller et al. stated, "In addition to existing computing resources available in the school of nursing and throughout the campus, a state-of-the-art microcomputer laboratory was dedicated to support the specialization in Nursing Informatics."[6]

The problem with the state of the art is that the development cycle for a new generation of a technological product, such as a microprocessor, is now approximately eighteen months.[7] However, the many new products now being marketed make the state of the art today old technology in a few months. With this in mind, this chapter presents a scenario of what today's environment could be like if current technology were used.

Hardware

Even in this era of downsizing, many companies may view their mainframe as the center of a large, corporatewide network. The mainframe is a hub connecting distributed minicomputers and PC/LAN (personal computer/local area network) clusters. It serves as an information reservoir, siphoning data to PCs, workstations, and minicomputers.[8] A minicomputer may be used to handle the needs of a large nursing department and may also serve as a hub connecting workstations and microcomputer-based LANs.

A LAN cluster is the focus of hardware for each nursing department. Workstations and microcomputers act as point-of-care technology centers at patients' bedsides. These computers can integrate computerized patient monitoring systems that measure ECG, arterial blood pressure, pulmonary artery pressure, temperature, chest drainage, urine, cardiac output, respiratory cycle, pulse, tidal volume, peak airway pressure, blood I/O, and fluid I/O.[9] These point-of-care computers would have color displays and be capable of 3-D graphics and full-motion video. Interaction would be via a pointing device—one's finger, a mouse, or a light pen. A camera would supply the capability for video interaction and monitoring. Finally, stacks of compact disc drives are attached to provide access to a neverending electronic library.

Software

State-of-the-art software centers around an open-systems model and a multitasking operating system. The open-systems approach seeks to integrate many different software environments, regardless of their hardware platforms. A multitasking operating system provides greater computing power and efficiency for the end user. The workplace is managed through a graphical user interface, and diverse automated systems are integrated and presented via interactive multimedia.

Interactive multimedia combine full-motion video, narration, art and animation, text, and stereo sound. They allow people to interact with information from multiple sources in new ways. The same information may be expressed simultaneously from many different points of view. This new medium will replace paper and printed information as we know them.[10]

Barriers to Computerization

The first barrier to overcome in dealing with computers is computer phobia. A general fear of change seems to exist within us all, and for some, being forced to work with computers elicits common reactions of apprehension and anxiety. The following are some tips for helping others to conquer computer phobia:[11]

- Do not procrastinate.
- Seek a nonthreatening environment, one in which everyone will feel comfortable.
- Maintain a positive attitude that learning will take place. Fear of not learning is a problem.
- Encourage hands-on opportunities.
- Indicate that knowing how to type is helpful but not essential.
- Do not allow the use of computer jargon. Use words that everyone understands.

- Insist that learning sessions last less than two hours and not cover too many subjects.
- Encourage note taking.
- Do not allow interruptions.
- Encourage assertiveness and requests for help.
- Encourage practice.
- Encourage everyone to relax!

Other reasons for computer phobia would be the fear of making mistakes and erasing data and the fear that jobs will be lost. Computer phobia can be overcome through proper management, education, and hands-on training.

Another barrier to using computers centers around the perception of cost versus benefit. The Health and Human Services Secretary's Commission on Nursing projected that health-care institutions allocate approximately 2.5 percent of their operating budget for information technology. In contrast, other service industries, such as banking and insurance, allocate from 7 percent to 10 percent. The inappropriateness of this low allocation of revenues is that health care is more information-intensive than the figures imply.[12]

Often administrators and nurses have a hard time believing that computer technology can enhance productivity and improve quality. Although some studies appear to show that computerized information systems are a time-saver, nurses may circumvent the information system, thus defeating the time savings. Even if time from paperwork is saved, there is concern that nurses will not use this time to focus on patient care.[13] Managers should become involved by researching information technology, installed or planned, and determining whether such technology is beneficial to nursing. Finding it so, they should inform others about its positive effects and advantages.

A final barrier relates to a system whose capabilities do not meet the organization's needs. Nurses who feel that the information system does not promote their clinical decision making and that it will detract from the amount of time spent doing patient care will not use it. This is usually a result of not involving staff nurses in the decision-making process from beginning to end. The solution seems to be to involve the staff in any decisions related to automation. Staff should be allowed to develop the system and fit it to the organization.

Ethical, Legal, and Security Issues

Certain ethical issues are involved in the use of technology in nursing. "Ethical" means conforming to professional standards of conduct. "Privacy means control over exposure of self or information about oneself and freedom from intrusion. Privacy denotes the right of an individual to decide how much personal information to share. It includes a right to secrecy of information and protection against the misuse or release of this information."[14] "Confidentiality" means being entrusted with the privacy of others. The relationship of the three terms can be expressed as a patient entrusting privacy to a professional who has an ethical responsibility to maintain the confidentiality of that privacy.

Legal issues associated with automation may involve the confidentiality of patient information and the risk associated with clinical decision making based upon computerized information. One method of addressing such issues is by maintaining professional standards. Information systems should be designed, developed, and implemented to validate patient outcomes and support professional nursing standards. This means that computer technology for nursing use needs to be based upon nursing input from start to finish. This requires the use of expert nurses who have sufficient clinical, theoretical, education, research, and management expertise to adequately represent professional standards. It also requires a unified nursing profession that can specify clear design criteria and professional standards guidelines.[15]

Nurses should be capable of assessing and managing the legal risks associated with automated information management. Computer data should be examined, analyzed, interpreted, and appraised. Forced selections and unclear logic should be questioned. Nurses should not hold as fact the belief that clinical decision making based upon the use of technology results in better patient care.

The American Nurses Association, the American Medical Records Association, and the Canadian Nurses Association offer the following guidelines and strategies for minimizing legal risks associated with automated charting:[16]

- Never give your computer password to anyone.
- Do not leave a computer terminal unattended after you've logged on.
- Follow procedure for modifying mistakes. Computer entries are part of the permanent record and cannot be deleted.
- Do not leave patient information displayed on a screen for others to see. Also, keep track of printed information about patients and dispose of it appropriately when it is no longer needed.
- Follow your institution's confidentiality policies and procedures.

Automation in nursing also involves security issues. "Security" means the level to which hardware, software, and information are safe from abuse and unauthorized use or access, whether accidental or intentional. From a management standpoint, professionals need to be aware that security must be overseen from physical, operational, and ethical viewpoints.

Physical security deals with the control of access to hardware, the assessment and determination of environmental threats, and the prevention of loss of information. Operational security deals with the threats to information and includes the assessment and prevention of unauthorized access or use of information, the policies and procedures governing the management of information, and the procedures required for recovery from loss of information. Ethical security deals with the individual's ability to conform to professional standards of conduct. This means that nurses have to respect the privacy of information and accept and enforce all guidelines that are imposed for the maintenance of physical and operational security of computer systems.

Nurses should be aware of various security measures that may be built into information systems. One of the first things they should have is the ability to perform auditing. This means leaving a trail of who did what, where, and when. Logs can record who, when, and where the system is accessed. This same information can be captured when vital information is created, modified, or deleted. Once this information is captured, standard procedures should be in place for the routine auditing of the information.

A significant amount of security may be associated with an individual's computer ID. Every individual should be assigned his or her own personal ID with the individual's name, title, department, security level, and menu linked to it. Each user should have a password that protects the user's ID and is known only by the user. Procedures should be in place to force users to change their password every thirty to ninety days and allow them to change their password more often as desired. Also, a number of each user's old passwords should be stored for comparison purposes, and users should not be allowed to reuse these passwords.

The security level should be implemented in a hierarchical manner from administrator to nursing assistant. It can be a range of numbers from largest to smallest that can be tested to determine who can perform particular functions. Menus that determine the capability to interact with the system should be developed and assigned based upon departmental and job requirements.

Exercise 21–1   You note that a nurse is accessing health-care records of other agency personnel. Outline a course of action to take to remedy this breach of ethics and confidentiality. (This may be done as a group exercise.)

GENERAL-PURPOSE MICROCOMPUTER SOFTWARE

Today's nursing management should be prepared to support increasing use of automation in all areas of nursing. Part of this support includes a greater interaction with microcomputers. Many nursing professionals come in contact with microcomputers daily. Nurses use microcomputers in such areas as patient-care documentation, budgeting, policy and procedure documentation, personnel records, patient and staff education, and inventory control. Some of the general-purpose programs available for nurses include spreadsheet programs, word-processing and desktop publishing programs, database management programs, graphics programs, communication programs, and integrated programs.

Spreadsheets

A spreadsheet is a tool used to record and manipulate numbers. Originally spreadsheets were paper ledgers used for business accounting, such as the recording of debits and credits. With the coming of the microcomputer, electronic spreadsheets were developed. An electronic spreadsheet is a software package that turns a microcomputer into a highly sophisticated calculator. Huge quantities of numbers can be recorded, manipulated, and stored quite simply and easily. A nurse could use the information from spreadsheets to maintain statistics (Exhibit 21–1), create graphics (Exhibit 21–2), and plan budgets (Exhibit 21–3).

Exhibit 21–1 Example Statistics for New Hires and Terminations

Nursing Orientation Statistics

Hires	Jan	Feb	Mar	Apr	May	Jun	Jul	Aug	Sep	Oct	Nov	Dec	Total
RNs	10	6	8	5	7	27	11	8	13	3	3	5	106
LPNs	3	3	6	1	2	11	5	2	7	4	2	1	47
USs	0	0	0	0	2	1	0	0	2	0	1	0	6
NAs	1	0	0	3	0	2	0	1	1	1	1	0	10
Terminations													
RNs	11	4	10	6	3	17	8	11	9	5	1	1	86
LPNs	2	5	4	1	3	8	3	5	3	5	1	1	41
USs	0	0	0	1	1	1	0	0	2	0	1	0	6
NAs	1	0	1	2	0	2	0	1	1	1	1	0	10

Exhibit 21–2 Example Pie Graph

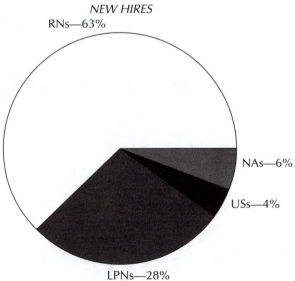

Nursing Orientation Statistics 19XX

NEW HIRES
RNs—63%
NAs—6%
USs—4%
LPNs—28%

Exhibit 21–3 Example Budget

Hospital Information Systems Budget
October 19xx–September 19xx

Pg 1: Oct 'xx–Jan 'xx

Sub Code	Description	Original Budget	Balance Available	Percent Used	Oct 'xx Current	Year	Nov 'xx Current	Year	Dec 'xx Current	Year	Jan 'xx Current	Year
1600	Student Wages	$12,000	($514)	104%	$373	$373	$786	$1,160	$1,612	$2,2771	$1,121	$3,892
1660	Accrued Salaries	$0	(567)	0%	$214	$214	$229	$443	$183	$626	(314)	$312
	Salaries	$12,000	($1,081)	109%	$587	$587	$1,015	$1,603	$1,795	$3,397	$807	$4,204
2110	Medical/Surgical Supplies	$100	$54	46%		$0		$0		$0		$0
2130	Drugs	$0	($8)	0%	$2	$2		$2		$2	$0	$2
	Medical/Surgical Supplies	$100	$46	54%	$2	$2		$2	$0	$2	$0	$2
2320	Office Supplies	$500	$291	42%	$35	$35	$3	$38	$23	$61	$6	$67
2330	Copying and Binding	$200	$97	51%	$14	$14	$3	$17	$6	$23	$43	$66
2340	Printing	$0	($64)	0%		$0		$0	$1	$1		$1
2400	Housekeeping Supplies	$0	($7)	0%		$0		$0		$0		$0
2500	Maintenance Supplies	$100	$100	0%		$0		$0		$0		$0
2700	Food Expense	$0	$0	0%		$0		$0		$0		$0
	General Supplies	$800	$418	48%	$49	$49	$6	$55	$30	$85	$49	$134
3110	Travel	$0	($220)	0%		$0		$0		$0		$0
3140	Local Travel	$0	($245)	0%	$18	$18	$34	$52	$4	$56	$13	$70
3160	Workshop and Training	$0	($68)	0%		$0		$0	$68	$68		$68
	Travel/Entertainment	$0	($535)	0%	$18	$18	$34	$52	$72	$124	$13	$138
3230	Contract Labor	$0	$0	0%		$0		$0		$0		$0
3290	Computer Software	$700	$340	51%		$0	$279	$279		$279		$279
3360	Equipment Maintenance/Repair	$500	$160	68%		$0		$0		$0		$0
3370	Maintenance Contracts	$1,560	$312	80%		$0		$0		$0		$0
3410	Equipment Rental	$0	($70)	0%		$0		$0		$0		$0
3650	Telephone Base	$100	$64	36%		$0	$31	$31	$5	$36		$36
3660	Telephone—Long Distance	$0	($4)	0%		$0		$0		$0		$0
3720	Books and Subscriptions	$0	($60)	0%		$0		$0		$0		$0
	Other Expenses	$2,860	$742	74%	$0	$0	$310	$310	$5	$315	$0	$315
5050	Minor Equipment (<$500)	$1,500	$707	53%	$0	$0	$450	$450	$139	$589	($139)	$450
	Minor Equipment Expenses	$1,500	$707	53%	$0	$0	$450	$450	$139	$589	($139)	$450
	Total Expenses	$17,260	$298	98%	$657	$657	$1,815	$2,472	$2,041	$4,513	$730	$5,243

Exhibit 21–3 Example Budget *(continued)*

Hospital Information Systems Budget
October 19xx–September 19xx

Pg 2: Feb 'xx–May 'xx

Sub Code	Description	Original Budget	Balance Available	Percent Used	Feb 'xx Current	Year	Mar 'xx Current	Year	Apr 'xx Current	Year	May 'xx Current	Year
1600	Student Wages	$12,000	($514)	104%	$1,087	$4,979	$984	$5,963	$1,046	$7,010	$1,103	$8,113
1660	Accrued Salaries	$0	($567)	0%	$21	$333	$76	$409	($20)	$389	$247	$636
	Salaries	$12,000	($1,081)	109%	$1,108	$5,312	$1,060	$6,372	$1,026	$7,399	$1,350	$8,749
2110	Medical/Surgical Supplies	$100	$54	46%	$2	$2		$2	$2	$4	$5	$8
2130	Drugs	$0	($8)	0%	$2	$2		$2		$2	$1	$3
	Medical/Surgical Supplies	$100	$46	54%	$2	$4	$0	$4	$2	$6	$6	$12
2320	Office Supplies	$500	$291	42%	$3	$70	$141	$211	$17	$228	$16	$244
2330	Copying and Binding	$200	$97	51%	$10	$76		$76		$76	$21	$97
2340	Printing	$0	($64)	0%	$39	$40		$40		$40	$6	$46
2400	Housekeeping Supplies	$0	($7)	0%	$2	$2		$2	$2	$4		$4
2500	Maintenance Supplies	$100	$100	0%		$0		$0		$0		$0
2700	Food Expense	$0	$0	0%		$0		$0		$0		$0
	General Supplies	$800	$418	48%	$53	$188	$141	$329	$19	$348	$43	$391
3110	Travel	$0	($220)	0%		$0		$0	$220	$220		$220
3140	Local Travel	$0	($245)	0%		$70	$53	$122		$122	$39	$162
3160	Workshop and Training	$0	($68)	0%		$68		$68		$68		$68
	Travel/Entertainment	$0	($533)	0%	$0	$138	$53	$190	$220	$411	$39	$450
3230	Contract Labor	$0	$0	0%		$0		$0		$0		$0
3290	Computer Software	$700	$340	51%		$279		$279		$279	$102	$381
3360	Equipment Maintenance/Repair	$500	$160	68%		$0	$8	$8	$68	$76		$76
3370	Maintenance Contracts	$1,560	$312	80%	$1,644	$1,644	$84	$1,728		$1,728	($891)	$838
3410	Equipment Rental	$0	($70)	0%		$0		$0		$0		$0
3650	Telephone Base	$100	$64	36%	$36	$36		$36		$36		$36
3660	Telephone—Long Distance	$0	($4)	0%		$0		$0	$4	$4		$4
3720	Books and Subscriptions	$0	($60)	0%		$0	$60	$60		$60		$60
	Other Expenses	$2,860	$742	74%	$1,644	$1,959	$152	$2,111	$72	$2,183	($788)	$1,395
5050	Minor Equipment (<$500)	$1,500	$707	53%	$15	$465	$119	$584	$0	$584		$584
	Minor Equipment Expenses	$1,500	$707	53%	$15	$465	$119	$584	$0	$584	0	$584
	Total Expenses	$17,260	298	98%	$2,822	$8,065	$1,525	$9,591	$1,340	$10,931	$650	$11,581

(continued)

Exhibit 21–3 Example Budget *(continued)*

Hospital Information Systems Budget
October 19xx–September 19xx

Pg 3: Jun 'xx–Sep 'xx

Sub Code	Description	Original Budget	Balance Available	Percent Used	Jun 'xx Current	Year	Jul 'xx Current	Year	Aug 'xx Current	Year	Sep 'xx Current	Year
1600	Student Wages	$12,000	($514)	104%	$1,019	$9,132	$1,818	$10,950	$1,564	$12,514		$12,514
1660	Accrued Salaries	$0	($567)	0%	($557)	$579	($325)	$254	$313	$567		$567
	Salaries	$12,000	($1,081)	109%	$962	$9,711	$1,493	$11,204	$1,877	$13,081	$0	$13,081
2110	Medical/Surgical Supplies	$100	$54	46%	$20	$29	$5	$34	$13	$46		$46
2130	Drugs	$0	($8)	0%	$5	$8		$8		$8		$8
	Medical/Surgical Supplies	$100	$46	54%	$25	$37	$5	$42	$13	$54	$0	$54
2320	Office Supplies	$500	$291	42%	($54)	$191	$16	$207	$2	$209		$209
2330	Copying and Binding	$200	$97	51%		$97	$3	$100	$3	$103		$103
2340	Printing	$0	($64)	0%		$46	$18	$64		$64		$64
2400	Housekeeping Supplies	$0	($7)	0%	$2	$6		$6	$1	$7		$7
2500	Maintenance Supplies	$100	$100	0%		$0		$0		$0		$0
2700	Food Expense	$0	$0	0%		$0		$0		$0		$0
	General Supplies	$800	$418	48%	($52)	$339	$37	$376	$6	$382	$0	$382
3110	Travel	$0	($220)	0%		$220		$220		$220		$220
3140	Local Travel	$0	($245)	0%		$162	$59	$220	$25	$245		$245
3160	Workshop and Training	$0	($68)	0%		$68		$68		$68		$68
	Travel/Entertainment	$0	($533)	0%	$0	$450	$59	$508	$25	$533	$0	$533
3230	Contract Labor	$0	$0	0%		$0		$0		$0		$0
3290	Computer Software	$700	$340	51%	$75	$456		$456	($97)	$360		$360
3360	Equipment Maintenance/Repair	$500	$160	68%	$64	$140		$140	$200	$340		$340
3370	Maintenance Contracts	$1,560	$312	80%	$137	$975	$137	$1,112	$137	$1,249		$1,249
3410	Equipment Rental	$0	($70)	0%	$70	$70		$70		$70		$70
3650	Telephone Base	$100	$64	36%		$36		$36		$36		$36
3660	Telephone—Long Distance	$0	($4)	0%		$4		$4		$4		$4
3720	Books and Subscriptions	$0	($60)	0%		$60		$60		$60		$60
	Other Expenses	$2,860	$742	74%	$346	$1,741	$137	$1,878	$240	$2,118	$0	$2,118
5050	Minor Equipment (<$500)	$1,500	$707	53%	$209	$793		$793		$793		$793
	Minor Equipment Expenses	$1,500	$707	53%	$209	$793	$0	$793	$0	$793	$0	$793
	Total Expenses	$17,260	$298	98%	$1,490	$13,071	$1,730	$14,801	$2,161	$16,962	$0	$16,962

A spreadsheet is made up of columns and rows of memory cells. These cells can be varied in size to allow for small or very large numbers. In addition to storing numbers, cells can store text and formulas. Text is used for titles, column and row headers, comments, and instructions. Formulas are used to perform the actual mathematical manipulation (addition, subtraction, multiplication, and division) of memory cells and their numbers, and even special math functions such as averages and standard deviations. Formulas are what really make a spreadsheet a powerful, number-crunching tool. Spreadsheets also have functions for copying, moving, inserting, and deleting cells. One of the most important spreadsheet functions is graphing, which allows numbers to be displayed in a graphic form. Exhibits 21–4 and 21–5 are examples of bar and line graphs, respectively.

Spreadsheets are the best tool to use in situations that require the management of a lot of numbers. For this reason, they are particularly pertinent to financial management, where they speed up such processes as budgeting, forecasting, and developing tables and schedules.

Exhibit 21–4   Example Bar Graph

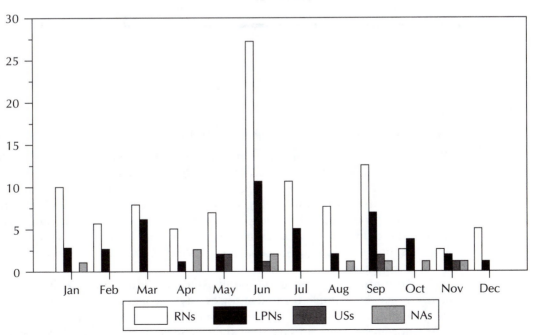

Nursing Orientation Statistics 19XX

NEW HIRES

Exhibit 21–5   Example Line Graph

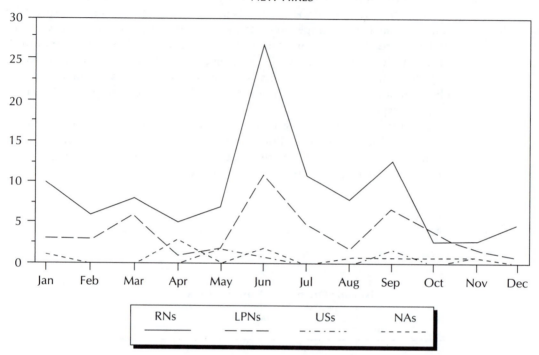

Nursing Orientation Statistics 19XX

NEW HIRES

| RNs | LPNs | USs | NAs |

Word Processing and Desktop Publishing

Word processing is the manipulation of words and special characters to produce a printed document. Desktop publishing is the manipulation of text and graphics to produce documents of publication quality. Five years ago, the difference between the two was vast. Today, each has incorporated aspects of the other. Among the documents that each can produce are memorandums and letters, policies/procedures, resumes, forms, envelopes and labels, instruction sheets, manuals, posters and signs, books, and newsletters. Exhibits 21–6 through 21–8 show a few examples.

Word-processing and desktop-publishing programs have facilities for the management of multiple document styles. Styles contain formatting codes that are grouped under a single structure. When applied to a section of text or an entire document, they can save time and ensure consistency.[17] A library of styles can be created and used among different documents. Styles can establish the following:

Exhibit 21–6   Example Memorandum

UNIVERSITY OF SOUTH ALABAMA
MEDICAL CENTER

HOSPITAL
INFORMATION
SYSTEMS

2451 FILLINGIM STREET
MOBILE, AL 36617
205-471-7679

September 13, 19XX

TO: Mr. Charles Jones
                Manager, Systems Programming

FROM: Richard J. Swansburg
                Management Systems Specialist

SUBJECT: Changes to Microcomputer Definition on 3745 Token-Ring

Please change the information related to Mr. Sanders' host connection via the 3745 Token-Ring network at USAMC. The old information is as follows:

Machine	Operating System	3270 Emulation	Token-Ring Address	Node I.D.	Logical Unit	Term I.D.	Home Printer	System Accesses
IBM 8590	OS/2	Communcations Manager	400004012590	B1011	H47LU02	AM6G	DPPG	CICS, HOSCICS, TSO

The new information is as follows:

Machine	Operating System	3270 Emulation	Token-Ring Address	Node I.D.	Logical Unit	Term I.D.	Home Printer	System Accesses
IBM 9552	DOS	PC3270	400004012552	B1011	H47LU02	AM6G	DPPG	CICS, HOSCICS, TSO

If you have any questions, please call.

Thank you.

Source: Reprinted courtesy University of South Alabama Medical Center, Mobile, Alabama.

- Font type, size, and style, such as `Courier 10-point normal`, *Times Roman 12-point italic,* **Helvetica 14-point bold,** or as small as ₄ to ₆ points.
- Spacing between lines and paragraphs.
- Margins and tabs.
- Page headers and footers.
- Footnote or outline formats.
- Paper size and type.

Exhibit 21–7   Example Policy Statement

UNIVERSITY OF SOUTH ALABAMA MEDICAL CENTER Hospital Information Systems	Approved by: Date: October 9, 19xx Page: 1 of 1

SUBJECT: Eating

Departmental employees will be allowed to eat within the department as long as the following guidelines are followed:

- All food and liquids will be consumed away from any computer equipment.
- No dishes, glasses, cups, silverware, trays, etc. will be brought out of the cafeteria. All dishes and silverware brought from home will be taken home in a timely manner.

- An appropriate trash container will be identified for the placement of all food and utensil waste disposal.
- Departmental personnel will be responsible for emptying the trash container as needed and at the end of each day.

Source: Reprinted courtesy University of South Alabama Medical Center, Mobile, Alabama.

Other tools that are often included in these programs are a spellchecker, a thesaurus, and a grammar checker. The speller contains a dictionary to which the text can be compared; words not in the program's dictionary can be added to a supplement. When the dictionary is invoked, words that it does not recognize are highlighted. A list of alternative words is generated, along with options to replace, edit, or add a word to the supplement. The thesaurus generates a list of synonyms and antonyms that can be used in place of selected words. The grammar checker is used to check the document for grammar and style errors. It will interpret the presentation of the subject and make recommendations for improvement.

Other utilities are available for performing block functions that operate on words, sentences, paragraphs, or pages within a document. These functions include copying, moving, deleting, italicizing, boldfacing, underlining, centering, and case conversion. Searching for and replacing particular words or phrases can be done by a simple request. Margins can be justified and words automatically hyphenated within set margins. Pages can be automatically defined and numbered.

Shell documents can be created where the main content of a document never changes but some areas are reserved for text that will change each time a new document is created from the shell. The best examples of this are in memorandums and letters, where the same memo or letter goes to many different destinations. The document and a list of variable information can actually be created separately and merged at printing time.

Exhibit 21–8 Example Form

SICK LEAVE

	E	U	B
Oct			
Nov			
Dec			
Jan			
Feb			
Mar			
Apr			
May			
Jun			
Jul			
Aug			
Sep			

TOTAL TIME

Reg | OT | Sick | Spec | Code

Calendar columns: SUN | MON | TUE | WED | THU | FRI | SAT

Legend:

8 Present (Enter Hrs Worked)
A Absent (No Pay)
(A) Absent on Hospital Business
S Sick (No Pay)
(S) Sick (Sick Leave Paid)
V Vacation
DO Day Off
H Holiday

HOLIDAYS

NY	MG	4TH	LD	TG	CH	PH1	PH2	PH3

VACATION

Remarks _____

Name _____
       Last,   First   Middle   Job Title _____

Address _____
       Department Perm/Temp Scheduled Hrs Department # Social Security # Employment Date

543

Database Management

A computer database is the electronic counterpart to the standard file cabinet and its contents. It is used to store data and can be manipulated for information much like paper files. Nurse managers could use a microcomputer and a database management program in place of a manual filing system to handle many of their information and record-keeping needs. Examples might include personnel records, education records, equipment inventory, and budget management.

A microcomputer database program allows for databases to be created by defining their record layouts and data fields. When a data field is defined, its length is set and the type of data that can be stored in it established. Data types can be character (allowing letters, numbers, and special symbols), numeric (allowing only numbers), logical (allowing only yes or no, true or false), or date (allowing only numbers in a date format). Exhibit 21–9 is an example of data fields, and Exhibit 21–10 is an example of actual data entry.

Once a database is created, procedures can be established to

- Create information.
- Modify information.
- Display information.
- Delete information.
- Generate printed reports.

Menus can be created to allow easy access to and execution of the procedures (see Exhibit 21–11 for an example). Most database tools have application generators that will lead the user through a series of steps to define a database, its procedures, and its menus. The greatest advantage to database management is the ease in maintaining information and the timely retrieval of this information in report format (illustrated in Exhibit 21–12).

The Nursing Management Minimum Data Set (NMMDS) is a research-based management data set available from the American Organization of Nurse Executives. NMMDS produces data for making nursing management decisions. It has seventeen elements clustered around three broad categories of environment, nurse resources, and financial resources. Implementing NMMDS empowers nurses with specific costs and quality data to answer questions related to such areas as outcomes of critical paths, turnover rates of personnel, nurse satisfaction, personnel ratings, budgets, and productivity. It provides data to compare time periods.[18]

Other databases include outcome measurement tools for rehabilitation that measure patients' levels of functional independence in the activities of daily living. They also measure progress and may be used to determine discharge to home, nursing home, or even back to the hospital, and other parameters of patient care.[19]

Exercise 21–2   Determine the extent to which databases are being used in the agency in which you work.

Exhibit 21–9   Example of Data Fields

TABLE=EMPLOYEE

******COLUMNS******

Column Name	Type	Length	Attributes
EMP_NAME	Character (Fixed)	30	Data required, Text
EMP_SSN	Character (Fixed)	9	Data required, Text
EMP_JOB_CODE	Character (Fixed)	1	Text
EMP_ASSIGN_NUM	Character (Fixed)	3	Text
EMP_POS_NUM	Character (Fixed)	6	Data required, Text
EMP_CLASS_CODE	Character (Fixed)	4	Text
EMP_CLASS_TITLE	Character (Fixed)	30	Text
EMP_JOB_STATUS	Character (Fixed)	2	Text
EMP_HIRE_DATE	Date		
EMP_TERM_DATE	Date		
EMP_PAY_ID	Character (Fixed)	1	Text
EMP_LIC_NO	Character (Fixed)	14	Text
EMP_LIC_REN_NO	Character (Fixed)	14	Text
EMP_LIC_DATE	Date		
EMP_LIC_EXP	Date		
EMP_LIAB_INS	Numeric	10	Integer
EMP_UNIT	Character (Fixed)	10	Text
EMP_SHIFT	Character (Fixed)	10	Text
EMP_ADDRESS_1	Character (Fixed)	30	Text
EMP_ADDRESS_2	Character (Fixed)	30	Text
EMP_CITY	Character (Fixed)	20	Text
EMP_STATE	Character (Fixed)	2	Text
EMP_ZIP	Character (Fixed)	10	Text
EMP_PHONE	Character (Fixed)	12	Text

Index Name:	EMPLOYEE
Duplicates Allowed:	No
Column Name	Order

Column Name	Order
EMP_NAME	Ascending
EMP_POS_NUM	Ascending

Graphics

Nurses can realize another valuable tool through the utilization of graphics programs. Such programs can produce graphics that can be used for presentations, illustrations, and teaching. Graphics can be printed, displayed to a monitor, or projected onto a screen for viewing by large numbers of people. They can also be converted to such presentation aids as overhead transparencies, videotapes, and slides.

In the past, graphics programs focused on the visual display of numerical data in the form of bar, line, and pie graphs. This relates to the early use of

Exhibit 21–10   Example of Data Entry

Change Employee Records

Name :   Swansburg, Richard J.   SSN :   987654321

Job Code :   P   Assignment # :   008   Position # :   00132
Class Code :   3187   Class Title :   Management Systems Spec II
Job Status :   11   Hire Date :   06-04-1979   Pay Code :   A

Address :   1110 Abilene Drive West
             —

City :   Mobile   State :   AL   Zip :   36695
Phone :   205 633 9172

Exhibit 21–11   Example of Database Menu

EMPLOYEE MENU

*** Select option with mouse or type letter for underlined option. ***

[Add Employee]

[Change/Display Employee]

[Change/Display Employee and Pay Period]

[Delete Employee]

[Print Employee Listing]

[Print Employee Pay Periods Listing]

[Print Selected Pay Period Listing]

graphics by business and management. Today, graphics systems can be used in a multitude of ways to visually illustrate almost anything. Features have been incorporated to display graphics like a slide show or with animation. Such presentation capability can be very helpful to the nurse trying to present information related to various clinical subjects. See Exhibits 21–13 and 21–14 for examples.

Graphics can be created in a number of ways. They can be created as part of the program in association with some numerical data; they can be scanned by a handheld or full-page scanner; they can be created freehand by the user; or they can be purchased as an add-on to the graphics program.

Exhibit 21–12 Example of Database Report

Employee Pay Periods Listing
Fiscal Year: 19xx–19xx

Employee Name	Pay Pd	Begin Date	Reg	OT	Hol	Vac	Sick	Other	Other	Other	Other	Vac Bal	Sick Bal	Comp Earned	Comp Taken	Comp Bal
Swansburg, Richard J.	01	09-20-19xx	78.25	—	—	—	1.75	—		—	—	172.58	828.39	3.00	—	78.50
	02	10-04-19xx	31.00	—	—	48.00	—	1.00	181	—	—	183.04	834.02	—	—	—
	03	10-18-19xx	64.00	—	—	8.00	—	8.00	181	—	—	140.28	836.72	—	—	—
	04	11-01-19xx	80.00	—	—	—	—	—		—	—	142.74	836.10	—	—	74.50
	06	11-29-19xx	80.00	—	—	—	—	8.00	181	—	—	163.66	849.37	—	—	—
	10	01-24-19xx	72.00	—	—	—	—	—		—	—	168.89	853.89	3.00	—	—
	11	02-07-19xx	80.00	—	—	—	—	—		—	—	174.12	848.75	—	—	81.50
	12	02-21-19xx	72.00	—	8.00	—	—	—		—	—	179.35	852.44	—	—	—
	13	03-07-19xx	80.00	—	—	—	—	—		—	—	184.58	856.13	—	—	81.00
	14	03-21-19xx	63.50	—	—	16.00	0.50	—		—	—	189.81	859.82	—	0.50	—
	15	04-04-19xx	75.50	—	—	—	3.00	1.50	181	—	—	179.04	863.01	3.00	—	—
	16	04-18-19xx	40.00	—	—	—	—	40.00	181	—	—	—	—	—	—	81.00
	17	05-02-19xx	24.00	—	—	56.00	—	—		—	—	173.51	839.40	—	—	81.00
	18	05-16-19xx	72.00	—	—	8.00	—	—		—	—	122.74	843.09	—	—	—
	19	05-30-19xx	80.00	—	—	—	—	—		—	—	119.97	846.78	—	—	81.00
	20	06-13-19xx	56.00	—	—	24.00	—	—		—	—	125.20	850.47	—	—	—
	21	06-27-19xx	70.00	—	8.00	—	—	2.00	181	—	—	106.43	854.16	—	—	84.00
	22	07-11-19xx	66.00	—	—	—	14.00	—		—	—	—	—	—	—	—
	23	07-25-19xx	80.00	—	—	—	—	—		—	—	116.90	845.55	—	—	—
	24	08-08-19xx	64.00	—	—	—	—	16.00	181	—	—	122.13	849.24	—	—	—
	25	08-22-19xx	80.00	—	—	—	—	—		—	—	—	—	—	—	—
	26	09-05-19xx	56.00	—	8.00	16.00	—	—		—	—	127.37	836.93	—	—	—

547

Exhibit 21–13 Example of Presentation Graphics to Discuss the Anatomy of the Ear

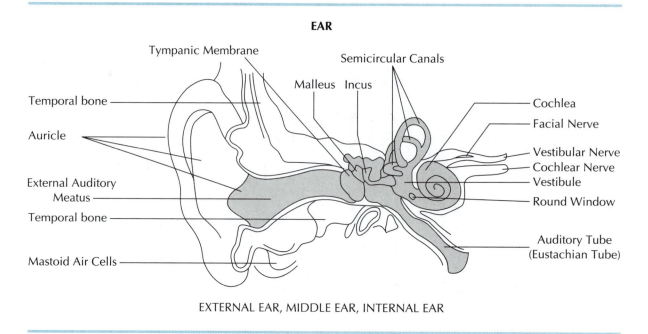

EXTERNAL EAR, MIDDLE EAR, INTERNAL EAR

Communications

Communications software permits nurses to access other computers for a variety of purposes. Such access may be in a dedicated manner (the link is maintained even when it is not in use), or it can be in a nondedicated manner (the link is maintained only while being used). Dedicated links can often be associated with access to the organization's information systems or access to resources on a LAN. Nondedicated links can be associated with access to various online services such as bulletin boards, support services, and remote information systems.

Communications can allow the nurse manager to support staff nurses in their interaction with information systems. The manager, when contacted about a problem, can access the system and mirror what the staff member is doing. The nurse manager can also use communications to move information in the form of a file transfer. This might be to transfer data to and from the host system (mainframe or minicomputer), across a LAN, or to another microcomputer, for example, a computer at home.

Integrated Software

Integrated programs seek to combine word processing, spreadsheets, database management, graphics, and communications. Such integration allows information to be readily moved among the components. A report being created in the

Exhibit 21–14   Example of Presentation Graphics to Discuss the Anatomy
of the Eye

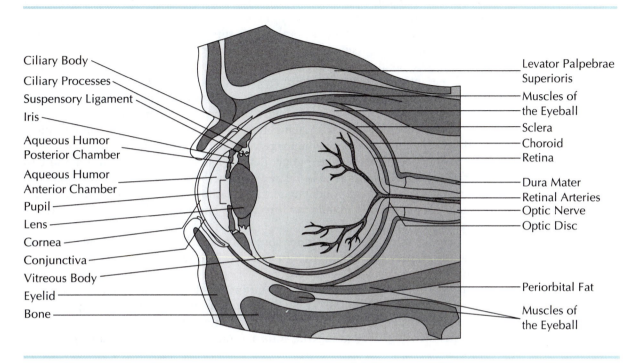

word processor can draw a table of numbers from the spreadsheet, draw a
graph from the graphics component, and add other information from a database.[20] The document can then be sent to another location via the communications component.

Such integration can simplify preparation and analysis of information.
However, integrated programs tend to lack the full functionality of programs in
the individual components' domains. The standard programs of today also provide excellent import and export facilities to most of the popular software in
other areas.

Exercise 21–3   Identify the software available to practicing nurses within your place of
employment. Is it current? If not, what can be done to make it current?

INFORMATION SYSTEMS

Nurses are beginning to find that the demands of working with automation
in nursing can be great. Nurses may be asked to interact with specialized and
generalized nursing information systems as well as with hospital information
systems.

Nursing Information Systems

Nursing information systems are software packages developed specifically for nursing usage. These programs may be explicit to a particular area of nursing application, or they may be general to the support of the nursing services division. Examples of nursing areas that can benefit from unique information systems support include mental health, neonatology, acute care, urology, enterostomal therapy, oncology, maternity, operating room, and infection control.

General nursing information systems have multiple programs, or modules, that are used to perform various clinical, education, and management functions. Most nursing information systems have modules for patient classification, staffing, scheduling, personnel management, and report generation. Other modules may be included, such as budget development, resource allocation and cost control, case mix and diagnosis-related groups (DRG) analysis, quality management, staff development, modeling and simulation for decision making, strategic planning, short-term demands for forecasting and work planning, and program evaluation.

Modules for patient classification, staffing, scheduling, personnel management, and report generation are often closely interrelated. Patients are classified according to established acuity criteria. The patient classification information is input into the staffing module, and staffing levels are calculated according to various workload formulas. Also, actual staffing is input, and a comparison of census, patient acuity, needed staffing, and actual staffing can be made. Schedules are then prepared using the information from the staffing and personnel records modules.

DRG analysis and quality management are done to associate patient acuity, quality of care, and DRG. This is helpful for establishing future guidelines and care needs for patients according to their DRGs. The budget is also supported by the census, patient acuity, and needed staffing patterns. This information is invaluable to support requests for additional full-time and part-time employees. The report generation module allows all of the stored information to be retrieved and output in a timely and presentable manner.

Nursing information systems can be used to make patient care more effective and economical. Clinical components include patient history and assessment, nursing care plans, nursing progress notes and charting, patient monitoring, order entry and results reporting, patient education, and discharge planning. This can all be done at the nurse's station or, with more progressive systems, from the patient's bedside.

Clinical nurses can use the nursing information system to replace manual systems of data recording. This may reduce costs while permitting improved quality of care as well as quality of work life. Clinical nurses can collect and input clinical data and use the computer to analyze it to formulate treatment plans. They can use quantitative decision analysis to support clinical judgments. Automated consultation can be applied to screen for adverse drug reactions, interactions, and preparation of correct dosages. Computers can be programmed to reject orders that could cause problems in these and other areas, thus preventing errors.[21]

Curtin reminds nurses to provide "high touch" in this inhuman high-tech world. Technology, computers, and information systems provide the knowledge to save lives or prolong them. Nurses can return to patients and families control over their lives when the latter have lost their freedom of action or understanding of events. Nurses can keep control of cybernetics through the exercise of human compassion.[22] High-tech includes the new scientific knowledge of microelectronics, computers, information, sensors, processors, displays, and education. Its objective is the solution of society's total problems, not just those of health care, including nursing.[23] Helping nurses provide high touch while using high-tech should be a primary goal of nurse managers.

Exercise 21–4   Identify the elements of the nursing information system in your place of work. How current is it? What improvement is needed?

Hospital Information Systems

Hospital information systems are large, complex computer systems designed to help communicate and manage the information needs of a hospital. They are tools for interdepartmental and intradepartmental use. A hospital information system will have applications for admissions, medical records, accounting, business services, nursing, laboratory, radiology, pharmacy, central supply, nutrition services, personnel, and payroll. Numerous other applications can exist for any department and for practically any purpose.

Admissions applications include patient scheduling, preadmission, admissions, discharges, transfers, and census procedures. Some medical records applications include master patient index maintenance, abstracting (diagnosis/procedure/DRG coding), transcription and correspondence, and medical record locator procedures. Business and accounting procedures include patient insurance verification, billing, billing follow-up, billing inquiry, accounts payable, accounts receivable, cash processing, and service master and third-party maintenance.

Applications in other areas, such as nursing (the nursing information system), laboratory, radiology, pharmacy, and central supply, may be so voluminous and complex that they have their own information systems. These systems stand alone and run independently of the hospital information system but are usually interfaced for information transfer.

Hospital information systems tend to be developed with mainframe and minicomputers in mind, although the trend today seems to be towards downsizing and distributed data networks. The advantages and disadvantages of each strategy should be weighed prior to information systems implementation. Selection, development, and implementation of information systems can take years. The time will vary depending on the system and the complexity of its applications. It may actually be a continuous process. The initial cost can be millions of dollars for the hardware and software. Continued yearly maintenance is required and can cost hundreds of thousands or even millions of dollars.

Implementation of Information Systems

Nurse managers should be involved in the implementation and development of information systems and the direction of their users. Implementation of an information system requires preparation of a management plan (see Exhibit 21–15). The first step is to form an implementation committee to assess the current system and what is wanted out of the proposed system. This assessment should lead to a strategic plan, as acquiring an information system requires expenditure of a large amount of human, material, and financial resources. It will include provision for continuous updates, a characteristic of a service economy in the information age.

Applications for Nursing Management

Many applications are available for nurse managers. In addition to those associated with the use of general-purpose microcomputer software, other applications might include a calendar of events, an employee database management system, and the use of interactive multimedia for staff and employee education.

A calendar can be useful in supplying clinical staff with dates and times of staff meetings, committee meetings, and educational events (see Exhibit 21–16). Educational events would include continuing education, annual reviews, and patient education. Information for the calendar can even be provided from the employee database.

An employee database management system can be an effective method of collecting and reporting nursing staff credentialing, special skills, and educational development. (See Exhibits 21–9 and 21–17 for examples of database field definitions.) Access to such information can identify employees' participation in education and employees with special skills or credentials. It can also identify employees facing credentialing renewal deadlines and those who need

---

Exhibit 21–15   Management Plan Worksheet

OBJECTIVE: Implement an information system

Activities	Target Dates	Person(s) Responsible	Accomplishments

Assessment
  Make strategic plan
  including a budget
	Sept. 1–15	Jay, Swansburg, Penne,
		  George, Gonzales,
		  Himmel	

Planning	Oct. 1–Nov. 15	Jay, Swansburg, Penne,
		  George, Gonzales,
		  Himmel	

Implementation	Jan. 1 _____	Swansburg and key users	
Evaluation (simultaneous)	Jan. 1 _____	Swansburg and key users	

Exhibit 21–16   Example Staff Development Calendar

Staff Development Calendar
October 19XX

Monday	Tuesday	Wednesday	Thursday	Friday
				1
4 Nursing Orientation Begins 8:00 AM Room 324 \n\n Nursing Assistant Course Intake/Output 7:30 – 8:30 AM 7:30 – 8:30 PM Room 334	**5** RNs and LPNs Understanding ECGs 7:30 – 8:30 AM 7:30 – 8:30 PM Room 334	**6** Diabetes Management Class 2:30 – 3:30 PM Room 334	**7** Diabetes Nutrition Class 2:30 – 3:30 PM Room 334	**8** RNs and LPNs Antibiotic Therapy 7:30 – 8:30 AM 7:30 – 8:30 PM Room 334
11 Nursing Assistant Course Body Mechanics 7:30 – 8:30 AM 7:30 – 8:30 PM Room 334	**12** RNs and LPNs Basic Genetics 7:30 – 8:30 AM 7:30 – 8:30 PM Room 334	**13**	**14**	**15** RNs and LPNs Understanding ECGs 7:30 – 8:30 AM 7:30 – 8:30 PM Room 334
18 ACLS Class Begins 8:00 AM Room 324 \n\n Nursing Assistant Course Intake/Output 7:30 – 8:30 AM 7:30 – 8:30 PM Room 334	**19** Annual Education Day Fire and Safety 8:00 – 11:30 AM Room 344 \n\n CPR 1:00 – 3:30 PM Room 354	**20** Diabetes Management Class 2:30 – 3:30 PM Room 334	**21** RNs and LPNs Antibiotic Therapy 7:30 – 8:30 AM 7:30 – 8:30 PM Room 334 \n\n Diabetes Nutrition Class 2:30 – 3:30 PM Room 334	**22**
25 Nursing Assistant Course Body Mechanics 7:30 – 8:30 AM 7:30 – 8:30 PM Room 334	**26**	**27** RNs and LPNs Basic Genetics 7:30 – 8:30 AM 7:30 – 8:30 PM Room 334	**28**	**29**

additional training. Exhibit 21–18 is an example of an employee education record. This information can also meet the reporting needs of the institution as to the requirements of the state board of nursing and the Joint Commission on Accreditation of Healthcare Organizations. Education components may include the following:[24]

- New employee orientation.
- Clinical specialty courses.
- Continuing education offerings.
- Competency validation of skills.
- Nursing station in-service education.
- Annual required reviews.

Exhibit 21–17   Example of Educational Course Data Fields

TABLE=EDCOURSE
******COLUMNS******

Column Name	Type	Length	Attributes
EDCOU_CODE	Character (Fixed)	6	Data required, Text
EDCOU_DESC	Character (Fixed)	35	Data required, Text
EDCOU_TYPE	Character (Fixed)	6	Data required, Text
EDCOU_CLAS_HRS	Numeric	5	Integer
EDCOU_CLIN_HRS	Numeric	5	Integer
EDCOU_CONT_HRS	Numeric	5	Integer

Index Name: EDTYPE
Duplicates Allowed: No

Column Name	Order
EDCOU_TYPE	Ascending
EDCOU_CODE	Ascending

TABLE=EMCOURSE
******COLUMNS******

Column Name	Type	Length	Attributes
EMCOU_CODE	Character (Fixed)	6	Data required, Text
EMCOU_POS_NUM	Character (Fixed)	6	Data required, Text
EMCOU_COMP_DATE	Date		
EMCOU_EVAL_CODE	Character (Fixed)	2	Text

Index Name: EMPOS
Duplicates Allowed: No

Column Name	Order
EMCOU_POS_NUM	Ascending

Exhibit 21–18   Example of Employee Education Record

EMPLOYEE EDUCATION RECORD
Employee Name   :   Jones, Mary L
Position Number :   353367
Nursing Unit   :   Med/Surg

Course Type	Description	Date Complete	Eval Code	Class Hours	Clinical Hours	Contact Hours
C	Antibiotic Therapy	10/08/93	S			1.0
	Basic Genetics	10/12/93	S			1.0
	Subtotal Continuing Education					2.0
I	Patient Monitoring	10/06/93	S	4.0		
	Infusion Pumps	10/06/93	S	1.0		
	Subtotal Inservice Education			5.0		
O	Personnel	10/04/93	S	2.0		
	Fire and Safety	10/04/93	S	3.0		
	Infection Control	10/04/93	S	3.0		
	Legal Issues	10/05/93	S	4.0		
	CPR	10/05/93	S	4.0		
	Information Systems	10/07/93	S	8.0		
	Unit Orientation	11/05/93	S		136.0	
	Subtotal Orientation			24.0	136.0	
S	IV Certification	10/08/93	S	3.0		
	Subtotal Skills Competency			3.0		
	Totals			32.0	136.0	2.0

Interactive multimedia are the educational medium of tomorrow. They have the capability of solving the problems related to education today.[25] They mix multiple media sources to provide interaction with the user. This method of instruction provides flexibility, independence for learners, reinforcement, and feedback. Students are able to control the presentation of content. They can work the program in any order and select and repeat segments as desired. The program provides students with immediate, individualized feedback based upon their answers to the program's questions.[26]

   The development and authoring of an interactive program involves a number of steps, the first of which is the determination of the content of the instructional program. The second step relates to the preparation of a script for the video components of the program. Next a flowchart is constructed to direct the authoring process. (Exhibit 21–19 is an example flowchart.) Finally, the computer programming is done using a software package developed specifically for interaction.[27] Such programs are commonly called authoring systems.

Exercise 21–5   Identify the elements of the agency information system that are helpful to nursing. How are they helpful? How can they be improved?

CURRICULUM AND CAREERS

It would appear that the time to start educating nurses about automation would be while they are in school. Exposing student nurses should begin at the undergraduate level by integrating informatics into the curriculum. This would include an introductory course in computer fundamentals, a course in the use of microcomputers and general-purpose software for enhancing per-

Exhibit 21–19   Example Flowchart

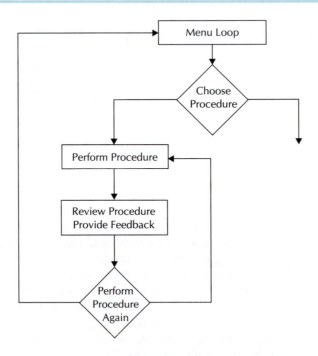

Source: Reprinted courtesy University of South Alabama Medical Center, Mobile, Alabama.

sonal productivity, and advanced incorporation of the computer into clinical education. The last two courses could be integrated into nursing courses and clinical experience.

A practice environment can be created with bedside terminals linked to an agency's or vendor's training system. The desire is to create a realistic effect by simulating an automated nursing station like those in hospitals today. Students can use the system to practice order entry, nursing assessments, care planning, and charting. They can learn how to combine high touch with high-tech.[28] Similar programs would be automated for long-term care and home health care.

This program could be taken a step further by collecting, analyzing, and organizing actual patient data into a clinical nursing abstract. Students could be taught nursing content based upon information from actual practice. For a particular diagnosis, students could study its interventions and outcomes. Assessment data could be accessed to examine etiologies, signs, symptoms, related medical diagnosis, and medical therapies.[29]

Today, there are several graduate programs with curricula for advanced degrees in nursing informatics. These programs are designed to provide specialized education for nurses interested in pursuing careers as nurse engineers, nursing information systems specialists, or systems nurses. These curricula should utilize an interdisciplinary approach. Courses would combine the study of nursing with theoretical and practical foundations of management and information sciences.[30]

A HUMAN RESOURCES INFORMATION SYSTEM

The management of human resources can be a formidable task for today's health-care organization. The collection and manipulation of information associated with such management can require significant time and personnel in itself. The development and implementation of a human resources information system can be a blessing to the organization and the professionals who manage these resources. Exhibit 21–20 is an example model of a human resources information system.

A couple of front-end systems can be established to analyze information related to all of the job applicants who apply to the organization and to analyze information related to the advertising and recruitment of these applicants. Some information needs to be retained on everyone who applies for any job position. This information can be useful for understanding the professional market. There are also concerns about equal opportunity based upon race or disability. The applications analysis system can show how many people apply for a position by these indicators. Exhibit 21–21 is an example applications analysis report. The advertising analysis system can provide recruitment information related to the method and placement of advertisements. Exhibit 21–22 is an example advertisement analysis report.

The central foundation of the human resources system is the employee database system. Individuals who are hired can be pulled from the applications analysis system and added to the employee system, which maintains all of the

Exhibit 21–20   An Example Human Resources Information System Model

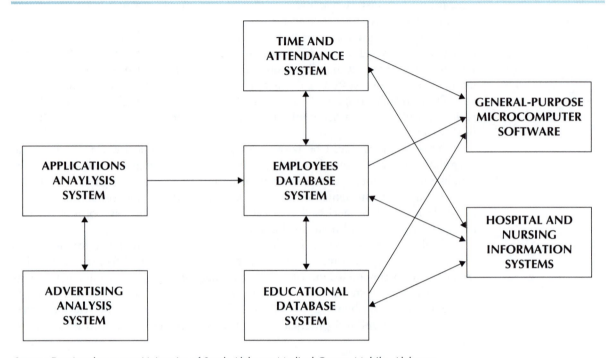

Source: Reprinted courtesy University of South Alabama Medical Center, Mobile, Alabama.

relevant information related to employees and their positions from the moment they are hired until they are terminated. See Exhibit 21–23 for an example of information placed on an ID card and Exhibit 21–24 for an example of a termination list. This part of the human resources system will be the basis for integrating additional components, such as an educational database system and a time and attendance system.

The educational system maintains all of the information associated with the education of employees (refer to Exhibit 21–18 for an example). The time and attendance system maintains the information associated with employees' work, vacation, holiday, and sick time. The information here produces timesheets (see Exhibit 21–25). From these systems, information can be exported and imported to the hospital and nursing information systems. It may also be exported to general-purpose microcomputer software for various purposes.

Exercise 21–6   Evaluate the agency's human resources information system where you are employed. What improvements, if any, are needed to make it state-of-the-art?

Exhibit 21-21 An Example Applications Analysis Report

Applications Analysis Report for the month of August 19xx

	POSITION	F	M	AM	AS	BA	CA	HI	PI	DIS	VET	DIS VET
01412	REGISTERED NURSE	3	0	0	0	2	1	0	0	0	0	0
02456	REGISTERED NURSE	2	0	0	0	1	1	0	0	0	0	0
02457	REGISTERED NURSE	6	2	0	1	2	4	1	0	0	0	0
11923	LICENSED PRACTICAL NURSE	7	0	0	0	5	2	0	0	0	0	0
15934	ASSISTANT ADMINISTRATOR	3	12	0	0	0	15	0	0	0	0	0
22921	UNIT SECRETARY	11	1	0	1	8	3	0	0	1	0	0
23110	EDUCATION SPECIALIST	5	2	0	0	2	5	0	0	0	1	0

Exhibit 21-22 An Example Advertisement Analysis Report

Advertisement Analysis Report for the month of August 19xx

ADD NUM	PLACEMENT	DATE	RN	LPN	PHR	PT	RT	CLK	MGR	OTH
1622	CHANNELS 4, 11	08/06/xx	3	2	0	0	1	0	0	5
1734	NEWSPAPER	08/08/xx	1	1	1	0	0	1	0	3
1622	CHANNELS 4, 11	08/13/xx	0	3	0	1	0	1	1	1
1734	NEWSPAPER	08/15/xx	5	0	0	0	1	3	0	2
1432	NEWSPAPER	08/15/xx	0	0	2	0	0	0	0	0
1622	CHANNELS 4, 11	08/20/xx	3	3	0	0	0	2	0	7
1734	NEWSPAPER	08/22/xx	8	3	0	2	3	0	1	3
1622	CHANNELS 4, 11	08/27/xx	0	1	0	0	0	1	0	1
1734	NEWSPAPER	08/29/xx	3	5	0	0	2	8	2	3

Exhibit 21–23   An Example Employee ID Badge

9/XX
EXPIRATION DATE

RICHARD J. SWANSBURG
NAME

MGMT SYSTEMS SPECIALIST
TITLE

HOSPITAL INFO SYSTEMS
DEPARTMENTT

SWANSBURG, RICHARD J.

Exhibit 21–24   An Example Employee Termination List

Employee Termination List for the month of August 19xx

POSITION	NAME	TITLE	DATE	REASON
00356	Johnson, Mary J.	Registered Nurse	08/26/xx	Q
10234	Armstrong, Helen M.	Licensed Practical Nurse	08/08/xx	Q
16212	Mims, Janet K.	Registered Nurse	08/13/xx	F
17335	Baker, Donald M.	Registered Nurse	08/05/xx	Q
17336	Smitherman, Carolyn S.	Registered Nurse	08/22/xx	R
18549	Jackson, Melanie J.	Unit Secretary	08/01/xx	Q
18675	Hanson, Marcus K.	Respiratory Therapist	08/29/xx	Q

Exhibit 21–25 An Example Employee Timesheet

Employee Timesheet Report 10/04/xx 07:40

Employee : 424345543   Johnson, Mary   Department : 51134 Medical/Surgical

DAY	DATE	IN	OUT	HOURS	DEPT	SCHED	REG	OT	HOL	VAC	SIC	OTHER	BREAK	TOT
SUN	09/19/xx	0700	1535	8.58		1	8.00						.50	8.00
MON	09/20/xx	0703	1537	8.57		1	8.00						.50	8.00
TUE	09/21/xx													
WED	09/22/xx	0659	1531	8.53		1	8.00						.50	8.00
THU	09/23/xx	0701	1523	8.37		1	8.00						.50	8.00
FRI	09/24/xx	0707	1528	8.35		1	8.00						.50	8.00
SAT	09/25/xx													
SUN	09/26/xx													
MON	09/27/xx	0655	1537	8.70		1	8.00						.50	8.00
TUE	09/28/xx	0706	1529	8.38		1	8.00						.50	8.00
WED	09/29/xx	0659	1529	8.50		1	8.00						.50	8.00
THU	09/30/xx	0701	1525	8.40		1	8.00						.50	8.00
FRI	10/01/xx													
SAT	10/02/xx	0707	1535	8.47		1	8.00						.50	8.00
	Totals						80.00	0.00	0.00	0.00	0.00	0.00	5.00	80.00

FUTURE TRENDS

Trends for the future include totally automated medical records, voice interaction, expert systems, and artificial intelligence, and the increased use of optical discs and robotics. A paperless medical record or budget sounds interesting and is probably possible today. This would allow for the immediate and complete access to patient information from many different locations. The use of voice interaction will eliminate the barriers associated with data entry.[31] Expert systems and artificial intelligence will enhance the process of clinical decision making. Robotics is already being used in surgery for the positioning of surgical instruments, in labs for the transport and placement of samples, and in nursing for the delivery of supplies and medications.

Other trends indicate information technology that is becoming easier to use and with greater end-user responsibility. Software is fast becoming more graphical and user friendly. Almost all software today has online help and is menu-driven. This means that users only have to select what they want to do from a list of items on the screen, and if a problem is encountered, help is only a keystroke or mouse click away. Many software development programs have instructions that are almost English-like. What used to take weeks and months to program can now be done in days or weeks.

Users are becoming more involved in designing applications and handling most things themselves. Expanded user involvement will occur as users become more knowledgeable about computer hardware and software. Software will continue to become easier for users to manipulate, and software vendors will provide greater support. The best examples are already evident in laboratory, pharmacy, central supply, and nursing information systems, where very little help is needed from information systems personnel.

Robotics

Robots will assist nurses in performing numerous tasks. The most practical use of robotics is electronic carts for storing and transporting drugs, linens, and other supplies. These carts can be remote-controlled and can actually follow predefined routes along the floor. Another example is robotic arms, which can do heavy lifting. Robotics seems destined for procedures that humans are unable to perform, such as delicate, microscopic eye, brain, or spinal surgeries or procedures where direct contact is contraindicated because of health hazards, such as a patient with a suppressed immune system or exposure to toxic chemicals or radioactive elements. Pharmacy robots fill prescriptions without error.

Voice Communication and Optical Discs

Voice communication will allow nurses to talk to their computers. Keyboards and bar-code readers will not be needed to enter or retrieve information. The computer will be requested to retrieve information or to record it by voice command. Optical discs will revolutionize information storage with their ability to store many times more information in the same space than on current storage media. Microcomputers today use removable floppy diskettes for limited information storage and nonremovable hard discs for volume information storage. New optical laser discs will be removable and, although the same size as floppy diskettes, will store many times more information than will a hard disc.

Conversant computers are widely used in industry. They tell airline baggage handlers which conveyor to put bags on and bank customers their account balances. Conversant computers can identify product deficiencies during manufacturing. They can maintain supply inventories, recording the voice print and processing a spoken reply. They are used to move cameras on spacecraft and turn on lights and roll up car windows. With use of conversant computers, productivity on assembly lines has increased by 25 percent to 40 percent.

Speaker-dependent machines use voice prints, so they must be programmed with the user's voice. Speaker-independent machines can understand any speaker. At present, voice communication is not 100 percent accurate. Even though computers have hardware to support voice technology, little software is available. Users have not responded well to computer-synthesized voices.[32]

Expert Systems and Artificial Intelligence

Other future trends in software are expert systems and artificial intelligence. Expert systems already exist. Nurses have access to a huge amount of information that can assist them in making everyday decisions. With expert systems, the nurse identifies the situation requiring a decision, the criteria defining the problem, and objectives for handling the situation. The expert system evaluates the information and provides a listing of alternative ways to manage the situation. The nurse then evaluates the alternatives and makes decisions.

Expert systems encode the relevant knowledge and experience of experts to make them available to less-knowledgeable and experienced persons. An example would be to take the total knowledge and experience of clinical nurse specialists in neuroscience nursing, encode them in a computer program, and make the program available to clinical nurses working in the neuroscience area. These nurses would consult the program to solve nursing-care problems.

With artificial intelligence, the machine is actually capable of "thinking" and acting on its own. The difference between artificial intelligence and an expert system is the fact that the machine with artificial intelligence would proceed to make the decision for handling the situation. In nurse staffing, for example, with an expert system, the nurse manager would describe the situation, and the machine would supply alternatives for handling the staff. With artificial intelligence, the machine could continuously monitor the patient's needs and manage staffing without human intervention. Some individuals do not believe artificial intelligence is possible, and at best it appears to be some years away.

Artificial intelligence attempts to develop ideas into computer operations duplicating human intelligence. Such systems use quantitative and qualitative data. Artificial intelligence is being used in robotics, the understanding of natural language, and expert systems.[33]

The industry is now capable of building computerized information systems to appeal simultaneously to the right and left sides of the brain. People share many judgments or assumptions and few symbolic numbers (symbols representing numbers and having a widely perceived meaning) and beliefs. They store facts, use them with a conceptual framework to connect them, and then identify them with a particular problem. The conceptual framework is called a schema, cognitive map, or conceptual model.

Conceptual models are compared with external physical representations by individuals such as artists and engineers. They change perceived differences in one or both conceptual model and external physical representation. People compare their conceptual models by sending them to others. Each model influences the other.

Conceptual models are created to solve organizational problems by identifying root causes. Market forces determine prices and quality of service. The Advocate Conceptualization/Communication/Creativity Support System can be used as a technological tool to manage communications and satisfy stakeholders. This concept will accelerate the corporate change to a systems world view. It will provide the linking corporate language. Ultimately, health care will use these systems.[34]

Exercise 21–7 Do a library search and identify expert systems available to nurses.

WEB ACTIVITIES

- Visit www.jbpub.com/swansburg, this text's companion website on the Internet, for further information on Nursing Informatics.
- The American Nursing Informatics Association is an organization offering information on Nursing Informatics; locate its site and review its offerings.
- Explore the Internet to locate various discussion areas and conferences on NMIS.

SUMMARY

Nursing can expect almost anything from computers but should not expect everything. No one should be concerned that somebody else is using state-of-the-art equipment and software, because if it really is state-of-the-art and beneficial, everyone will soon be using it.

The intent of this chapter is to provide an overview of nursing and computers. The computer is a necessary information-handling tool, and most people feel the impact of it on their daily lives. In fact, the computer is now a necessity in managing the complex financial structure of today's health care.

Computers are used to support and run highly complex information systems that have tremendous capabilities for manipulation and storage of information. Almost any nursing application can be implemented through an information system. There are systems that assist nursing in doing patient-care documentation, order processing, clinical decision making, and patient and professional education.

Other general-purpose microcomputer software is also available for personal productivity enhancement. Nurses have needs for document preparation, number crunching, and record keeping. Nurse managers should find graphics, multimedia, and communications invaluable tools for presentations and educational support.

In the future, more and more will be accomplished through computers. All nurses will have to be able to interact with these machines. Nurse managers are finding themselves in crucial positions. Nursing schools are incorporating the use of the computer into the nursing curriculum. New positions are being developed for nurses in computer education and support.

The computer has come of age. These machines are tools that already assist most of us in performing numerous tasks. They are excellent for the management of all types of information.

NOTES

1. F. R. Vlasses, "Computerized Documentation Systems: Blessings or Curse?" *Orthopaedic Nursing,* January/February 1993, 51–52.
2. S. W. White, "The Universal Computer," *National Forum,* summer 1991, 2.
3. R. L. Axford, "Implementation of Nursing Computer Systems, A New Challenge for Staff Development Departments," *Journal of Nursing Staff Development,* summer 1988, 125–130.
4. *Webster's New World Dictionary of the American Language* (New York: Simon & Schuster, 1979).
5. C. A. Romano, "Preparing Nurses for the Development and Implementation of Information Systems," NLN Publication 14-2234, 1988, 83-92.
6. B. R. Heller, C. A. Romano, L. R. Moray, and C. A. Gassert, "The Implementation of the First Graduate Program in Nursing Informatics," *Computers in Nursing,* September/October 1989, 209–213.
7. B. Nadel, "The Cyrix Plan: Catch Up, Then Lead," *PC Magazine,* 27 April 1993, 126.
8. J. Rothfeder, "Is Big Iron Good for You?" *Beyond Computing,* May/June 1993, 24–27.
9. K. Andreoli and L. A. Musser, "Computers in Nursing Care: The State of the Art," *Nursing Outlook,* January/February 1985, 16–25.
10. "Swords Speak in First Interactive Multimedia Novel," *San Antonio Light,* 19 October 1992, E8.
11. C. Buszta, "Conquering Computer Phobia—Advice from Someone Who Did It," *RN,* December 1989, 57.
12. C. T. Barry and L. K. Gibbons, "Information Systems Technology: Barriers and Challenges to Implementation," *Journal of Nursing Administration,* February 1990, 40–42.
13. K. Abbott, "Student Nurses' Conceptions of Computer Use in Hospitals," *Computers in Nursing,* March/April 1993, 78–89.

14. C. A. Romano, "Privacy, Confidentiality, and Security of Computerized Systems," *Computers in Nursing,* May/June 1987, 99–104.

15. L. K. Woolery, "Professional Standards and Ethical Dilemmas in Nursing Information Systems," *Journal of Nursing Administration,* October 1990, 50–53.

16. P. Iyer, "Computer Charting: Minimizing Legal Risks," *Nursing,* May 1993, 86.

17. *WordPerfect Version 5.2 Reference.* (Orem, Utah: WordPerfect Corporation, 1993), 541.

18. D. Huber, L. Shumaker, and C. Delaney, "Nursing Management Minimum Data Set (NMMDS)," *Journal of Nursing Administration,* April 1997, 42–48.

19. "Outcomes Management Tools Can Boost Your CM Efforts, Enhance Better Patient Oversight," *Care Management Advisor,* April 1994, 45–49.

20. S. A. Finkler, "Microcomputers in Nursing Administration, A Software Overview," *Journal of Nursing Administration,* April 1985, 18–23.

21. H. W. Gottinger, "Computers in Hospital Care: A Qualitative Assessment," *Human Systems Management,* fall 1984, 324–345.

22. L. Curtin, "Nursing: High Touch in a High-Tech World," *Nursing Management,* July 1984, 7–8.

23. P. McKenzie-Sanders, "The Central Focus of the Information Age," *Business Quarterly,* winter 1983, 87–91.

24. J. E. Robinette and P. S. Weitzel, "Design and Development of a Computerized Education Records System," *Journal of Continuing Education in Nursing,* July/August 1989, 174–182.

25. M. Rogers, "MTV, IBM, Tennyson and You," *Newsweek Special Issue,* fall/winter 1990, 50–52.

26. A. R. Redland and C. Kilmon, "Interactive Video, Rational and Practicalities of One Experience," *Computers in Nursing,* March/April 1986, 68–72.

27. M. A. Sweeney and C. Gulino, "From Variables to Videodiscs, Interactive Video in the Clinical Setting," *Computers in Nursing,* August 1988, 157–163.

28. R. L. Simpson, "Closing the Gap Between School and Service," *Nursing Management,* November 1990, 16–17.

29. J. C. McCloskey, "The Nursing Minimum Data Set: Benefits and Implications for Nurse Educators," NLN Publication 41-2199, 1988, 119–126.

30. C. A. Romano and B. R. Heller, "Nursing Informatics: A Model Curriculum for an Emerging Role," *Nurse Educator,* March/April 1990, 16–19.

31. L. Lancaster, "Nursing Information Systems in the Year 2000: Another Perspective," *Computers in Nursing,* January/February 1993, 3–5.

32. N. Madlin, "Conversant Computers," *Management Review,* April 1986, 59–60.

33. F. L. Luconi, T. W. Malone, and M. S. Scott Morton, "Expert Systems: The Next Challenge for Managers," *Sloan Management Review,* Summer 1986, 3–14.

34. L. C. Charalambides, "Systematic Organizational Communications," *Human Systems Management,* April 1985, 309–321.

Appendix 21–1 Glossary of Commonly Used Computer Terms

ABEND: Abnormal end of task.

Algorithm: A prescribed set of rules for the solution of a problem in a finite number of steps.

Artificial intelligence: The capability of a machine that can proceed or perform functions that are normally concerned with human intelligence, such as learning, adapting, reasoning, self-correction, automatic improvement.

Authoring: A structured approach to combining all the media elements in an interactive production.

Authoring system: Software that integrates the multimedia components of an interactive production. To include the computer, CD-ROM, sound, etc.

Bar code reader: An optical scanning unit that can read documents encoded in a special bar code. A laser scanner.

Batch processing: A systems approach to processing where similar input items are grouped for processing during the same machine run.

Binary: (1) The number system based on the number 2 and (2) pertaining to a choice or condition where there are two possibilities.

Bit: The smallest unit of data, a binary digit of 0 or 1.

Buffer: Intermediate storage, used in input/output operations to temporarily hold information.

Bug: A mistake or error in a computer program.

Byte: A set of eight adjoining bits thought of as a unit.

Cache: A storage buffer that contains frequently accessed instructions and data.

Central processing unit (CPU): The part of the computer that contains the circuits that calculate and perform logic decisions based on a set of instructions.

Character: A letter, digit, or other symbol that is used as part of the representation of data. A byte.

Compact disk (CD): A type of disk storage that used magnetic optical recording and lasers.

CRT (cathode ray tube): Cathode ray terminal. A display terminal used as an input/output station.

Data: Representation of information in a form suitable for processing.

Database: A collection of files or tables.

Disc: A round, flat, data medium that is rotated in order to read or write data.

DOS: Disc operating system.

Downtime: The elapsed time when a computer is not available for use, may be scheduled for maintenance or unscheduled because of machine or program problems.

Expert systems: Systems that rely on large amounts of information to provide assistance in decision making.

Field: A unit of information within a record.

File: A collection of related data with a given structure.

Forecasting: Describing the possible future, anticipating the impact of present decisions or actions on future activities of nursing. Forecasting uses simple techniques, such as graphs and hand calculators, and complicated mathematical models that can be developed using desktop computer software packages.

GUI (graphical user interface): Graphical software that allows you to interact with and perform operations on a computer.

Hard copy: Printed computer output: reports, listings, documents.

Hardware: The physical computer equipment.

Hospital Information System (HIS): A system designed to facilitate the day-to-day needs of a hospital; a system that stores and manipulates information for interhospital communication and decision support.

Input/Output (I/O): The transfer of data between an external source and internal storage.

Interface: The point at which independent systems or computers interact.

Key field: A field within a record that makes that record unique with respect to other records in a file.

Kilobyte (KB): 1,024 bytes or characters.

Laser scanner: A type of device that utilizes a laser to recognize and receive input.

Local area network (LAN): Two or more computers connected for local resource sharing.

Mainframe computer: A large computer capable of being used and interacted with by hundreds of users, seemingly simultaneously.

Management information system (MIS): A system designed to manipulate information to assist in management decision making.

Megabyte (MB): Approximately 1,000,000 bytes.

Appendix 21–1 Glossary of Commonly Used Computer Terms *(continued)*

Microcomputer: A small computer built around a microprocessor.

Minicomputer: A medium-size computer, smaller than a mainframe but larger than a microcomputer.

Modeling: Development of mathematical equations that can be used to fit and balance relationships between or among variables. Forecasting uses models. Managers decide which variables to include and the form of the model. In management there are budget models, inventory models, production process models, cash-flow models, models for work-force planning, models of distribution systems, linear programming resource allocation models, and many others.

Modem: A device that converts digital data from a computer to an analog signal that can be transmitted on a telecommunications line and that converts received analog transmissions to digital data.

Multimedia: The combination of different elements of media, such as text, graphics, audio, video, animation, and sound.

Multitasking: A mode of operation that provides for concurrent performance of two or more tasks.

Number crunching: A process of taking numbers and performing mathematical functions on them.

Nursing Management Information System (NMIS): A type of information system geared towards assisting nurse managers in performing their management functions.

Online processing: A form of input processing where information is input and updated at that time.

Operating system: An organized collection of techniques and procedures combined into programs that direct a computer's operation.

Optical disc: Same as a compact disc.

Printer: A terminal or peripheral that produces hard copy or printed output.

Program: A set of computer instructions directing the computer to perform some operation.

Random access: A storage technique whereby a record can be addressed and accessed directly at its location in the file.

Record: A group of related fields of information treated as a unit.

Robotics: Machines that work automatically and perform physical movements.

Scenario projection: Use of a scenario, or set of planning assumptions, to describe and plan for the possible future state of the environment at a point in time and considering the economic, political, social, technological, and natural effects. Scenario projections use trends and trend analysis.

Sequential access: A storage technique whereby a record can be addressed and accessed only after all those before it have been.

Simulation forecasting: Risk analysis, a procedure that mimics possible or probable business conditions to describe the possible future of each. Simulations stress model structure.

Software: A program or set of programs written to tell the computer hardware how to do something.

Spreadsheet: A specialized type of software for manipulation of numbers.

Table: A collection of related data with a given structure.

Trend: Systematic pattern of change (increase or decrease) over time based on history or a particular theory. *Example:* an increase in the acuity level of patients over a one-year period.

Trends extrapolation forecasting: Describing the possible future by projecting the systematic pattern of change (increase or decrease) using the prevailing tendencies of a time series.

Trend impact analysis: Analysis of the impact or consequences of the pattern of change (increase or decrease) over time. *Example:* How will the increased acuity level of patients over a one-year period affect operational costs, use of resources, cash flow, etc?

Trend line: A straight line fitted to a graph plotting trends in a time series. It shows the pattern of change (increase or decrease) over time.

User-friendly (software): Easier to use because of menu and help facilities.

Voice communication: Interaction with a computer by voice recognition.

Word processing: The manipulation of words within documents by a computer.

Word processor: A specialized type of software for manipulation of printed material.

STAFF DEVELOPMENT

by Nancy C. McDonald, EdD, RN
Associate Professor, School of Nursing,
Auburn University at Montgomery
Montgomery, Alabama

"Nursing students and nurses are adults whose learning is based upon principles of adult learning embodying critical thinking."

OBJECTIVES

- Distinguish among characteristics of the adult learner.
- Explain the staff development process.
- Describe the andragogical approach to program design.
- Differentiate among characteristics of learning.
- Describe the role of the teacher in adult education.
- Describe the role of the learner in adult education.
- Use evaluation procedures in adult education.
- Apply the critical thinking/learning model in staff development.

KEY CONCEPTS

staff development
adult education
andragogy
critical thinking
evaluation

Manager behavior: Provides orientation and staff development programs needed as determined by the staff development coordinator.

Leader behavior: Recognizes that staff development is an investment in human capital and applies the critical thinking/learning model to involve personnel in all aspects of a staff development system.

Staff development is based on a philosophy of adult education and utilizes teaching/learning principles and concepts of adult education. Adult learners are people who have a "formal education, a career or employment commitment, identified areas of interest, and family and financial responsibilities."[1] Nurses are adult learners who practice in an environment of rapid change that requires them to update their knowledge and skills or prepare themselves for a different area of expertise.

PHILOSOPHY OF ADULT EDUCATION

Staff development programs are designed to motivate adult learners to consider the learning process as a natural part of living. People are born into society devoid of knowledge. From the day they are born until the day they die, they are part of a society whose institutions are constantly changing. People are capable of learning during this entire life span. Cross believes that "lifelong learning means self-directed growth. It means acquiring new skills and powers—the only true wealth which you can never lose. It means investment in yourself. Lifelong learning means the joy of discovering how something really works, the delight of becoming aware of some new beauty in the world, the fun of creating something, alone or with other people."[2]

Lifelong learning is essential in nursing because of the rapid changes in the health-care delivery system and the changing roles of nursing within that system. Knowledge acquired in basic nursing education programs quickly becomes obsolete. Nursing is influenced by public policy, technology, and societal and economic changes.

Technology, which continually increases in complexity and scope, is a major force motivating nurses to pursue lifelong learning. Nurses use computers while working in specialty units and caring for critically ill patients with artificial hearts, heart transplants, and other types of advanced surgical techniques. Nurses adjust quickly to the demands associated with high-tech skills in many areas such as these. Staff development programs respond to the needs of nurses practicing under these increased demands.

Nurses also have lifelong learning needs related to the processes of physical, cultural, political, and spiritual maturation. One of the weaknesses of staff development programs has been their narrow emphasis on the major field of study. Continuing education that focuses on education of the whole person will promote the development of free, creative, and responsible nursing personnel.

Staff development programs to educate the whole person are aimed at building competencies for performing various roles in life, such as friend, citizen, individual (self), family member, worker, and leisure-time user.[3] For example, nurses are adult citizens of the communities in which they live. Educational systems should show them how to participate in social institutions and how to assume their responsibilities, rights, and privileges. Nurses learn to be people who strive to attain high standards in the institutions in which they actively participate.

Boshier interviewed 453 adult-education participants and found that the leading motivators for those adults were to become better citizens, participate in group activity, relieve boredom, and live in a more satisfying way.[4]

THE STAFF DEVELOPMENT PROCESS

Staff development may be defined as "a management program to aid staff in developing skills and knowledge which adds to their professional goals and at the same time increases their value as employees."[5] Staff development is a comprehensive program that includes orientation, in-service education, continuing education programs, and job-related counseling. Orientation introduces employees to new situations and includes content related to philosophies, goals, policies, procedures, personnel benefits, role expectations, and physical facilities. Employees need orientation each time their roles change.

In-service education provides learning experiences in the work setting for the purpose of refining and developing new skills and knowledge related to job performance. These learning experiences are usually narrow in scope and brief because they are aimed at only one competency or knowledge area. For example, a learning experience might be developed to introduce nursing staff in cardiac care to a new, more sophisticated monitor.

Continuing education programs are planned and organized around learning experiences that focus on competencies and knowledge that can be used by employees in a variety of settings. Continuing education offerings often give employees new approaches to health-care delivery. Examples of continuing education activities are workshops, conferences, self-learning modules, and seminars. Continuing education is required for licensure to promote continued competency to practice nursing.

Staff development also includes job-related counseling, which involves promoting professional growth of employees by helping them give their best job performance. It involves counseling about promotion possibilities and assistance in obtaining formal training.

Philosophy of the Staff Development Program

An organization needs a statement of beliefs about how it will accomplish its staff development program. The staff development philosophy should relate to the mission and philosophy of the organization of which it is a part. The statement of philosophy should be written by a representative group, not by an individual, and be accepted by both staff and administrators.

In writing a philosophy for staff development for health-care professionals, the group needs to address its beliefs with regard to the following areas:

- How learning takes place.
- Teaching methods.
- Responsibility of employees for their own learning.
- Organization's responsibility for providing staff development.
- Clients' right to health care.

Exhibit 22–1 is an example of a staff development statement of philosophy.

Organization of Staff Development

A staff development program can function under many organizational models depending on the philosophy of the agency. A centralized model would have an agencywide staff development department, and the educational staff might consist of nurses or educators who are not nurses. In this model, all departments collaborate in determining and planning job needs of their staff. The centralized model facilitates scheduling and use of equipment and may prevent duplication of efforts. The main criticism of this model is separation

Exhibit 22–1 Department of Nursing Service Staff Development Philosophy Statement

Philosophy

The philosophy of Staff Development is in agreement with the philosophy of the Department of Nursing Service.

We recognize that quality health care depends to a large degree on the knowledge, skills, attitudes, and activities of practicing health care personnel. An effective Staff Development program is necessary to assist nursing personnel to maintain and improve competency as new knowledge, technology, and environmental changes continue to emerge.

We believe that the responsibility for identifying learning needs, providing opportunities for meeting these needs, and evaluating the effectiveness of learning activities lies not only with the learner but also with Nursing Service Administration. The Department of Staff Development should provide support services in assisting the staff in becoming more knowledgeable and competent in fulfilling role expectations.

Staff Development supports decentralization of education programs. We acknowledge that the development of personnel is best accomplished through the provision of informal as well as formal learning opportunities. Individual competencies and expertise should be utilized in educational programs. The development and implementation of programs may be carried out by, or in collaboration with, nursing staff clinicians whenever possible.

We believe that education is a continuous process that begins with graduation and entry into practice. We recognize that much adult learning involves changes in attitudes and self-image and assisting the learner to accept change and be a change agent. We believe that Staff Development should strive to inculcate nursing personnel with an awareness of the commitment to and value of continuous learning, professional accountability, and professional involvement.

November 19xx
Revised November 19xx
Revised November 19xx

Source: Courtesy University of South Alabama Medical Center, Mobile, Alabama.

---

of education staff from nursing staff and perpetuation of the us-against-them attitude.

In a decentralized model, the nursing department has its own organized inservice or staff development department. The nursing staff development department may then adopt a centralized or decentralized model. The strength of a decentralized model is that the specific needs identified by an area can be addressed. The major areas of concern in decentralization are the use and scheduling of classrooms, potential duplication of efforts, and the cost of providing multiple small programs. There is a trend toward decentralization of as many functions as possible in health-care organizations.

Exercise 22–1   Write a philosophy of staff development for your unit or organization.

Staff Development Personnel

Nursing service administrators are responsible for staff development to promote quality client care. The following are among their responsibilities:

- Providing financial and human resources.
- Establishing policies for staff development.

- Providing release time, finances, or both for staff to attend continuing education offerings.
- Motivating employees to assume responsibility for their own professional development.
- Providing mechanisms to identify staff growth needs.
- Evaluating the effects of staff participation in continuing education offerings on quality of client care.

The staff development coordinator is an administrator and a teacher who is able to communicate and establish trust, has knowledge and skills in adult education, has knowledge of training resources and subject matter, and understands the program planning process.

The professional development staff are selected by the coordinator to work in the planning, implementing, and evaluation of staff development programs. The size of the staff depends on the size of the agency. In small agencies, the coordinator may be the only staff member. These personnel may be totally decentralized to unit level.

Advisory Committees

An advisory committee can be useful for identifying needs and resources and for planning programs. Members of the committee should represent all fields of practice in the agency. Other members may include people with needed expertise. Committee members may increase participation because they can communicate the purpose of staff development programs directly to the people they represent.

Budgets for Staff Development

The amount of budget allocation for staff development depends on staff size, expected number of new employees, and existing resources.[6] The staff development coordinator is responsible for developing and implementing the budget, with input from staff. The agency administration will demonstrate a commitment to staff development by allocating adequate funds for salaries, staff time for training, periodicals, books, audiovisuals, and outside education resources.

Exercise 22–2   Staff development programs should be aimed at preparing individuals for various life roles and for maintaining competence in those roles. Identify three roles filled by nurses and give examples of staff development programs that will assist them in coping with these social roles and related tasks.

ANDRAGOGICAL APPROACH TO PROGRAM DESIGN

The characteristics of adult learners require an andragogical approach to curriculum development and teaching in staff development programs. Andragogy is the art and science of helping adults learn, in contrast to pedagogy, the teaching of children. This approach assumes that the learners themselves are the facilitators who create a climate that motivates their own achievement.[7]

Mutual Diagnosis of Needs

Effective staff development programs begin with a needs assessment of the learners. For adults to be interested and motivated, they enter educational programs because of perceived needs they have identified. Adult learners have a perception of the level of competency they want to achieve and the knowledge they need for better performance in their personal lives or work settings. If adult learners' needs differ from those perceived by the planners, participation in the educational offerings will be decreased or nonexistent. A training program is a waste of time and money if it does not increase the efficiency and effectiveness of workers.[8] As a result, educational needs assessment is the first step in adult education programming.

Needs Assessment Methods

Staff development planners decide on a method of assessment that will meet their purposes. The following factors should be considered before designing a needs assessment survey:

1. Target population.
2. Development time.
3. Cost.
4. Financial and human resources.
5. Analysis time.
6. Anonymity.
7. Objectivity.

The needs survey should address content, design of learning activities, and learners' backgrounds.[9] Content relates to the specific topics of interest to the learners. Design of learning activities covers such areas as planning when individuals can attend courses and what kind of learning options (such as workshops or modules) would best facilitate their learning.

When considering a method of assessment, it is important to address the needs of the organization as well as those of the learner. Organizational needs are influenced by such factors as the standards of the Joint Commission for Accreditation of Healthcare Organizations (JCAHO), the American Nurses Association Standards for Continuing Education, consumer needs, standards of practice, and the philosophy and objectives of the institution. If staff developers ignore these needs, they may lose the support of the sponsoring organization.

Questionnaire or Survey. A questionnaire is perhaps the most frequently used method for assessing needs. Questions on the survey tool may be either forced choice, which allows selection of one of several categories of context needs, or open-ended, which allows more freedom of response. An example of the latter is a statement such as, If I could learn more about stress management, I would like to learn. . . . The survey tool should be designed with a combination of the two types of questions.

A pilot test of the survey is done to ensure that questions are clear and that the data gathered are complete and relevant. Individuals completing the pilot survey are asked to comment on whether they understood the questions, how long it took them to complete the questionnaire, and whether other areas should be added. Their responses are then analyzed by a group and necessary changes made to the questionnaire.

The advantages of the questionnaire include ease and convenience of administration and easily computed results. Disadvantages include the cost of data collection and analysis. Also, if a mailed questionnaire yields a low return, the data may not result in a representative sample. Exhibit 22–2 is one example of a broad-scale questionnaire.

Exhibit 22–2   Broad-Scale Questionnaire

How can Staff Development help meet your needs over the next year? Please answer the following questions. This is an anonymous survey.
Check most appropriate.

1. I am:
   _____ a. RN
   _____ b. LPN
   _____ c. NA
   _____ d. WC

2. I work in the following type of nursing area:
   _____ a. Medical
   _____ b. Surgical
   _____ c. Orthopedic/Neuro
   _____ d. Obstetrical
   _____ e. Pediatric
   _____ f. Neonatal
   _____ g. Emergency room
   _____ h. Operating room
   _____ i. Other (specify)_____

3. I have worked in my nursing area for:
   _____ a. less than 3 months
   _____ b. 4 to 11 months
   _____ c. 1 to 3 years
   _____ d. 4 to 6 years
   _____ e. over 6 years

4. What is the best time of day for you to attend in-service programs?
   _____ a. mornings
   _____ b. afternoons
   _____ c. evenings

5. What is the best day for you to attend in-service programs?
   _____ a. Monday
   _____ b. Tuesday
   _____ c. Wednesday
   _____ d. Thursday
   _____ e. Friday
   _____ f. Saturday

Circle the most appropriate response, according to your interest, for the following in-service education programs:
4 = I am highly interested.
3 = I am interested.
2 = I am somewhat interested.
1 = I have no opinion or don't know.
0 = I have no interest.

6. 4 3 2 1 0   Respiratory care
7. 4 3 2 1 0   Wound management
8. 4 3 2 1 0   Stress management
9. 4 3 2 1 0   Nursing and the law
10. 4 3 2 1 0   Communication skills
11. 4 3 2 1 0   Nursing process
12. 4 3 2 1 0   Use of computers in nursing
13. 4 3 2 1 0   Death and dying
14. 4 3 2 1 0   Body image
15. 4 3 2 1 0   Cost care
16. What other topics would you like included in in-service education programs? _____
   _____
   _____

Observation.   When used with other methods, observation is an effective way to assess needs. A nurse manager or clinical specialist can observe personnel and perhaps identify learning needs. The effectiveness of this technique is increased if a standardized observation guide is used.

A disadvantage of this method is that observations are subjective and can produce incomplete data. For instance, a nurse observed to be charting incorrectly may be doing so because of lack of time, not faulty knowledge of the procedure.

Interview.   Interviewing of a sample representing the target population is a method that can be used to gather valuable information about need. Interviews can clarify ambiguous data gathered through surveys. Respondents often feel more comfortable expressing feelings verbally than in writing. A disadvantage is that data collected are difficult to sort, measure, and report.

Open Group Meetings.   Learning needs can be assessed in group discussions if a resource person is available with questions to focus the group on the topic. The resource person should be skilled in group process technique so that all group members can be aided in clearly expressing their learning needs. This method can be time-consuming and of limited value if group members are hesitant about speaking out.

Analysis of Professional Literature.   A systematic review of the previous six months to a year of pertinent journals is an excellent means to identify trends and to compare national information with the leader's own setting. This method is inexpensive and can be present- or future-oriented. On the negative side, a review of literature is time-consuming because it involves analyzing and synthesizing many articles to find trends. Also, a time lag is involved in publication.

Competency Model.   A competency model is a valuable means for discovering needs of an individual. In building a competency model, a series of statements are developed that identify expected performance or behavior. After the competencies are refined to small units that reflect only single behaviors, individuals can then compare their performance to each behavior. Staff developers can help individuals identify gaps between their level of competency and the desired level. Individuals can then participate in learning activities to close the gaps.

Employee Performance Appraisals.   The performance appraisal can be an effective method for identifying needs if done in a positive way. Appraisals should avoid confrontation, be meaningful instead of demeaning, and be a worthwhile activity that develops staff. People should be encouraged to state their own hopes and aspirations and identify their learning needs. Both the rater and the ratee have a clear picture of duties and demands of the job and current abilities and level of performance. They then identify gaps between the desired and the actual levels of performance. Staff development programs are then designed to improve performance or prepare the employee for a new position.

Exercise 22–3 Staff development planners do careful needs assessments before designing programs. Locate a needs survey done in your organization. Is it adequate? How has it been used? What would you do to improve it?

Mutual Planning

Once needs are identified and priorities set, appropriate learning experiences are designed. Adult learners are able to help plan the educational offerings. Professional nurses are more committed to an activity when they have been involved in the decision-making process. They see themselves as self-directed, whereas they may resist a staff development program that is imposed on them by the establishment. A committee that represents all subgroups is one mechanism for mutual planning. The nursing service administrator or the education coordinator is responsible for appointing the planning committee.

Translating Learning Needs into Goals

The planning committee should be involved in setting goals for the learning experience. The staff development director will assist the committee in developing these goals, because this is often a difficult part of the planning process.

Goals provide intent and direction for movement.[10] Goals are important in providing a basis for planning learning activities, selecting methods and materials, and defining and organizing content. For goals to serve as workable tools, certain guidelines should be followed.

1. Goals should be centered on the learner, not the teacher. For example, "The student will understand selected concepts of shock"—not "The instructor will present selected concepts of shock."
2. Goals do not dictate specificity but may simply indicate a general aim. They may be inexact and imprecise as long as intent is provided.
3. One overall goal may be sufficient for a training program if it is stated broadly. For example, an appropriate goal for a program on care of patients with gastrostomy tubes could be "The learner will employ care and critical thinking in addressing specific human needs of the patient and family dealing with a gastrostomy tube."

Exercise 22–4 Locate the goals of two staff development programs for your unit or organization. If they are not learner-centered, change them to make them so.

CRITICAL THINKING/LEARNING MODEL

A model for teaching adult learners that emphasizes collaboration between teacher and learner was developed by N. C. McDonald. The conceptual base for this model, called a Critical Thinking/Learning Model, is an open system of simultaneous interaction between teacher, learner, and the teaching/learning environment (see Exhibit 22–3). The model shows continual influence from each

Exhibit 22–3 Critical Thinking/Learning Model

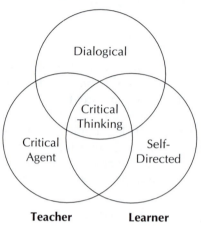

Teaching/Learning Environment

Dialogical

Critical Thinking

Critical Agent

Self-Directed

Teacher   **Learner**

component to all other components even when there is no overt interaction taking place. This represents a departure from the linear interaction of traditional teaching, in which response from the student occurs as a result of stimulus from the teacher. The Critical Thinking/Learning Model shows a balance of influence from all components, with no single component dominating the exchange. Core elements are considered central to each component and are necessary for the outcome of critical thinking to occur. Each component contains five basic characteristics, as seen in Exhibit 22–4.

Teaching/Learning Environment

The core element in the teaching/learning environment is dialogical. This concept uses the process of dialogue as the central focus in the classroom, as opposed to the traditional lecture method (see Exhibit 22–5). To arrive at the desired outcome of critical thinking, students must be able to relate their new ideas and experiences to previous knowledge. They must be able to share, justify, and validate their new understanding. Dialogue implies a struggle for insight into possible alternatives and a consideration of new perspectives. The development of critical thinking involves the acting upon and sharing of knowledge through discourse. This rational process takes place in the creative and unpredictable environment that occurs with dialogic classes.

Five characteristics are necessary for the provision of a teaching/learning environment that supports the process of critical thinking and learning.

Comfort.   When a working adult student arrives at class to participate in learning activities, demanding work schedules and responsibilities are already surrounding the learning experience. The teacher must take into consideration such

Exhibit 22–4   Characteristics of the Components in the Critical Thinking/Learning Model

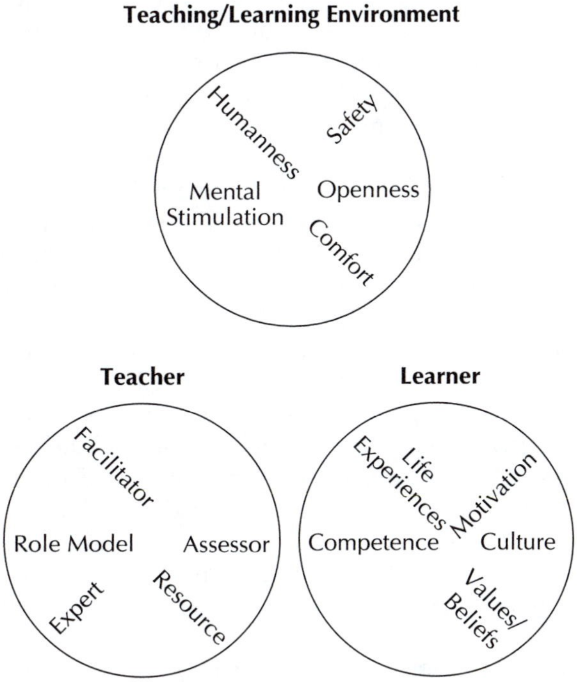

Teaching/Learning Environment

Humanness   Safety
Mental
Stimulation   Openness
Comfort

Teacher

Facilitator
Role Model   Assessor
Expert   Resource

Learner

Life
Experiences   Motivation
Competence   Culture
Values/
Beliefs

Exhibit 22–5   Comparison of Traditional, Stimulus/Response Interaction and Critical Dialogue
(● = teacher/○ = student)

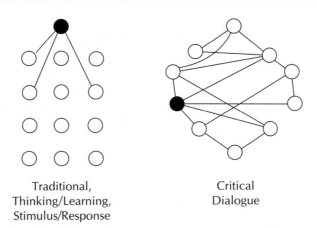

Traditional,
Thinking/Learning,
Stimulus/Response

Critical
Dialogue

Source: Created by Nancy McDonald for research study, "The Measurement of Selected Aspects of Critical Thinking."

factors as fatigue and distraction, or simply the role change that accompanies adult learners to the classroom. An environment that provides for comfort is a first step in promoting collaboration between teacher and student.

Comfortable seating, good lighting, access to beverages, and thermostat control can make a difference between actively attending to learning activities and simply enduring a class session, particularly in the longer class sessions that are typical of programs structured for adult learners.

Openness. Establishment of a community in the classroom creates free and open interaction between teacher and student. A circular seating arrangement for students and teacher promotes a nonlinear sharing of power. The dialogue that is central to critical thinking occurs more easily when all members of the class are visible to one another.

Activities that encourage sharing among students are appropriate at the initial class session. If students are asked to repeat other students' names and name their favorite foods and fun activities, attention is more likely to be focused away from self. The teacher should be included in this ice-breaking exercise, which offers valuable information related to the culture, background, and values of the students. The experience that each adult learner brings to the classroom can be identified during these get-acquainted exercises and later used as a resource among students. Unique experiences and life skills can contribute to the teaching/learning process, as well as enhance the confidence of the participants.

Mental Stimulation.   Classes that begin with a mental warm-up assist with the transition of adults from working professionals to students. The following activities stimulate thinking:

1. Round-robin sessions in which students name things involving threes (*examples:* triangles, butcher-baker-candlestick maker, French hens).
2. Round-robin sessions in which students name things involving time (*examples:* ETA, time-out, Greenwich mean time).
3. Nine-dots experiment in which students try to draw four continuous straight lines through dots (• • •)
   (• • •)
   (• • •)
4. A Mensa genius quiz (*example:* Five men raced their cars on a racing strip. Will did not come in first. John was neither first nor last. Joe came in one place after Will. James was not second. Walt was two places below James. In what order did the men finish?)

Involving students in problem solving can be facilitated through the use of small groups to encourage participation from each member and provide an opportunity for students to get to know one another. By having participants form groups by counting off by twos or threes around the room, dependent partners are separated (all the number ones become a group, all the number twos become a group, and so on). This minimizes visiting and promotes individual involvement. Students who have not had the opportunity to talk can then engage in dialogue and learn from one another.

The infusion of humor and pleasure into the learning experience can minimize stress and stimulate learning. Humor in the classroom promotes a community atmosphere as well as a sense of ease and relaxation. Care should be taken to establish an environment safe from ridicule. Humor is funny only when self-esteem is not threatened.

Safety.   Adult learners, as do all other students, need to build personal confidence in classroom performance and to feel comfortable as part of the group. Students are often fearful that expressing thoughts or asking questions might reveal inadequacies or inappropriate thinking. A technique helpful in reducing this fear or discomfort is to have each student respond to a specific concept by writing the answer and then sharing the answer with a classmate. Working in pairs initially enables students to test ideas and questions, modify responses, and develop confidence before interacting with the larger group. Pairing each student with a different classmate for several of these exercises establishes a known support base and provides a network with other students.

An environment that is safe and nonthreatening is essential to the development of critical thinking. The response of the teacher to each student and to the group must convey respect, caring, and support. A student who fears reprisal, humiliation, or embarrassment will be unlikely to voice opinions or engage in dialogue. Adult learners are often fearful of the unknown and are usually anxious to establish credibility and make a good impression. The learning environment must be supportive of the efforts of adults while providing an atmosphere that supports humor and enjoyment of the learning experience.

Humanness.   A person-centered approach to the teaching/learning process means emphasizing the competence of the learners. Teachers who are not afraid to show that they are human value each student's personal choice, responsibility, and contribution to the process of learning. Humanness pervades all interactions within the teaching/learning environment. Human qualities that are essential for the teacher to possess include valuing the student as a fellow human being regardless of the quality or quantity of classwork, trusting the student to engage in self-discovery, being genuine in responses and interactions, and offering empathic understanding.

The Learner

Self-direction is the core element for the learner in the Critical Thinking/Learning Model. The element of self-direction is intimately related to critical thinking and must be present for the student to be a critical thinker. Responsibility for the internal process of cognition rests with the learner and is a precondition for the development of understanding and knowledge. Each learner who participates in the critical thinking/learning process brings life experiences, competence, motivation, culture, and values/beliefs to the educational experience.

Life Experiences.   Adult learners are individuals who have accumulated experience, skills, and wisdom through the process of living. These students are not as malleable as twenty-year-olds and may be more resistant to change. In the Critical Thinking/Learning Model, reciprocal interaction occurs in a continuous process in which the teacher learns from the student, and vice versa. Life experiences of adult students are a valuable resource for the teaching/learning process, and teachers who recognize and use this resource enrich the process and help to build the self-esteem of the learners.

Competence.   The educator of adults who subscribes to the concept of critical thinking and learning must assume that each student is competent to engage in active learning unless individual performance over time proves otherwise.

Creative thinking is an inherent characteristic of human beings, although it may have been suppressed by rigid and punitive methods encountered in previous educational experiences. Development of competence to assume individual responsibility for learning may be necessary before students can become responsible for personal learning. The teacher should challenge the tendencies toward convergent thinking, give positive feedback for risk taking or creative thinking, and encourage consideration of alternative solutions.

Brainstorming is a process that develops competence in self-discovery and critical thinking. No response generated during the exercise of brainstorming can be seen as incorrect, no viewpoint or statement has to be justified, and all members of the group are given the opportunity to participate. This process frees students from censoring others' or their own responses. Divergent rather than convergent thinking is encouraged by rewarding uninhibited and outrageous responses.

Strategies such as brainstorming encourage and release the competence for active learning that is present in the nature of human beings.

Motivation.   Adult learners return to the classroom for various reasons. Identifying these motivators can help the learner develop and maintain the initiative needed to engage in critical-thinking activities. Insight into extrinsic and intrinsic aspects of motivation to learn can promote integration of new ideas and highlight the approaches best suited for the exploration of these ideas. Understanding individual motivators can enable teacher and student to anticipate and adjust to the stress and anxiety that may accompany new learning experiences.

Styles of learning can be diagnosed through tools and measurement scales such as those previously described. Students who can understand personal methods of learning are more able to choose approaches that facilitate critical thinking/learning. Preferences, habits, and aptitudes of each student ideally should be identified so as to enable both teacher and student to select effective strategies for learning.

Culture.   The cultural background of an individual is the basis for many of the assumptions, values, and beliefs held by that individual. Political stances, life choices, and much of behavior in general are grounded in the time and place of birth and maturation. During the process of becoming aware of personal choices, students must examine the scripts inherited from acculturation.

Students may experience for the first time the basis of personal choices when engaging in critical thinking/learning. In this process, students question and challenge rules that have governed their past actions. The disruption and discomfort that result from this process are part of the examination of previously held assumptions.

The open interchange of the Critical Thinking/Learning Model indicates that self-directed learning includes the learner's right to challenge both the teacher's assumptions and the learner's personal assumptions. This interchange should never be conducted in an autocratic or intimidating manner by either teacher or student.

When familiar assumptions such as those resulting from cultural influence are the launching point for the critical thinking/learning process, students are able to respond specifically and with familiarity. Easily identifiable areas of questioning will be more readily broached than sophisticated or complicated conceptual areas.

Values/Beliefs.   Many individuals believe that absolute truths exist, and some individuals are certain of what these truths are. The emotional responses that result from challenging personal values and beliefs may be difficult for individual students, the group, and the facilitator or teacher. An environment of safety, trust, and caring must exist for adult learners to engage in critical thinking/learning related to personal commitments.

As with all groups of people, the classroom will have individuals who are more developed or mature and who more readily exhibit skepticism, analysis, and divergent thinking. Those students who have not yet reached this level of self-discovery cannot be forced into using imaginative thought. The teacher of adults can only support, challenge, and offer alternatives to those learners who are resistant to the process. Acceptance of the values and beliefs of others must be role-modeled by the teacher, who continues to offer students ways to achieve insight into their own values and beliefs.

The Teacher

The teacher involved in the critical thinking/learning process must consistently function as a critical agent. The teacher is the catalyst for the process of critical thinking and must function as a critical agent to provide diversity of thinking, disagreement, and the challenging ideas in the classroom. Leading students toward critical thinking requires that the teacher engage in activities that identify and challenge the assumptions of students and assist students in imagining and exploring alternatives. This must be done without unnecessary criticism or unrealistic utopianism.

Facilitator.   Effective listening skills are crucial to the collaborative process between student and teacher in the Critical Thinking/Learning Model. Attention to body language and nonverbal communication is as important as attending to the spoken interchanges between fellow students and between student and teacher. Effective listening assists the students to clarify concepts and to problem-solve. Responding specifically and thoughtfully to a student's viewpoint indicates that the teacher values that individual, which enhances the individual's self-esteem.

Learning can be facilitated through specific classroom activities, such as the use of case studies, team learning, or role playing. Case studies can be developed by students whose life experiences apply to the concepts being studied. Dialogue then involves the entire class in examining and analyzing the application of the case study to class content.

Team learning is a process using groups of students who are assigned specific areas of content and then share the concepts with the class. Assignments can be made sufficiently in advance to allow the teams to plan and organize the presentation. All students are given the opportunity to contribute knowledge and expertise. This exercise also develops cooperative work and leadership ability.

Role playing involves assigning a subject or content to be studied and acted out. Several students can participate as a group in the center of a circle of classmates. Observers may chart the interaction of role players, then participate in an assessment and discussion at the conclusion of the activity to provide both learning and feedback.

Role Model.   One of the most common means of teaching is by role modeling. Educators of students of all ages are aware of the influence exerted by behavior and of the importance of demonstrating positive qualities in the teaching/learning environment.

In the application of critical thinking to role modeling, positive behaviors demonstrated by teachers include encouraging criticism of their actions, refusing to evade difficult questions, and being flexible in changing requirements or behaviors as a result of student input.

Resource.   The role of teacher as resource begins with the collaboration process in which learning projects and contracts are identified in the learning environment. Once goals are established, the teacher serves as a resource and then guides the student toward other resources appropriate for achievement of those goals. Student learning styles can be used as a basis for selecting human and nonhuman resources, as well as the methods needed to promote goal achievement. Emphasis should be placed on adjusting resource selection to meet individual strengths and weaknesses.

Resources for personal communication include friends, faculty, and other students, as well as experts in the area to be examined. Professional journals, textbooks, videotapes, and cassettes are also available as resources. Teachers should guide students toward appropriate methods for achievement of goals while individualizing resources for the learning environment. Methods for meeting goals range from random approaches to trial-and-error methods and from sequential to structured approaches. Management plans are often useful in assisting students to map goals, presentations, and resources or for simply organizing time.

Expert.   Lecture is rarely used in the Critical Thinking/Learning Model, but if deemed necessary by the teacher, it can be appropriate if limited to time frames of ten to twenty minutes. Lecturing frees students from active learning and, if lengthy, is not assimilated. Activities that promote student involvement in the learning process are crucial to critical thinking. The teacher as expert in the teaching/learning process uses methods to minimize passivity and promote activity in the learning process.

Assessor.   A needs assessment conducted at the first class session provides information related to the classroom. Students are given the opportunity at this time to recognize and appreciate the knowledge brought by themselves and fellow students to the learning experience. The teacher in the role of assessor may then explore ways to use student expertise for teaching/learning.

The motivation or willingness to learn is an area that the teacher must address in the role of assessor. If the adult learner has already identified the need to learn, goal achievement will be more likely to occur. Motivation may be intrinsic or extrinsic. When the student engages in learning for the sake of learning, motivation is intrinsic and occurs for personal motives. Extrinsic motivation is based on external, or social, motives and occurs when the student engages in learning for other than personal reasons.

During evaluation procedures, the teacher functions as assessor, although the role may be simplified if grade contracts are used. Students and teacher may collaborate to set standards of evaluation or may evaluate the abilities of students against set criteria. Self-analysis is another method of evaluation that students may use to assess goal achievement. Targeting areas and expertise that need developing and/or improving should follow assessment by teacher and students.

TEACHING METHODS

To maximize learning, staff should be aware of several important aspects involved in teaching adult learners.

1. Collaboration between teacher and student is essential for active learning to occur. Learning should be a shared activity in which both the teacher and the students have responsibilities. If students are active participants, learning is more apt to take place. Teaching as a collaborative effort may be viewed as negotiating meaning rather than imparting ready-made knowledge.[11]

2. Critical thinking may be seen as a basic principle of adult education. This process is one of logical reasoning that involves the recognition of assumptions underlying beliefs and behaviors and justification for ideas and actions.[12] Information should be analyzed to make sense out of external experiences.[13] Critical thinking demands comprehension. Students are conditioned to be passive when a teacher begins to lecture. Lecture should not be used as a way to challenge a student's thinking.

The wealth of experience brought to the classroom by adult learners can be incorporated into critical-thinking activities that result in greater involvement with the learning experience.

3. Self-directed learning has an important place in the educational activities of adults. Adults have a deep need to be self-directing, which involves being able to make decisions and manage personal experiences. The teacher should determine what the students already know and must be open about the intent to share responsibility for learning.

EVALUATION PROCEDURES

Evaluation is essential to provide staff with information to improve programs or to determine whether training programs should be continued or dropped. Each course, seminar, class, or workshop is evaluated when it is completed to see whether the program met the needs it was designed to meet. Evaluation includes the learner as well as the program.

Learner Evaluation

Adult learners should have a sense of progress toward their goals and should be involved in evaluating their learning. Teachers should involve learners in developing mutually acceptable criteria and methods for measuring progress toward the learning objectives. If objectives are written in behavioral terms, the standard for evaluation is included in each objective. It can then be observed whether the knowledge, skill, attitude, or practice is accomplished.

When measuring learning, a before-and-after approach should be used so that learning can be related to the training program. If possible, learning should be measured objectively, such as by a written test. Also, if practical, a control group should be compared with the experimental group that receives the training.

Several types of techniques can be used to evaluate learning.

1. Observation of skills or behavior is often useful. Observation guides need to be developed, and observers need to be told specifically what they should be scrutinizing. Validity may be a problem if learners perform in a particular way because they are being observed or if the perception of the observer is incorrect.

2. Paper-and-pencil methods, such as true/false, multiple-choice, or fill-in-the-blank tests are frequently used. Pretesting and posttesting should be done so that comparisons can be made. For some students, tests produce anxiety, which may contribute to poor test results.

3. Unobtrusive measures, when used with other evaluation data, can be valuable. Examples of unobtrusive measures are chart reviews, audits, wear of textbook pages, or numbers of staff using self-directed learning modules.

Program Evaluation

The content, process, and method of a program should be evaluated. A survey or questionnaire is often used to elicit participants' reactions to the program. The following information can be obtained by a survey:

1. What the participants liked or disliked about the program.
2. Whether the faculty or speakers were prepared.
3. Whether objectives were met.
4. How well the program was organized.
5. Whether the facilities were adequate.
6. Suggestions for improvements.
7. Suggestions for future programs.

Problems can arise if the questionnaires are too long or unwieldy for the participants to complete or for the person who must tabulate them. The following guides are useful for preparing questionnaires:

1. Determine what you want to find out and avoid unnecessary questions.
2. Design the form so that most reactions can be tabulated by a computer.
3. Make the form anonymous.
4. Give participants the opportunity to make additional comments.
5. Pilot-test the questionnaire on a simple target audience.

Exhibit 22–6 is an example of an evaluation questionnaire.

Exercise 22–5   Design a questionnaire to evaluate an in-service or continuing education program presented in your workplace. Use it and analyze the results.

Use of Evaluation Data

Evaluation data can point out needed changes in the program or can indicate future educational needs. Evaluation can demonstrate whether a program is worthwhile and whether it justified the expenditure of time and energy. Funding sources, board members, and administrative superiors require evaluation data for making decisions about support of staff development programs.

Evaluation data can be used as a public relations marketing tool to enhance the image of the program. Favorable participant comments can be published.

Evaluation studies can be published in journals so that others who are planning similar programs can learn from the data. Comparison data can be beneficial for future program planning.

Exercise 22–6   Refer to the Critical Thinking/Learning Model in Exhibit 22–3 and Exhibit 22–4 and the accompanying text. Evaluate a staff development program using this model as a standard. Analyze the results and make a management plan to correct any deficiencies.

Exhibit 22–6   Evaluation Questionnaire

Purpose
To provide feedback to program planners so presentations can be improved.

Complete the following anonymously.
Evaluation of the Burn Therapy course, August 12. Circle the number representing your feelings about each statement.

	Strongly Disagree	Disagree	Agree	Strongly Agree	No Opinion
1. The content presented is applicable to my work.	1	2	3	4	5
2. The goals of the program were clear to me.	1	2	3	4	5
3. The content presented reflected the goals.	1	2	3	4	5
4. The content presented was what I expected.	1	2	3	4	5
5. The content was valuable to me.	1	2	3	4	5
6. The instructor's presentation was clear and informative.	1	2	3	4	5
7. The instructor made good use of audiovisuals.	1	2	3	4	5
8. The level of presentation was too theoretical.	1	2	3	4	5
9. The level of presentation was not practical.	1	2	3	4	5

Please respond to the following questions:

10. What were the most positive aspects of this presentation?

11. What did you like best about the presentation?

12. Please make any other comment or suggestion.

13. Suggestions for future presentations.

WEB ACTIVITIES

- Visit www.jbpub.com/swansburg, this text's companion website on the Internet, for further information on Staff Development.
- What organizations or journals could you search for information on staff development?
- What sites would you recommend for more information on the role of the teacher in adult education?

SUMMARY

The purposes of staff development include the improvement of care given to clients and the improvement of participants' quality of life. Nurses who present successful staff development programs understand and apply principles of adult education. Staff members, as adult learners, are self-directed and want to be involved in diagnosing their learning needs, developing objectives, and evaluating their own learning. They have a wide variety of experiences on which to build new learning, and they are looking for experiential types of teaching techniques that allow them to share their knowledge. They want educational programs that are problem-centered and can be applied in their work or life roles. Nurses as teachers in staff development programs are facilitators of learning. This role is enhanced if the educator possesses certain attributes such as openness, flexibility, and spontaneity.

NOTES

1. C. E. Smith, "Planning, Implementing and Evaluating," *Nurse Educator,* November–December 1978, 31–36.
2. K. Cross, *Adults as Learners* (San Francisco: Jossey-Bass, 1982), 16.
3. M. Knowles, *The Adult Learner: A Neglected Species,* 2d ed. (Houston: Gulf Publishing, 1978).
4. R. Boshier, "Motivational Orientations of Adult Education Participants: A Factor Analytic Exploration of Howle's Typology," *Adult Educational Journal,* February 1971, 3–26.
5. G. Morrow-Winn. "Elements of Staff Development," *Journal American Health Care Association,* September 1981, 19–26.
6. Ibid.
7. M. Knowles, *Andragogy in Action* (San Francisco: Jossey-Bass, 1984).
8. M. Moore and P. Dutton, "Training Needs Analyses," *Academy of Management Review,* July 1978, 532–545.

9. P. Yoder Wise, "Needs Assessment as a Marketing Strategy," *Journal of Continuing Education in Nursing,* September/October 1981, 5–9.

10. J. E. Gould and E. O. Bevis, "Here There Be Dragons," *Nursing and Health Care,* March 1992, 126–133.

11. P. C. Candy, *Self-Direction for Lifelong Learning* (San Francisco: Jossey-Bass, 1991).

12. S. D. Brookfield, "Passion, Purity, and Pillage: Critical Thinking About Critical Thinking," *Adult Education Research Conference Proceedings* (University of Georgia): 25–30.

13. D. R. Garrison, "Critical Thinking and Adult Education: A Conceptual Model for Developing Critical Thinking in Adult Learners," *International Journal of Lifelong Education,* October/December 1991, 287–303.

MANAGING CONFLICT

by Enrica Kinchen Singleton, DrPH, MBA, RN
Chair and Professor, Division of Nursing
Dillard University
New Orleans, Louisiana

OBJECTIVES

- Analyze causes of conflict.
- Make plans to manage conflict.
- Use techniques or skills for managing conflict.

KEY CONCEPTS

conflict
quality circles
assertiveness
conflict management

Manager behavior: Imbues all employees with the viewpoint that all conflict is negative behavior and must be avoided.

Leader behavior: Manages conflict through appropriate application of discipline, through communication and assertiveness training, and by applying known conflict management skills.

Any organization in which people interact has a potential for conflict. Health-care institutions include many interacting groups: staff with staff, staff with patients, staff with families and visitors, staff with physicians, and so on. These interactions frequently lead to conflict.

Conflict relates to human feelings, including feelings of being neglected, being taken for granted, being treated like a servant, not being appreciated, being ignored, and being overloaded. Conflict is related to ignoring an individual's worth. The individual's feelings build into anger to the point of rage. This results in such overt behaviors as brooding, arguing, or fighting. The individual can let feelings and behavior get in the way of work. Productivity declines, sometimes purposefully, and mistakes are made.

Rapid changes in health care, including the dismantling of the status quo in health-care organizations, uncertainties advanced by changes in roles and role relationships among traditional health-care personnel, and uncharted relationships with new categories of health-care workers, create an atmosphere of uncertainty in the health-care environment. Under these conditions, conflict is a certainty. Conflict is defined as

> an expressed struggle between at least two interdependent parties, who perceive incompatible goals, scarce rewards, and interference from the other party in achieving their goals. [The parties] are in a position of opposition in conjunction with cooperation.[1]

CAUSES OF CONFLICT

Organizational Conflict

According to Barker, "Organizational conflict arises because of rapid and unpredictable rates of change, new technological advances, competition for scarce resources, differences in cultures and belief systems, and the variety of human personalities."[2] Managers need to understand the concept of conflict, its antecedents, its impact on personnel relationships, and its management and resolution.

Bennis indicates that conflict in organizations is inevitable. Conflict can be destructive or useful, depending upon the leader's handling of it. Conflict derives from misinformation and misperception: One party or group has information that the other does not have, or the parties have different information. Bennis states that "leaders do not avoid, repress, or deny conflict, but rather see it as an opportunity. . . . They don't feel threatened, they feel challenged."[3]

Stevens indicates that the three most often cited potential sources of conflict are "human shortcomings, interpersonal failure, and the nature of an organization (not of the people in it)."[4] Also, individuals as well as departments often oppose one another to gain prestige, power, or resources or to show dominance.[5]

Marriner-Tomey states that conflict arises because individuals have divergent views of their own power and authority and ambiguous jurisdictions. Conflict increases with the need for consensus, the number of organizational levels, the number of specialties, an increase in the degree of associations, and the degree of dependence of some parties on others. When separation in time and space exists, factionalism is fostered, and communication barriers impede understanding. Even though policies, procedures, and rules regulate behavior, make relationships more predictable, and decrease arbitrary decisions, they impose controls over individuals that are likely to be resisted by those who value autonomy.[6]

Sources of Conflict

Conflict may develop from a number of sources:[7]

1. Incompatible goals.
2. Distribution of scarce resources, when individuals have high expectations of rewards.

3. Regulations, when individuals' needs for autonomy conflict with others needs for regulating mechanisms.
4. Personality traits, attitudes, and behaviors.
5. Interest in outcomes.
6. Values.
7. Roles, when two individuals have equal responsibilities but actual boundaries are unclear or when they are required to simultaneously fill two or more roles that present inconsistent or contradictory expectations.
8. Tasks, when outputs of one individual or group become inputs for another individual or group or when outputs are shared by several individuals or groups.

Nurses and Conflict

Nurses are now "experiencing increased competition for status from a proliferation of allied health professionals, many of whom enjoy higher standards of education, pay, and autonomy."[8] Conflict can arise between (1) the nurse and the hospital as employer, as attested to by nurses going on strike; (2) nurses and physicians, because of overlapping roles and nurses' desire for collegiality and also because of changing role relationships as nurses achieve increased levels of education; (3) nurses and lawyers, as nurses act as expert witnesses and are increasingly named defendants in malpractice litigation; (4) nurses and patients; (5) nurses and families; (6) nurses and other disciplines; (7) nurses and assistive personnel; and (8) nurses and nurses.

Nurses and Intradisciplinary Conflict.   Intradisciplinary conflict has the potential to be a serious problem for nurse administrators. The overriding cause of conflict among nurses stems from their major knowledge-assessing modes: (1) the empirical mode, which uses the senses and inductive reasoning; (2) the noetic mode, which uses intuitive feelings and abductive reasoning; and (3) the rational mode, which uses defined standards or rules and deductive reasoning. Each individual has a predisposition to use a particular style or a combination of the three styles. One research study indicates a resulting dissimilar interpretation of reality that may lead to conflict between nurse managers and clinical nurses. Failure to resolve intradisciplinary conflict in nursing will "inevitably debilitate both profession and patients."[9]

Intrapersonal Conflict and Redesign of Delivery Systems.   Nurses are expected to experience intrapersonal conflict as delivery systems are restructured. Their education or employment experiences may cause them to have a preference for a particular nursing delivery modality. For example, they may have learned primary nursing in school and used that modality in the work setting. Acceding to the use of another modality challenges their values and their comfort. Research studies that evaluated outcomes from using functional, team, primary, and modular models were inconclusive and often contradictory.[10]

Currently, nurses are involved in project management, also referred to as product-line management, service-line management, or program management. This decentralized organizational approach uses teams of specialists to achieve specific objectives in a specified time, especially when rapid change is needed. Team membership may cross vertical and horizontal lines. Oncology, with its multiple disciplines, specialists, treatments, and types of cancer, is appropriate as a product line.[11] As rapid changes in health-care delivery continue, the incidences of project management should increase.

Nurses and Other Disciplines: Interdisciplinary Conflict. Studies suggest that interdisciplinary team members see themselves "primarily as representatives of their respective disciplines rather than members of a whole that transcends individual disciplines. Perspectives are splintered rather than united. . . . In the conflictual situations that were described, the perspective of a more technical and high status discipline (psychology) prevailed."[12]

Conflict Between the Patient's Family and Hospital Staff

Abramson et al. discussed the conflict that may arise within families during the course of discharge planning. They indicated that the impact of illness on the lives of patients and families is a major factor in the development of disagreements. Responses depend on the life stage of the family, the age of the patient, the degree of change required in the social situation of the family, the family's capacity for role flexibility, and their problem-solving skills.[13]

Attention to staff input into discharge planning is particularly important if the patient is to have a minimal hospital stay. According to Lowenstein and Hoff, "nurse administrators face major challenges in establishing care delivery systems that emphasize and encourage creative nursing approaches to discharge planning."[14] In their study of registered nurses' involvement in discharge planning in eight hospitals, the nurses were divided in their perception of whether nurses or social workers had primary responsibility for discharge planning. Only eighty-eight nurses (39 percent) had attended an interdisciplinary team meeting. In this situation, nurses are probably experiencing role ambiguity and confusion. Inherent in this situation is the potential for conflict within nursing and between nurses and other disciplines.

Nursing Dislocation and Redesign

According to Porter-O'Grady, many hospital and nursing leaders are indifferent about the centrality of nursing and strongly advocate a decreased nursing leadership role in favor of a multidisciplinary integrated approach. Porter-O'Grady says:

> At times, there appears to be a tacit embarrassment regarding any concerted effort to enumerate the critical role of nursing and nurses in leading change in institutional settings. There has even been discussion suggesting that the creation of a universal, nonaligned care giver might be in the best interest of the health care system. This thinking . . . is flawed. There must be someone who is concerned with the integration and continuum of patient services.[15]

This would include attention to continuous quality improvement, cost containment, and patient-focused care.

Clearly, the role of the nurse will continue to change, as will the various modalities for restructuring patient care. However, the lack of role clarity will continue to be a major source of conflict as health-care personnel establish different roles and relationships. Since resistance is a definitive part of the change process, it may become a major tactic for nurses as they perceive their influence diminishing within the developing interdisciplinary framework.

Defiant Behavior

Defiant behavior can create conflict. It produces guilt feelings in the person to whom it is directed. The nurse should take the position that the person expressing defiance is responsible for the conflict. Defiance is a threat to rational dialogue; it violates the acceptable protocols for adult interaction. The defiant person challenges the authority of the nurse leader through obstinate and intransigent behavior. This behavior may be both verbal and nonverbal.

Murphy describes three versions of the defier. The first of these is the Competitive Bomber, who simply refuses to work. Such people mutter statements that translate into "go to the devil." They scowl and will even walk away from the nurse leader or walk off the job.[16] Competitive defiers can be aggressive underminers who plan deliberate assaults. They comment about unfair and terrible working conditions, manipulation, and lousy schedules. These behaviors are acted out to provoke managerial response. If they do not elicit a response, the competitive defier sulks and pouts to win the pity of peers or even higher management.

The second defier is the Martyred Accommodator, who uses malicious obedience. Such persons work and cooperate but do so mockingly and contemptuously. They complain and criticize to enlist the support of others.

A third category of defier is the Avoider. These defiers avoid commitment and participation. They do not respond to the nurse leader. When conditions change, they avoid participation.[17]

Stress

Conflict leads to stress, fear, anxiety, and disruption in professional relationships. These conditions can, in turn, increase the potential for conflict. Stressors include "having too little responsibility, lack of participation in decision making, lack of managerial support, having to keep up with increasing standards of performance, and coping with rapid technological change."[18] Stress results in decreased productivity from errors, illness, and injuries. Stress costs are billions of dollars per year.

Confrontation, disagreements, and anger are evidence of stress and conflict, which are caused by poorly expressed relationships among people, including unfulfilled expectations.

Stress in patients leads to iatrogenic ailments, complications, and delayed recovery. It may be created by depression and anxiety. Stressed staff cannot cope with stressed patients, and this leads to inefficiency, job dissatisfaction, and insensitive care. Ultimately, the staff are provoked into conflict. They, too, can develop iatrogenic ailments, just like their patients. Families of patients can add to stress if the families are not managed appropriately. Increased stress for patients and staff decreases effective use of staff time. Such problems increase patient care costs because they increase the length of the illness and decrease nursing efficiency and effectiveness. The next time, the patients may go elsewhere for care, whether on their own initiative or on the recommendations of physicians, relatives, friends, or acquaintances.[19]

Space

When nurses have to work in crowded spaces, they must interact constantly with other staff members, visitors, and physicians. This is particularly true in crowded critical care units. Such conditions cause stress that leads to burnout and high turnover.

Physician Authority

Physicians are trained to be in authority over nurses. Today's nurses want to be more independent, to have professional responsibility and accountability for patient care. They spend more time with patients than physicians do and often have valid proposals for altering therapeutic measures. Physicians sometimes ignore nurses' suggestions, indicating they do not want feedback. Nurses become angry as their feelings of self-worth diminish. Communication, particularly two-way communication, fails.[20]

Beliefs, Values, and Goals

Incompatible perceptions or activities create conflict. This is particularly evident when nurses hold beliefs, values, and goals different from those of nurse managers, physicians, patients, visitors, families, administrators, and so on. Nurses' values may boil over into conflicts related to ethical issues involving such matters as do-not-resuscitate orders, callous statements that belittle human worth, abortion, abuse, and AIDS. Personal goals frequently conflict with organizational goals, particularly with regard to staffing, scheduling, and the climate within which nurses work.

Nurses who have to violate their personal standards will lash out at the system. This is demeaning to them and can cause loss of self-esteem and emotional stress. Nurses must know that they are valued, that their beliefs, values, and personal goals are respected. Like other people, nurses act to protect their personal or public image when confronted or invaded. They respond in terms of other people's expectations of them, as they want approval. They will defend their rights and their professional judgments. The ego is easily bruised and becomes a big problem in conflict. Defense becomes more heated when one or both parties to conflict are uninformed or manipulated. When nurses are not recognized or respected, they feel helpless, and they feel hopeless when they are unable to control the situation.[21]

Other Causes

The following are some other causes of conflict:[22]

- Change when people are not prepared for change; such change threatens.
- Conflicting rules of different managers.
- Inadequate orientation and training and poor communication.
- Off-the-job problems, including marital discord, drug use, alcoholism, mental stress, and financial problems.
- Age. Aging nurses can fear not being able to compete with younger nurses and build up resentment against them.
- Pressures related to cost containment, effectiveness of patient care, collective bargaining, consumer awareness and involvement, regulating agencies, entry-level qualifications, scope of practice, and mandated continuing education.
- Computers, ad hoc forces, project teams, and small, autonomous business units, downsizing, decentralization and fewer levels of management, and increased accountability and more demanding performance evaluations.
- Discrimination and prejudice; racial minorities sensitized to real or imagined slights.

Characteristics of Conflict

The following are characteristics of conflict:[23]

1. At least two parties (individuals or groups) are involved in some kind of interaction.
2. Mutually exclusive goals or values exist, either in fact or as perceived by the parties involved.
3. Interaction is characterized by behavior destined to defeat, reduce, or suppress the opponent or to gain a mutually designated victory.
4. The parties face each other with mutually opposing actions and counteractions.
5. Each party attempts to create an imbalance or relatively favored position of power vis-à-vis the other.

CONFLICT MANAGEMENT

Discipline

In using discipline to manage or prevent conflict, the nurse must know and understand the organization's rules and regulations on discipline. If they are not clear, the nurse should seek help to clarify them. Discipline is the last resort in correcting undesirable employee behavior. Rules and regulations must be reasonable and work-related. Rules that are unreasonable or reflect personal bias invite infractions.

The following rules will help in managing discipline:[24]

1. Discipline should be progressive.
2. The punishment should fit the offense, be reasonable, and increase in severity for violation of the *same* rule.
3. Assistance should be offered to resolve on-the-job problems.
4. Tact should be used in administering discipline.
5. The best approach for each employee should be determined. Managers should be consistent and should not show favoritism.
6. The individual and not the group should be confronted. Disciplining a group for a member's violation of rules and regulations makes the other members angry and defensive, increasing conflict.
7. Discipline should be clear and specific.
8. It should be objective, sticking to facts.
9. It should be firm, sticking to the decision.
10. Discipline produces varied reactions. If emotions are running too high, a second meeting should be scheduled.
11. The nurse performing the discipline should consult with the supervisor. One should expect to be overruled sometimes. Knowing the boundaries of authority and the supervisor will avoid most overrulings.
12. A nurse should build respect, trust, and confidence in her or his ability to handle discipline.

Communication

Communication is an art essential to maintaining a therapeutic environment. To promote communication that prevents conflict, the nurse leader/manager should do the following:[25]

1. Teach nursing staff effective communication and their role in it.
2. Provide factual information to everyone—be inclusive, not exclusive.
3. Consider all aspects of a situation—emotions, environment considerations, verbal and nonverbal messages.
4. Develop basic skills of
   a. Reality orientation, by direct involvement and acceptance of responsibility in resolving conflict.
   b. Physical and emotional composure.
   c. Having positive expectations that generate positive responses.
   d. Active listening.
   e. Giving and receiving information.

Assertiveness Training

Assertive nurses, including managers, will stand up for their rights while recognizing the rights of others. They are straightforward, being free to be themselves. Assertive nurses know they are responsible only for their own thoughts, feelings, and actions. They can help others deal with their anger and thus prevent conflict. They know their strengths and limitations. Rather than attack or defend, assertive nurses assess, collaborate, support, and remain neutral and nonthreatening. They can then accept challenges.

Assertiveness can be taught through staff development programs in which nurses are taught to make learned, thoughtful responses. Nurses learn to accept responsibility rather than blame others. They learn when to say no, even to the boss. They learn to hold people to a standard. When they are dissatisfied, they do something to increase their satisfaction. Most of these assertive behaviors can be learned with case studies, role playing, and group discussion.

When they finish their training, assertive nurses will use positive comments to reinforce their expectation that others do their job. Praise and consideration promote wellness and positive individual behavior, which are linked to effective management and communication. Nurse managers learn that direct communication of support to the staff increases staff job satisfaction.

Assertive nurses focus on data and issues when offering constructive criticism to the boss or constructive feedback to the staff. This encourages dialogue and produces solutions rather than conflict. Assertive nurses ask for assistance or for delay when it is needed.

People usually respond positively to assertion and negatively to aggression, although some people respond negatively to assertion.[26]

Assessing the Dimensions of Conflict

Greenhalgh has developed a system for assessing the dimensions of conflict.[27] His view is that conflict may be considered to be managed when it does not interfere with ongoing functional relationships. Participants in a conflict have to be persuaded to rethink their views. A third party must understand the situation empathetically from the participants' viewpoints. The conflict may be the result of a deeply rooted antagonistic relationship.

Greenhalgh's Conflict Diagnostic Model has seven dimensions, each with a continuum from "difficult to resolve" to "easy to resolve." Once the dimensions of the conflict have been assessed, those viewpoints that fall in the difficult-to-resolve domain should be shifted to the easy-to-resolve domain (see Exhibit 23–1).

The following paragraphs discuss the seven dimensions of Greenhalgh's model.

The Issue in Question.   It has already been stated that values, beliefs, and goals are difficult issues to bring to a reasonable compromise. Principles fall into the same category, since they involve integrity and ethical imperatives. The third party must persuade the conflicting parties to acknowledge each other's legitimate point of view. How can principles be maintained and the organization and employees be saved?

The Size of the Stakes.   The size of the stakes can make conflict hard to manage. If change threatens somebody's job or income, the stakes are high. The third party must try to keep egos from being hurt, postponing action if necessary.

Exhibit 23–1   Conflict Diagnostic Model

	Viewpoint Continuum	
Dimension	*Difficult to Resolve*	*Easy to Resolve*
Issue in question	Matter of principle	Divisible issue
Size of stakes	Large	Small
Interdependence of the parties	Zero sum	Positive sum
Continuity of interaction	Single transaction	Long-term relationship
Structure of the parties	Amorphous or fractionalized, with weak leadership	Cohesive, with strong leadership
Involvement of third parties	No neutral third party available	Trusted, powerful, prestigious, and neutral
Perceived progress of the conflict	Unbalanced: One party feeling the more harmed	Parties having done equal harm to each other

Source: L. Greenhalgh, "Managing Conflict," *Sloan Management Review,* summer 1986, 47. Reprinted by permission. Copyright © 1986, Sloan Management Review Association. All rights reserved.

What will the parties settle for? Precedents create potential for future conflicts: If I give in now, what will I have to give up in the future?

Interdependence of the Parties.   People must view resources in terms of interdependence. If one group sees no benefits from the distribution of resources, it will be antagonistic. A positive-sum interdependence of mutual gain is needed.

Continuity of Interaction.   Long-term relationships reduce conflict. Managers should opt for continuous, not episodic, interaction.

Structure of the Parties.   Strong leaders who unify constituents to accept and implement agreements reduce conflict. When informal coalitions occur, strong leaders involve their representatives to find and implement agreements.

Involvement of Third Parties.   Conflicts are difficult to resolve when participants are highly emotional and resort to distorting nonrational arguments, unreasonable stances, impaired communication, or personal attacks. Such conflicts can be solved with a prestigious, powerful, trusted, and neutral third party. The third party can be an outside consultant, mediator, or arbitrator. The inside manager who acts as judge or arbitrator polarizes the participants; inviting a third party makes the conflict public. Third parties have to be involved when the nurse manager, as party to a conflict, cannot resolve it.

Perceived Progress of the Conflict.   Parties should be convinced that the score is equal and enough suffering has occurred.

TECHNIQUES OR SKILLS FOR MANAGING CONFLICT

Aims

When involved in managing conflict, the nurse manager should aim for broadening of the understanding of the problems. The nurse manager should help the parties to see the big picture rather than the limited perspectives of each party. He or she should aim to increase the possible number of alternatives in resolving the conflict. If possible, the nurse manager should encourage conflicting parties to voice several possibilities acceptable to each party and then work on a compromise. This stimulates the parties' interaction and involvement, another aim of conflict management. Still other aims include better decisions and commitment to decisions that have been made.

Strategies

The following are some strategies for managing conflict:[28]

Avoidance. Avoidance is a strategy that allows conflicting parties to cool down. The nurse involved in a conflict can sidestep the issue by saying, "Let's both take time to think about this and set a date for a future talk." This approach allows both parties to cool down and to gather information. Avoidance can be used when the issue is not critical or when the potential damage of immediate confrontation outweighs the benefits. In the latter case, a third party may have to be involved. Certainly the nurse manager as third party can tell the parties to a conflict, "I want you both to go on with your work while I take time to determine the facts and analyze them." Then the nurse manager should set a not-too-distant date for the future meeting.

Accommodation. The nurse who is a party to the conflict can accommodate the other party by yielding and placing the other's needs first. This is a particularly good strategy when the issue is more important to the other person. It maintains cooperation and harmony and develops subordinates by allowing them to make decisions.

Competition. A nurse manager as supervisor can exert position power at a subordinate's expense. This enforces the rule of discipline. It is an assertive position that fosters competition rather than commitment to conflict resolution on the part of the subordinate.

Compromise. Taking a middle ground may resolve a conflict. It should be a temporary strategy when time is needed to work out a permanent satisfactory position. A compromise that leaves both parties dissatisfied is not a good one.

Collaboration. When both parties collaborate to resolve conflict, they will both be satisfied. This is especially true of important issues. There should be integration of insights. This takes time and energy. A consensual solution wins full commitment. Collaboration leads to satisfaction among nurses.

Resolving Conflict Through Negotiation

Negotiation is probably the most rapidly growing technique for handling conflict. According to Hampton, Summer, and Webber, negotiation includes bargaining power, distributive bargaining, integrative bargaining, and mediation. These terms are defined as follows:[29]

1. *Bargaining power* refers to another person's inducement to agree to your terms.
2. *Distributive bargaining.* What either side gains is at the expense of the other. Most labor-management bargaining falls into this category.
3. *Integrative bargaining.* Negotiators reach a solution that enhances both parties and produces high joint benefits. Each party looks out for his or her own interests, with the focus shifting to problem solving—from reducing demands to expanding the pool of resources.
4. *Mediation.* Mediators attempt to eliminate surrender as a demand. They encourage each party to acknowledge that each has injured the other but is also dependent on the other.

Specific Skills

The following is a list of skills (many of which are preventive) to use in managing conflict.[30]

1. Establish clear rules or guidelines and make them known to all.
2. Create a supportive climate with a variety of options. This makes people feel comfortable about making suggestions. It energizes them, promoting creative thinking and leading to better solutions, and strengthens relationships.
3. Tell people they are appreciated. Praise and confirmation of worth are important to everyone for job satisfaction.
4. Stress peaceful resolution rather than confrontation. Build a bridge of understanding.
5. Confront when necessary to preserve peace. Do so by educating people about their behavior. Describe the behavior you perceive and tell the person what is wrong with the behavior and how it needs to be corrected.
6. Play a role that does not create stress or conflict. Do not play an ambiguous and fluctuating role that creates confusion among employees.
7. Judge timing for communication that is best for all. Do not postpone indefinitely.
8. Keep the focus on issues and off personalities.
9. Keep communication two-way. Tune in to the message, to correct interpretation, and to the feeling level of the employee. Reassure peo-

ple by listening to them unload and dump. Determine what is the real problem.

10. Emphasize shared interests.
11. Separate issues and confront those that are important to both parties.
12. Examine all solutions and accept the one most acceptable to both parties.
13. Avoid overriding your better judgment, becoming defensive, reprimanding the individual, cutting off further expression of feelings, and monopolizing the conversation. Such responses increase frustration and are ineffective management techniques.
14. If conflict is evident at decision-making or implementation stages, work to reach an agreement. Commit to a course of action serving some interests of all parties. Seek agreement rather than power.
15. Understand barriers to cooperation or resolution and focus on the dynamics of conflict to resolve it.
16. Distinguish between defiant behavior and normal on-the-job mistakes. Defiance is usually an individual behavior. Determine who the defier is and prepare emotionally and intellectually for the confrontation. Deal with one defiant person at a time. Establish authority and competence. Interview privately; teach, evaluate, resolve, guide, and deal with the defier. Do this immediately and follow up in two days. Discuss behavior and consequences, including possible termination, keeping calm and steady. Assume adults have a sense of courtesy and cooperation. When challenged, respond on the spot and stand your ground. Then move to a private area or remove yourself from the scene.
17. Be a sponge to a charge by an angry person.
18. Determine who owns the problem. Take responsibility for it as if you own it and say thanks.
19. Determine needs that are being ignored or frustrated and need recognition and nurturing.
20. Help distinguish demands from dreams.
21. Build trust by listening, clarifying, and allowing the challenges to unwind completely. Give feedback to make sure you understand. Let people know you care and that you trust them. Recognize other viewpoints and be willing to work to improve the relationship. Be factual. Ask for feedback. Work out a common bridge of "must" items. If another employee has a valid point, recognize it, apologize if necessary, and be genuine.
22. Renegotiate problem-solving procedures to forestall further anger, distrust, and defensiveness.

RESULTS OF CONFLICT MANAGEMENT

If attention is given to the role of the nurse manager in creating a climate for productive work by nurses, many of the causes of conflict will be eliminated. Knowledge of and skill in managing conflict when it occurs is an active role of nurse managers.

Conflict can be a positive source of energy and creativity; it can be constructive when properly managed. Otherwise, conflict can become dysfunctional and destructive, draining energy and reducing both personal and organizational effectiveness.

Conflict can destroy initiative or creativity; cause hostile and disruptive behavior, loss of team spirit, and loss of the desire to work toward common goals; and result in deadlocks and stalemates. Managed conflicts do not escalate.[31]

Exercise 23–1

For the following three case studies, form groups of five to eight students or employees. Select a leader for each group to keep the group moving and a recorder to write the plan or report. Refer to the chapter for techniques or skills in assessing and managing conflict. Outline a plan to deal with each case study using the following format:

1. What is (are) the cause(s) of the conflict?
2. Assess the dimensions of the conflict using Greenhalgh's Conflict Diagnostic Model.
3. Decide on aims, strategies, and specific skills for resolving the conflict. List them.

Case Study #1
You are called to a unit to resolve a conflict between an RN and an LPN. The nurses are shouting at each other in the hallway. The RN is the LPN's supervisor. As you approach them, you hear the following dialogue:

RN: I asked you to get Mr. W. ready to go to x-ray, and you ignored me. The transport person was here and left because you would not help him.

LPN: I was busy with Mrs. L. and could not leave. Why didn't you get Mr. W. ready? You apparently knew about it.

RN: It was your job. I assigned Mr. W. to you.

LPN: I do my own work and part of yours. You are the RN. You are supposed to be the leader in this hall.

RN: Don't get sarcastic with me. I don't have to put up with it. I'm going to call the supervisor and report you for your insolence.

LPN: My insolence! Go ahead and report me! I'll tell the supervisor what a lazy —— you are!

Case Study #2
During p.m. change-of-shift report, an RN calls in ill, and the staffing office says she cannot be replaced. This leaves only one RN, Mrs. K, for twenty-six patients. Mrs. K. says, "If you do not get another RN for this unit, I am going to quit this job. I will do it this shift, but I will not put up with this constant shortage of help. I don't care whether or not it's an RN, but I should have people with some skills to get the patients cared for. The reason everyone quits around here is because they are overworked and underpaid and the hospital management does not give a hoot. The place needs to be investigated."

(continued)

Exercise 23–1
(continued)

Case Study #3
A surgeon and a scrub nurse get in an argument during an operation. The surgeon tells the scrub nurse she is stupid and he does not want her to ever scrub for him again. The scrub nurse says that she is totally competent but that he expects her to read his mind. She says, "If you don't quit badgering me, I'm going to sue you and this hospital!" This comment escalates the dialogue into a shouting match.

Exercise 23–2

Describe a recent instance of a conflict in which you were involved. Was it resolved satisfactorily? Can the group help in finding a better solution? Discuss.

Exercise 23–3

Do an Internet search on conflict management. Prepare an abstract on two recent reports. The abstract should describe the value of the report to dealing with conflict among nurses.

WEB ACTIVITIES

- Visit www.jbpub.com/swansburg, this text's companion website on the Internet, for further information on Managing Conflict.
- Explore the Internet to locate various discussion areas on managing conflict.
- Search for discussion groups or organizations that help indivduals develop assertiveness. What can you find?

SUMMARY

The interrelationships among nurses and other personnel, patients, and families offer great potential for conflict. For this reason, nurse managers and leaders should know how to manage conflict.

Causes of conflict include defiant behavior, stress, crowded space, physician authority, and incompatibility of values and goals.

Conflict can be prevented or managed by discipline, communication, assertiveness training for nurses, and assessment of the dimensions of the conflict.

Aims of conflict management include broadening understanding about problems, increasing alternative resolutions, and achieving a workable consensus on decisions and genuine commitment to decisions made. Specific strategies include avoidance, accommodation, competition, compromise, collaboration, and negotiation. In addition, nurse managers and leaders can learn and use specific skills to prevent and manage conflict.

Conflict management keeps conflict from escalating, makes work productive, and can make conflict a positive or constructive force.

NOTES

1. J. H. Frost and W. W. Wilmot, "Making Conflict Work for You," in *Contemporary Leadership Behaviors: Selected Readings,* ed. E. C. Hein and M. J. Nicholson (Philadelphia: J. B. Lippincott, 1944), 338.
2. A. M. Barker, *Transformational Nursing Leadership: A Vision for the Future* (Baltimore: Williams & Wilkins, 1990), 47.
3. W. Bennis, *Why Leaders Can't Lead* (San Francisco: Jossey-Bass, 1990), 158.
4. B. S. Stevens, *The Nurse as Executive,* 3rd ed. (Gaithersburg, Md.: Aspen, 1985), 214.
5. J. M. Richardson, "Management of Conflict in Organizations," *Physician Executive,* January–February 1991, 41.
6. A. Marriner-Tomey, *Guide to Nursing Management and Leadership* (St. Louis: C. V. Mosby, 1996), 314–317.
7. P. J. Decker and E. J. Sullivan, *Nursing Administration: A Micro/Macro Approach for Effective Nurse Executives* (Norwalk, Conn.: Appleton & Lange, 1992), 551.
8. L. G. Bertinasco, "Strategies for Resolving Conflict," *The Health Care Supervisor,* July 1990, 35–37.
9. K. A. Noble and R. Rancourt, "Administration and Intradisciplinary Conflict within Nursing," *Nursing Administration Quarterly,* summer 1991, 36–42.
10. C. L. Anderson and E. Hughes, "Implementing Modular Nursing in a Long-Term Care Facility," *Journal of Nursing Administration,* June 1993, 29–35.
11. M. K. Hermann, J. Alexander, and J. T. Kiely, "Leadership and Project Management." in *Nursing Administration: A Micro/Macro Approach for Effective Nurse Executives,* ed. P. J. Decker and E. J. Sullivan ed. (Norwalk, Conn.: Appleton & Lange, 1992), 571.
12. R. G. Sands, J. Stafford, and M. McClelland, "'I Beg to Differ': Conflict in the Interdisciplinary Team," *Social Work in Health Care* 14, no. 3 (1990): 55–72.
13. J. S. Abramson, J. Donnelly, M. A. King, and M. D. Mallick, "Disagreements in Discharge Planning: A Normative Phenomenon," *Health and Social Work,* February 1993, 58–59.
14. A. Lowenstein and P. S. Hoff, "Discharge Planning: A Study of Nursing Staff Involvement," *Journal of Nursing Administration,* April 1994, 45–50.
15. T. Porter-O'Grady, "The Real Value of Partnership: Preventing Professional Amorphism," *Journal of Nursing Administration* 24, no. 2 (1994): 11–15.
16. E. C. Murphy, "Managing Defiance," *Nursing Management,* May 1984, 67–69.
17. Ibid.
18. D. R. Faulconer and V. B. Goldman, "Managerial Stress," *Nursing Administration Quarterly,* winter 1983, 32.
19. E. C. Murphy, "Communication and Wellness: Managing Patient/Staff Relationships," *Nursing Management,* October 1984, 64–68.
20. G. S. Wlody, "Communicating in the ICU: Do You Read Me Loud and Clear?" *Nursing Management,* September 1984, 24–27.

21. M. B. Silber, "Managing Confrontations: Once More into the Breach," *Nursing Management,* April 1984, 54, 56–58.

22. E. C. Murphy, "Practical Management Course," *Nursing Management,* March 1987, 76–77; American Hospital Association, *Role, Functions, and Qualifications of the Nursing Service Administrator in a Health Care Institution* (Chicago: AHA, 1978); R. Zemke, "The Case of the Missing Managerial Malaise," *Training,* November 1985, 30–33; M. A. Palich, "What Supervisors Should Know About Discipline," *Supervisory Management,* October 1983, 21–24; L. Greenhalgh, "SMR Forum: Managing Conflict," *Sloan Management Review,* summer 1986, 45–51.

23. A. C. Filley, "Types and Sources of Conflict," in *Management for Nurses: A Multidisciplinary Approach,* ed. M. S. Berger, D. Elhart, S. C. Firsich, S. B. Jordan, and S. Stone (St. Louis: C. V. Mosby, 1950), 154–165.

24. M. A. Palich, op. cit.

25. E. C. Murphy, "Communication and Wellness," op. cit.

26. C. C. Clark, "Assertiveness Issues for Nursing Administrators and Managers," *Journal of Nursing Administration,* July 1979, 20–24.

27. L. Greenhalgh, op. cit.

28. H. K. Baker and P. I. Morgan, "Building a Professional Image: Handling Conflict," *Supervisory Management,* February 1986, 24–29.

29. D. R. Hampton, C. E. Summer, and R. A. Webber, *Organization Behavior and the Practice of Management* (Glenview, Ill.: Scott Foresman, 1987), 635–639.

30. H. K. Baker and P. I. Morgan, op. cit; E. C. Murphy, "Practical Management Course," op. cit.; R. Lamkin, "Communicating Effectively," *B & E Review,* July 1984, 16; H. K. Baker and P. Morgan, "Building a Professional Image: Using 'Feeling Level' Communication," *Supervisory Management,* January 1986, 20–25; E. C. Murphy, "Managing Defiance," op. cit.; L. Greenhalgh, op. cit.; M. B. Silber, op. cit.

31. H. K. Baker and P. I. Morgan, "Building a Professional Image: Handling Conflict," op. cit.

24

CONTROLLING OR EVALUATING

OBJECTIVES

- ▪ Define "controlling" or "evaluating."
- ▪ Describe the relationship of controlling (evaluating) to the other major functions of management: planning, organizing, and directing (leading).
- ▪ Illustrate the use of controls as a management tool.
- ▪ Illustrate the use of standards for controlling or evaluating.
- ▪ Demonstrate controlling (evaluating) techniques.
- ▪ Use a set of standards to evaluate the controlling (evaluating) function of a nursing agency or unit.

KEY CONCEPTS

controlling
standards
benchmarking
controlling techniques

Manager behavior: Uses policies and procedures as standards for the controlling or evaluating process, including the standards of Medicare, Medicaid, and the Joint Commission on Accreditation of Healthcare Organizations.

Leader behavior: Provides opportunities for clinical nurses to input into all controlling or evaluating activities—standards, techniques, and applications—of the agency.

The final element of management defined by Fayol was control, which he defined as

> verifying whether everything occurs in conformity with the plan adopted, the instructions issued, and principles established. It has for its object to point out weaknesses and error in order to rectify them and prevent recurrence.[1]

Controlling or evaluating was defined by Urwick as "seeing that everything is being carried out in accordance with the plan which has been adopted, the orders which have been given, and the principles which have been laid down."[2] Urwick referred to three principles:[3]

1. The principle of uniformity ensures that controls are related to the organizational structure.
2. The principle of comparison ensures that controls are stated in terms of the standards of performance required, including past performance. In this sense, controlling means setting a mark and examining and explaining the results in terms of the mark. Today this is called benchmarking.
3. The principle of exception provides summaries that identify exceptions to the standards.

It is important that controlling be done on a factual basis. When issues arise, people should be made to meet with each other and settle them through direct contact. To stimulate cooperation, they need to participate from the beginning. Nurses can teach people to cooperate across departmental lines and to let reason and common sense prevail.[4] Management authors, including nurses, have described the controlling process as follows:[5]

1. Establish standards for all elements of management in terms of expected and measurable outcomes. These standards are the yardsticks by which achievement of objectives are measured.
2. Apply the standards by collecting data and measuring the activities of nursing management, comparing standards with actual care.
3. Make any improvements deemed necessary from the feedback.
4. Keep the process continuous for all areas, including
   a. Management of the nursing division and each subunit.
   b. Performance of personnel.
   c. Nursing process/product.

This process may be expressed as a formula:

$$Ss + Sa + F + C \rightarrow I$$

(Standards set + Standards applied + Feedback + Correction will yield Improvement.)

According to Peters, vision, symbolic action, and recognition make up a control system in the truest sense of the word. Peters also stated that "what gets measured gets done."[6]

CONTROLLING AS A FUNCTION OF NURSING MANAGEMENT

Control is "the management function in which performance is measured and corrective action is taken to ensure the accomplishment of organizational goals."[7] Control includes coordination of numerous activities—decision making related to planning and organizing activities and information from directing and evaluating each worker's performance. Control is also viewed as being concerned with records, reports, organizational progress toward aims, and effective use of resources. Control uses evaluation and regulation; controlling is identical to evaluation.[8] Koontz and Weihrich defined controlling as "the measurement and correction of the performance in order to make sure that enterprise objectives and the plans devised to attain them are accomplished."[9]

Systems Theory

Feedback and adjustment make up the control element of nursing management. Output is described or defined in terms of the patient in the patient-care model and is measured by quality indicators. In case management, these indicators are predicted and met on a timed basis. Discharge planning will take note of them. When the outcomes or indicators fall short, the information is fed back to the clinical nurses, who make adjustments in the case management plan and the process controlled by the critical path. Both the patient and the nurse are system inputs, while throughput consists of nursing actions related to patient outcomes and managerial actions related to setting goals for nurses' behavior. Quality management is the process by which the nursing product or process is measured and action prescribed to correct deficiencies.

Similarly, systems theory can be applied to performance evaluation of the registered nurse as output. Input is still the patient and the nurse, with throughput the managerial actions related to goals for nurse behavior. A performance results contract between clinical nurse and nurse manager spells out agreed-upon performance goals or results. When they are not being met, the nurse manager discusses the deficiency with the clinical nurse and they agree upon corrective actions. In an open system the process is continuous.

An effective control system has standards, measuring tools, and a surveillance process culminating in corrective action. A quality control program for measuring patient care will have these same components.[10]

Controlling is the second physical act of administration, the first physical act being directing or leading. It is the fourth and final element of the administrative composite process (ACP), planning and organizing being the conceptual acts. All functions of management—planning, organizing, directing, and controlling—occur simultaneously. Inputs would include resources other than the clinical nurse, such as supplies, equipment, and plant, plus all of the direct and indirect cost elements used in achieving the outputs.[11] Nurse managers will use staffing reports, budget status reports, and other information to control the functioning system. These reports are both monitoring devices and feedback to the clinical nurses and care managers.

Controls as Management Tools

In the process of measuring the degree to which predetermined goals are achieved and of applying necessary corrective actions to improve performance, policies and procedures are used as standards. Also, observations, questions, patient charts, patients, and health-care team members serve as sources of data. Corrective actions can be corroborative, disciplinary, or educational.[12] In the process of feedback, a positive experience will stimulate motivation and contribute to the growth of employees.[13]

Controls are management tools for improving performance. Among the controls are rules that are needed to let people know what is expected of them and how functions are to be coordinated. Communication of information is essential to control. Self-control is essential to managerial control, as it is the highest form of control. Self-control includes being up-to-date in knowledge, giving clear orders, being flexible, understanding reasons for behavior, helping others improve, increasing problem-solving skills, standing calm under pressure, and planning ahead. People should be told the facts in language that they understand and words that have the intended meaning. Effective nursing managers set limits and make them known to their employees. Then, when the line is crossed, the appropriate disciplinary action can be taken. The latter is achieved by corrective action consistently applied after checking the facts.[14]

The following are ten characteristics of a good control system:[15]

1. Controls must reflect the nature of the activity.
2. Controls should report errors promptly.
3. Controls should be forward looking.
4. Controls should point out exceptions at critical points.
5. Controls should be objective.
6. Controls should be flexible.
7. Controls should reflect the organizational pattern.
8. Controls should be economical.
9. Controls should be understanding.
10. Controls should indicate corrective action.

Nurses will remain cognitive that the best way of ensuring the quality of nursing services provided in the patient units is to establish philosophy, standards of care, and objectives. At least two of these, philosophy and objectives, involve planning, further evidence that the major functions of management take place simultaneously.[16] Controlling mechanisms also include accreditation procedures, consultants, evaluation devices, rounds, reports, inspections, and nursing audits.[17]

Nurses activate the processes of control. This function involves the use of power and should be used by nurses to promote openness, honesty, trust, competence, and even confrontation. It involves value systems, ethical decision making, self-control, professional self-regulation, and control by an aggregate of professionals. It is emerging as a system of quality control programs. The dimensions of quality management programs are quality of care, including accessibility, beliefs, and attitudes of patients about health care; structure of health care; processes of care; professional competence; outcomes of care; and self-regulation. Audits and budgets are the major techniques of control.[18]

STANDARDS

A prime element of the management of nursing services is a system for evaluating the total effort, including evaluation of the management process as well as the practice of nursing and all nursing care services. Evaluation requires standards that can be used as yardsticks for gauging the quality and quantity of services. The key source for these standards, which are available for both management and practice, is the ANA, whose publications include *Scope and Standards for Nurse Administrators* and *Standards of Clinical Nursing Practice*. Several functional yardsticks can be developed using these source documents. They can be of assistance in developing the objectives of the division of nursing and of each unit and clinic. Objectives are developed into operational or management plans, and systematic and periodic review of accomplishment of these objectives will be part of the evaluation system. In addition, a management evaluation system can be developed with a similar format. Further evaluation can be effected through development of criteria for nursing rounds by the nurse executive and other nurse managers. Performance standards can be used for individual performance, and criteria can be developed for collective evaluation of patient care. The latter may include the standards for use during nursing rounds as well as criteria for the quality management program.

Standards are established criteria of performance, planning goals, strategic plans, physical or quantitative measurements of products, units of service, labor hours, speed, cost, capital, revenue, program, and intangible standards.[19] They have also been defined as "an acknowledged measure of comparison for quantitative or qualitative value, criterion, or norm, . . . a standard rule or test on which a judgement or decision can be based." Nursing managers develop, in collaboration with clinical nurses, the "clinical nursing criteria against which to measure patient outcomes and the nursing process."[20] These standards are stated as patient outcomes and as nursing care processes. Eight categories of standards are physical standards, cost standards, capital standards, revenue standards, program standards, intangible standards, goals as standards, and strategic plans.[21]

Hospitals use the Joint Commission's Quality Cube as a model to illustrate the relationship between dimensions of performance and important functions and a range of patient populations and services provided. The cube is a tool that can help stimulate thought about and focus measurements related to improvement priorities. It can be entered at any point and can be used for global or very specific analysis (see Exhibit 24–1).[22]

Schoessler described a process for preparing documentation for a JCAHO (Joint Commission on Accreditation of Healthcare Organizations) visit, including a system for maintaining ongoing documentation that is being adapted to changes in JCAHO standards. Such a system assures that standards are kept up-to-date and prevents last-minute crisis preparation for JCAHO visits. Exhibit 24–2 is an example of a program grid for addressing staff education standards.[23]

Self-study is also a method of meeting JCAHO safety requirements. Employees are held accountable for meeting the standards and are tested to verify competency.[24] Programs are written and distributed by education personnel. Records are maintained on education cards or by computer. Self-study methods can be used to meet other standards.

Measuring productivity is a function of the controlling process. To do this, management establishes a measurement of productivity as the standard for each department and unit. Inputs are computerized and reported to appropriate cost-center managers each month. Productivity measurement tools should be developed, with input from the people being measured. This may be done locally or through consultation. Nursing departments with computerized patient classification systems often have accurate productivity indexes and reporting. Tools to evaluate productivity of independent nurse practitioners are available.[25]

Exhibit 24–1 The Quality Cube: A Model for Assessing the Quality of Health Care

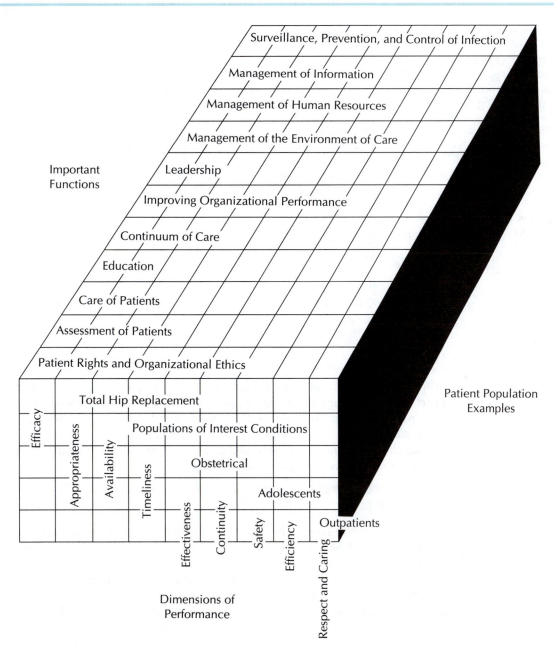

Source: © *1995 Comprehensive Accreditation Manual for Hospitals* (Oakbrook Terrace, Ill.: Joint Commission on Accreditation of Healthcare Organizations, 1994), 32. Reprinted with permission.

Exhibit 24–2 Program Grid

Program	Maintain Competence	Develop New Competence	Respond to QA Findings	Needs Assessed Through*	Evaluation Occurred Through†	Staff Contribute Through‡
Oncology Workshop	X			I/N	S/E	I/P/D
Advanced Life Support	X			I/P	S/E/P	I
Critical Care Residency		X		I/N	S/E/P	I/P/D
Discharge Planning		X	X	C	S/Q	I

*P = Pretest	†P = Posttest	‡I = Identifying needs of staff
I = Interview	S = Skill demonstration	P = Planning and presentation
N = Needs survey	Q = QA audit	D = Directing unit-based programs
C = Changed or new procedure	E = Evaluation form	S = Sharing information from out-of-house workshops

Source: M. Schoessler, "Preparing Documentation for a JCAHO Visit," *Journal of Nursing Staff Development,* September/October 1991, 217. Reprinted with permission of J. B. Lippincott.

Exhibit 24–3, "Operational Plan," is an example of an evaluation or controlling plan for nursing services.

CONTROLLING TECHNIQUES

Although evaluation operational plans are controlling techniques, other specific controlling techniques can be developed, including planned nursing rounds by nurse managers from all levels, checklists from ANA *Scope and Standards for Nurse Administrators,* ANA *Standards of Clinical Nursing Practice,* JCAHO *Accreditation Manual for Hospitals,* and other published standards of third-party payers, such as Medicare and Medicaid.

Nursing Rounds

An effective controlling technique for nursing managers is planned nursing rounds, which can be placed on a schedule and can include all nursing personnel. Rounds cover such issues as patient care, nursing practice, and unit management. To be effective, the results should be discussed with appropriate nursing personnel in a follow-up conference. Part of the evaluation process takes place as a result of the communication occurring during the rounds. Exhibit 24–4 shows a protocol for planned monthly nursing rounds.

Nursing Operating Instructions

Nursing operating instructions or policies become standards for evaluation as well as controlling techniques (see Exhibit 24–5 on p. 618).

Exhibit 24–3 Operational Plan

Mission Statement to Which Objective Applies
The division of nursing has a stated philosophy and has objectives. Personnel of each department or unit within the division will have their own philosophy and will set up their own objectives. The objectives will be continuously evaluated and a written statement as to progress will be sent to the chair's office each August and February.

Philosophy Statement to Which Objective Applies
We believe that a continuous evaluation of the activities of the division of nursing is necessary to assess how effectively the needs of the patients are being met and to take action to improve nursing service when indicated. Research must be performed, and the results must be analyzed, adapted, and implemented to modify nursing procedures and practices for the attainment of more effective patient care.

Objective 6
The patient benefits from close nursing supervision of all nonprofessional personnel who give patient care, and the patient benefits from continuous evaluation of the nursing care given and of performances of all nursing service personnel based on professional standards.

Plans for Achieving Objective	Action and Accountability	Target Dates	Accomplishments
1. Plan and execute a system of continuous evaluation and appraisal of nursing services.	1. Make complete rounds throughout the hospital at least once a day from nursing office. Establish a system of formal nursing rounds by chair, assistants, and clinical nursing coordinators monthly.	Apr. 23, 19XX	Being done.
	2. Do a monthly nursing audit. Have committee chair brief the chair of the division of nursing afterward.	Dec. 1, 19XX	Criteria for major nursing diagnosis outcomes completed. Committee combined with other disciplines. Criteria applied to four nursing diagnosis outcomes with retrieval by medical records personnel and corrective actions taken.
	3. Develop standards for patient care. Use ANA Standards of Clinical Nursing Practice for evaluating patient care. Obtain copies for all head nurses.	Jan. 1, 19XX	Obtained. Being incorporated into system by committee of staff nurses. Will cross-check with job performance standards.
	4. Develop standards for personnel performance.	Dec. 31, 19XX	Completed for clinical nurses I, II, and III, charge nurse, inservice education coordinator, clinical coordinator, chair and assistants, operating room supervisor and staff nurses, public health nurse, and rehabilitation nurse.

(continued)

Exhibit 24–3 Operational Plan *(Continued)*

Plans for Achieving Objective	Action and Accountability	Target Dates	Accomplishments
	5. Set up a system whereby managers attend a. Change-of-shift reports. b. Unit conferences c. Unit in-service programs.	July 1, 19XX	Receiving reports and need to plan for their use. Will discuss with managers.
	6. Review and use ANA *Scope and Standards for Nurse Administrators*	Dec. 1, 19XX	
2. Study organization.	1. Reorganize as needed. Have organization chart printed.		
	2. Write policy on unit policies and procedures.	July 1, 19XX	Done as hospital policy.
3. Establish a counseling program for all nursing personnel.	1. Program counseling sessions for all head nurses. Have them do the same for those they supervise.	July 1, 19XX Jan. 1, 19XX	Done as nursing operating instruction 160-2-4. All done once by Jan. 1, 19XX.
	2. Use the job performance standards.		

The ANA *Scope and Standards for Nurse Administrators* can be developed into a checklist for evaluating the management processes of nursing services. Exhibit 24–6 shows a format for converting these standards into a usable control tool.

The ANA *Standards of Clinical Nursing Practice* can be implemented in several ways. One way is to convert them into a checklist as in Exhibit 24–6. The entire set of standards can be developed into a checklist along these lines. Written protocols should be developed to implement a program for the evaluation process. Another way these protocols may be implemented is by using them to develop the evaluation standards as shown in Exhibit 24–7.

Gantt Charts

Early in this century, Henry L. Gantt developed the Gantt chart as a means of controlling production. The chart, which is usually used for production activities, depicted a series of events essential to the completion of a project or program.

Exhibit 24–8 shows a modified Gantt chart that could be applied to a major nursing program or project. The five major activities identified are seg-

Exhibit 24–4   Protocol for Planned Monthly Nursing Rounds

1. The chair, assistant chair, and other appropriate nursing personnel will make nursing rounds monthly.

2. Time is 10:00 to 11:00 a.m. unless otherwise indicated.

3. Schedule:

Unit	Day
1F	1st Tuesday
2A	1st Wednesday
2B	1st Thursday
2F	2nd Tuesday
ICU	2nd Wednesday
4A	2nd Thursday
3A	2nd Friday
3-OB	3rd Tuesday 10:30 to 11:30 a.m.
3F	3rd Wednesday
4B	3rd Thursday 11:00 a.m. to 12:00 noon
5A, CCU	4th Tuesday
5B	4th Wednesday

4. All unit nursing personnel are welcome to attend these rounds with their head nurse. Patient-care needs come first. The following areas will be covered as rounds are made to each patient's bedside:
   a. Nursing histories
   b. Nursing care plans
   c. Nursing notes
   d. Nurses' signatures on necessary documents

5. Other management areas of note will be discussed after bedside rounds:
   a. Equipment and supplies
   b. Staffing and assignments
   c. Narcotic registers

---

ments of a total program or project. The chart could be applied to a project such as implementing a modality of primary nursing or implementing case management. The following are possible nursing activities for a project:

1. Gather data.
2. Analyze data.
3. Develop a plan.
4. Implement the plan.
5. Evaluate, give feedback, and modify the plan as needed.

Exhibit 24–8 is only an example. Application of this controlling process by nurses would be specific to the project or program, and the time elements for the various activities would vary. Also, these five major activities could be modified by using subcategories of activities with estimated completion times. The nurse manager's goal is to complete each activity or phase *on or before* the projected date.

Exhibit 24–5   Operating Instructions

1. Special care units will maintain policies and procedures relative to their mission. (These procedures will be reviewed, updated, and signed at least annually.)
   a. Intensive care unit
   b. Critical care unit
   c. Newborn/intensive care unit nursery
   d. Renal dialysis
2. Special care units will maintain a list of equipment needed to achieve their mission.

3. Supplies and equipment
   a. Blount resuscitator will have percent adaptor to increase oxygen concentration.
   b. Ambu resuscitator will have tail on to increase oxygen concentration.
   c. Humidification will not be used with oxygen with Ambu resuscitator.
   d. Trays from Central Sterile Supply will be returned as soon as used so that instruments will not be lost or misplaced.

Exhibit 24–6   Format for Converting the ANA *Scope and Standards for Nurse Administrators* into a Usable Control Tool

Standard No. _____ :

_____

Measurement Criteria   Yes   No

(List)

Exhibit 24–7   Standards for Evaluating the Controlling (Evaluating) Function of Nursing Administration of a Division, Service, or Unit

1. An evaluation plan exists and is used for each nursing department, service, or unit.
2. Each evaluation plan is specific to the needs and activities of the individual department, service, or unit.
3. Evaluation findings are given in immediate feedback to subordinate nursing personnel.
4. Standards are accurate, suitable, and objective.
5. Standards are flexible and work when changes are made in plans and when unforeseen events and failures occur.

6. Standards mirror the organizational pattern of the nursing division, service, or unit.
7. Standards are economical to apply and do not produce unexpected results or effects.
8. Nursing personnel know and understand the standards.
9. Application of the standards results in correction of deficiencies.

Exhibit 24–8 Modified Gantt Chart

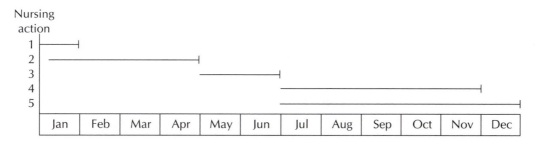

Note: Five nursing actions are needed to complete a program planned to start in January and end in December. In Exhibit 24–9, these five actions are translated into milestones and critical control points.

Critical Control Points and Milestones

Master evaluation plans should have critical control points, specific points in the production of goods or services at which the nurse judges whether the objectives are being met, qualitatively and quantitatively. Critical control points tell whether the plan is progressing satisfactorily. They pinpoint successes and failures and their causes. Critical control points tell nurses whether they are on target with regard to time, budget, and other resources. Milestones are segments or phases of specific activities of a project or program that are projected to occur within a time frame.

Exhibit 24–9 represents a modified Gantt chart with networks of milestones and critical control points.

The critical path is $1 \to 2 \to 3 \to 4 \to 5 \to 6 \to 7 \to 8 \to 9 \to 17 \to 18$. Line 5 represents evaluation of all other nursing actions. This is a simplified illustration of control techniques. Case management also uses critical paths with milestones and control points. Any major nursing program could have dozens or even hundreds of milestones and critical control points. This system may also be known by the name PERT (program evaluation and review technique).

Program Evaluation and Review Technique (PERT)

The program evaluation and review technique (PERT) was developed by the Special Projects Office of the U.S. Navy and applied to the planning and control of the Polaris weapon system in 1958. It worked then, and it still works, and it has been widely applied as a controlling process in business and industry.

PERT uses a network of activities, each of which is represented as a step on a chart. A time measurement and an estimated budget should be worked out that includes the following:[26]

Exhibit 24–9   Milestones and Critical Control Points

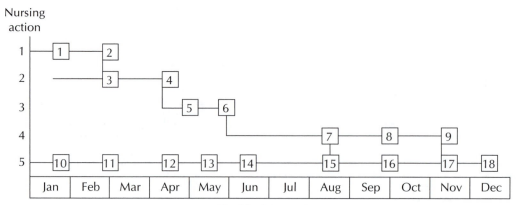

Modified Gantt chart
with milestones and critical control points
and network of milestones

1. The finished product or service desired.
2. The total time and budget needed to complete the project or program.
3. The starting date and completion date.
4. The sequence of steps or activities that will be required to accomplish the project or program.
5. The estimated time and cost of each step or activity.
6. Three paths for steps 4 and 5:
   a. The optimistic time.
   b. The most likely time.
   c. The pessimistic time.
7. Calculation of the critical path, the sequence of the events that would take the longest time to complete the project or program by the planned completion date. The reason this is the critical path is that it will leave the least slack time.

Benchmarking

Benchmarking is an offshoot of quality management and is a technique whereby an organization seeks out the best practices in its industry so as to improve its performance. It is a standard, or point of reference, in measuring or judging such factors as quality, values, and costs. The following are examples of benchmarks that could apply to nursing:[27]

▪ Establishment of a skill mix of nursing employees to obtain the highest quality of patient care at the lowest cost. This is called vertical leveraging. Horizontal leveraging uses cross-training to boost productivity. If the average for the industry is a ratio of 60 percent RNs to 40 percent other nursing personnel, the institution's management would make a decision to meet or exceed this ratio.

- An OR utilization rate of 80 percent or higher if the industry rate is 75 percent.
- An average turnover time between cases of 15 minutes if the industry rate is 20 minutes.
- A reduction of 10 percent from the average for industry cost of supplies per patient day.
- A reduction of 30 percent from the average for industry rate of hospital-acquired infections.

Standards of practice and standards of care are the benchmarks for nursing practice in all domains. Standards of care define the levels of care that a patient can expect to receive in a given situation or on a given nursing unit. They are clinical benchmarks and are the foundation for quality improvement programs. Quality occurs when personnel meet the established standards.

Structure standards describe the environment in which care is delivered.

Process standards describe a series of activities, changes, or functions that bring about an end or result.

Clinical standards, a subgroup of process standards, are developed to include clinical issues specific to areas of practice. They include both standards of care and standards of professional practice. According to the American Nurses Association, standards of care are authoritative statements describing a competent level of practice. Standards of professional practice are authoritative statements describing a competent level of behavior in the professional role.[28] Outcome standards are the results to be achieved.

Standards of practice to be achieved are used to structure the quality management program. They are linked to policy and procedure development and to job descriptions and performance appraisal. Implementation of standards is done through use of generic nursing care plans and the computer. The latter provides generic nursing care plans and nursing diagnoses. Exhibit 24–10 is an example of a generic nursing care plan.[29]

Benchmarking is enhanced when quality teams perform at the highest level of service by sharing their best practices and processes with similar committee teams in other institutions and organizations. Quality management is a necessary element of benchmarking. The following are some benefits of benchmarking:

- Setting goals and objectives and obtaining full team support to meet them.
- Continual improvement of practices, processes, and outcomes.
- Commitment and accountability for excellence.
- Seeking out, learning about, and adapting new approaches.

The benchmarking program includes planning during team meetings, collection of specific data, analysis of data to determine gaps, integration through keeping all team members informed, action, and follow-up and monitoring.[30]

Exhibit 24–10   Generic Nursing Care Plan

ST. JOHN MEDICAL CENTER
Medical Excellence • Compassionate Care

GENERAL SURGERY

Date	Nursing Diagnosis/Problems	Init	Interventions/ Discharge Plans	Goals	Date Reslv'd
	☐ Anxiety related to fear of surgical procedure as evidenced by ☐ call light on frequently ☐ multiple questions ☐ inability to sleep ☐ _____ _____ _____		☐ Preoperative teaching method _____ _____ _____ ☐ Provide reassurance and comfort _____ _____ _____		☐ Patient will express feelings of comfort and decreased anxiety
	☐ Alteration in comfort related to surgical procedure as evidenced by ☐ protecting the surgical site ☐ inability to stand upright ☐ shallow respiration ☐ _____ _____ ☐ _____ _____		☐ Position for comfort _____ _____ _____ ☐ Instruct patient on splinting of incision ☐ Anticipate patient's needs for analgesics _____		☐ Pain is minimized/ controlled with good muscle relaxation and ventilation

Source: M. McAllister, "A Nursing Integration Framework Based on Standards of Practice," *Nursing Management,* April 1990, 31. Reprinted with permission.

MASTER CONTROL PLAN

A master control or evaluation plan can be used by nurse managers to fulfill this important management function. It can be a general plan for all, with each manager adding specific items for his or her own management area. A sample basic master control plan is depicted in Exhibit 24–11.

Exhibit 24–11 Master Control Plan

Objective 1

Inspect for and identify the presence of written, current, and practical statements of mission, philosophy, vision, and objectives for the division of nursing and each of its component units. The statements should reflect the purposes of the health-care organization and give direction to the nursing care program.

Actions

1. The written statements of mission, philosophy, and objectives were current (reviewed or revised within past year).
2. They existed for the division of nursing and for each department, ward, unit, and clinic.
3. They were written by appropriate nursing personnel, representative of people who will accomplish them.
4. The philosophy reflected the meaning of clinical practice.
5. The philosophy was developed in collaboration with consumers, employees, and other health-care workers.
6. The objectives were specified, written in behavioral terms, and achievable.
7. They guided the process of implementing the philosophy.
8. They were used for orientation of newly assigned personnel and were otherwise widely distributed and interpreted.
9. They supported the mission, philosophy, and objectives of the institution.
10. Nursing personnel knew the rights of individuals and served as advocates for these rights.

Objective 2

Inspect for and identify the presence of written operational or management plans for accomplishment of the objectives of the division of nursing and each of its component units.

Actions

1. The written operational or management plans were current (entries within past 30 days).
2. They existed for the division of nursing and for each department, ward, unit, and clinic.
3. They included specific actions to be taken to achieve objective, target dates, and names of personnel assigned responsibility for each action.

4. They were used to evaluate progress; accomplishments were listed.

Objective 3

Inspect for and identify the presence of an organizational plan for the division of nursing and each of its component units.

Actions

1. The organizational plan was current; it agreed with actual organization when checked.
2. It existed for the division of nursing and for each department, ward, unit, and clinic.
3. It showed the relationships among component parts, spelling out the major functions of each, and it showed relationships with other services.
4. The organizational plan supported the mission assigned to personnel.
5. All nursing functions were managed by the nurse administrator.

Objective 4

Inspect for and identify the presence of adequate policies and procedures for guidance of personnel of the division of nursing and each of its component units.

Actions

1. Policies and procedures of the division of nursing and of each department, ward, unit, and clinic were current (reviewed within past year).
2. Policies and procedures did not duplicate those of higher echelons.
3. Policies and procedures were not obsolete, restrictive, or inappropriate in context.
4. Content of location of policies and procedures was known by people who needed this information.
5. Policies and procedures for special care units included
   a. Function and authority of unit director.
   b. Admission and discharge criteria.
   c. Criteria for performance of special procedures, including cardiopulmonary resuscitation, tracheostomy, ordering of medications, administration of parenteral fluids and other medication, and the obtaining of blood and other laboratory specimens.
   d. The use, location, and maintenance of equipment and supplies.

(continued)

Exhibit 24–11   Master Control Plan *(Continued)*

e. Respiratory care.

f. Infection control.

g. Priorities for orders for laboratory tests.

h. Standing orders, if any.

i. Regulations for visitors and traffic control.

6. The nursing annex to the disaster plan was current and included

a. Recall procedures.

b. Assignment procedures.

c. Training plan.

Objective 5

Inspect for and identify the presence of job descriptions and job standards for all personnel throughout the division of nursing.

Actions

1. Job descriptions and job standards existed and were current throughout the division of nursing (reviewed within past year).

2. Nursing personnel participated in formulating them.

3. Nursing personnel were classified according to competence, and salaries were commensurate with qualifications and positions of comparable responsibility within the agency and the community.

4. Job descriptions were used for purposes of counseling and helping employees to be productive.

5. They were used for orientation of newly assigned personnel.

6. They described the functions, qualifications, and authority of each position identified in the organizational plan.

7. They were readily available and known to each employee.

8. There was a designated nurse leader for the division of nursing who was a registered nurse with educational and experiential qualifications in nursing practice and the administration of nursing services.

Objective 6

Inspect for and identify the presence of a master staffing plan for the division of nursing and each of its component units.

Actions

1. A master staffing plan existed and was current for the division of nursing and each department, ward,

unit, or clinic. It showed authorized versus assigned personnel and was reviewed at least monthly.

2. Adequate personnel policies existed to give guidance to nursing personnel in the planning of time schedules and to allow for mobility so that personnel could be matched to jobs.

3. Avenues of communication existed to give input from nursing personnel to the nurse administrator regarding staffing problems.

4. An active plan existed for sponsoring newly assigned personnel and for identifying their special training and experience and their desired assignments.

Objective 7

Inspect for and identify the presence of a planned counseling program for all personnel of the division of nursing.

Actions

1. The nurse executive had a planned program for counseling with managers, including charge nurses.

2. Counseling occurred at least every six months on a scheduled basis.

3. Charge nurses counseled with individual staff members on a scheduled basis at least once every six months.

4. The counseling process included discussion of progress toward personal objectives, and revisions resulted from the sessions. Job standards were reviewed, and special educational and experience goals were discussed and acted on.

5. Records of counseling sessions were available and were reviewed.

6. A career progression plan was operational.

Objective 8

Inspect for and identify the presence of a system of evaluation of nursing activities in the division of nursing and each of its component units.

Actions

1. A system for evaluation of the division of nursing and each of its departments, wards, units, and clinics was in operation.

2. Change-of-shift reports and ward conferences were being periodically evaluated (at least once every six months).

Exhibit 24–11   *Master Control Plan (Continued)*

3. Management plans indicated current evaluation of accomplishment of objectives (within past 30 days).
4. Management personnel, including the nurse executive, made planned ward rounds at least monthly and checked all aspects of department, ward, unit, or clinic management, including
   a. Narcotic registers
   b. Nursing histories
   c. Nursing care plans
   d. Nursing notes
   e. Drug levels and security
   f. Supplies and equipment
   g. Assignment procedures
   h. Patient records
5. The quality assurance program was in effect, and at least one problem per month had been evaluated since June 1.
6. There was provision for inclusion of other health-care disciplines and consumers in evaluating the nursing care programs.
7. Results of evaluation were used to assess planning for change.

Objective 9
Inspect for and identify the representation of division of nursing personnel on institutionwide and departmental boards, committees, and councils.

Actions
1. The division of nursing was represented on institutionwide boards, committees, and councils whose activities affected nursing personnel directly.
   a. Social actions
   b. Personnel boards such as awards and benefits
2. Nursing service committees had specific objectives.
3. Membership was current and representative of all appropriate segments of the nursing staff.
4. Minutes of meetings reflected progress toward objectives and follow-up of problems.

Objective 10
Inspect for and identify the existence of a working public relations program that serves as a means of communication between personnel of the division of nursing and the community they serve.

Actions
1. Evaluation programs existed to tell consumers of the nursing services available to them and to receive feedback from consumers on the types of services they needed.
2. There was a planned program to publicize nursing activities and recognize contributions and accomplishments of nursing personnel.

Objective 11
Inspect for and identify the existence of a planned program for training and continuing education for all division of nursing personnel.

Actions
1. Written statements of mission, philosophy, and objectives existed and were current (reviewed within past year).
2. An operational or management plan for the accomplishment of objectives was current (entries made within past 30 days).
3. The plan listed activities, set priorities and target dates, assigned responsibility, and provided for continuous evaluation.
4. The plan provided for identification of training and continuing education needs, including input from participants, translation of needs into objectives, and the accomplishment of objectives.
5. An orientation program existed and included philosophy and objectives of organization and nursing service, personnel policies, job descriptions, work environment, clinical practice policies and procedures, and operational policies and procedures.
6. Supplemental classes were taught to meet on-the-job training needs.
7. Training programs were documented.
8. The program supported career advancement.

Objective 12
Inspect for and identify the existence of procedures and policies for providing needed primary nursing care to patients.

Actions
1. Collection of data on each patient was sufficient to permit identification and assessment of the patient's needs and to institute an individual plan of care. Included were admission data and patient's nursing history.
2. The nursing care plan included the nursing diagnosis, prescription for care, and patient's teaching needs.

(continued)

Exhibit 24–11 Master Control Plan *(Continued)*

3. The plan was used to provide care to the patient, and there was an ongoing reassessment of the patient's needs with appropriate changes made in the plan of care.

4. There was evidence that nursing actions required by physicians' orders, nursing care plans, and hospital policies were accomplished appropriately. Observations of patient's progress and response to actions were made and recorded.

5. There was evidence of interpretation and implementation of the ANA *Standards of Clinical Nursing Practice.*

6. Nursing administration had a plan for reviewing the requirements for giving credentials to individuals and health-care organizations and for participating in their implementation.

7. Guidelines existed for assignment of personnel based on level of competence.

8. There were policies to use unit managers and ward clerks to perform clerical, managerial, and indirect service roles.

9. Nursing administration provided resources to accomplish primary nursing care to patient: facilities, equipment, supplies, and personnel.

WEB ACTIVITIES

- Visit www.jbpub.com/swansburg, this text's companion website on the Internet, for further information on Controlling or Evaluating.
- Use your favorite search engine to obtain further information about "benchmarking."
- What organizations or journals could you search for information on controlling and evaluating?

SUMMARY

Controlling or evaluating is an ongoing function of nursing management occurring during planning, organizing, and directing activities. Through this process, standards are established and then applied, followed by feedback that leads to improvements. The process is kept continuous.

Each nurse manager should have a master plan of control that incorporates all standards related to these actions. This plan can be applied to obtain immediate feedback and meet the objectives of control established for the unit, department, or division. The plan will verify results, provide instructions, and apply principles of uniformity, comparison, and exception.

Controls include policies, rules, procedures, self-control or self-regulation, discipline, rounds, reports, audits, evaluation devices, quality control, and benchmarking. They should reflect the nature of the activity and be forward looking, objective, flexible, economical, and understandable. They should lead to continuous action.

Standards are the yardsticks for evaluation and include ANA *Scope and Standards for Nurse Administrators* and *Standards of Clinical Nursing Practice*. Other standards include management plans, goals, programs, costs, revenues, and capital. Physical standards use Gantt charts, critical control points, milestones, and PERT. Each nurse manager should have a master evaluation plan.

Exercise 24–1   With a group of your peers or colleagues, use Exhibit 24–7 and Exhibit 24–11 to discuss development of a new evaluation plan for a nursing cost center. Incorporate the standards from both exhibits. How can the standards be measured? Modify them if need be. Use your final product to evaluate the cost center.

NOTES

1. H. Fayol, *General and Industrial Management* translated by C. Storrs (London: Sir Isaac Pitman & Sons, 1949), 107.
2. L. Urwick, *The Elements of Administration* (New York: Harper & Row, 1944), 105.
3. Ibid., 107–110.
4. Ibid., 113–117.
5. H. Koontz and H. Weihrich, *Management,* 5th ed. (New York: McGraw-Hill, 1990), 394–395; R. M. Hodgetts, *Management: Theory, Process, and Practice,* 5th ed. (Orlando, Fla.: Harcourt Brace 1990), 226–229; H. S. Rowland and B. L. Rowland, *Nursing Administration Handbook,* 4th ed. (Gaithersburg, Md.: Aspen, 1997), 15–16, 35–44; P. F. Drucker, *Management: Tasks, Responsibilities, Practices* (New York: Harper & Row, 1973), 495–505; A. Marriner-Tomey, *Guide to Nursing Management and Leadership,* 5th ed. (St. Louis: C. V. Mosby, 1996), 379; D. C. Mosley, P. H. Pietri, and L. C. Megginson, *Management: Leadership in Action,* 5th ed. (New York: HarperCollins, 1996), 492–512.
6. T. Peters, *Thriving on Chaos* (New York: Harper & Row, 1987), 587, 593.
7. H. S. Rowland and B. L. Rowland, op. cit., 40.
8. T. Kron and A. Gray, *The Management of Patient Care: Putting Leadership Skills to Work,* 6th ed. (Philadelphia: W. B. Saunders, 1987), 100.
9. H. Koontz and H. Weihrich, op. cit., 393.
10. B. S. Barnum and M. Kerfoot, *The Nurse as Executives,* 4th ed. (Gaithersburg, Md.: Aspen, 1995), 229.
11. C. Arndt and L. M. D. Huckebay, *Nursing Administration: Theory for Practice with a Systems Approach,* 2d ed. (St. Louis: C. V. Mosby, 1980), 22–46.
12. P. Franck and M. Price, *Nursing Management,* 2d ed. (New York: Springer Publishing, 1980), 135.
13. M. L. Holle and M. E. Blatchly, *Introduction to Leadership and Management in Nursing* (Monterey, Calif.: Wadsworth Health Services Division, 1982), 178–185.
14. A. Levenstein, *The Nurse as Manager,* ed. M. J. F. Smith (Chicago: S-N Publications, 1981), 17–33.
15. R. M. Fulmer and S. G. Franklin, *Supervision: Principles of Professional Management,* 2nd ed. (New York: MacMillan, 1982), 216–217.

16. I. G. Ramey, "Setting Standards and Evaluating Care," in *Management for Nurses,* eds. S. Stone et al. (St. Louis: C. V. Mosby, 1976), 79.

17. H. M. Donovan, *Nursing Service Administration: Managing the Enterprise* (St. Louis: C. V. Mosby, 1975), 160–169.

18. M. Beyers and C. Phillips, *Nursing Management for Patient Care,* 2d ed. (Boston: Little, Brown, 1979), 109–141.

19. H. Koontz and H. Weihrich, op. cit., 394–395.

20. J. M. Ganong and W. L. Ganong, *Nursing Management,* 2d ed. (Gaithersburg, Md.: Aspen, 1980), 191.

21. H. Koontz and H. Weihrich, op. cit., 396–398.

22. *1995 Comprehensive Accreditation Manual for Hospitals.* (Oakbrook Terrace, Ill.: Joint Commission on Accreditation of Healthcare Organizations, 1994), 31–32.

23. M. M. Schoessler, "Preparing Documentation for a JCAHO Visit," *Journal of Nursing Staff Development,"* September/October 1991, 215–219.

24. A. Haggard, "Using Self-Studies to Meet JCAHO Requirements," *Journal of Nursing Staff Development,* July/August 1992, 170–174.

25. D. R. Kearnes, "A Productivity Tool to Evaluate NP Practice: Monitoring Clinical Time Spent in Reimbursable Patient-Related Activities," *Nurse Practitioner,* April 1992, 50, 52, 55.

26. H. Koontz and H. Weihrich, op. cit., 424–428; R. M. Hodgetts, op. cit., 240–242.

27. P. Patterson, "Benchmarking Study Identifies Hospitals Best Practices," *OR Manager,* April 1993, 11, 14–15.

28. American Nurses Association, *Standards of Clinical Nursing Practice* (Washington, D.C.: American Nurses Publishing 1991), 21.

29. M. Mc Allister, "A Nursing Integration Framework Based on Standards of Practice," *Nursing Management,* April 1990, 28–31.

30. J. A. Murray and M. H. Murray, "Benchmarking: A Tool for Excellence in Palliative Care," *Journal of Palliative Care* 8, no. 4 (1992): 41–45.

TOTAL QUALITY MANAGEMENT

"Improve quality (and) you automatically improve productivity. You capture the market with lower price and better quality. You stay in business and you provide jobs. It's so simple."[1]

W. Edwards Deming

OBJECTIVES

- Describe the elements of total quality management.
- Discuss Deming's fourteen points of a theory of management.
- Discuss Deming's seven deadly diseases related to his theory of management.
- Distinguish among examples of common causes and special causes of variation.
- Apply the Deming (Shewhart) cycle.
- Make a Pareto diagram using categories and measures of your choice.
- Do a fishbone diagram to isolate the causes of a problem.
- Identify nursing's internal and external customers.
- Prepare a total quality matrix related to current culture examples within your place of work.
- Form and use a quality circle to identify, analyze, and solve a problem within your place of work.

KEY CONCEPTS

Total quality management (TQM)
Customers
Theory Z
Quality circles

Manager behavior: Provides basic resources needed for developing a total quality management program.

Leader behavior: Provides all resources needed for developing a total quality management program and participates in the activities to ensure a successful outcome.

In total quality management (TQM), quality is a state of mind, a work ethic involving everyone in the company.[2] TQM has been described "as a way of life that [business leaders] believe can ensure the survival of American business."[3]

Among its elements are decentralization and participatory management—the process of making decisions at lower levels in the organizational hierarchy. This process involves every employee in making management contributions; it allows them to fix things instead of being treated like robots. TQM reduces or eliminates adversarial relationships.[4] Other elements of TQM are matrix management and management by objectives (MBO), statistical analyses, team building, quality circles, and Theory Z.

Many U.S. managers blame workers, taxes, government regulations, and the decay of society, among other things, for productivity problems. W. Edwards Deming, an early advocate of the principles of management for quality, found that 80 percent to 85 percent of problems are with the system; only 15 percent to 20 percent are with workers. Workers should be told this and should be given the freedom to speak and contribute as thinking, creative human beings. Deming's theory of management includes fourteen points (see Exhibit 25–1). Deming also warned against the seven deadly diseases that decrease productivity and profitability because they destroy employee morale (see Exhibit 25–2).

APPLICATION OF DEMING'S THEORY

According to Piczak, General Douglas MacArthur summoned W. Edwards Deming to set up quality circles for the Japanese in 1950.[5] When Deming presented the quality methods to forty-five Japanese industrialists, the Japanese applied the methods. "Within six weeks, some of the industrialists were reporting gains of as much as 30 percent without purchasing any new equipment."[6]

Using Deming's methods, managers and workers have a natural division of labor: The workers do the work of the system, while the managers improve the system. Thus, the potential for improving the system is never-ending. Since workers know where the potential for improving the system lies, consultants are not needed. Managers know that the system is subject to great variability and that problem events occur randomly. The common language for managers and workers is elementary statistics, which all workers learn.[7]

The Language Is Statistics

Variation.   Deming used and advocated the use of the language of statistics to identify which problems are caused by workers and which by the system. The most-used statistical tool is that of variation, which measures whether an activity is under control or, if not, to what degree it is out of control. Statistics enable workers to control variation by teaching them to work more intelligently. The common language of statistics stimulates discussion between workers and bosses at quality circle meetings.[8] Variation is the concept that distinguishes normal routine changes in a process from unusual, abnormal changes that can be attributed to specific causes. Variations in performance are mostly attributable to the system. Deming, in examples, found 400 percent variation in performance attributable to the system.[9]

Exhibit 25–1   Deming's Fourteen Points

1. Create constancy of purpose toward improvement of product and service. Everyone should have a clear goal every day, month after month. Satisfy the customer and reduce variation so all employees do not have to constantly shift their priorities.
2. Adopt a new philosophy by learning how to improve systems in the presence of variation, thus reducing variation in materials, people, processes, and products. End tampering and overreacting to variation.
3. Cease dependence on inspection to achieve quality by thoroughly understanding the sources of variation in processes and working to reduce variation.
4. End the practice of awarding business on the basis of price tag alone. Instead, minimize total cost by working with a single supplier.
5. Improve constantly and forever every process for planning, production, and service. Everyone uses PDCA (plan-do-check-act) cycle.
6. Institute training on the job. Know methods of performing tasks and standardize training. Accommodate variation in ways people learn.
7. Adopt and institute leadership. Work to help employees do their jobs better and with less effort. Learn which employees are within the system and which are not. Support company goals, focus on internal and external customers, coach, and nurture pride in workmanship.
8. Drive out fear, including fear of reprisal, fear of failure, fear of providing information, fear of not knowing, fear of giving up control, and fear of change. Fear makes accurate data nonexistent.
9. Break down barriers among staff areas, between departments. Promote cooperation. What is the constant, common goal?
10. Eliminate slogans, exhortations, and targets for the work force. Improvement requires changed methods and processes. Leaders change the system.
11. Eliminate numerical quotas for the work force and numerical goals for management. All people do not work at the same level of speed. There will be variation. Use realistic production standards. Eliminate management by objectives and use a system that rewards people's efforts toward improvement.
12. Remove barriers that rob people of pride of workmanship. Eliminate the annual rating or merit system.
13. Institute a vigorous program of education and self-improvement for everyone. This can be any education that improves self-esteem and potential to contribute to improvements in existing processes and advances in technology.
14. Put everyone in the company to work to accomplish the transformation.

Source: Reprinted from *Out of the Crisis* by W. Edwards Deming by permission of MIT and the W. Edwards Deming Institute. Published by MIT, Center for Advanced Engineering Study, Cambridge, MA 02139. Copyright 1986 by the W. Edwards Deming Institute. Dr. Deming rejected the concept of TQM, saying it was undefined.

Exhibit 25–2   Deming's Seven Deadly Diseases

1. Lack of constancy of purpose.
2. Emphasis on short-term profits.
3. Evaluation of performance, merit rating, or annual review.
4. Management by use of only visible figures.
5. Mobility of management.
6. Excessive medical costs.
7. Excessive costs of liability.

Source: Reprinted from *Out of the Crisis* by W. Edwards Deming by permission of MIT and the W. Edwards Deming Institute. Published by MIT, Center for Advanced Engineering Study, Cambridge, MA 02139. Copyright 1986 by the W. Edwards Deming Institute.

According to Deming, Shewhart, and others, there are chance (common) causes and special (assigned) causes of variation. Chance causes are common causes that are the fault of the system. They are system variations (such as process inputs or conditions) that are ever-present and cause small, random shifts in daily output. They occur in 90 percent of cases and require fundamental system change by management. Chance causes are controlled causes. A system totally influenced by controlled variation or common causes is said to be in statistical control.

A special, or assigned, cause is specific to a particular group of workers, an area, or a machine. It is an uncontrolled variation resulting from an assignable cause or source. Special causes occur in less than 10 percent of cases. They require finding the source and the taking of preventive action by the local workforce. Special causes require obtaining timely data to effect changes that will prevent bad causes and keep good causes happening (see Exhibit 25–3).

Management by action uses the Deming (Shewhart) cycle (see Exhibit 25–4). The cycle should be kept in constant motion and used at all levels of the organization. Reports should conform to the new system.[10]

Training in statistical process control takes the guesswork out of what is really happening in the operation. Statistical process control aims to prevent errors by identifying where they occur. The process is then tightened to improve the outcome. In looking at safety systems, Smith indicated that 85 percent to 90 percent of problems have common causes (the system), while only 10 percent to 15 percent of problems have special causes (employees). Using control charts to determine whether the causes of accidents are common or special leads to development of methods to prevent accidents. Employees can then set goals to reduce the special causes.[11]

Variation is a part of everything—of the supplies used by workers and of employee performance and many other activities. Causes exist other than common and special causes. One is tampering or making unnecessary adjustments to compensate for common-cause variation. Another is structural variation caused by seasonal patterns and long-term trends.[12]

Exhibit 25–3 Assigning Responsibility for Variation

Type of Variation	Frequency of Occurrence	Characteristic	Action Needed	Responsibility
Common cause	High (> 90%)	Fault of the system	Fundamental system change	Management
Special cause	Low (< 10%)	Traceable to an assignable cause	Find the source and take preventive measures	Local work force

Source: Reprinted with permission from A. E. Francis and J. M. Gerwels, "Building a Better Budget," *Quality Progress,* October 1989, 71.

Exhibit 25–4   The Deming (Shewhart) Cycle

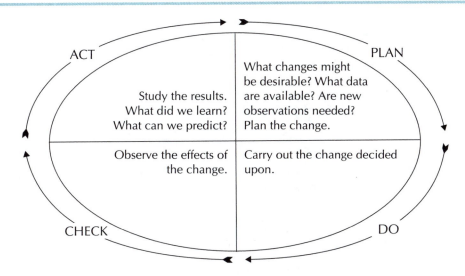

ACT	PLAN
Study the results. What did we learn? What can we predict?	What changes might be desirable? What data are available? Are new observations needed? Plan the change.
Observe the effects of the change.	Carry out the change decided upon.
CHECK	DO

Source: Reprinted with permission from A. E. Francis and J. M. Gerwels, "Building a Better Budget," *Quality Progress,* October 1989, 73.

Data Analysis.   Quality is not just another fad. Just as business and industry must have the high quality to compete in international markets, the U.S. health-care industry's institution of TQM at every level of the process will support the industry's expansion to provide at least an affordable safety net for all citizens. Deming states that quality must be defined and employees trained to deliver quality products and services. According to Deming, we should "measure the variations in a process in order to pinpoint the causes of poor quality and then how to gradually reduce those variations."[13]

Quality control should be online rather than end-of-line. This is achieved by sampling products during the process to determine how to correct those variations if the product deviates from the acceptable range. Quality improves as variability decreases.[14] Statistical charts are used to plot variations from the ideal in the production process and determine the right course to correct those variations.

Pareto charts are one example of control charts (see Exhibit 25–5). The Pareto principle states that most effects come from relatively few causes. Eighty percent of rework costs come from 20 percent of the possible causes. The Pareto principle is one of the most powerful decision tools available. Among the data that can be plotted on Pareto charts for nursing services are wasted time, number of jobs that have to be redone, customer inquiries, and number of errors, accidents, incidents, infections, and complications.[15]

Exhibit 25–5   Generalized Pareto Diagram

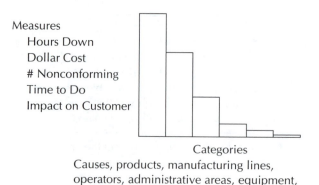

Measures
  Hours Down
  Dollar Cost
  # Nonconforming
  Time to Do
  Impact on Customer

Categories
Causes, products, manufacturing lines,
operators, administrative areas, equipment,
cost centers

Source: J. T. Burr, Center for Quality and Applied Statistics, Rochester Institute of Technology, One Lomb Memorial Dr., P. O. Box 9887, Rochester, NY 14623-9887. Reprinted with permission.

When constructing Pareto diagrams, one should place the most frequent cause at the left and arrange the remainder in descending order of occurrence. The impact on the system becomes obvious, as does the priority for fixing it. A double Pareto diagram can be used to contrast two areas, for example, the use of flexible work shifts before and after improvement. One must recognize what data are useful. Group consensus should be used to identify important causes and problems. Nominal group technique may be used:[16]

1. Give each person ten 3" by 5" cards.
2. Have each person write problems and causes on cards, one pair for each card.
3. Have each person rate causes by importance (10 = most important to 1 = least important).
4. Compile numbers for each cause.
5. Construct a Pareto chart.

Pareto charts may be used to plot reasons why nurses leave an agency. Reasons may be constructed using the National Commission on Nursing report or a career resource book and exit interviews.

Calculating system variations on process data allows control limits to be set, with variations being expected in the process as a result of aggregate common causes. Data may be plotted on a graph to show upper control limits (UCL) and lower control limits (LCL). If all points fall within these lines, variations are due to common causes, and one should not tamper with them (see Exhibit 25–6).

It is common but incorrect to treat all causes of variance as special and to tamper with them although the special causes of variation are but 10 percent of all causes. One should plot all data on control charts, including performance

Exhibit 25–6   Statistical Control Chart: All Points Falling within Control Limits

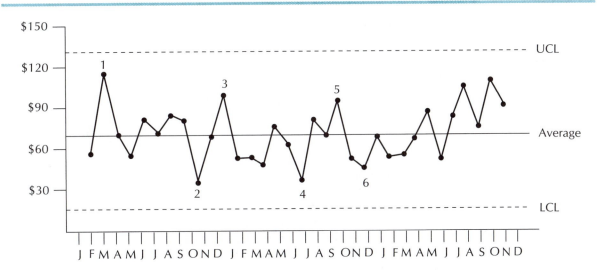

appraisals, which are often based on a system of common-cause variation. Plotting data reveals who performs at a level outside the system—above (UCL) or below (LCL) the control limits. One should learn what causes an employee to perform outside the system (below the control limits) and correct the cause by fixing the system. One should dispense with praise-and-blame sessions, study the performance appraisal system, find the special causes, and prevent them from recurring. If all causes are common causes, one should study ways to improve the variation in the system so that all employees work in an environment that facilitates their being able to improve by correcting special causes of variation. One also must remember to remove such barriers to pride of workmanship as annual or merit ratings.[17]

Fishbone analysis can be used in conjunction with Pareto analysis, although each may be used separately. Fishbone analysis has been successfully used at the Rotor Clip Company, Somerset, New Jersey, as a problem-solving technique as follows:[18]

1. Involve all employees having knowledge of the problem/product/service.
2. Express the problem in the simplest terms possible.
3. Divide the problem into potential problem areas. Draw a fishbone structure (see Exhibit 25–7).
4. Use brainstorming techniques to identify reasons for the problem (refer to chapters 13 and 15). Assign reasons to appropriate problem areas.
5. Review all the causes and decide on and test the solution.

Exhibit 25–7   A Fishbone Diagram

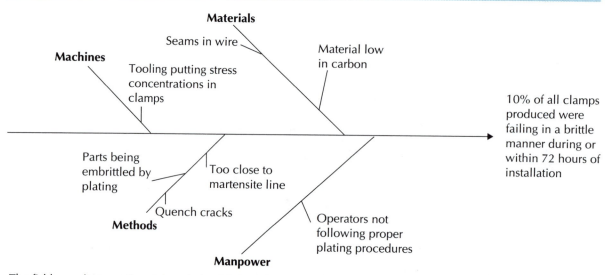

The fishbone diagram shown here helped Rotor Clip isolate the cause of defective parts. Seams in the wire turned out to be the culprit.

Source: B. Rudin, "Simple Tools Solve Complex Problems," *Quality,* April 1990, 50. Reprinted with permission from *Quality,* a publication of Hitchcock/Chilton Publishing, a Capital Cities/ABC, Inc., Company.

Exercise 25–1   Using a team representing nurse managers and clinical nurses, examine the purpose of a nursing division. How long has the purpose existed? Has the purpose been constant over time? Does it need changing? Examine a definition of total quality management and decide whether a change in purpose is needed. Will the change affect nursing services? Is this desirable? Make a management plan for accomplishing the agreed-upon purpose and for communicating it to all employees.

Exercise 25–2   Using a team representing nursing leaders within the organization, identify a major problem. Decide on the data to be collected and the statistical methods to be applied. Proceed to gather the data, analyze it, and solve the problem.

CUSTOMERS

The customer is the focus of TQM philosophy. One should first find out what the customer wants, then describe it, then meet it exactly. The service that meets the customer's needs provides the income to the supplier, be it an educational institution or a health-care agency. Quality is freedom from waste, trouble, and failure. One endeavors to meet and exceed customers' needs and expectations, then continues to improve.[19]

Internal and External Customers

In TQM, there are both internal and external customers, all of whom should be given service. In nursing, the external customers are patients, employers, and the community. These customers will be satisfied by quality care that produces a patient improved to the point of being discharged and able to get on with his or her life. A patient facing death wants a quality of care to make his or her remaining time peaceful. The employer wants knowledgeable and skilled workers; the community wants a productive citizen.

Internal customers are those who interact with each other within and among departments and disciplines. Internal customers to nursing are those departments that contribute to patient care, such as pharmacy, radiology, and medical laboratory. Clinical nurses are customers of nurse managers, admission services, and others. For each organization, the goal of quality care is defined by each self-managed team and possibly by an interdepartmental team. Quality takes time. It is here to stay. The customer should be satisfied quickly and economically if nurses are to stay in business. Business, including that of nursing, focuses on core customers and learns from them. This core of customers includes those who generate a profit and inspire nurses to their best ideas and highest motivation.[20]

The focus of TQM is harmony, not competition or adversarial relations. The optimal system of delivering patient care is achieved when all workers function as teams. The next shift in nursing is also an internal customer. Quality control focuses on satisfying such customers, not confronting them. The continual quest for improvement would reduce variation caused by confrontation, adversarial relationships within and among departments, and disharmony. This can be done by developing information and using statistical tools to analyze it.[21]

Quality improves nursing services because it reduces costs and keeps customers happy. Even in a recession, customers buy quality products and services.

Quality is not a program but a philosophy and a way of life. It is a survival issue. Traditional management is out. Quality management is customer-oriented, decentralized, empowering, and quality-focused.[22] Quality nurses aim for a world-class quality of care. This entails learning to deal with the most difficult of patients and families. Nurse managers would facilitate the capability of clinical nurses to deal with difficult customers.

Successful customer relations requires constant training and education programs. The need for staff development will continue to increase as nursing deals with improved technology, greater product reliability, a customer-service orientation, and flexibility in adapting to change. Nurse managers will continue to move decisions down the chain of command to all associates or team members. An educated and well-trained workforce is a nursing imperative. Every team member will need the skills of reading, understanding math, and conveying ideas.[23]

Each nursing associate will know the status of the work entering the nursing station, how to handle the customer in the workstation, and what the next internal customer requires. Such a quality system requires massive and continuous training to prevent errors. Authority and responsibility for quality of nursing care reside in the workstation, where associates take pride in craftsmanship and group output as well as ownership of the process.[24]

According to Peters, three percent of gross revenues should be spent on training to produce quality products and services. CEOs who put customers first put employees first. The latter will keep learning new skills and knowledge to be marketable.[25]

Exercise 25–3   Using a team that represents both nursing leaders within the organization and customers, construct a questionnaire for measuring external customer satisfaction. If such a questionnaire is currently available, review it and make changes only if changes are needed. Use the questionnaire to measure external customer satisfaction with nursing. Analyze the results using statistical applications and plan for changes to improve external customer satisfaction.

Exercise 25–4   Using a team that represents nursing leaders within the organization and internal customers of nursing, identify problems and make plans to fix them. Aim for cooperation and win-win fixes.

LEADERSHIP

Although leadership is treated in chapter 18, its importance to TQM requires mention here. Leadership is an essential element of the theory and philosophy of TQM. It transcends the process, requiring a people-oriented leadership style, cooperation in all ventures, and win-win relationships.[26] Such leadership will include all persons who work in nursing.

TQM requires total commitment by top management. It is long-range, focusing on the achievement of top quality in every relationship with every customer. Leadership will make each worker a "business person" with commitment to total responsibility for patient care. Every worker will be cross-trained and have access to all information. Every worker will have customers and be a manager.[27]

Long-term leadership is needed to achieve continuous improvement of productivity and services for the consumer. These require innovation and investment in research and education, long-range planning, and focus on the future. Long-term leadership is needed to maintain constancy of purpose and common purpose, part of which is to stay in business and provide jobs. Leadership oversees the mental revolution required when TQM becomes the process, with its constant focus on training and instruction. Leadership focuses goals and conserves productive energy by efficient direction; it builds quality with every stage of production, beginning with the purchase of high-quality raw materials.[28]

If managers do not attend to quality in today's health-care environment, they will lose their leadership to someone else. Deming indicates that leadership aims to improve performance of person and machine, improve quality, increase output, and provide pride of workmanship. According to Bryce, Juran states that leadership will be of the hands-on type and leadership will provide the breakthroughs.[29]

Leaders have a clear set of values and the integrity to institutionalize them. This occurred at LTV Steel, where integrated process management was the model of the quality process improvement implemented. As a result, LTV Steel went from a bottom-quality steel producer to a top-quality company. It did this by establishing a culture in which workers were obsessed with customer satisfaction, innovation became the norm, people were turned on throughout the organization, and common-sense systems were used.[30] Successful nursing leadership will change climate and culture to foster TQM.

CULTURE AND CLIMATE

TQM requires a favorable environment for total quality behavior in which values are shared as worthwhile or desirable and beliefs as truth. All employees in such an environment, including top management, believe in focusing on customers, both internal and external. They believe in an employee focus, teamwork, safety, and candor. There is total involvement because individual employees are empowered to identify and solve problems. A process focus exists that prevents errors and problems rather than fixes them.[31]

The total quality culture exists in a warm, friendly climate in which employees feel good about themselves, others, and their work. Employees in such a culture trust managers, who facilitate their work and treat them as equals who have intelligence and creative abilities. Fear has been driven out through leadership that has promoted teamwork, respect, and trust. All employees feel empowered to speak freely and to suggest changes. The heroes of the culture include employees who accept blame even though they are not at fault, who frequently defend employees of other departments or units, and who model total quality behavior to all customers. Myths and artifacts that may be eliminated include all titles from name tags, business cards, and nameplates. Rites and rituals that may be changed in a total quality culture include the abolition of reserved parking and the increased visibility of managers throughout the workplace. Management has spent great effort to create a strong total quality culture that has thickness, breadth, and clarity of ordering.[32]

Linkow suggests changing the culture through a total quality culture matrix tool (see Exhibit 25–8) that follows these steps:[33]

1. Describe the current culture through group brainstorming and interviewing.
2. Establish seven core total quality values and beliefs.
3. Correlate core values and beliefs with current culture.
4. Determine the strength of the current culture.

Exhibit 25–8 Total Quality Culture Matrix

Cultural Media	Current Culture Examples	Customer Focus	Employee Focus	Teamwork	Safety	Candor	Total Involvement	Process Focus	Symbols
Heroes	Employee who got out of a hospital bed for important meeting with a client	●	△	△	△				
	Person who left his family on vacation to work with client	●	△	△					
	Understudy steps in at last minute for sick "star" and makes resoundingly successful presentation to tough clients	●		○					● = highly correlated
Myths and Artifacts	No titles on business cards		○	○			○		
	Stories of failures with clients are told with relish		○			●			○ = correlated
	Employees do whatever it takes to satisfy the client	●	△						
Rites and Rituals	Anyone may be interrupted at any time		△	○			○		△ = negatively correlated
	When a problem is identified a list of solutions is brainstormed by a group			●			○		
	CEO walks through headquarters many afternoons asking, "What are you working on?"		○	●			○		

Strength of Culture									
Thickness		●	△	○	△	○	○	△	● = high
Extent of Sharing		●	○	●	△	●	○	△	○ = medium
Clarity of Ordering		●	○	●	△	○	○	△	△ = low

Source: Reprinted with permission of P. Linkow, Interaction Associates, Cambridge, Massachusetts.

5. Identify targets for culture change. These will be core values and beliefs with negative or nonexistent correlation or that are low in strength.
6. Use group to change culture.
7. Use external threats to mobilize internal forces of change.

O'Boyle indicates that U.S. managers of Japanese plants are frustrated with the Japanese concepts of consensus building and shared decision making. Over 350,000 Americans work for Japanese companies in the United States. In the corporate culture of these plants, the workers are called "associates" or "team members." Teamwork, harmony, and consensus are stressed. Presidents have the same kinds of metal desks as secretaries and in the same offices. There are no executive dining rooms, reserved parking, special bonuses, or stock options.

When business is poor, the employer educates workers in analytical and statistical procedures. Productivity is up 50 percent and costs down 55 percent. Almost 100 percent quality has been achieved. Factories are immaculate, well-lit, ergonomically designed, and air-conditioned. Warm-up exercises are used to eliminate back or wrist injuries. Workers rotate jobs every two hours and maintain output. There are twenty-four-hour child-care facilities. Bosses provide direction, guide group decision making, and facilitate continuous improvement.[34]

Florida Power & Light went from the worst to the best electric utility in the United States through TQM. Its middle managers became "facilitators" who coaxed team members to look for and solve problems. In a major training effort, 230 employees were trained in a five-week course in advanced statistical process control. Eight hundred employees studied basic statistics, and all 15,000 employees learned how to interpret data. The company launched a policy deployment management system of strategic planning, budgeting, and management with short- and long-range goals set at every level by consensus and involvement of every employee. It held expos to share solutions and awards banquets. It went for the Deming prize and got it![35]

Exercise 25–5 Using a team representing nursing leaders within the organization, describe the culture of the organization. Decide which beliefs and values need to be changed. Make a plan for changing them.

THEORY Z ORGANIZATIONS

Theory Z organizations focus upon consensual decision making. The leadership style of such organizations is a democratic one that includes decentralization, participatory management, employee involvement, and an emphasis on quality of life. Leaders are managers who concentrate on developing and using their interpersonal skills. This theory has been attributed to William Ouchi.[36]

Theory Z management and TQM are closely interrelated. Both start with planning that includes emphasis on staff development to improve quality of staff and their work. They start with a statement of philosophy that embodies the elements of both theories and proceed to the training of managers. Theory Z and TQM both require a long-term relationship between the organization and the employees. The organization invests in the employee by caring, by focusing on career needs, and by assisting employees to integrate their work and home lives through child-care centers, wellness programs, recreation, shift options, counseling, and opportunities for career development. Results have included production of generalists who can do more than one job, reduced turnover rate from 30 percent to 4 percent, unity because of the greater independence of nurses, reduced interdepartmental conflicts, reduced costs, improved risk management, and improved quality.[37]

QUALITY CIRCLES

Quality circles (QCs) are a participatory management technique that uses statistical analysis of activities to maintain quality products. The technique was initiated in Japan after World War II through the teaching of W. Edwards Deming, an American. The concept is to use statistical analysis to make quality improvements. Workers are taught the statistical concepts and use them through trained, organized, structured groups of four to fifteen employees, called quality circles. Group members share common interests and problems and meet on a regular basis, usually an hour a week. They represent other employees from whom they gather information to bring to the meetings.[38]

Quality circles should meet successful group design guidelines, including the following:[39]

1. Participation groups possess or have access to the necessary skills and knowledge to address problems systematically. All actors in the process receive training. Support people participate only as needed.

2. Formalized procedures enhance the effectiveness of the group. Systematic records are kept, and formal schedules of meetings adhered to.

3. To promote communication, participation groups are integrated horizontally and vertically with the rest of the organization. Accomplishments are publicized through awards dinners and publicity in in-house newspapers. Organized higher-level support groups hear the ideas of lower-level groups. All are limited by usual formal and informal communication mechanisms and routes.

4. Groups are a regular part of the organization and not a special or extra activity. They are composed of members of natural work groups. Results are measured in terms of ongoing organizational objectives and goals.

5. Normal accountability processes operate using the same skills, habits, and expectations as general organizations.

6. Groups manage themselves and are assisted by leaders and facilitators who are peer group members.

7. Participation occurs in such areas as decisions about job enrichment, hiring, training in problem-solving skills, management skills, and business conditions, pay based on skill mastery, gain sharing, and union management relationships based on mutual interests.

Research indicates that productivity and morale improve strongly when employees participate in decision making and planning for change. It is important that participation include goal setting, because participation will lead to higher levels of acceptance and performance. This research has been supported by meta-analysis. Research also shows that highly nonparticipatory jobs cause psychological and physical harm. *It is an ethical imperative to prevent harm by enabling employees to participate in work decisions.* Mental health is positively influenced by feelings of interest, a sense of accomplishment, personal growth, and self-respect.[40] Nurse managers will use this knowledge in managing clinical professional nurses.

According to Piczak, Deming set up QCs for the Japanese in 1950. QCs are focus groups and often survive in hostile environments. They are not an end in themselves. In 1985, over 90 percent of Fortune 500 companies were using QCs. In Japan, QCs use statistical methods, meet on their own time, and are given financial rewards. In the United States, QCs are voluntary, share an area of responsibility, and meet, discuss, analyze, and propose solutions to quality goals or problems and other programs.

Exercise 25–6   Make a plan for a quality circle using the guidelines described in this chapter.

APPLICATION OF TQM TO NURSING

Before deciding to apply the principles of TQM to nursing, top managers should learn the theory of TQM. TQM can be implemented in nursing with or without implementation in the total organization. If there is a source of knowledge of TQM theory within the organization, it may be tapped first. This will give recognition to employees as experts within their own organization. Schonberger suggests that using outside persons to interpret quality is not effective.[41]

The lead team should all read *Out of the Crisis,* in which Deming describes his theory of total quality management and the deadly diseases of management and recommends a management philosophy. Then the team can write its management plan for implementing TQM. The process will be never-ending, because quality is a complicated construct and producing high-quality nursing services is a complicated process.

The first goal of a nursing management plan is to write the stated purpose of nursing service so that it is constant and provides a clear goal for everyone for every day, month after month. This is the first of Deming's fourteen points (refer to Exhibit 25–1). All fourteen points should be discussed by the lead team. The management plan should list activities to achieve each of these points. Teams can be assigned to develop plans for assessing the culture and climate and making plans to change them, for planning training in statistical methods with particular emphasis on variance, for improving supplier relationships, for breaking down interdepartmental barriers, for developing realistic production standards, and for transforming the entire nursing organization.

Quality management should be decentralized so that practicing nurses own quality and apply the processes needed to deliver quality nursing service. Nurses would develop quality methods to check the application of nursing process to patients, check process and outcomes, and fix any deficits (variance) in the process. When necessary, these nurses subject the nursing process to Pareto and fishbone analysis. They may repeat the process at more specific levels to identify the solution to a problem. They will "commit to 'do right' principles: maintain control of every process, post quality evidence on the walls, brook no compromises, find a way to check every unit (where checks are necessary), fix their own mistakes, and assess continual involvement in quality improvement projects."[42]

Traditional American management theory "motivates employees by fear (principally of losing their jobs), by requiring them to meet quotas, and by attempting to maximize their merit increases. Deming's principles require a fundamental change in American habits."[43]

Habits are based on immediate consequences of behavior, on short-term success. Their long-term consequences and subsequent problems have been very destructive. Management habits often cause problems. Well-established destructive habits of management can be changed. The following are some principles for making changes:[44]

1. The individual manager or leader must perceive a need to change, must genuinely admit and accept that he or she must change, and must commit to the change. Unfortunately, managers or leaders often do not perceive a need for change unless their business is in serious trouble.
2. The change must be voluntary, not coercive.
3. The change process requires a philosophical base, a statement of beliefs about how people will be managed. If TQM is to be implemented, the philosophical base may be a statement of beliefs that include all or some of Deming's fourteen points. The leader who implements this change process acts as teacher and planner and is the object of a process called "transference."
4. The change process requires the support of others participating in the same process. Thus, a group interacts, shares insights and feelings, and provides social support while implementing a philosophy of TQM.
5. The process should be broken into steps that can be accomplished in sequence. The nurse leader or manager should aim for at least one quick success, make a road map or plan, and provide education and communication.

Today's manager is "a high-tech management-trained individual with a focus on profitability through quality and a sensitive, but widely encompassing, utilization of work force talent."[45] Committed to TQM, this manager leader knows that if quality is improved, productivity will be improved. The following are some goals for this new breed of nurse leader:

1. Change management style and operating climate.
2. Do the job right the first time to meet and exceed customers' expectations.

3. Stop producing waste, stop sorting good from bad to avoid poor services to customers, stop paying people to produce waste. Innovate and excite the customer with high-quality services.

4. Look at the waste standards and spoilage problems of nursing.

5. Identify and eliminate performance inhibitors and continuously improve productivity.

6. Use process data to change methods, techniques, and technology to create improvements.

7. Replace boss-imposed solutions with group interaction.

8. Eliminate as many layers of management and support personnel as possible. Replace with integrated, self-governing work teams.

9. Train managers to be coaches, trainers, and information resources.

10. Reach out and involve customers and suppliers.[46]

11. Recognize that all improvements take place project by project.

12. Publish quality goals with names of projects and names of team members to fix responsibility and give rights to teams. Review progress on projects.[47]

13. Constantly work to improve the work system for employees by providing better tools and raw materials and building a culture of trust.

14. Scrap quality control departments, numerical goals, and quotas. Give workers the right to shut down the production line if the quality of the product is in jeopardy. Spot and fix defects in process. Give authority to practicing nurses.

15. Drive out fears by throwing out or simplifying worker performance evaluations.

16. Learn to live without enemies. Get workers to cooperate, not compete.[48]

17. Use plan-do-check-act (PDCA) cycle

Exhibit 25–9 summarizes several successful applications of TQM in U.S. organizations.

One estimate is that 40 percent of operating costs of service industries is spent on errors.[49] Hospital and nursing administration make the commitment and create the environment for making quality improvement happen.

TQM has its detractors, including managers involved in downsizing and restructuring U.S. business and industry. Executives who are committed to TQM are making it work (Xerox, Motorola, Federal Express, and Harley-Davidson, among others). Many executives claim that TQM costs more than it is worth. The theory of TQM is solidly integrated into the theory of human resources development as the management theory that will produce the most motivated and productive workers. It takes true leadership to make it work.

The literature abounds with examples of application of TQM in healthcare systems. Rush-Presbyterian-St. Luke's Medical Center in Chicago started implementing TQM in 1987. Its program centered on the establishment of professional standards for clinical services. Rush examined various industrial models of quality management to identify the elements of the model that would strengthen its own quality initiatives. The employees were trained in TQM

(text continues on p. 649)

Exhibit 25–9 Examples of TQM in U.S. Organizations

Department of Veterans Affairs, Philadelphia

Initiated TQM with concept of veterans as customers. Established cross-functional teams and involved middle management so they were not threatened by new ideas and won their trust. Start-up training costs were $75,000: 2-hour orientation class for every employee run by division managers; 40-hour quality improvement course in group dynamics, analytical tools, hypothetical problem solving for 50 percent of employees; 24-hour course for team members to act as team facilitators; and series of 2-hour modules teaching clerks and staffers to welcome change, and suggest new ideas. Teams with IDs listing team and members' names. Success: $168,000 saved on loan default processor improvements; people believe their ideas are being heard, and people relate to other's jobs.

Source: E. Penzer, "A Philadelphia Story," *Incentive,* July 1991, 33–34, 36.

Brazosport Memorial Hospital

Brazosport Memorial Hospital established a quality improvement process of quality orientation, continuous process improvement, and total employee involvement. A quality improvement council of top administrators developed a policy with employee input: "It is our commitment at BMH to promote genuine pride in excellence among our employees and other professionals in order to continuously improve the quality and value of the services provided to achieve customer satisfaction." A definition of quality states: "Providing health care services which are continuously improved to meet the needs and expectations of our patients, physicians, employees, payers and the community we serve." Employees are encouraged to speak freely about hospital operations and generate ideas for improvement. They are encouraged to collect and analyze data in process improvement. Questionnaires are sent every six months to 300 former patients to assess quality. Process includes quality improvement teams, training, changes including management style, commitment, stress on ideas, and networking among others.

Source: M. L. Lynn, "Deming's Quality Principles: A Health Care Application," *Hospital & Health Services Administration,* spring 1991, 111–120.

Publishers Press

Assessed the organization's working environment through employee surveys. Provided three-week train-

ing course in SPC for all middle managers. All employees trained in Deming's philosophy. Process improvement team (PIT) members were trained to change the work culture to eliminate fear and lack of communication. Because employee input and experience was considered important, the culture was changed to make the employees want to get involved. Teams of owners and experts met 1–2 hours a week to determine internal customers and suppliers of the process chosen for study. Teams decided where process began and ended, applied process components, measured process input, and made change as needed. They validated prioritized objectives and diagrammed process control charts. Brainstorming led to action plan for improvement. New PITs form, old PITs disband when processes improve. Statistical improvements take months. Had 17 percent error reduction in order entry and 20 percent in film spoilage. Process requires coach, not judge, and interaction between managers and employees.

Source: G. A. Ferguson, "Printer Incorporates Deming—Reduces Errors, Increases Productivity," *Industrial Engineering,* August 1990, 32–34.

General Motors

Adopted Deming's philosophy to transform GM's culture. Results included decreased parts transport from 5 days to 31 hours and with 35 percent fewer shipping racks and fewer rail cars. Applied successfully to re-engineering an engine to decrease variance.

Source: J. P. White, "No More Excuses," *The Wall Street Journal,* 21 November 1991, 1, A6.

Ingersoll Machine Tool

"But in the machine tool segment of manufacturing, Ingersoll has faced hard times and has shown that top management's involvement in a quality program can keep a company competitive in world markets."

Ingersoll made an unstinting investment in new technology. They expanded during recession by integrating computers into manufacturing systems. They expanded production capacity and made a commitment to employees, thus preparing for a business upturn. They kept a skilled and knowledgeable work force intact, as well as a shop full of new, modern, updated, and accurate machines. Everyone learned to work a little more effectively. Through planning and commitment to quality on a long-term basis, they sold machines to Hitachi, Fuji, and Honda and competed worldwide.

Exhibit 25–9   Examples of TQM in U.S. Organizations *(continued)*

Ingersoll has a philosophy of original design. Their mission is defined in the quality policy statement "we achieve quality . . . when we successfully design and build to specifications that accurately . . . define our customers' needs." Ingersoll spent money to develop inspection equipment. They developed supplier evaluation programs, annual quality improvement programs, continuous training of workers to upgrade quality skills, and process evaluations for SPC.

Source: J. Wolak, "From the Top," *Quality,* August 1988, 14–15.

Levi Strauss

Levi Strauss will attempt to keep its plants in the U.S. by restructuring. Assembly lines will be replaced by self-managed teams of 30 to 50 workers who will make an entire product. Team members will learn a variety of skills. The restructuring process requires much time and training. Workers will help make decisions, and they will make the teamwork system successful because they believe in it. They will run the factories, hire colleagues, set their own hours, and purchase their own thread and equipment: empowerment and flattened organizational structure with the workers in control. There will be programs to help workers pay for child care. Dress will be informal and managers will be called by their first names in a casual culture. They will provide quality products for satisfied customers. There will be decreased injuries and increased profits.

Mission Statement. The mission of Levi Strauss & Co. is to sustain responsible commercial success as a global marketing company of branded apparel. We must balance goals of superior profitability and return on investment, leadership market positions, and superior products and service. We will conduct our business ethically and demonstrate leadership in satisfying our responsibilities to our communities and to society. Our work environment will be safe and productive and characterized by fair treatment, teamwork, open communications, personal accountability, and opportunities for growth and development.

Aspiration Statement. We all want a Company that our people are proud of and committed to, where all employees have an opportunity to contribute, learn, grow, and advance based on merit, not politics or background. We want our people to feel respected, treated fairly, listened to, and involved. Above all, we want sat-

isfaction from accomplishments and friendships, balanced personal and professional lives, and to have fun in our endeavors.

When we describe the kind of LS&CO we want in the future, what we are talking about is building on the foundation we have inherited: affirming the best of our Company's traditions, closing gaps that may exist between principles and practices, and updating some of our values to reflect contemporary circumstances.

What type of leadership is necessary to make our aspirations a reality?

Teamwork and Trust. Leadership that exemplifies directness, openness to influence, commitment to the success of others, willingness to acknowledge our own contributions to problems, personal accountability, teamwork and trust. Not only must we model these behaviors but we must coach others to adopt them.

Diversity. Leadership that values a diverse workforce (age, sex, ethnic group, etc.) at all levels of the organization, diversity in experience, and a diversity in perspectives. We have committed to taking full advantage of the rich backgrounds and abilities of all our people and to promote a greater diversity in positions of influence. Differing points of view will be sought; diversity will be valued and honesty rewarded, not suppressed.

Recognition. Leadership that provides greater recognition—both financial and psychic—for individuals and teams that contribute to our success. Recognition must be given to all who contribute: those who create and innovate and also those who continually support the day-to-day business requirements.

Ethical Management Practices. Leadership that epitomizes the stated standards of ethical behavior. We must provide clarity about our expectations and must enforce these standards throughout the corporation.

Communication. Internally, leadership that builds an environment in which information is actively shared, sought, and used in ways that lead to empowerment that works, improved performance, and meaningful feedback. Externally, leadership that strengthens our corporate reputation with key stakeholders. All communications should be clear, timely, and honest.

Empowerment. Leadership that promotes ways of working in which responsibility, authority, and accountability for decision making are held by those closest to

(continued)

Exhibit 25–9 Examples of TQM in U.S. Organizations *(continued)*

products and customers, and every employee has the necessary perspective, skills, and knowledge to be successful in his or her job. We all share responsibility for creating the environment that will nurture empowerment at all levels of the organization.

In an interview with Robert Howard for the *Harvard Business Review,* Robert Haas, the CEO of Levi, stated, "A company's values—what it stands for, what its people believe in—are crucial to its competitive success." He went on to say, "Because we value open and direct communication, we give people permission to disagree."

Note: Mission Statement and Aspiration Statement used courtesy Levi Strauss Associates, Inc., San Francisco, California. Updated November 1995.

Source: J. Kever, "People Power," *San Antonio Light,* 12 July 1992, A1, A10–12; Editorial, "Levi's Plan to Tailor Production Fits U.S. Manufacturing Needs," *San Antonio Light,* 6 February 1992, C8; P. Konstam, "Levi's New System Can Save U.S. Jobs," *San Antonio Light,* 5 February 1992, D1; R. Howard, "Values Make the Company: An Interview with Robert Haas," *Harvard Business Review,* September/October 1990, 133–144.

Mars

Mars, Inc., is a multibillion-dollar, world-class company that is a leader in candy, pet food, rice, and other products. At the Mars company there are no assigned parking spaces for anyone. There are no offices or partitions between desks. Offices have a concentric structure, with the president and staff at the center and others fanning outward. Senior officers are totally visible and accessible. Time clocks are at doors, and everyone, including owners, punches in. An employee who punches in on time gets a 10 percent punctuality bonus.

Communications at Mars are personal and immediate. Memos are not written and electronic mail goes unused. Factories are spotless and shining, with efficient, high-speed lines. Employees, including managers, wear white uniforms and white hats in production areas. Otherwise dress is casual for all. Employees are highly paid, nonunion, loyal, and proud. Quality is an obsession and is everyone's responsibility. All Mars employees get the same annual step increase. There are only six pay levels, with vice presidents all receiving approximately the same salary. People can be easily transferred from business unit to business unit and from function to function.

Mars is a true quality culture. It maintains state-of-the-art technology. Equipment is valued at replacement cost. The company uses a unique equation called ROTA (return on total assets) that accounts for inventory turns and asset utilization.

The business acumen of the Mars family has created great personal wealth for them. They are listed in *Fortune,* June 28, 1993, as among the world's 101 richest people.

Source: C. J. Cantoni, "Quality Control from Mars," *The Wall Street Journal,* 27 January 1992, A10.

USAA

USAA, which is based in Texas, is a Fortune 500 insurance and financial services company whose chairman of the board, Robert F. McDermott, is a septuagenarian. Over 10,000 employees work in San Antonio, TX. Another 5,000 work in other branches of the United Services Automobile Association in Atlanta, GA; Colorado Springs, CO; Norfolk and Reston, VA; Sacramento and San Diego, CA; Seattle/Tacoma, WA; Tampa, FL; and several overseas locations where there are high concentrations of military officers.

USAA was started in 1922 by military officers. McDermott came as CEO in 1968, lured away from his post as dean of the United States Air Force Academy. At that time 40 percent of employees quit each year. Many jobs were mundane and low-paying, and management was untrained. McDermott believed that technology had to be developed to make dull jobs easier. Also, employees "had to be made to feel they were part of something special if they were to make the company's customers feel the same way."

In 1994, the corporate culture of USAA includes the following:

• A community recreation complex where employees leave work to play softball on two manicured diamonds; soccer on a lush, green field; basketball on two outdoor courts outfitted with scoreboards and bleachers; tennis courts; and volleyball courts.
• A sense of community, enthusiasm, not-too-serious competition, a sense of sportsmanship, and a given sense of purpose.
• An employee health clinic.
• Encouragement of employees to participate in the external community as mentors to students.
• A 286-acre "campus."

Exhibit 25–9 Examples of TQM in U.S. Organizations *(continued)*

- A structure that rivals the Pentagon in square footage and consumes more than $4 million in gas and electricity per year.
- A work experience that gives pleasure, satisfaction, and psychic income.
- Stress on teamwork and common goals, even though the organization is highly structured and insists on adherence to protocol.
- A take-care-of-its-own attitude reflected in its pay, benefits, perks, and working conditions, including a four-day work week.
- A state-of-the-art plant and equipment. The computer operation handles 8 million transactions a day and is linked via cable and satellite with field offices in other cities.
- Training and conference rooms that include the company's own television production facility, the latest in video technology, production of video press releases, training videos, a USAA news program that runs on its own closed-circuit network, documentaries for use by the insurance industry, and 50 to 60 hours a month of teleconferencing.
- Comfortable workstations and high-tech equipment.
- Facilities to increase fitness and improve wellness.
- First-rate cafeterias. Employees are offered a "dinner express" from 3 to 6 P.M. They take home 3,000–4,000 dinners each week.
- A credit union and the USAA Federal Savings Bank.
- College courses; job-related courses have tuition paid by USAA.
- A company-owned store for employees.
- A local post office branch, which processes 350,000 pieces of mail daily.
- A day-care facility serving 300 employees' children up to age 5 will be opened by USAA in 1995. "Having a well-adjusted child in a quality day-care arrangement reduces stress on employees who have children."**

The whole idea is to make employees happy and productive. They are! Turnover is down to 8.5 percent a year. USAA's customers are happy and the company is highly profitable and expanding. It is poised for the future.* A new CEO, General Robert Herres, has replaced McDermott, who has retired.

Source: *M. Tolson, "USAA, TX 78228," *San Antonio Light,* 23 September 1990, A1, A12; **L. Hicks, "USAA to Erect Day Care Facility," *San Antonio Express-News,* 12 May 1994, 1E.

Dialysis Center, Lincoln, Nebraska
At the Dialysis Center of Lincoln, NE, after implementation of TQM the following changes occurred:

	1987–1988	1990–1991
Employee satisfaction survey	40%	92%
Staff turnover	70%	5%
Absenteeism	8 days/yr/ employee	2.5 days/yr/ employee
Medicare statement of deficiencies	7 pages	3 pages

Source: M. Churchill, "Employees Are Also Our Customers," *ANNA Journal,* April 1992, 152.

Motorola
Motorola is one of the best-managed companies in the world. Part of this is due to their commitment to TQM, termed "six sigma quality." With only 3.4 mistakes per one million parts produced. Motorola attempts to measure every task performed by its 120,000 employees. It calculates $1.5 billion saved by reducing defects and simplifying procedures during 1993.

Source: R. Henkoff, "Keeping Motorola on a Roll," *Fortune,* 18 April 1994, 67–68, 70, 72, 74, 77–78.

concepts and empowered to make improvements in their work. The corporation required a cultural change that focused on a vision and unrelenting pursuit of the realization of that vision.

To accomplish a change in the culture of this organization, a combined emphasis was placed on training, measurement, and communications. Among the improvements noted were a reduction in the preparation time to pick up a neonatal infant from a referring hospital, a reduction in the number of incomplete medical records following hospital discharge, a reduction in the x-ray repeat rate, and a reduction in patient delays in radiology. Rush management acknowledges that total quality management has worked because the employees were willing to try something new.[50]

McEachern, Schiff, and Cogan outline the application of continuous quality improvement (CQI) to direct patient care. The goal of the CQI process is to improve direct patient care. The principles used are the customer's knowledge level, process focus, and statistical-mindedness. Three methods of developing direct patient-care teams are (1) following the interest of an individual who usually becomes the team leader, (2) organizing the top twenty-five diagnosis-related groups (DRGs) by functional body systems or major functional processes, and (3) team formation by clinicians.[51]

Health-care institutions are finding that between 40 percent and 60 percent of all therapeutic effects can be attributed to placebo and Hawthorne effects. Kindness prevents malpractice suits. Quality of life is improved by esteem-enhancing interventions. Attention, information in the form of follow-up summaries of visits, and surroundings all contribute to improved quality of care and life.[52]

WEB ACTIVITIES

- Visit www.jbpub.com/swansburg, this text's companion website on the Internet, for further information on the Theory of Quality Management.
- Try searching under the names of some of the theorists and theories discusses in this chapter. What do you find?
- The W. Edwards Deming Institute is an organization offering information on Deming's teachings, publications, and theories; locate its site and review its offerings.

SUMMARY

Total quality management is fast replacing old concepts of management. It is a system that empowers the worker. TQM has evolved from the work of W. Edwards Deming who found that 85 percent to 90 percent of problems are due to the system (common causes) and only 10 percent to 15 percent are due to employees (special causes). Through the use of statistical concepts such as variation, the common causes can be separated from the special causes, and workers can themselves fix the special causes during the process of production. Application of the philosophy and theory of TQM leads to increased productivity and profitability.

Among the data analysis tools that are used to fix causes are Pareto charts or diagrams and fishbone diagrams.

TQM focuses upon customer satisfaction and includes the notion of internal and external customers. If the customer is going to radiology for a special procedure, the nurse's next internal customer is radiology. Clients, families, and communities are external customers.

Leadership is the paramount qualification for success in TQM. It is leadership that will change the culture and the climate of the business to give workers the training they need to participate in planning, make decisions, be creative, and improve productivity through improvement of quality of products and services. It is leadership that fosters self-esteem and eliminates formal barriers to cooperation such as job titles, unfair pay practices and performance appraisals, and divisive perquisites of office.

TQM is the new wave of nursing management. It is a proven theory waiting for broad application.

NOTES

1. J. Oberle, "Quality Gurus: The Men and Their Message," *Training,* January 1990, 47–52.
2. J. J. Kaufman, "Total Quality Management," *Ekistics* May–August 1989, 182–187.
3. P. Konstam, "'Quality Should Begin at Home," *San Antonio Light,* 1 March 1992, D1.
4. Ibid; R. Boissoneau, "New Approach to Managing People at Work," *The Health Care Supervisor,* July 1989, 67–76.
5. M. W. Piczak, "Quality Circles Come Home," *Quality Progress,* December 1988, 37–39.
6. M. Tritus, "Deming's Way," *Mechanical Engineering,* January 1988, 28.
7. Ibid., 26–30.
8. Ibid.
9. W. J. Duncan and J. G. Van Matre, "The Gospel According to Deming: Is It Really New?" *Business Horizons,* July–August 1990, 3–9.
10. A. E. Francis and J. M. Gerwels, "Building a Better Budget," *Quality Progress,* October 1989, 70–75.
11. T. A. Smith, "Why You Should Put Your Safety System Under Statistical Control," *Professional Safety,* April 1989, 31–36.
12. B. L. Joiner and M. A. Gaudard, "Variation, Management, and W. Edwards Deming," *Quality Progress,* December 1990, 29–39.
13. L. A. Heinzlmeir, "Under the Spell of the Quality Gurus," *Canadian Manager,* spring 1991, 22–23.
14. Ibid.
15. J. T. Burr, "The Tools of Quality Part VI: Pareto Charts," *Quality Progress,* November 1990, 59–61.
16. Ibid.
17. B. L. Joiner and M. A. Gaudard, op. cit.
18. B. Rudin, "Simple Tools Solve Complex Problems," *Quality,* April 1990, 50–51.
19. M. Schrage, "Fire Your Customers," *The Wall Street Journal,* 16 March 1992, A12.
20. D. Schaaf, "Beating the Drum for Quality," *Quality,* March 1991, 5–6, 8, 11–12.
21. G. Rex Bryce, "Quality Management Theories and Their Application," *Quality,* January 1991, 15–18.

22. "What's Next on the Quality Agenda?" *Quality,* March 1991, 42.
23. P. Konstam, "Making Productivity Grow Takes Work," *San Antonio Light,* 1 January 1992, 1E.
24. J. J. Kaufman, op. cit.
25. T. Peters, "Plenty Left to Do for U.S. Economy," *San Antonio Light,* 14 January 1992, B9.
26. Ibid.
27. T. Peters, "Turn Your Workers into Business People," *San Antonio Light,* 26 November 1991, E3.
28. W. J. Duncan and J. G. Van Matre, op. cit.
29. G. R. Bryce, op. cit.
30. R. H. Slater, "Integrated Process Management: A Quality Model," January 1991, 27–31.
31. P. Linkow, "Is Your Culture Ready for Total Quality?" *Quality Progress,* November 1989, 69–71.
32. Ibid.
33. Ibid.
34. T. F. O'Boyle, "Two Worlds," *The Wall Street Journal,* 27 November 1991, 1.
35. L. Dusky, "Anatomy of a Revolution," *Executive Excellence,* May 1991, 19–20.
36. W. G. Ouchi, *Theory Z* (Reading, Mass.: Addison-Wesley, 1981).
37. M. N. Adair and N. K. Nygard, "Theory Z Management: Can It Work for Nursing?" *Nursing & Health Care,* November 1982, 489–491.
38. The theory of quality circles was actually developed by Frederick Herzberg and F. Edwards Deming of the United States 50-plus years ago. S. Johnson, "Quality Control Circles: Negotiating an Efficient Work Environment," *Nursing Management,* July 1985, 34A–34B, 34D–34G; A. M. Goldberg and C. C. Pegels, *Quality Circles in Health-Care Facilities* (Gaithersburg, Md.: Aspen, 1984).
39. S. A. Morhman and G. E. Ledford, Jr., "The Design and Use of Effective Employee Participation Groups: Implication for Human Resource Management," *Human Resource Management,* winter 1985, 413–428.
40. M. Sashkin, "Participative Management Remains an Ethical Imperative," *Organizational Dynamics,* spring 1986, 62–75.
41. R. J. Schonberger, "The Quality Concept: Still Evolving," *National Productivity Review,* winter 1986–87, 81–86.
42. Ibid., 82.
43. B. Carder, "Kicking the Habit," *Quality Progress,* March 1991, 87–89.
44. Ibid.
45. W. C. Lamporter, "The New Breed," *American Printer,* July 1991, 28–31.
46. Ibid for goals 1–10.
47. "Quality Can't Be Delegated," *Supervision,* May 1988, 6–7 for goals 11–12.
48. B. Richmond, "Auto Advice Is Good School of Thought," *San Antonio Light,* 11 January 1992, 1B for goals 13–16.
49. F. F. Jespersen, "Once More with Feeling: Quality Starts at the Top," *Business Month,* August 1989, 65–66.
50. M. E. Sinioris, "TQM: The New Frontier for Quality and Productivity Improvement in Health Care," *Journal of Quality Assurance,* September/October 1990, 14–17.
51. J. E. McEachern, L. Schiff, and O. Cogan, "How to Start a Direct Patient Care Team," *Quality Review Bulletin,* June 1992, 191–200.
52. T. Peters, "Good Service Vital to Health Care, Too," *San Antonio Light,* 10 November 1992; B2.

26

QUALITY MANAGEMENT

by Linda Roussel, DSN, RN
Consultant in Nursing

OBJECTIVES

- Define quality management.
- Differentiate among components of a quality management program.
- Describe the structure of a quality management program.
- Differentiate among tools for collecting and analyzing quality management data.
- Differentiate among elements of a risk management program.

KEY CONCEPTS

quality management	**Manager behavior:** Provides resources to meet the requirements of accreditation and legal entities for quality management.
structure audit	
process audit	
outcome audit	
risk management	**Leader behavior:** Supports accountability of nurses through education and assurance that they deliver quality patient care.
incident report	

As discussed in Chapter 24 on controlling, a master evaluation or control plan is needed to evaluate the total program of any nursing department, service, or unit. One of the most critical components of such a plan will be a quality management program. A key element of quality management is continuous improvement. As the costs of hospital and all aspects of health care continue to grow, it becomes essential that quality management programs truly establish standards to maintain and, indeed, deliver quality care. A primary assumption is that nursing must be accountable to the client for the care rendered by its practitioners.

Quality assurance (QA) programs began in hospitals in the 1960s with voluntary implementation of nursing audits. Initially, nursing QA programs were designed to set standards for nursing care delivery and establish criteria by which to evaluate these standards. The term has emerged in the health-care field as a synonym for evaluation, or as a significant evaluative activity. Kirk describes the relationship between QA, quality control (QC), and quality improvement (QI). QA defines performance measurements and compares actual processes and outcomes to clinical and satisfaction indicators. QC involves performance management and maintenance and includes systematic methods of ensuring conformance to a desired standard or norm. QI is concerned with performance development and is ongoing, involved with fixing now, preventing future costly mistakes, and fostering breakthroughs.[1]

QA, QC, and QI are integrated and now include additional focal points of service quality and customer satisfaction. These elements must be incorporated into any QA program if it is to be a success. Matching the expectation of the service with that which is actually experienced by the customer defines the link between service quality and customer satisfaction. In other words, if the customer's perception is that the expectation of the service has been met or exceeded, the service is generally considered a quality one, and thus one has a satisfied customer.[2] Being ever-watchful of client satisfaction of services provided is essential in all QA programs.

The Joint Commission on Accreditation of Healthcare Organizations (JCAHO) purports that from its initial form of retrospective, time-limited audits, the process has evolved to its current form of ongoing monitoring using well-chosen process and outcome indicators. In the same vein, the quality improvement process must be a never-ending cycle.[3] According to Deming, this cycle must employ statistical quality control, and the development of a "bedrock philosophy of management" is critical to ensure an enduring process of quality improvement.[4] It is the blending and balancing of caring and providing such care around which a well-thought-out quality management program is built. This is a major part of the evaluation phase of the nursing management process.

Part of evaluation involves the understanding of the vision and the purpose the organization serves for its clients, employees, and customers and the community. The leadership role in providing this vision is ultimately critical to how well management's vision is translated into well-written and understood objectives and outcomes. In addition, one would be remiss if efficiency (the cost of achieving objectives) were not considered in the model. Quality assurance not only incorporates evaluation but also involves its use to secure improvement.

COMPONENTS OF A QUALITY MANAGEMENT PROGRAM

A quality management program is composed of the following components:

1. Clear and concise written statements of purpose, philosophy, values, and objectives.
2. Standards or indicators for measuring the quality of care.
3. Policies and procedures for using such standards for gathering data. These policies define the organizational structure for the program.
4. Analysis and reporting of the data gathered, with isolation of problems and variances.
5. Use of the results to prioritize and correct problems and variances.

6. Monitoring of clinical and managerial performance and ongoing feedback to ensure that problems stay solved.
7. Evaluation of the quality management system.

These components may be conceptualized in many different ways. Continuous quality improvement (CQI), the essence of quality management, can be conceptualized to illustrate how one component builds on another. Batalden and Stoltz describe a framework for the continual improvement of health care (Exhibit 26–1) that incorporates underlying knowledge, policy for leadership, tools and methods, and daily work applications.[5] Underlying knowledge incorporates professional and improvement knowledge. Such knowledge includes knowledge of a system, knowledge of variation, knowledge of psychology, and theory of knowledge. The mission, vision, guiding principles, and integration of values are critical to the policy for leadership. "For the continual improvement of health care, tools and methods are available that can accelerate building and using knowledge and communicating that understanding to others."[6] Tools and methods can be grouped into four major categories: process and system, group process and collaborative work, statistical thinking, and planning and analysis. Daily work applications include developing models for testing change and making adjustments as well as reviewing the improvements. Conceptualizing QA and CQI provides the nurse with tools for assisting the nursing department with the overall process.

Exercise 26–1 Examine the quality management program of a health-care agency. How does the program address the components previously outlined?

Exhibit 26–1 The Framework for the Continual Improvement of Health Care

Underlying Knowledge	Policy for Leadership	Tools and Methods	Daily Work Applications
Professional knowledge: • subject • discipline • values	Mission, vision, and quality definition Guiding principles	Process, system Group process and collaborative work	Models for testing change and making improvement Review of improvement
Improvement knowledge: • system • variation • psychology • theory of knowledge	Integration with values	Statistical thinking Planning and analysis	

Source: P. B. Batalden and P. K. Stoltz, "A Framework for the Continual Improvement of Health Care: Building and Applying Professional and Improvement Knowledge to Test Changes in Daily Work," *Joint Commission Journal on Quality Improvement,* October 1993, 426. Oakbrook Terrace, Ill.: Joint Commission on Accreditation of Healthcare Organizations, 1993, p. 426. Reprinted with permission.

Statement of Purpose, Philosophy, and Objectives

The initial planning of a quality management program includes the development of clear and concise statements of purpose, philosophy, and objectives. The program's purpose and philosophy go hand in hand with the organizational purpose and philosophy and should be interwoven with the value the organization places on quality and continual improvement of the services provided. The JCAHO gives specific guidelines designed to assess and improve quality of client care. In addition, quality improvement theories are recommended to health-care organizations to better conceptualize the entire quality management program. Such quality improvement theories include those of Deming, Crosby, Juran, and Senge.[7] An organization need not limit itself to one theory and may incorporate concepts from a wide variety to develop a framework that best fits the organization's purpose, philosophy, and objectives. Every quality management program needs well-articulated objectives, and every study a purpose (Exhibit 26–2 gives example mission and purpose statements).

Exercise 26–2   Examine the statements of purpose, philosophy, and objectives of a health-care agency. What elements of quality management are evident?

Standards for Measuring the Quality of Care

Standards define nursing care outcomes as well as nursing activities and the structural resources needed. They are used for planning nursing care as well as for evaluating it. Outcomes include positive and negative indexes. Standards are directed at structure, process, and outcome issues and guide the review of systems function, staff performance, and client care.

A number of health-care organizations issue indexes. The Health Care Financing Administration (HCFA) annually discloses projected and actual hospital mortality rates by diagnosis-related groups. The HCFA outlines physical quality indexes. The JCAHO has issued clinical and organizational performance

---

Exhibit 26–2   Mission and Purpose Statements

Mission
The mission of the Quality Assurance Plan of the University of South Alabama Medical Center is directly reflective of the mission of the University of South Alabama Medical Center. As stated in the policy, "Functional Plan of Organization of the University of South Alabama Medical Center" (from Mission Statements), the Department of Quality Assurance "ensures that the quality of patient care at the University of South Alabama Medical Center is optimal

through a unified program for patient care evaluation activities."

Purpose
The purpose of the Quality Assurance Plan of the University of South Alabama Medical Center is to ensure that all patients receive the optimal quality of care.

Source: Courtesy University of South Alabama Medical Center, Mobile, Alabama.

measures and outcomes under the auspices of quality assessment and improvement. It requires that the organization have a written plan for assessing and improving quality that describes the objectives, organization, scope, and mechanisms for overseeing the effectiveness of monitoring, evaluating, and improving activities. Such activities include quality of patient care, clinical performance with clinical privileges, pharmacy and therapeutics functions, infection control, utilization review, and risk management. Scoring guidelines are identified, and the organization is judged against its own criteria from individual guidelines.

Other organizations collecting data for quality measurement are the American Hospital Association, Voluntary Hospitals of America, National Committee for Quality Healthcare, and the National Association of Health Data Organizations. These organizations will gather, analyze, and publish data on quality of health care for consumers, employers, and the federal government. The standards will include performance standards for providers (see Exhibit 26–3). The objectives are to achieve improvement in the health status of clients, reduce unnecessary utilization of health-care services, and meet specifications of clients

---

Exhibit 26–3   Standards for Nursing

Definition of Nursing Care
Based on the University of South Alabama Hospital's mission, USAMC philosophy of Nursing, rules of Alabama State Board of Health Division of Licensure and Certification, and Nurse Practice Act, nursing care at the University of South Alabama Medical Center is defined as those acts received by the patient/significant other from nursing to assist the patient/family to reach the optimal level of wellness. Nursing care is further defined as being under direction of or provided by a Registered Nurse on a 24-hour basis and supports the nursing process as evidenced by documented actual or potential patient/family problems, planned interventions, nursing care provided, and results of interventions for the stated actual/potential problem. Nursing practice is defined by departmental policies, procedures, and standards which direct nursing care within the hospital.

I.   POLICY STATEMENT
Using the nursing process, patients receive nursing care within the guidelines of the following Standards of Care and Standards of Practice. These standards apply to all settings in which nursing care is provided: Medical Surgical Units: 8th, 7th, 6th, 5N, 5S; Labor and Delivery; Post-Anesthesia Care Unit; Operating Room; Special Care Units (SICU, NTICU, SINU, CCU, MICU, CCU II, MINU, ICN/Premature,

Burn Center); Obstetrics: High-Risk/Antepartum, Mother-Baby; Newborn Nursery; and Ambulatory Surgery.

II.   PURPOSE
1. To guide the provision of nursing care.
2. To provide the means by which nursing personnel are evaluated in the provision of nursing care.
3. To provide the means by which to measure the end results of nursing care through patient outcomes.

III.   GENERAL INFORMATION
1. Nursing standards are used to monitor, evaluate, and initiate actions to improve the delivery of care through quality assessment and improvement.
2. Standards for Nursing serve as the foundation for the development of policies and procedures.
3. Standards for Nursing identify important aspects of care; standards of practice; concurrent process; retrospective process; standards of care; concurrent outcome; and retrospective outcome.

Source: Courtesy University of South Alabama Medical Center, Mobile, Alabama.

and purchasers. These standards will address improvement of health care quality, functions, and processes that must be carried out effectively to achieve good patient care outcomes, patient care, governance, and management. Theory of quality management has been applied in the form of identifying common causes and special causes of performance variation.[8] Outcomes or indexes serve as measures of the value, rank, or degree of excellence (see Exhibit 26–4 and Appendix 26–1).

Exercise 26–3	Examine the standards for quality management of a nursing entity. How do they meet the outcomes listed in Exhibit 26–4?

Policies and Procedures

The third component of a quality management program is the development of policies and procedures for using standards or indicators for gathering data to measure the quality of care. Batalden and Stoltz describe guiding principles that reflect the organization's assumptions about the responsibilities and desired actions of leaders leading to the creation of a positive work environment. It is essential to integrate the leadership policy with the values common to health professionals and underlying health-care work; this contributes to shared ownership of the policy by everyone in the organization.[9] The policies and procedures define the organizational structure for the quality management program and will prescribe the tools for gathering data.

ORGANIZATIONAL STRUCTURE

The organizational structure of a quality assurance program is defined by organizational policy encompassing every department and the medical staff. If the organization is large enough, it will have a quality management department. Otherwise, a full-time or part-time person will be assigned to oversee the pro-

---

Exhibit 26–4   Measurable Outcomes to Achieve with Verification from Automated Documentation

1. Admission assessment within 24–48 Hours
2. All diagnosis and treatment orders fulfilled
3. Discharged in safe physical, emotional and mental health
4. Discharged with stable vital signs
5. No abnormal diagnostic findings left unattended
6. Normal fluid hydration
7. Continent (urinating and defecating appropriately)
8. Mobile, steady gait without threat of falls
9. Without drug interactions
10. Comfort achieved to the extent possible
11. Without decubitus ulcers and oral mucosal membrane ulcers
12. Capable of bathing, toileting, feeding and dressing self
13. No nosocomial infection
14. No purulent or blood drainage from wounds
15. Patient understands home treatment plan and was satisfied with care given by nursing staff

Source: K. A. McCormick, "Future Data Needs for Quality of Care Monitoring, DRG Considerations, Reimbursement, and Outcome Measurements," *IMAGE: Journal of Nursing Scholarship,* spring 1991, 32. Reprinted with permission.

gram. Quality management programs are designed to meet the needs of the organization and to accomplish the organization's program objectives. The program should have an organizational and functional scheme, which is generally outlined in the policy (as in Appendix 26–1). QA committees often function at the level of both the organization and the nursing department. Each level should have representation from practitioners, since the major focus concerns the quality of patient care and patient-care delivery systems.

Committees will usually be defined by policy that includes the purpose, membership, and functions designed to support the quality management program. Clinical nurses generally have hours assigned to accomplish their QA committee function.

TOOLS FOR COLLECTING QUALITY DATA

Tools for collecting quality data should incorporate standards to be measured into the quality control and appropriateness measures. Standards alone are not evaluation instruments. Quality assessment and improvement (QAI) are both a staff and a line function. QAI entails both quality control and appropriateness measures. Cotter defines quality control measurement as evaluation of the effectiveness of a nursing strategy that incorporates efficiency, timeliness, and congruence with established criteria describing performance.[10] Cotter defines appropriateness measurement as the determination of the necessity of a specific nursing intervention through the evaluation of the client's clinical condition in comparison with objective, predetermined indicators for nursing interventions.[11] With regard to operative and other procedures, JCAHO standard for determining the appropriateness of a procedure for each patient is based on a review of the patient's history, physical status, and diagnostic data; the risks and benefits of the procedures; and the need to administer blood or blood components.[12] Nursing judgments must weigh standard procedures and immediate appropriateness in providing individualized care that restores, stabilizes, or improves the client's health status.[13] Quality control, appropriateness, and standards are essential to a comprehensive quality assessment program. Various standardized instruments are available. If the QA committee decides to develop new tools, reliability and content validity will need to be determined prior to implementation.

Nursing Audits

A basic form of quality data collection is the nursing audit. An audit is essentially an examination, a verification, or an accounting of predetermined indicators. There are three basic forms of nursing audits: structure audits, process audits, and outcome audits.

Structure Audits.   Structure audits focus on the setting in which care takes place. They include physical facilities, equipment, caregivers, organization, policies, procedures, and medical records. Standards or indicators are measured by a checklist that focuses on these categories. Structure can include such content as staff knowledge and expertise in addition to policies and procedures for nursing practice. Content related to specific nursing care to meet established standards are included in nursing process audits.

Process Audits.   Process audits implement indicators for measuring nursing care to determine whether nursing standards are met. They are generally task-oriented. Process audits were first used by Maria Phaneuf in 1964 and were based upon the seven functions of nursing established by Lesnick and Anderson. The Phaneuf audit is retrospective, being applied to measure the quality of nursing care received by the client after a cycle of care has been completed and the client discharged. The Phaneuf audit has seven subsections:

1. Application and execution of physicians' legal orders.
2. Observations of symptoms and reactions.
3. Supervision of the client.
4. Supervision of those participating in care (except the physician).
5. Reporting and recording.
6. Application and execution of nursing procedures and techniques.
7. Promotion of physical and emotional health by direction and teaching.

The Phaneuf model uses a Likert scoring system. It does not evaluate care recorded.[14]

The Quality Patient Care Scale (Qual PacS) is a process audit that measures the quality of nursing care concurrently with the cycle of care being given. Its six subsections are

1. Psychosocial—individual.
2. Psychosocial—group.
3. Physical.
4. General.
5. Communication.
6. Professional implications.

In this audit, the nurse is evaluated by direct observation in a nurse-client interaction. A 15 percent sample of nurses on a unit is considered adequate.

Both the Phaneuf and the Qual PacS process audits use the performance of the first-level staff nurse as a standard for safe, adequate, therapeutic, and supportive care.[15]

The Qual PacS audit was developed from the Slater Nursing Competencies Rating Scale. The Slater model references five staff nurses from best to poorest, contains eighty-four questions, and takes two and one-half to three hours to administer per nurse-client interaction. Qual PacS reduced the questionnaire to sixty-eight items.[16] Higgins and associates, using a modified version of the Qual PacS, found that such outcome measures did prove to be a useful and cost-effective method of evaluating patient care inasmuch as they identify problems at the unit level where they can most easily be resolved.[17]

Other open system audits include the Commission on Administrative Service in Hospital (CASH) Scale and the Medicus Corporation Nurses' Audit. They also measure or monitor intervention, assessment, and clinical skills.

Outcome Audits.   Outcome audits can be either concurrent or retrospective. They evaluate nursing performance in terms of establishing client outcome criteria. The National Center for Health Services developed an outcome audit based on Orem's description of nine categories of self-care requirements:

1. Air.
2. Water/fluid intake.
3. Food.
4. Elimination.
5. Rest/activity/sleep.
6. Social interaction and productive work.
7. Protection from hazards.
8. Normality.
9. Health deviation.

These categories are evaluated in terms of the following:[18]

1. Evidence that the requirement is met.
2. Evidence that the client has the necessary knowledge to meet the requirement.
3. Evidence that the client has the necessary skill and performance abilities to meet the requirement.
4. Evidence that the client has the necessary motivation to meet the requirement.

Outcome criteria are set for selected topics. They can evaluate specific aspects of nursing care for particular groups, such as AIDS clients, residents with brain injury, and long-term care residents. Evans and Ruff describe three measurable consumer-driven variables when evaluating rehabilitation outcomes achieved in acquired brain injury. These variables are identified as residential-setting status, living assistance, and productive activity. Residential-setting status is rank-ordered of independent functioning from least to most restrictive. Living assistance refers to the amount of time per twenty-four-hour period for which the client requires supervision or assistance from others, such as a professional, paid attendant, or family member. Productive activity as a measurable outcome is the primary productive activity in which the client is engaged and includes competitive employment or degree-directed academic or vocational training. It may also include homemaking, volunteer service, avocational activities, or no productive activity.

The outcome variables as described by Evans and Ruff have face validity as outcomes of functional utility, and their value can be reliably assessed using descriptive statistics. These variables are considered important rehabilitation outcomes by clients, family members, and financial providers and have an impact on long-term functioning.[19]

Morbidity, disability, and mortality during and following provision of health-care services are nationally recognized outcomes of health care. Nursing assessment and intervention may make a significant difference in the outcome variables, such as nosocomial infection rates in high-risk clients.[20] McCormick illustrates the direction of outcomes that patients can take related to the assessment and treatments carried out. The outcome of improvement, stabilization, or deterioration can be facilitated through an automated system if patient data can be quantified in relation to days (refer to Exhibit 26–4).

While using an automated system may improve production time, the benefits to nursing are still a challenge with regards to describing health-care costs, accessibility, and outcomes of care. McCormick illustrates a model for computerization of quality assurance that incorporates nursing inputs to affect quality outputs (see Exhibit 26–5). Such inputs include essential elements in a hospitalized patient's nursing record, including demographic information, patient history, physical information, nursing problem list, recovery progress, medication administered, interactions, and drug errors.[21]

Another method of developing outcome criteria is the grouping of items for efficiency: DRGs, specific protocols for treatment, life stages, and like standards. A determination is made as to whether the outcomes are met. If outcomes are not satisfactorily met, deficiencies are identified, corrected, and followed up.

More on Tools

Four major categories of tools and methods that can accelerate building and using knowledge of continual quality improvement of health care are process and system, group process and collaborative work, statistical thinking, and planning and analysis. Exhibit 26–6 illustrates a system map as a graphic tool that may display the various components of a system, such as a whole organization, a department or unit within the organization, or even a system of clinical care.

The flowchart is the most commonly used process analysis tool. It can be helpful in revealing repetitive activity, steps with little or no value, and the needless complexity and ambiguity of a process.

Group process and collaborative work, such as brainstorming, problem solving, and decision making, can also lead to streamlining a process, enhancing project plans, and improving teamwork. Examples are multiple voting and rank ordering, which promotes understanding and consensus during the selection process so that a final alternative is representative of the best judgment of the knowledgeable group and increases the likelihood of success.

Statistical methods can be simple, and workers can be taught to use them correctly at every level in the organization. Such tools include the checksheet, Pareto chart, time plot or run chart, and scatter diagram. With a degree of skill in the use of these tools and methods, workers can obtain and analyze data to validate their ideas about potential improvements and later test the results of changes implemented.[22] Exhibit 26–7 is an example of a run chart illustrating the effect of a process change on emergency-room triage time.

Planning and analysis are conceptual methods that were generally thought to be limited to top-level management. Given the tools and methods to plan and analyze data, all levels of workers are equipped to manage a critical aspect of quality improvement. A central obligation for top leaders is the creation of conceptual space so that health-care professionals may redesign their own work for the overall improvement of health care. A large part of creating conceptual space is inviting exploration or nurturing curiosity. "Creating opportunity for new learning and nurturing curiosity about improvement in the midst of the places we work may be the most fundamental contribution leaders can make toward better health care."[23]

Exhibit 26–5   A Model for Computerization of Quality Assurance

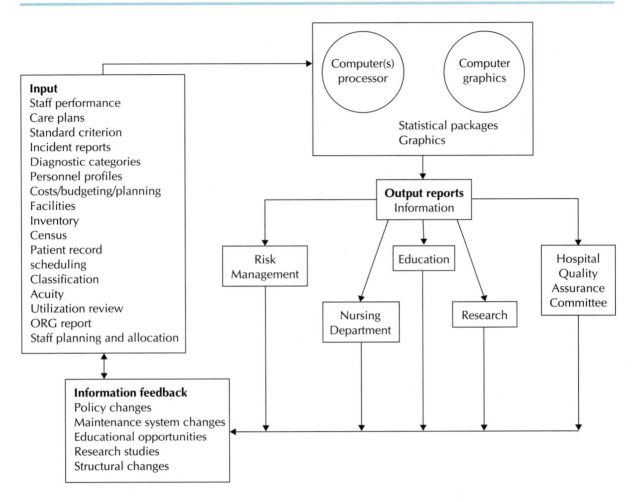

Source: K. A. McCormick, "Future Data Needs for Quality of Care Monitoring, DRG Considerations, Reimbursement, and Outcome Measurements," *IMAGE: Journal of Nursing Scholarship,* spring 1991, 32. Reprinted with permission.

Quality Improvement Teams

One method of implementing a quality improvement (QI) program is through a QI team or council. This team functions with a team leader, team members, and a facilitator. The team supports management in developing and implementing a QI program and may follow the group dynamics described in chapter 15, "Committees and other Groups".[24] The ANA Guidelines for Review of Nursing Care at the local level is pertinent in today's evaluation of outcomes environment (see Exhibit 26–8).

Exhibit 26–6 A System Capable of Continual Improvement

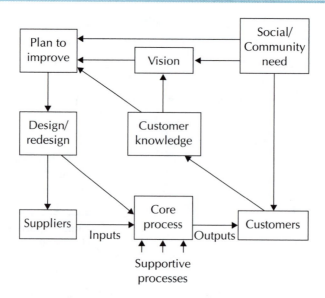

Source: P. B. Batalden and P. K. Stoltz, "A Framework for the Continual Improvement of Health Care: Building and Applying Professional and Improvement Knowledge to Test Changes in Daily Work," *Joint Commission Journal on Quality Improvement,* October 1993, 428. Oakbrook Terrace, Ill.: Joint Commission on Accreditation of Healthcare Organizations, 1993. Reprinted with permission.

Exhibit 26–7 Example of a Run Chart: The Effect of a Process Change on Emergency-Room Triage Time

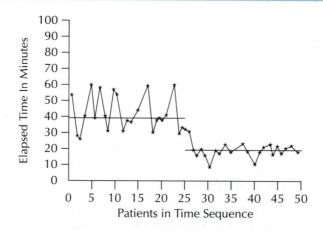

Source: P. B. Batalden and P. K. Stoltz, "A Framework for the Continual Improvement of Health Care: Building and Applying Professional and Improvement Knowledge to Test Changes in Daily Work," *Joint Commission Journal on Quality Improvement,* October 1993, 436. Oakbrook Terrace, Ill.: Joint Commission on Accreditation of Healthcare Organizations, 1993. Reprinted with permission.

Exhibit 26–8   Guidelines for Developing Sets of Outcome Criteria Statements

1. Screening criteria are a crucial factor that, if not met, may indicate a significant deficiency in nursing care.
2. The purpose of screening criteria is to survey a large number of cases and quickly determine acceptable levels of patient outcomes.
3. The outcome stated in the criteria must be possible to achieve.
4. Criteria should be statements of specific outcomes representing optimal achievement.
5. Criteria should be written as specifically as possible, including the time when they are to be measured and the measurement to be used to determine if the criteria have been met.
6. In establishing criteria, one should select the most critical time for the measurement of the identified outcome for a particular patient population.
7. Criteria must be appraisable. However, the ease of measurement should not be used as the sole basis for accepting or rejecting potential criteria. If criteria are important, some assessment can usually be obtained.
8. Criteria should be stated to yield a dichotomous distinction (yes-no).
9. Criteria should be phrased in positive terms (presence of) rather than negative terms (absence of), when applicable.
10. Criteria should be pertinent to the particular patient population under consideration. For example, for the ambulatory patient receiving photocoagulation of the eye, skin care is not a priority. Hence, criteria would not be written for skin care.
11. Criteria should be free from bias. Each patient to whom criteria are applied should be equally likely to be able to meet the criteria. For example, the skin condition of an aged patient and a youth might require different criteria.
12. A set of criteria applicable to a specific patient population may include criteria for outcomes of care for members of the family or significant others.

Establishing criteria is a "pencil and eraser" operation. Criteria will change as values and scientific knowledge change and as health care practices change. Thus criteria should be revised at regular intervals.

Source: ANA Guidelines for Review of Nursing Care at the Local Level. © 1977, American Nurses' Association, Washington, D.C.: 21–22. Reprinted with permission.

Triad Models

Some nursing quality management models employ a triad of structure, process, and outcome. Measurement criteria are referenced by code to specific structural, process, or outcome standards. A modular approach has been used in which client conditions were related to five areas: client rights, developmental stage of client, social groups, therapy-associated needs, and medical diagnoses. Standards for each client group were developed and used to construct the evaluation tool.

The modular design for QA provides discrete components that can be used independently or in different combinations. This design has three modules:[25]

1. Client care standards.
2. Outcome, process, structure trail.
3. The standard, with derived measurement criteria.

Outcome indicators also include mortality rates, infection rates, and incident reports.

Exercise 26–4	Identify the tools used for audits in a nursing organization. Use one of them and analyze your results.

PROBLEM IDENTIFICATION

Analysis and reporting of the data gathered from the evaluation process lead to problem identification and isolation. Evidence comes from primary sources, such as the client and nursing personnel, and from secondary sources, including the client's chart and family. Active client and family participation should be part of the process. Quality management addresses current problems. Nurses look for patterns or trends of deviation from normal. They also identify deficiencies relating to other departments that affect nursing care. If one takes a systems approach, problem identification is a team approach, with the client and family as major team players.

PROBLEM RESOLUTION

Once problems have been defined and isolated, plans are made to solve them on a priority basis. Those problems that are critical are addressed first, and plans are immediately made and implemented to resolve them. Those involving the safety and welfare of the client take first priority. Other factors used in determining priority will include severity, frequency, benefit, cost-effectiveness, elimination, reduction, association with professional liability, and impact on accreditation. The first consideration is always based on the impact on client care.[26]

Solutions and corrective action for problems will be assigned to appropriate nursing departments, services, and units. The need is to resolve problems, not just evaluate them.

MONITORING AND FEEDBACK

The quality management process is cyclic and requires monitoring of clinical and managerial performance and feedback to ensure that problems stay solved. Follow-up can be expensive and difficult. Its breadth should determine what should be covered. Problems of a multidisciplinary nature, such as those involving occupational therapy, physical therapy, speech pathology, and nursing, can be one consideration.

The cyclic process will continue to set standards of care, take measurements according to those standards, evaluate care from multiple sources, recommend improvements, and, above all, ensure that improvements are carried out.

SYSTEM EVALUATION

Although nurses defend their right to define and regulate the quality of care, they often do not pursue QA activities. A study of nurse managers, staff development nurses, and clinical nurses in ten metropolitan hospitals found that most nurses believed that QA involved all levels of nursing personnel but was not part of their daily work. Twenty-five percent viewed QA as an accreditation requirement. Peer review and patient-care audits ranked low against direct patient-care activities. Less than 50 percent of respondents wanted to participate in these activities.

Nurses with formal QA experience were more likely to want to write standards for their specialty, participate in peer review, and be on QA committees. They were more interested in QA associated with direct patient care.[27]

FOCUS-PDCA Model

Several models for quality program evaluation have been developed, including the FOCUS-PDCA model. The FOCUS-PDCA model is an adaptation of the Deming cycle (Plan-Do-Check-Act) and provides a systematic method to study a work process for improvement. It includes the following steps:[28]

1. Find a process to improve.
2. Organize a team that knows the process.
3. Clarify current knowledge of the process.
4. Understand causes of process variation.
5. Select the process improvement.
6. Plan the improvement.
7. Do data collection, data analysis, and improvement.
8. Check data for process improvement and customer outcomes.
9. Act to maintain and continue improvement.

The FOCUS-PDCA model has been cited as an example of how such a model can prove effective in streamlining a system and improving client satisfaction in the emergency room. Clarifying the process was done through flow-charting, which highlighted the number of events that occurred prior to the physician's examination of the patient. In addition, flowcharting helped to outline the steps that a client proceeded through from actual entrance into the emergency room, assessment, intervention, evaluation, and eventual treatment and discharge or admittance.[29]

PROCESSES INVOLVED IN QUALITY MANAGEMENT

Quality management is important to accountability of nurses who want to control their practice arena. Many groups are seeking evidence that outcomes of nursing care are of good quality and represent a cost-effective use of resources. An excellent example of this is the dialogue currently being maintained with legislators regarding the advanced practice nurse's role in health-care reform. Nursing's Agenda for Healthcare Reform has been accepted by the President's Committee on Healthcare Reform, and such goals as universal coverage and access to affordable and portable health care will be paramount to any health-care plan adopted. Statistics have been frequently cited along with anecdotal reports of nursing's outcomes of quality care (shorter hospital stays, healthier babies, decreased infection) and improved client satisfaction.

Notwithstanding, accountability for nursing practice is still diffused by the employment environment, and this fact must be addressed and corrected by nurses.

Involvement of Practicing Nurses

Practicing nurses can be stimulated to increase their positive attitudes about quality management by direct behavioral experience. Nurse managers should find out the reasons these nurses view QA unfavorably. This author found that from her own personal experience as a nurse executive, reasons for negative connotations existed as a result of lack of executive administrative support, viewing the process as an academic exercise without changes in practice noted, and physicians' overall lack of involvement in quality health care. Correcting and changing this viewpoint may be managed by a variety of strategies that include the following:

1. Having practicing nurses choose QA topics.
2. Providing release time for practicing nurses to participate in QA activities, including attendance at committee meetings and time for QA audits.
3. Providing rewards, such as performance results achievement records, that can lead to pay raises, promotions, educational opportunities, or special assignments.
4. Targeting QA to patient-care outcomes, the very essence of nursing practice.
5. Involving clinical nurses in management through such techniques as quality circles, employee involvement programs, participatory management, decentralization, adhocracy, and quality of work life.
6. Establishing a peer review program involving nursing staff at all levels of patient care. Such a program's expectation is to identify outcome criteria based on established standards for nursing practice. Peers determine whether outcomes have been met based on ongoing and retrospective audits. Corrective action is determined by peers based on the outcome being adequately met.

Resources

Quality management programs are labor intensive, requiring efficient and effective use of resources that include personnel, physical plant, supplies, equipment, policies, and procedures. Nurses should be selective in determining areas to be evaluated, considering time and difficulty as well as safety and urgency. They should sample the standards rather than dogmatically evaluate every one. This will require placing priority on standards and even making a decision whether to eliminate some that are not critical.

Efficiency

Efficiency is concerned with the cost/benefit ratio. Can the appropriate standard be met with a cost acceptable to both consumer and provider?[30] The computer is a labor-saving device for developing and conducting a QA program. Nurse managers will use it and teach other practicing nurses to use it. The computer can be used to track the QA process.

Standards will be kept up-to-date and accessible to all units. A loose-leaf notebook or the computer memory is efficient for easy access. Standards should be cross-referenced.

Charts can be labeled so as to be easily retrieved for nursing QA evaluation. They can be coded by nursing diagnosis or nursing-care standards.[31] In addition, using the long-term care minimum data set (MDS) can be an efficient QA tool for nursing homes. The MDS is a collection of baseline data (physical, social, psychological factors) that can be used to assess, analyze, and plan care for residents in nursing homes. Its specific elements were mandated by the 1987 Omnibus Budget Reconciliation Act.[32]

The following are some other elements of efficiency and effectiveness:

1. Identification of the impact of nursing care on the health of the patient—results or outcomes measured in terms of the patient's health status. Do the notes meet such a standard?
2. A program practical enough to be used in all clinical nursing settings.
3. Random, unannounced samples.
4. Nursing personnel who serve on committees long enough to be proficient.
5. Grading by each person administering criteria.
6. Higher patient acuity combined with shorter hospital stays.
7. Interdisciplinary programs so that nurses will not do the work of other disciplines. Nursing is ethically and operationally interdependent with other groups and organizations.
8. Planning for uncertain future by blueprinting scenarios for managing the future, changing the culture of nursing organizations, developing interpersonal skills, and making a creative response to risk taking.[33]
9. Each nurse should be held responsible for self-improvement and for delivering a high standard of patient care.

Customer Satisfaction

Customers will be involved in all aspects of a quality management program, including discharge planning. They know what they want and are demanding quality with economy. A study of consumers' perspectives of quality nursing care found that patients' and families' descriptions of quality nursing care fell into two major attributes: (1) practice attributes and (2) nurse attributes. A smaller number of patients and families did identify a third type, practice-setting (structural) attributes. Practice attributes included holistic care, nurse-patient interaction, and effective communication. Nurse attributes identified were personal qualities (kind, nice, friendly, helpful), proficiency, professional character, and commitment to excellence. Practice-setting attributes, although of smaller significance, were effective organization, management, and patient environment. Overall, the customer expressed a close relationship and frequent contact with the nurse as synonymous with quality nursing care. Consumer satisfaction as an outcome of QA can be assessed through methods such as patient, family, and nurse interviews or surveys and observation checklists of nurse-patient interactions.[34]

Training and Communication

Training and communication are important elements of a total quality program. Training includes interpersonal skills, stress management, and conflict management. Learning is a cyclic or continuous process. Nurse managers who play educator roles develop self-awareness by applying learning principles to their own behaviors. Patient education requires an interdisciplinary team approach.

Communication of QA findings, including problems, resolution of problems, and results, must be clear. Both physicians and nursing employees need to be kept up-to-date. Quality must be provided and communicated to be successful. This means that providers as well as consumers will know the status of the quality of care being rendered.

Quality in the health-care marketplace is defined by employers, employee benefit consultants, physicians, and consumers—not by providers (even though physicians are providers, as are hospitals, nurses, and other caregivers). The reason physicians determine quality is that they have control over all orders for diagnosis and treatment procedures. Only one-half of consumers, employers, and employee consultants ever differentiate between high- and low-quality hospitals. Two-thirds of physicians do.[35]

Good employee relations and consumer relations programs are necessary for success in the health-care marketplace, and their good quality must be communicated. Consumers want quality factors in this order:[36]

1. Warmth, caring, concern.
2. Expert medical staff who are concerned, thorough, and successful.
3. Up-to-date technology/equipment.
4. Specialization/scope of services available.
5. Outcome.

RESEARCH AND QUALITY MANAGEMENT

Nursing quality assurance programs can be combined with research programs. Nursing research is being done in clinical settings to improve patient-care outcomes. Research can be sold to nurse managers because it provides prestige, advanced knowledge for nursing professionals, and a database for clinical nursing practice.[37]

Nursing research can be used to evaluate management issues such as staffing, cost management, and staff retention. It produces new knowledge of the relationship between process and outcome. Combining quality management with research makes efficient use of personnel and other resources to link research with a mandatory process, increase the probability that research will relate to patient care, and increase sharing of successful quality management programs with others outside the institution.[38] Research and quality management complement each other.

RISK MANAGEMENT

Risk management can be defined as a "process that centers on identification, analysis, treatment and evaluation of real and potential hazards."[39] Risk management has its beginnings in transportation and industry, with the present concepts being formed from investigations into aviation and traffic accidents. The primary reason for the investigations was to determine patterns or causative factors in the accidents and then to eliminate, or at least control, as many factors as possible.[40]

Hayden describes risk management as the risk of financial loss. Specifically, she addresses control of financial loss resulting from legal liability. Financial loss and legal liability can be best understood by the following steps:

1. Identifying patterns and trends of risk through internal audits and claims.
2. Reporting individual risk-related incidents and taking steps to reduce the liability related to them.
3. Developing and engaging in product evaluation systems with appropriate informed-consent protocols.
4. Vigilant evaluation of patient-care settings to determine risks.
5. Preventing those occurrences that are likely to be a liability to the organization.

Hayden goes further and describes three aspects of risk identification that should be monitored on a continuous basis:

1. Clinical settings, clinical problems, personnel, and specific incidents involving patients, employees, and visitors.
2. Safety management.
3. Procedures for evaluation and follow-up on identified risks.

In addition, review of pertinent documents such as medical records, incident reports, pharmacy logs, infection control, and utilization review reports is paramount to a successful risk management program. Excellent communication skills are essential when interacting with medical and administrative staff as well as with clients. Substandard communication skills are often the root of a complaint or claim.[41]

The JCAHO recommends the establishment of an integrated risk management/quality assurance program that would provide a more efficient and cost-effective method of evaluation than having two separate functions. The following parameters are incorporated into the JCAHO model for risk management:[42]

1. Continuing education and in-service training.
2. Use of data from a variety of sources, such as patient surveys and feedback from other providers (referring or referral facilities).
3. Improvement of credentialing protocols for practitioners.
4. Development and enforcement of rules, regulations, policies, and procedures.
5. Establishment of written criteria to evaluate risk factors, including follow-up on conclusions reached.

Bennett further describes the importance of both quality improvement and risk management, identifying issues associated with quality patient care, collecting and analyzing data, making recommendations, and evaluating outcomes to prevent recurrences and to upgrade quality. Avoidance of costly malpractice litigation is as important as providing safe and quality patient care.[43]

Five common reasons for malpractice litigation are injuries to patients resulting from the following:[44]

1. Errors or failures in safety of care that result in patient falls.
2. Failure to identify and document pertinent information (omissions of significant data).
3. Failure to correctly perform treatments or nursing care.
4. Failure to communicate significant data to patients or other therapists.
5. Errors in medication.

Adhering to standards of care (general and specialty nursing) can provide a model for risk management. It is significant to note that quality nursing care is concerned, compassionate, and nurturing. It is often within the context of a therapeutic nurse-patient relationship that problems are solved and errors avoided. Effective communication is a cornerstone to a therapeutic relationship and is enhanced by active listening, empathy, understanding, and positive reinforcement. When the patient and family truly feel cared about, errors that do occur are considered in the context of this relationship. In addition, the following primary responsibilities of every nurse are essential in preventing malpractice litigation:[45]

1. Practice safety—deliver quality nursing care to all patients.
2. Incorporate effective patient rapport in nursing practice.
3. Keep accurate and complete records.
4. Act reasonably—as all other professional nurses would in the community, the state, and the nation—to give standard nursing care.

The risk manager uses carefully planned public relations, makes private explanations, apologizes when necessary, and collects, prepares, and presents evidence.[46] The risk manager's job duties are further outlined in Exhibit 26–9.

Risk Management Process

The following process describes an effective risk management program:[47]

1. Identify areas within the organization that expose it to loss.
2. Evaluate the potential loss those exposures represent.
3. Treat the exposure through two broad categories: risk financing and risk control.
4. Reduce the severity of the loss through such risk control strategies as hospital bill write-offs or early investigations of the event.

Employing these strategies is a joint effort of the risk management department along with health-care providers, as it is everyone's responsibility to provide a safe environment for the patient. Such strategies include early warning systems, documentation, informed consent, and patient relations.[48]

Early Warning Systems.   Early warning systems include strategies that involve acquiring early information and knowledge of an untoward event. Early reporting provides an opportunity to evaluate the incident while the circum-

Exhibit 26–9 Risk Manager Competencies

1. Keep an up-to-date manual, including policies, lines of authority, safety roles, disaster plans, safety training, procedures, incident and claims reporting, procedures, and schedule, and description of retention/insurance program.
2. Update programs with changes in properties, operations, or activities.
3. Review plans for new construction, alterations, and equipment installation.
4. Review contracts to avoid unnecessary assumptions of liability and transfer to others where possible.
5. Keep up-to-date property appraisal.
6. Maintain records of insurance policy renewal dates.
7. Review and monitor all premium and other billings and approve payments.
8. Negotiate insurance coverage, premiums, and services.
9. Prepare specifications for competitive bids on property and liability insurance.
10. Review and make recommendations for coverage, services, and costs.
11. Maintain records and verify compliance for independent physicians, vendors, contractors, and subcontractors.
12. Maintain records of losses, claims, and all risk management expenses.
13. Supervise claim-reporting procedures.
14. Assist in adjusting losses.
15. Cooperate with director of safety and risk management committee to minimize all future losses involving employees, patients, visitors, other third parties, property, and earnings.
16. Keep risk management skills updated.
17. Prepare annual report covering status, changes, new problems and solutions, summary of existing insurance and retention aspects of the program, summary of losses, costs, major claims, and future goals and objectives.
18. Prepare annual budget.

stances are still very clear. "Early reporting also allows the organization to secure medical records related to the event and equipment that may have malfunctioned and contributed to the event."[49] With computerization, a formal information system may be put in place, with labels for generic screens or occurrence screens that serve as a set of criteria and list the kinds of red-flag occurrences that indicate a loss.

The nurse manager and the clinical staff are often the key players in reporting early warnings. Claims management can be included in the early warning systems. It includes analysis of risk for possible loss frequency and severity—the assessment of potential claims based on data analysis. This information (written and verbal reports) is used to investigate potentially compensable events and losses and their causes, thereby determining liability and settlement value.

Documentation. Documentation strategies are essential to an effective risk management program. The medical record generally serves as a means of determining whether a deviation existed in the standard of care. Contradictions, inconsistencies, and unexplained time gaps in the medical records signal potential problems during litigation. It is recommended that documentation take place as soon after the occurrence as possible and that a minute-by-minute recording be done during the emergency. When time is of the essence, brief notes with times, interventions, and other relevant information should be written on a pad of paper and transferred to the medical records as soon as the crisis is over. Any corrections to the medical records should be made with a thin line drawn through the original entry, dated, and initialed. Information should be documented as a factual recording, and objectivity should be practiced. Documentation of any instructions given to the patient should also be recorded.

Informed Consent.   Informed consent does not involve just the signing of a consent form. This procedure has little relation to the patient's understanding of the procedure to be performed. Informed consent is the provision of enough information to patients to enable them to make a rational decision whether or not to undergo the treatment. The form that is signed, however, is indicative that adequate information has been given to the patient and that understanding and consent have been duly explained. Exceptions to the rule are emergency treatments and situations where such disclosure could potentially adversely affect the patient's medical condition. Informed consent may be sought for diagnosis, nature and purpose of proposed treatment, risks and consequences of the proposed treatments, and feasible treatment alternatives.

Patient Relations.   Patient relations are important; often the deterioration of the professional-to-patient relationship leads to many malpractice claims. Many large health-care organizations employ patient representatives who provide such services as orientation of patients and their families to organization policies, procedures, and services provided; resolution of complaints; making phone calls and mailing letters; and daily follow-up. Volunteers often assist the patient representative.[50]

Exercise 26–5   Interview a risk manager. How do the manager's job duties compare to those outlined in Exhibit 26–9? What risk-prevention strategies does the manager use? What has been the cost of losses caused by negligence during the past year?

INCIDENT REPORTING

Incident reporting is an effective technique of a good risk management program. The tool itself should be constructed to collect complete and accurate information, including the name, address, age, and condition of the individual involved; exact location, time, and date of the incident; description of the occurrence; physician's examination data; bedrail status; reason for hospitalization; names of witnesses; and extent of out-of-bed privileges.

Use of the Incident Report

Incident reports are used to collect and analyze future data for the purpose of determining risk-control strategies. They are prepared for any unusual occurrence involving people or property, whether or not injury or damage occurs. Blake describes the use of a multiple causation model in incident report investigation. This theory purports that causes, subcauses, and contributing factors weave together in particular sequences to cause incidents. An incident may have many concomitant causes; therefore, seeking out as many causes as possible and rating them to their proximate or primary influence upon the incident may be useful in reducing the chance of the incident's recurring. Proximate causes are often referred to as unsafe acts and conditions and are generally the most apparent and closest cause of the incident. Primary causes are procedural in nature, and such causes are discovered through backtracking from the proximate cause. Blake identifies six principles of risk management related to incident investigation:[51]

> *Principle I:* Each cause of an incident reflects a management problem.
> *Principle II:* One can predict that sets of circumstances will produce incidents. These circumstances can be identified and controlled.
> *Principle III:* In any given group or array, a relatively small number of items will tend to give rise to the largest proportion of results.
> *Principle IV:* The purpose of incident investigation is to locate and define the operational errors that allow incidents to occur.
> *Principle V:* Accountability is the key to effective incident investigation and analysis.
> *Principle VI:* The past performance of an organization or unit tends to forecast future performance.

Preparation of the Incident Report

The incident report is discoverable by the plaintiff's attorney. For this reason, it should be prepared by the involved employee(s) in a timely manner to ensure accuracy and objectivity of reporting. It must be complete and factual. The incident report is corrected in the same manner as any other medical record and should not be altered or rewritten. It should contain no comments criticizing or blaming others. To keep the incident report from being discoverable, it must be sent directly from preparer to attorney to assure confidentiality. Nurse managers frequently insist on reviewing the report, although they can obtain accurate information from the patient's chart and from conversations with the preparer. The incident report should be prepared in a single copy and should never be placed on the patient's medical record. Exhibit 26–10 lists the do's and don'ts of incident reporting.

Attorneys can prepare abstracts of data from collective incident reports. Thus, they identify the number of occurrences of particular incidents. The information will be used by the risk manager to do his or her job, including trend analysis to establish patterns and education and training of personnel.[52]

While it may be institutional policy to send the incident report to the risk manager, an alternative method of notification is better. The preparer can call the risk manager and the nurse manager and give them verbal information on the need to investigate and evaluate deviations from the standard of care and for making corrections. To accomplish this, managers will have to establish a climate of trust that supports incident reporting by nurses. The JCAHO requires incident reporting.

Exercise 26–6   Examine the incident reporting program in a health-care agency. What are its strengths? Its weaknesses? How can it be improved?

Exhibit 26–10   DOs and DON'Ts of Incident Reporting

DOs	DON'Ts
• Report any event involving patient mishap or serious expression of dissatisfaction with care. • Report any event involving visitor mishap or property. • Be complete. • Follow established policy and procedure. • Be prompt. • Act to reduce fear by the nursing staff. • Correct in the same manner as any medical record. • Include names and identities of witnesses; record their statements on separate pages. • Report equipment malfunctions, including control numbers. Remove equipment from service for testing. • Keep the report confidential. • Report to nurse manager. • Confer with risk manager. • Work to provide nursing care to meet established standards. • Attend all staff development programs. • Confirm all telephone orders in writing.	• Place blame on anyone. • Place report on the patient's chart. • Make entry about an incident report on the patient's chart. • Alter or rewrite. • Report hearsay or opinion. • Be afraid to consult, ask questions, or complete incident reports. They can be part of your best defense and protection. • Prescribe in the M.D.'s domain. • Be cold and impersonal to patients, families, or visitors.

Accidents

Incidents involving employees are frequently referred to as accidents. The accident report preparer should follow the same principles as for incident reporting. These will usually be covered by institutional policy and procedure. Perceptions vary too much to require personnel to discriminate between incident and accident. An accident is an incident, and many incidents are accidents.

INFECTION CONTROL

A major area for quality control and risk management is infection control. Infections acquired in hospitals are termed *nosocomial infections*. Many hospitals have full-time infection control nurses who investigate all reported nosocomial infections. A source of data is the medical laboratory. It is good policy to have all laboratory reports positive for infectious diseases routed to the infection control nurse. The diseases will be investigated and procedures implemented to prevent their spread and future development. Staff development is a major function of infection control. Standards followed are those of the Centers for Disease Control.

DISCHARGE PLANNING

Schuman, Ostfeld, and Willard studied discharge planning in an acute care hospital. The need for this function was recognized in 1944, and thirty-two years later, studies indicated that it was still being poorly done. The research team indicated that the nurse manager supervises the function of discharge planning by nurses and supports their communication with physicians.[53] The competency required of the nurse manager is to supervise staff nurses, who need to provide discharge planning that makes patients aware of necessary precautions related to diagnosis and therapy; their medical regimens, including times to take medications and dietary restrictions related to their medications; and how to get needed help. The fact is that patients suffer decreased functional capacity after discharge, and discharge planning decreases hospital readmission rates by fostering compliance with therapy. Instructions increase the importance of therapy in the eyes of the patient. Schuman and associates suggested that "nurses tend to be the most qualified personnel to delineate a patient's nursing needs following discharge and tend also to be aware of the patient's need for ancillary services."[54]

WEB ACTIVITIES

- Visit www.jbpub.com/swansburg, this text's companion website on the Internet, for further information on Measuring Quality.
- What resources are available through the Internet for risk management?
- Is there any information available from government agencies concerning quality?

SUMMARY

Quality management programs make certain that the patient care delivered meets established standards. QA programs have as their objective the determination of whether the actual service provided matches predetermined criteria of excellence. Quality management also involves continuous action to eliminate deficiencies in meeting standards.

QA is a management process that provides a sound basis for decision making and problem solving. Management of care by competent clinical nurses and nurse managers ensures the quality of that care.

NOTES

1. R. Kirk, "The Big Picture: Total Quality Management and Continuous Quality Improvement," *Journal of Nursing Administration,* April 1992, 24–31.
2. J. B. Patterson, "The Client as Customer: Achieving Service Quality and Customer Satisfaction in Rehabilitation," *Journal of Rehabilitation,* October/November/December 1992, 16–21.
3. P. B. Batalden and P. K. Stoltz, "A Framework for the Continual Improvement of Health Care: Building and Applying Professional and Improvement Knowledge to Test Changes in Daily Work," *Joint Commission Journal on Quality Improvement,* October 1993, 424–450.
4. W. E. Deming, *The New Economics for Industry, Education, Government* (Cambridge, Mass.: MIT, Center for Advanced Engineering Study, 1993).
5. P. B. Batalden and P. K. Stoltz, op. cit.
6. Ibid., 434.
7. W. E. Deming, *Out of the Crisis* (Cambridge, Mass.: MIT Press, 1986); P. B. Crosby, *Quality Without Tears* (New York: McGraw-Hill, 1984); J. M. Juran, *Juran on Planning for Quality* (New York: Free Press, 1988); P. M. Senge, *The Fifth Discipline: The Art and Practice of the Learning Organization* (New York: Doubleday, 1990).
8. "Using Standards and Indicators to Measure and Improve Performance," *1997 Comprehensive Accreditation Manual for Hospitals* (Oakbrook Terrace, Ill.: JCAHO, 1997), US 1-1 to US 1-8.
9. P. B. Batalden and P. K. Stoltz, op. cit., 434.
10. K. Cotter, *Quality Review Strategies for Clinical Nursing Practice* (North Hampton, N.H.: InterQual, 1989), 10.
11. Ibid.
12. *Comprehensive Accreditation Manual for Hospitals,* updated 1998, TX36.
13. M. R. Ventura, J. Rizzo, and S. Lenz, "Quality Indicators: Control Maintains—Propriety Improves," *Nursing Management,* January 1993, 46–50.
14. B. J. Curtis and L. J. Simpson, "Auditing: A Method for Evaluating Quality of Care," *Journal of Nursing Administration,* October 1985, 14–21.
15. Ibid.
16. Ibid.
17. M. Higgins, D. McCaughand, and M. Carr-Hill, "Assessing the Outcomes of Nursing Care," *Journal of Advanced Nursing,* May 1992, 561–568.
18. B. J. Curtis and L. J. Simpson, op. cit.
19. R. W. Evans and R. M. Ruff, "Outcome and Value: A Perspective on Rehabilitation Outcomes Achieved in Acquired Brain Injury," *Journal of Head Trauma,* December 1992, 24–36.
20. E. Larson, I. Oram, and E. Hedrick, "Nosocomial Infection Rates as an Indicator of Quality," *Medical Care,* July 1988, 676–684.
21. K. A. McCormick, "Future Data Needs for Quality Care Monitoring, DRG Considerations, Reimbursement and Outcome Measurements," *Image: Journal of Nursing Scholarship,* spring 1991, 29–32.
22. P. B. Batalden and P. K. Stoltz, op. cit., 434–438.
23. Ibid., 438.
24. H. S. Rowland and B. L. Rowland, eds. *Nursing Administration Handbook,* 4th ed. (Gaithersburg, Md.: Aspen, 1997), 405–428.
25. L. Edmunds, "A Computer Assisted Quality Assurance Model," *Journal of Nursing Administration,* March 1983, 36–43; A. DeLotto, "Examining Quality of Care Becomes Top Industry Priority," *Amherst Quarterly,* winter 1988, 1–3.

26. H. S. Rowland and B. L. Rowland, eds. "Quality Assurance," *Hospital Legal Forms, Checklists, and Guidelines* (Gaithersburg, Md.: Aspen, 1988), 26:1–26:14.

27. S. R. Edwardson and D. I. Anderson, "Hospital Nurses' Evaluation of Quality Assurance," *Journal of Nursing Administration,* July–August 1983, 33–39.

28. E. Street and D. Alvis, "A Quality Improvement Process Team," in *Continuous Quality Improvement in Nursing,* ed. J. Dienemann (Washington, D.C.: American Nurses Association 1992), 107–114.

29. Ibid.

30. H. S. Rowland and B. L. Rowland, *Nursing Administration Handbook,* op. cit., 424.

31. L. Edmunds, op. cit.

32. J. Spuck, "Using the Long-Term Care Minimum Data Set as a Tool for CQI in Nursing Homes." in *Continuous Quality Improvement in Nursing* ed. J. Dienemann (Washington, D.C.: American Nurses Association, 1992), 95–105.

33. R. Allio, "Forecasting: The Myth of Control" (interview with Donald Michal), *Planning Review,* May 1986, 6–11.

34. A. G. Taylor, K. Hudson, and A. Keeling, "Quality Nursing Care: The Consumers' Perspective Revisted," *Journal of Nursing Quality Assurance,* January 1991, 23–31.

35. D. C. Coddington and K. D. Moore, "Quality of Care as a Business Strategy," *Healthcare Forum Journal,* March/April 1987, 29–34.

36. Ibid.

37. E. Larson, "Combining Nursing Quality Assurance and Research Programs," *Journal of Nursing Administration,* November 1983, 32–34.

38. Ibid.

39. Intravenous Nurses Society, "Revised Intravenous Nursing Standards of Practice," *Journal of Intravenous Nursing,* 1990, 13(suppl), s91.

40. J. T. Rogers, *Risk Management in Emergency Medicine* (Dallas: Emergency Medicine Foundation—American College of Emergency Physicians, 1985), 2.

41. L. S. Hayden, "Risk Management Strategies," *Journal of Intravenous Nursing,* September/October 1992, 288–290.

42. R. Wilkinson and B. J. Moore, eds., *Quality Assurance in Ambulatory Care,* 2d ed. (Chicago: Joint Commission on Accreditation of Healthcare Organizations, 1990), 25.

43. B. Bennett, "Quality Care Through Risk Management," *Orthopaedic Nursing,* May/June 1993, 54–55.

44. G. Troyer and S. Salman, *Handbook of Health Care Risk Management* (Germantown, Md. Aspen, 1986).

45. B. Bennett, op. cit.

46. D. Joseph and S. K. Jones, "Incident Reporting: The Cornerstone of Risk Management," *Nursing Management,* December 1984, 22–23.

47. T. A. Goldman, "Risk Management Concepts and Strategies," *Journal of Intravenous Nursing,* May/June 1991, 199–204.

48. Ibid.

49. Ibid.

50. Ibid.; "QAs Pave the Way: The Quest for Quality," *Hospital Profiles,* Alabama Hospital Association, December 1987/January 1988, 1, 4–5.

51. P. Blake, "Incident Investigation: A Complete Guide," *Nursing Management,* November 1984, 37–41.

52. G. W. Poteet, "Risk Management and Nursing," *Nursing Clinics of North America,* September 1983, 451–465. K. H. Henry, ed., *Nursing Administration and Law Manual* (Gaithersburg, Md.: Aspen, 1985), 9:1–9:39.

53. J. E. Schuman, A. M. Ostfeld, and H. N. Willard, "Discharge Planning in an Acute Hospital," *Archives of Physical Medicine and Rehabilitation,* July 1976, 343–347.

54. Ibid.

Appendix 26–1 Quality Assessment and Improvement Program

University of South Alabama Medical Center
Department of Nursing
Quality Assessment and Improvement Program

I. POLICY STATEMENT

The University of South Alabama Medical Center Department of Nursing will monitor the provision of nursing care and the results of nursing care in an ongoing and systematic manner following the Quality Assessment and Improvement Program for the Department of Nursing. This program is designed to improve care based on the monitoring and evaluation of structure, practice (process), and care (outcome) standards, and is consistent with the Quality Assessment and Improvement Plan for the University of South Alabama Medical Center.

Nursing quality assessment and improvement activities are reports to the QAI Executive Committee of the University of South Alabama Medical Center.

II. PURPOSE

1. To ensure that the quality of patient care is optimal through a unified program.
2. To provide the process by which the provision of nursing care and end results (patient outcomes) are measured and evaluated against Standards for Nursing.
3. To integrate efforts of physicians and nurses in Special Care Units to continuously improve patient care.
4. To maintain quality care in current use.

III. GENERAL INFORMATION

Structure Standards describe the environment in which safe, effective and appropriate care takes place, i.e., organization, management, resources, care delivery, productivity, and turnover rate. Structure standards are a form of productivity reporting and are used for management information. Nurse Managers receive daily productivity/variance reports from Nursing Information Systems to assist in monitoring and evaluating structure standards.

Standards of Practice describe the nature and sequence of health care activities and are based on identified important aspects of care. Policies and procedures describe how important aspects of care are carried out.

Standards of Care describe nursing care results for the major patient populations and those patients who receive high-risk, high-volume nursing care.

Care Plans define and describe individual patients' nursing care and expected results.

Quality Care Framework (Exhibit A26–1) clarifies Integration of Standards for Nursing into Quality Assurance.

Nursing staff members participate, by way of the Nursing Practice Committee and unit meetings, in the identification of the important aspects of care, identifying the indicators, planning action to improve care, and evaluating the results. All nursing departments participate on CQI teams as assigned.

Each nursing department develops and follows an annual plan for QAI that is maintained on each unit, and copies of which are located in the office of Nursing Administration. The JCAHO ten-step process is the method used to accomplish improvements. Each unit plan is assisted by a matrix—used to simplify and clarify information pertinent to each indicator.

IV. PROCEDURE

Responsibility. The Nurse Manager is responsible for ensuring the completion of QAI activities.

Scope of Care. This is a 406-bed, level I trauma center that provides nursing care by RNs, LPNs and NAs 24 hours a day to patients requiring emergency services, interfacility transportation, aeromedical transportation, surgical services, post-anesthesia care, labor and delivery, obstetrics, intensive care nursery, neonatal transportation, premature nursery, newborn nursery, medical-surgical nursing, burn center, neuro-trauma intensive care, surgical intensive care, renal dialysis, medical intensive care, coronary intensive care, and intermediate nursing care. Medical-surgical pediatric patients are located on 6th and 5th South nursing units. Pediatric patients also receive nursing care in the Burn Center, CCU, and, less frequently, in SICU/NTICU. The scope of care is based upon the needs and expectations of the high-risk and high-volume patient who is admitted (Special Care Units) or discharged from each nursing unit. High volume is determined by annual review of diagnoses (DRGs) and by categorizing the diagnoses according to similar patient needs. The largest categories or patient

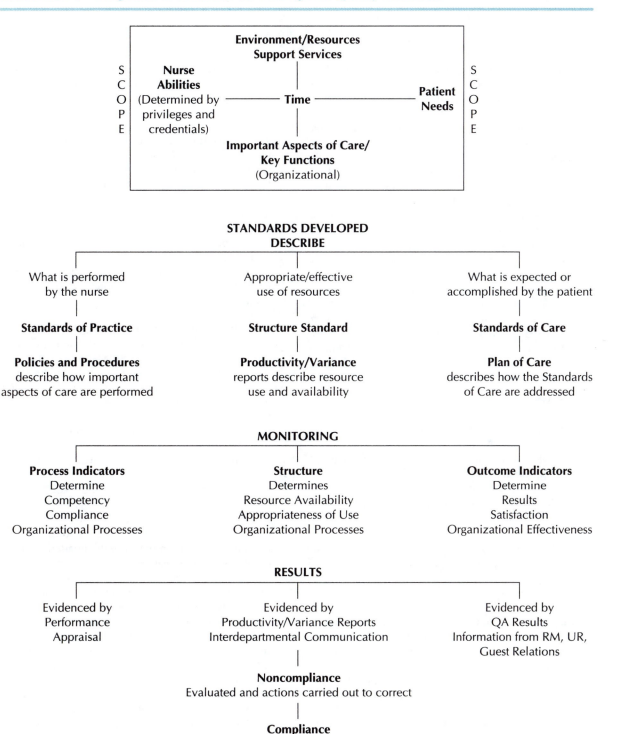

S C O P E

**Environment/Resources
Support Services**

**Nurse
Abilities**
(Determined by
privileges and
credentials)

———— **Time** ————

**Patient
Needs**

S C O P E

**Important Aspects of Care/
Key Functions**
(Organizational)

**STANDARDS DEVELOPED
DESCRIBE**

What is performed by the nurse	Appropriate/effective use of resources	What is expected or accomplished by the patient
Standards of Practice	**Structure Standard**	**Standards of Care**
Policies and Procedures describe how important aspects of care are performed	**Productivity/Variance** reports describe resource use and availability	**Plan of Care** describes how the Standards of Care are addressed

MONITORING

Process Indicators Determine Competency Compliance Organizational Processes	**Structure** Determines Resource Availability Appropriateness of Use Organizational Processes	**Outcome Indicators** Determine Results Satisfaction Organizational Effectiveness

RESULTS

Evidenced by Performance Appraisal	Evidenced by Productivity/Variance Reports Interdepartmental Communication	Evidenced by QA Results Information from RM, UR, Guest Relations

Noncompliance
Evaluated and actions carried out to correct

Compliance
Evaluated and actions carried out to improve

Appendix 26–1   Quality Assessment and Improvement Program *(Continued)*

populations having similar needs based on diag- noses are designated as high volume. Patients iden- tified as at-risk are determined by the history of complications within certain groups of patients or for individual patients. In addition to the needs and expectations of the major patient populations, sub- categories are identified to reflect those patients who receive problem-prone nursing care and those patients who are at risk to develop complications due to their biophysical status.

Important Aspects of Care are identified in address- ing the high-volume and/or problem-prone (present a risk to the patient or nurse) nursing care activities. From the important aspects of care, standards are devel- oped: Standards of Practice, Concurrent Process, Retrospective Process, Standards of Care, Concur- rent Outcome, and Retrospective Outcome. Policies and procedures are based on standards determined by the requirements of the major patient populations.

The following generic key functions are impor- tant to patient care at the University of South Alabama Medical Center:

    Assessment/Reassessment
    Care Plan
    Implementation/Evaluation
    Continuity of Care
    Safety/Universal Precautions/Infection Control
    Appropriateness
    Teaching/Emotional and Spiritual Support
    Medication Administration/Treatments
    Discharge Preparation
    Confidentiality
    IV Therapy

Each Nursing Unit has identified aspects of care related to generic standards for quality assessment and improvement.

Indicators. Elements of the high-volume, problem- prone nursing activities that provide evidence as to whether or not the care provided is of quality are developed into statements called Indicators for each nursing unit. The Indicator Development Form (Exhibit A26–2) is used to operationalize indicators as needed.

Process Indicators measure how well depart- ments and individuals meet stated standards for practice, use the nursing process, and doc- ument care.

Outcome Indicators measure specific patient outcomes and direct departments in needed action and changes towards meeting standards of care.

Thresholds for Evaluation. A numerical value is placed on each indicator to assist in determining if opportunity for improvement exists. The Threshold for Evaluation (TFE) shall not be less than 85 per- cent and reflects expected variations, as well as the importance of the indicator used by each nursing unit. Any indicator that is evaluated as demonstrat- ing opportunity to improve is remonitored within thirty days and at least monthly thereafter until compliance is sustained for at least three months. Each Nursing Unit has identified thresholds for evaluation for each indicator.

Collection and Organization of Data. The Nurse Manager or designee sets up an annual Quality Assessment and Improvement Matrix that specifies the sequence and the data to be collected for mon- itoring. At least two aspects and indicators related to outcomes are monitored for sustained (minimum three months) compliance. Data sources include patient charts and questionnaires. Process monitor- ing may involve staff observation/interview, and outcome monitoring may involve patient/family interview/observation.

In addition to the aspects and indicators selected for continuous (ongoing) monitoring, focus studies will be performed as planned. Noncompliant indi- cators incurred during the focus studies will be monitored at least monthly until quarterly (three- month) average is reached.

Special Care Nursing Units (SICU/NTICU, CCU/ MICU, Burn Center, ICN) and medical staff of Special Care Units monitor joint aspects of care and patients, integrating efforts to improve patient care. Nursing concurrently monitors patients applicable to the cho- sen joint aspect and supplies the medical record number to the medical staff Quality Assurance Coor- dinator for physician review. Department heads and medical directors discuss findings and opportunities to improve via the Critical Care Committee.

Documentation review classes will be held on Committee Day, the first Tuesday of each month. RNs will be assigned to participate in retrospective review of documentation. Generically, Nursing will

(continued)

Exhibit A26–2 Indicator Development Form

I. Indicator Statement: _____

_____

II. Definition of Terms: _____

_____

III: Type of Indicator: Rate based _____   Process _____

                            Sentinel event _____   Outcome _____

IV: Rationale

    A. Why useful? _____

    B. Supportive references: _____

    C. Components of quality assessed: _____

V. Description of Indicator Population

    A. $\dfrac{\text{(Numerator)}}{\text{(Denominator)}}$: _____

    B. Subcategories: _____

VI. Indicator Data Collection Logic

    Data Elements   Data Source

VII. Underlying Factors

    A. Patient factors: _____

    B. Practitioner factors: _____

    C. Organization factors: _____

Appendix 26–1   Quality Assessment and Improvement Program *(Continued)*

monitor 5 percent of patient admissions for appropriate documentation. Please refer to the generic matrix (Exhibit A26–3) for documentation indicators and related information.

Concurrent monitoring is performed on each nursing unit each month as part of assignments to the nursing staff. Results of monitoring and any adverse effects to the patient as a result of individual performance are addressed and followed up through Nurse Credentialing as part of the Performance Appraisal.

The staff nurse follows Staff Nurse Guidelines for Quality Monitoring (Exhibit A26–4) in using a quality review worksheet or concurrent data sheet for monitoring.

Evaluate. The data is initially evaluated by the Nurse Manager who further involves the staff in evaluation through staff meetings and Nurse Practice Committee Meetings. Evaluation may consist of more intensive review of specific cases or continued monitoring. Concurrent monitoring is advantageous in that the staff nurse who takes corrective action at the time of review is involved in the initial evaluation.

Actions to Improve Care. Methods to resolve problems and improve care identified through monitoring include staff meetings, individual counseling, education, problem solving with other departments, developing standards, modifying documentation tools, changing departmental/organizational process and related policies, and revision of Quality Assessment. Actions taken will specify who will do what and when.

Specific problems may be referred to standing committees within the department. Problems identified by any staff member that involve any department or activity are documented on a Quality Assurance Problem Reporting Sheet (Exhibit A26–5, p.688) and attached with follow-up to the monthly narrative analysis report.

Assess Actions/Document Improvement. A time frame for assessing effectiveness for action is determined. Subsequent findings are reviewed at that time and further recommendations for action are made if necessary. The QAI Report Grid is completed monthly for all indicators monitored during the report interval. The Nurse Manager or designee uses instructions for completion of the Report Grid (Exhibit A26–6, p. 689) to complete the form.

Communicate Relevant Information. Information obtained from staff nurse data collection is communicated appropriately as per the established communication system (Exhibit A26–7, p. 691).

Monitoring results of Special Care Units are communicated through the Critical Care Committee and signed by the Medical Director. All nursing units forward monthly QA reports to the Clinical Administrator for Nursing Practice.

Each quarter the Clinical Administrator for Nursing Practice summarizes each unit's specific report into a Division Report that is signed by the Director of Nursing and the Assistant Administrator for Nursing. Signed original quarterly reports are maintained in the office of Nursing Administration and copies are maintained by the hospital QAI Department.

V. ANNUAL EVALUATION

Quality Assurance for the Department of Nursing and Standards for Nursing are reviewed at least annually and revised as needed by the Nurse Practice Committee and Nurse Managers. Review and revision of Standards considers:

1. Patient requirements and the effectiveness of the staffing plan.
2. Ability to attract and retain the numbers and types of nursing personnel required.
3. Variance reports that indicate the staffing plan's adequacy or inadequacy to meet patient needs.
4. Monitoring information that relates to the staffing plan.
5. The consistency for the provision of nursing care between units based on Standards.
6. The staff's ability to pursue activities to promote innovation and/or improvement of nursing care.

The annual report will identify any opportunities to improve care, care that improved, and revisions to the plan.

VI. CONFIDENTIALITY STATEMENT

Quality assessment and improvement documents and activities are privileged and confidential for the USAMC Quality Management Program and are prepared and maintained pursuant to the Code of Alabama 1975: 6-5-333, 22-21-8, and 34-24-58.

Source: Reprinted courtesy University of South Alabama Medical Center, Mobile, Alabama.

Exhibit A26–3 Quality Assessment and Improvement Matrix and Generic Documentation

Department: __Nursing__   Date: __December 21, 19XX__   Revised: __September 19XX__

Key Function/ Important Aspect	Quality Indicators	Reason for Assessment	Type of Indicator	Age-Specific Consideration*	Sample Size	T.F.E.	Collection Schedule	Collection Method	Reporting Schedule	Others Involved
DOCUMENTATION										
Nursing Process	1. Completion of admission assessment and reassessments	High volume	Rate-based/ process	None	5%	92%	1 day per month	Retrospective Structured Chart Review Class	Per Division scheduled to report to hospital QA Committee. One Nursing Division each month will report.	
	2. Developmental assessment for patients age <13	High risk	"	Indicator		"				
	3. Completion of care planning	High volume	"	None		"				
	4. Completion of implementation and evaluation of care planning	High volume	"	None		"				
Safety	5. Appropriate safety measures documented	High risk	"	None		"				
Teaching/ Emotional Support	6. Teaching and emotional support provided	Problem prone	"	None		"				Dietary/PT Social Services
	7. Results of teaching/ emotional support	Problem prone	Rate-based/ outcome	None		"				"
Medication Administration	8. Completion of Medication Administration Record	High volume, high risk and problem prone	Rate-based/ process	None		100				

Exhibit A26–3 Quality Assessment and Improvement Matrix and Generic Documentation *(Continued)*

Department: Nursing   Date: December 21, 19XX   Revised: September 19XX

Key Function/ Important Aspect	Quality Indicators	Reason for Assessment	Type of Indicator	Age-Specific Consideration*	Sample Size	T.F.E.	Collection Schedule	Collection Method	Reporting Schedule	Others Involved
Treatments /Blood Transfusion	9. Completion of Blood Transfusion Report	High risk and problem prone	Rate-based/ process	None		100				
Discharge Planning	10. Completion of discharge planning	High volume and problem prone	Rate-based/ process	None		92				Dietary/PT Social Services "
	11. Effectiveness of discharge planning	High volume and problem prone	Rate-Based/ outcome	None		"				
IV Therapy/ I&O	12. Documentation of IV assessment	High risk and high volume	Rate-based/ process	None		100%				
	13. Complete I&Os	High risk and high volume	Rate-based/ process	None		100%				
Pre-op/ Perioperative Care	14. Appropriate documentation of circulating nurse	High risk and high volume	Rate-based/ process	None		100%				
	15. Pre-op nursing assessment/ checklist complete	High risk and high volume	Rate-based/ process	None		100%				

*Applies to all or "age specific" indicator.

Exhibit A26–4   *Staff Nurse Guidelines for Quality Monitoring*

Quality Assurance monitoring is documented on unit-specific data retrieval sheets by the assigned staff nurse each month. The data retrieval sheets are located on each nursing unit in a QA notebook or in the employee file for QA.

The data retrieval sheets monitor two different aspects of nursing: (1) Standards of practice are monitored by process indicators. Practice/process measures what the nurse does (nursing practice, nursing process) and is stated in terms of "The nurse will. . . ." (2) Standards of care are monitored by outcome indicators. Care/outcome measures the final picture of the patient as a result of nursing/interdepartmental care and is stated in terms of "The patient will . . ." or "The patient can expect. . . ."

The staff nurse retrieves the QA data sheets from the book or file and monitors a patient/chart according to the indicators during a month specified by the Nurse Manager or designee.

The staff nurse uses the column beside the indicator to designate the results of the patient/nurse/chart that is monitored. Each time the indicator is monitored, the adjacent column is used. The month in which the monitoring takes place is written at the top of the page.

The result of monitoring is documented using the following key:

+   Results are compliant

–   Results are not compliant

J   Results are not compliant but are justified

N/A   Results do not apply

When justification (J) is used, the justifier must be written below the standard to which it applies.

Example: The patient was not wearing identification band because of injuries to the extremities—BUT, *the I.D. band was taped to the head of the bed.*

Example: The nurse did not document confirmation of the enteral feeding tube insertion because M.D. inserted it and started feedings—BUT *the M.D. documented in the progress notes the confirmation of the feeding tube.*

Not applicable (N/A) is used when a specific indicator does not apply for that patient. Examples would be a patient who has no IV tubing to be changed because the patient has an INT, or the patient is discharged without medications needed at home. In these instances, indicators for IV tubing changed or verbalizing understanding of discharge medications would be N/A.

The staff nurse should seek out the patient populations for which the Standard of Care applies versus monitoring one patient for all outcome indicators.

Examples: An abdominal surgery patient is found to monitor the outcome for abdominal surgery patients; a seizure patient is monitored for outcome of seizure patients; a cardiac patient is found to monitor outcome of cardiac patients; a patient with an IV is found to monitor outcomes for IV therapy; a patient who has been discharged, or is in the process of being discharged, is monitored for discharge criteria and discharge teaching.

This process assures that the standards are applicable in the majority of situations.

At the end of each month the Nurse Manager or designated staff nurse compiles the information from each data sheet and then returns this sheet to the file or QA book. Indicators are monitored every month until they reach quarterly compliance. At that time another standard and/or indicators may be added by the Nurse Manager or designated staff nurse, depending on problems identified.

The staff nurse participates in identifying standards and indicators by way of staff meetings, the Nursing Practice Committee, or one-to-one conferences with the Nurse Manager or designated staff nurse.

Exhibit A26–5   Quality Assurance Problem Reporting Sheet

Department: _____   Date: _____

Initiated by: _____   To: _____

Problem or concern studied:

_____

_____

_____

How identified and why important (data sources) impact on patient care:

_____

_____

_____

_____

Contributing factors:

_____

_____

Quality goal (after study is completed):

_____

_____

_____

_____

Departments involved:

_____

_____

Referred to department: _____   Action taken: _____

_____

_____

_____

Follow-up plan or recommendations:

_____

_____

_____

Please respond by: _____   To: _____

Thank you very much. _____(signature)

Exhibit A26–6 Report Grid

Department: _____   Reporting period: ___ Nov., Dec., Jan. ___

F/U Date	Quality Indicators	Findings					Conclusions/ Recommendations	Actions	Evaluation of Action Report Due
		TFE	Sample	Met	Not Met	%			
	List the aspect of care and indicators on which you are reporting. You must report on all indicators that were monitored.	This column should be stated clearly and succinctly:					In this column you should talk about what your findings mean (conclusions). Are they improved or worse than previous reports?	What actions, based on your recommendations, do you plan to take? Who will do it? When will it be done?	State the date that your next report on this particular indicator is due
	If this is an evaluation of the action of a previous report, please state.	*TFE:* Threshold for evaluation							
		Sample: The number monitored					e.g.: Staff nurse participation in chart review has been effective (or has not)	Options could include continued monitoring	
	Nursing has added this column to the left to assist in standardization and compliance.	*Met:* Write in the number met or number compliant						Changing the indicator to be more valid	
		Not Met: Write in the number not met or noncompliant					Several orientees have affected results as there was no improvement	Dropping the indicator	
	If the indicator is one requiring follow-up (action has been stated previously), then put the date (month/year) that actions were reported.	%: Write in the percentage of compliance					Nurses are not performing IV assessment	Staff education	
							Is there a trend? Progressively better or worse?	Changing a process or procedure, etc.	
							Are findings meaningless? Why?	Be specific	
							You should also discuss recommendations for improvement of findings.		

(continued)

Exhibit A26–6 Report Grid *(Continued)*

Department: _____   Reporting period: _____Nov., Dec., Jan._____

F/U Date	Quality Indicators	Findings				Conclusions/ Recommendations	Actions	Evaluation of Action Report Due
		TFE	Sample	Met	Not Met %			
	Appropriateness: TED hose and SCD cuff is removed each day and bath/skin care is provided beneath the devices	100%	16	9	7 56%	Nine patients received proper skin care. This has improved from October by 2%. Two new NAs stated that they were not aware of proper procedure. All other NAs were compliant. Educate new NAs. Incorporate correct procedure into NA orientation.	CNS has completed floor-to-floor classes. NM has contacted CNS and set up classes for these new NAs on 12/16. CETN also monitoring these patients. NM informed Clinical Consultant (Staff Dev) of recommendations. Continue to monitor the procedure.	April
						Develop policy.		
		100%	10	10	0 100%	Education and communication of new policy/procedure has been effective. Communicate to staff. Remonitor Aug. quarter.	NM will hold staff meeting on 12/24 to communicate results.	N/A

Signatures: _____   _____   _____   _____
                        Department Head/Nurse Manager   Date   Assistant Administrator   Date

Source: Courtesy University of South Alabama Medical Center, Mobile, Alabama.

Exhibit A26–7   Communication System

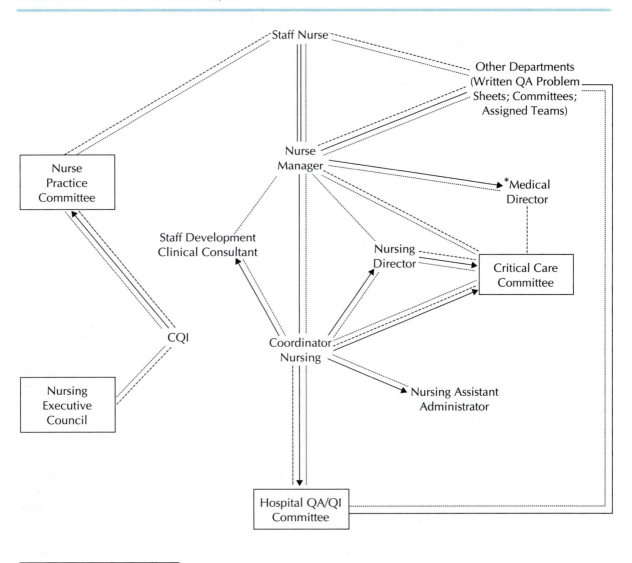

Staff Nurse

Other Departments
(Written QA Problem
Sheets; Committees;
Assigned Teams)

Nurse
Manager

Nurse
Practice
Committee

*Medical
Director

Staff Development
Clinical Consultant

Nursing
Director

Critical Care
Committee

CQI

Coordinator
Nursing

Nursing
Executive
Council

Nursing Assistant
Administrator

Hospital QA/QI
Committee

Key:
Data ═══════
Written ──────
Verbal ------------
Feedback ··············
Special Care
   Units Only*

PERFORMANCE APPRAISAL

OBJECTIVES

- Define performance appraisal.
- Illustrate purposes for performance appraisal.
- Differentiate among standards for performance appraisal.
- Illustrate training approaches for performance.
- Distinguish among performance appraisal methodologies.
- Illustrate performance appraisal problem areas.

KEY CONCEPTS

Performance appraisal
Performance standards
Job analysis
Job description
Job evaluation
Feedback
Self-rating
Peer rating

Manager behavior: Oversees implementation of a performance appraisal system that meets all official requirements.
Leader behavior: Involves employees in developing a performance system they view as fair in its standards, application, and outcomes.

Performance appraisal is a control process in which employees' performances are evaluated against standards. The literature on performance appraisal is voluminous, indicating its value to management. Considerable research has been done on various aspects of the performance appraisal process.

Neither employees nor managers like performance appraisal. Some employees view performance appraisal as being more valued by top management than by themselves and their supervisors. Some managers do not like to do performance appraisals because it makes them feel guilty: Did I do justice by the employee? As writers of performance appraisals, managers are concerned that they may "cast something in stone" that is inaccurate, be criticized for written grammar and spelling, say something illegal about the ratee, or may not be able to substantiate their comments.[1] Other managers are afraid of employees' reactions to ratings. Also, performance appraisal requires careful planning, information gathering, and an extensive formal interview—a time-consuming process. Managers perform activities of short duration, attend ad hoc meetings, perform nonroutine functions, and focus on current information—all short-term activities in comparison with ongoing performance appraisal.[2] The process is usually not interactive, moves slowly, is passive, is isolated, and is not people-oriented.[3]

Measurement of performance is imprecise. Often the focus is upon the format, not the people. In some organizations, the human resources department sends the rating forms to the departments shortly before the end of the fiscal year. The forms have to be completed immediately and are done with little or no training and preparation of either rater or ratee. The result is distrust by employees and dread by managers.

A survey of Fortune 1300 companies (1000 industrial and 300 nonindustrial) indicated that 29 percent of hourly workers are not evaluated by a formal appraisal system. Thirty-nine percent of respondents indicated that where used, performance appraisal systems are "extremely effective" or "very effective." Performance appraisal systems are underappreciated.[4]

Performance appraisal systems require top management commitment. They can be tied to the planning cycle by relating them to personnel budgets or including them as a management plan. They are most helpful when managers commit to using them for purposes beneficial to both employees and the organization.

Research in performance appraisal domains has little effect on the process or the outcome. A suggestion is that research and practice focus on fair and accurate performance appraisal as a process before attempting to use it to improve performance.[5]

Performance appraisal literature published between 1985 and 1990 indicates the following results:[6]

1. U.S. industry uses performance appraisal systems for an average of eleven years. Performance appraisal systems had little input from line managers, employees, and customers.
2. Most formats use management by objectives for executives, managers, and professional employees. Trait-based rating scales are the norm for nonexempt employees. Behaviorally anchored rating scales (BARS), forced-choice scales, or mixed standard scales are little used. Executives and hourly employees are least likely to be evaluated.
3. Supervisor ratings are most common. Self, peer, and subordinate ratings are seldom used.
4. Very few organizations allow decisions about performance appraisal policies or practice to be made at the level at which they are executed.
5. While some raters receive rater training, employees are seldom involved.
6. Only 25 percent of raters are held accountable for managing the appraisal process.
7. Few employees' opinions about the appraisal process are solicited.
8. Managers are concerned with fairness, justice, and future performance.
9. Sixty percent to 70 percent of an organization's workforce are rated in the top two performance levels.
10. A more comprehensive theory of the performance appraisal process is needed.

PURPOSES OF PERFORMANCE APPRAISAL

Performance appraisal may be a nurse manager's most valuable tool in controlling human resources and productivity. The performance appraisal process can be used effectively to govern employee behavior in order to produce goods and services in high volume and of high quality. Nurse managers can also use the performance appraisal process to govern corporate direction in selecting, training, doing career planning with, and rewarding personnel. The Fortune 1300 survey indicated that 80 percent used appraisal systems to justify merit increases, provide feedback, and identify candidates for promotion—all considered short-range goals. These goals were linked to long-range goals of performance potential for succession planning and career planning but could be much more useful in strategic planning. Fifty-eight percent used performance appraisal to identify strengths and weaknesses, while 39 percent used it for career planning. Eighty-nine percent used it for general guidelines for salary increases, while only one percent used it for forced distribution for bonuses. Forced distribution sets a limit on the number of high-level ratings.[7]

In addition to being used for promotions, counseling, training and development, staff planning, retention, termination, selections, and compensations, performance monitoring has been found to make employees effective. It is a managerial tool that can facilitate performance levels that achieve the company's mission and objectives.[8]

Appraisal systems are needed to meet legal requirements, including those for standardized forms and procedures, clear and relevant job analysis, and trained raters. When they do not meet such requirements, disciplinary actions, including termination, do not stand up in court.[9]

Motivation

A goal of performance appraisal is to stimulate motivation of the employee to perform the tasks and accomplish the mission of the organization. Promotions, assignments, selection for education, and increased pay are some of the employee goals that stimulate this motivation. If performance appraisal is to improve performance, the science of behavioral technology as described in chapter 4 should be employed.

Salary Problems. Performance evaluation is used to determine and provide equitable salary treatment. Jobs within groups of professionals such as engineers, physicians, chemists, physicists, and nurses have the same basic characteristics. Differences exist in the complexity of jobs. One could say that the job of a nurse assigned to a special care unit is more complex than that of one assigned to an intermediate care unit. This could be true to the extent that the depth of complexity exists. Contrast this with the complexity of managing the care of an active, intermediate care unit of twenty to forty-five patients. The *breadth* of complexity of the nursing care of many patients with differing problems who are treated by many physicians directing many medical care plans and many nonprofessional workers appears to be equivalent to the *depth* of complexity of intensive nursing care. In fact, some nurses want to be assigned to special care units not because of the dynamics of the situation but because their sphere of operations is encapsulated. Is one entitled to more salary than another? The job analysts say yes if special training is required, if complicated specialized equipment is being used, and if the nurse is required to make more independent and critical judgments.

Certainly the jobs of all professionals can be evaluated using the yardsticks of conventional performance appraisal techniques. However, arguments abound regarding the relationship between performance appraisals and salaries and promotion. Some writers say keep performance appraisals well away from times of salary increases and promotions.[10] In a survey of 875 companies, 32 percent experimented with some form of performance-based pay,[11] a concept discussed in the following chapter.

Kirkpatrick recommends separating appraisals for merit salary increases from appraisals for performance improvement. Those used for merit salary increases look backward at past performance, look at total performance, compare one individual to others doing the same job, are subjective, and are done in an emotional climate. Appraisals done for performance improvement look ahead; are concerned with detailed performance; are compared with what is expected in standards, goals, and objectives; and are conducted in a calm climate.[12]

For performance reviews related to salary administration, nurse managers would explain to subordinates the basis of decisions. The reviews would be fair and would be totally understood by the managers, who would allow employees to react even to the point of discussing them with higher management. If a high salary increase results, the nurse manager communicates the good news to the employee. Three months should elapse between appraisals for salary administration and those for improved performance.[13]

Expectancy theory states that "the greater a person's expectancy (i.e., subjective probability) that effort expenditure will lead to various rewards, the greater the person's motivation to work hard."[14] Rewards of high value should be obtainable and related to job performance. Employees will repeat rewarded behavior, and they will be retained, thus maintaining productivity.

Research indicates that productivity increases in a range of 29 percent to 63 percent with output-based pay plans versus time-based pay plans. Also, individual incentive plans are better than group incentive plans.[15]

Pay is the most powerful motivator of performance, and people will not work without it. Other financial incentives such as shift differentials, education pay, and certification pay also are positive motivators. Research has shown that productivity actually drops with time-based rewards and hourly wages. Good employees will leave rather than work with poorly performing ones. Rewards should be related to job performance. The results can be seen by correlating rewards across individual performances. There should be substantial differences in the rewards.

Kopelman suggests a mixed-consequence system: rewards for good performance, deductions for poor performance. The latter requires coaching, training, counseling, reassigning, or terminating. Important job responsibilities and behaviors deserving of high rewards can be determined from job analysis. They should be related to difficult performance standards or goals.[16]

The Xerox Experience.   Prior to 1983, Xerox had a traditional appraisal system, tying merit pay increases to performance rating. Employees were dissatisfied with the lack of an equitable rating distribution. Ninety-five percent of employees were at the level 3 or 4 in a four-level rating system. Forced distribution was used to control the numbers of employees above or below a specific level. There were no preplanned objectives, the focus being on the summary rating. A task force was used to develop a performance feedback and development process with the following characteristics:

1. Objectives were set between manager and employee.
2. The evaluation was documented and approved by a second-level manager.
3. An appraisal review was held at the end of six months, with review and discussion of objectives and progress. The written report was signed by both manager and employee.
4. A final review was held at one year.
5. The process emphasized performance feedback and improvements.
6. A merit increase discussion was held one to two months later.
7. There was agreement on personal goals related to communications, planning, time management, human relations, and professional goals (specialty and job).
8. There were financial and human resource management objectives.
9. Managers were trained in the process.

Regular surveys of the Xerox system indicated that 81 percent of employees understood their work group objectives better, 84 percent considered appraisals fair, 72 percent understood how merit pay was determined, 70 percent met personal and professional objectives, and 77 percent favored the system.[17]

DEVELOPING AND USING STANDARDS FOR PERFORMANCE APPRAISAL

Performance Standards

Performance standards are derived from job analysis, job descriptions, job evaluation, and other documents detailing the qualitative and quantitative aspects of jobs. They are established by authority, which may be the agency in which they are used or a professional association, such as the American Nurses Association (ANA). They are measuring sticks for qualitative and quantitative evaluation of the individual's performance. They should be based on appropriate knowledge and practical enough to be attained. Like other documents, they must be kept up-to-date.

Job or performance standards for the nurse manager may be developed using the ANA *Scope and Standards for Nurse Administrators*. Performance standards are written for a job and are used to measure the performance of the individual filling the job. Employees should know that these standards are being used and know what they are. They may be asked to bring copies of the standards to their supervisor for scheduled counseling. They may also be asked to list their accomplishments in relation to the standards. This makes performance counseling less of a threat and allows employees to recognize and discuss their accomplishments. Employees may be guided into recognition of areas where their performance falls short and to be encouraged to voice goals for improvement in these areas. This method of using performance standards has been found to be effective.

The ANA Congress for Nursing Practice has developed and published standards of practice in several specialty areas. The ANA *Standards of Clinical Nursing Practice* can be used in the development of performance standards. Exhibit 27–1 is an example of performance standards for a clinical nurse.

A standard is "a unit of measurement that can serve as a reference point for evaluating results."[18] Clinical nurses develop these units of measurement as both process and outcome criteria.

Accuracy and fairness of performance appraisal come from having an objective, standards-oriented performance appraisal plan. The plan should have objectively defined task standards that can be measured in terms of output and observable behavioral change. These performance standards will relate to both the quantity and quality of work, the who, how, when, where, and what are produced. They will include production standards.[19]

Performance evaluation includes standards for experience, complexities of job, trust level, and understanding of work and mission. Friedman recommends developing job standards based on four to eight core responsibilities. For nurse managers, these core responsibilities could be in the major management functions of planning, organizing, directing (leading), and controlling (evaluating). They could also be related to the roles of clinician, teacher, administrator, consultant, and researcher. Finally, they could be related to self-development. Desired behaviors, outputs, or results under each core responsibility are then developed as performance objectives. Objectives are related to or combined with behaviors as standards for performance evaluation.[20]

Job analysis, job descriptions, and job evaluations are important sources of standards for performance evaluation.

Job Analysis

Edwards and Sproull list objective performance dimensions, developed by management and employees as a necessity for effective performance appraisal and developed from job analysis. "Performance criteria should be: (1) measurable through observation of behaviors of the job, (2) clearly defined, and (3) job-related."[21] Nurse managers and nursing employees would agree on the meaning and priority of each measurement. These standards need not be quantifiable but must be keyed to observable behavior:

Observable Behavior → Job Analysis → Job Standards

Exhibit 27–1   Performance Standards—Clinical Nurse

Performance Standards

1. *Type of work:* Nursing care of patients
   Major duty: Performs the primary functions of a professional nurse (50 percent of working hours).
   a. Obtains nursing histories on all newly admitted patients.
   b. Reviews nursing histories of all transfer patients.
   c. Uses nursing histories to make nursing diagnoses determining patients' needs and problems. Using this information:
   d. Initiates a nursing care plan for each patient.
   e. Lists goal(s) for each nursing need or problem.
   f. Writes nursing prescription or orders for each patient to meet each need or problem and goal.
   g. Applies the plan of care, giving evidence of knowledge of scientific and legal principles.
   h. Executes physicians' orders.

2. *Type of work:* Management of nursing personnel
   Major duty: Plans nursing care of patients on a daily basis (14 percent of working hours).
   a. Rates each patient according to number and complexity of needs and goals.
   b. Knows abilities of each team member.
   c. Makes a daily assignment for each team member.
   d. Discusses assignment with each team member at the beginning of each shift.
      (1) Listens to taped report with team members.
      (2) Sees that team members review physicians' orders and nursing care plans.
      (3) Answers questions arising from these activities.
   e. Confers with charge nurse and ward clerk periodically to ascertain whether there are any new orders.
   f. Plans for a team conference at a specific time and place and tells team members.
   g. Incorporates division and unit philosophy and objectives into team activities.
   h. Assists with assignment of LPN and RN students, including them as active team members according to their backgrounds and learning needs.

3. *Type of work:* Management of nursing personnel
   Major duty: Supervises team activities (10 percent of working hours).
   a. Makes frequent rounds to assist team members with care of patients. At the same time, talks to and observes patients to determine

   (1) New needs or problems.
   (2) Progress. Confirms these observations with patient if possible.
   b. Conducts 15- to 20-minute team conference using a specific agenda that has been made known to team members at previous day's conference.
      (1) Involves all team members.
      (2) Solicits comments on new problems or special problems of patients and updates selected nursing care plans as needed.
      (3) Assigns roles for next day's team conference.
   c. Writes nursing progress notes and updates remaining nursing care plans.
      (1) Assists technicians with writing notes as needed for training. Otherwise reads and countersigns their notes. Writes own notes.
      (2) Updates those nursing care plans not done at team conference. Recognizes this is a professional nurse's responsibility.
      (3) Reads notes of LPNs and RNs.
   d. Communicates nursing service and hospital policies to team members on a daily basis through referral to such information as daily bulletins, minutes of meetings, and changes in regulations.

4. *Type of work:* Management of equipment and supplies
   Major duty: Identifies needs, plans and submits requests for new and replacement equipment and supplies to charge nurse (1 percent of working hours).
   a. While working with team members identifies malfunctioning equipment and supply shortages and reports same to charge nurse and ward clerk on a daily basis.
   b. Submits requests for new equipment and supplies to charge nurse on a quarterly basis.

5. *Type of work:* Training
   Major duty: Identifies training needs of team members and plans activities to meet needs (5 percent of working hours).
   a. Identifies specific training needs of individual team members through daily observation of their performance and interviews.
   b. Evaluates performance through use of performance standards. Makes these standards known to each team member and holds each responsible for meeting standards.

Exhibit 27–1 Performance Standards—Clinical Nurse *(Continued)*

c. Plans counseling and guidance of each team member on an individual basis and at least quarterly.

d. Plans and conducts unit in-service education programs at least monthly. Involves team members.

e. Recommends team members for seminars, short courses, college programs, and correspondence courses.

f. Thoroughly orients all new team members. Conducts skill inventory during initial interview and plans on-the-job training for those needed skills in which team member is not proficient.

g. Annually submits budget requests for training materials and programs to charge nurse.

h. Makes reading assignments and allows time for team members to use library resources.

6. *Type of work:* Planning patient care.
   Major duty: Coordinates nursing resources essential to meeting each patient's total needs and goals (5 percent of working hours).

   a. Consults with patients' physicians daily.

   b. Requests consultations of clinical nurse specialists. This may include clinical nurse specialists in pediatrics, mental health, medical/surgical, radiology, public health, and rehabilitation.

   c. Consults with other personnel as needed, including chaplain, social worker, recreation worker, occupational therapist, physical therapist, pharmacist, and inhalation therapist. Coordinates with physicians and charge nurse as needed.

   d. Supports philosophy of having ward clerks assume nonnursing activities by assisting with their training as needed on a daily basis to help them become proficient in their duties.

   e. Aggressively pursues having ward clerks do administrative tasks and nursing team members perform the primary functions of nursing. The latter most commonly occurs at patients' bedsides.

7. *Type of work:* Teaching patients
   Major duty: Teaches patients to care for themselves after discharge from the hospital (5 percent of working hours).

   a. Plans teaching as a major rehabilitation goal for each newly admitted patient. Includes it as part of nursing assessment and enters it on the nursing care plan.

   b. Daily reviews and updates teaching plans.

   c. Involves resource people in teaching program.

   d. Refers cases to visiting nurse for follow-up.

   e. Makes follow-up appointments for assessment of progress toward nursing goals with a clinical nurse.

   f. Involves families in teaching as indicated.

8. *Type of work:* Evaluation of care process
   Major duty: Conducts audits of nursing care (3 percent of working hours).

   a. Audits nursing records on a daily basis.

   b. Performs bedside audit on a weekly basis.

   c. Audits closed charts of discharged patients on a monthly basis.

   d. Reviews patient questionnaires.

   e. Discusses results of all audits with team members as a group and on an individual basis.

9. *Type of work:* Personnel administration
   Major duty: Rates performances of team members (2 percent of working hours).

   a. Writes performance reports.

   b. Discusses reports with individuals to learn their personal goals.

10. *Type of work:* Self-development
    Major duty: Pursues a program of continuing education activities (5 percent of working hours).

    a. Sets own goals for self-development, including a reading program and a set of educational goals for short courses, conventions, workshops, college courses, and management courses.

    b. Participates in division and departmental in-service education programs.

    c. Participates in nursing service committee activities.

    d. Participates in research projects.

    e. Participates as a citizen in the community through involvement in professional organizations and service projects.

    f. Assumes responsibility for knowledge of, progress in, and utilization of community resources such as

    (1) Health groups

    (2) Civic groups

    (3) General education groups

    (4) Nursing recruitment

    (5) Others

Basing performance appraisal on job analysis makes it more relevant and establishes content validity.[22] Job analysis systematically gathers information about a particular job. It "identifies, specifies, organizes, and displays the duties, tasks, and responsibilities actually performed by the incumbent in a given job."[23] It begins with identification of the domain or universe of content to be measured. The domain or universe of content may be stated in terms of the tasks to be performed, the knowledge base required, the skills or abilities needed for the work, or personal characteristics deemed necessary.[24] Exhibit 27–2 is a format for gathering data for doing a job analysis.

Recent downsizing and demassing of organizations have caused managers to plan and restructure the work of those employees remaining. This includes eliminating, simplifying, and combining steps, tasks, or jobs to make work easier and enjoyable. One goal is to get rid of stress by eliminating unneeded rules, procedures, reviews, reports, and approvals. Oryx, a Dallas-based oil and gas company, used teams to eliminate 25 percent of internal reports and reduced signatures for capital expenditures from twenty to four. It reduced the annual budget time from seven months to six weeks and saved $70 million in operating costs in one year.

Another goal is to redesign physical work by analyzing jobs using the overall process described in Exhibit 27–3. Money is saved by eliminating ineffective

Exhibit 27–2   Job Analysis Questionnaire

Title: Nurse Manager

Check here if you ever do the task in your present job:	Relative time spent	Training emphasis
_____ 1. (List DTRs)	\<Lo>\<Avg>\<Hi>	\<Lo>\<Avg>\<Hi>
_____ 2.	\<123456789	123456789

Source: Modified from E. P. Prien, I. L. Goldstein, and W. H. Macey, "Multidomain Job Analysis: Procedures and Applications," *Training and Development Journal,* copyright August 1987, pp. 68–72. American Society for Training and Development. Reprinted with permission. All rights reserved.

Exhibit 27–3   Step-by-step Process for Eliminating, Simplifying, and Combining

Step 1   Observe and understand current decision-making process.

Step 2   Document decisions by using a flow chart.

Step 3   Critically evaluate each step of the current decision-making process and any proposed changes in it.

Step 4   Implement the change.

Step 5   After sufficient time has passed, revise the decision-making steps when and as necessary.

Source: D. K. Denton, "Redesigning a Job by Simplifying Every Task and Responsibility." Reprinted from *Industrial Engineering,* August 1992, 47, 25 Technology Park/Atlanta, Norcross, GA 30092 (404) 449-0461. Copyright © 1992.

bureaucracy. Sometimes money is saved by adding employees and slowing the production process to improve quality.[25]

Job analysis leads to a job description of the work expected by the institution and to a job description that can be used for performance appraisal.

Job Descriptions

The Job Description as a Contract.   A job description is a contract that should include the job's functions and obligations and tell the incumbent to whom he or she is responsible. It is a written report outlining duties, responsibilities, and conditions of the work assignment. It is a description of a job and not of the person who happens to hold that job. "That many executives recognize the importance of obtaining good position descriptions is reflected in a survey made several years ago by the American Management Association. In this study, seventy firms reported a median fee of $20,000 paid to management consultants for preparation of their job descriptions. Most significantly, 95 percent of the respondents reported that the expenditure was 'definitely worth-while.' In two instances the fee paid for this service approached $100,000."[26] Most formats include a job title, statements of basic functions (one sentence), scope, duties, responsibilities (areas in which achievements are measured), organizational relationships (for communication), limits of authority, and criteria for performance evaluation. Job descriptions should be one to two pages in length.[27]

What Are Job Descriptions Used For?   Job descriptions are used for many purposes including the following:

1. Establishing a rational basis for the salary structure.
2. Clarifying relationships between jobs.
3. Analyzing employees' duties.
4. Defining the organizational structure.
5. Reassigning and fixing functions and responsibilities in the entire agency.
6. Evaluating job performance.
7. Orienting new employees.
8. Assisting in hiring and placement.
9. Establishing lines of promotion.
10. Identifying potential training needs.
11. Critically reviewing existing work practices.
12. Maintaining continuity of all operations.
13. Improving the work flow.
14. Providing data as to proper channels of communication.
15. Developing job specifications.
16. Serving as a basis for planning staffing levels.

Many changes in the dynamic environment of a health-care agency, such as changes in personnel, departmental or agency objectives, budget, and technology, create the necessity for periodic review and revision of job descriptions. Job descriptions should be available to all personnel so that they will know the dimensions of their jobs, who in the agency can help them in their work, how their performances will be evaluated, and the opportunities for advancement. To make the data more useful, numerical values may be assigned to the important elements of the specific duties, as in Exhibit 27–1.

To avoid bias, data for job descriptions should be gathered from several sources. Data may be collected by interviewing the job incumbent, having an incumbent keep a log of duties performed during a specific time period, observation, and a questionnaire (job analysis).

It is important to consult with all employees and allow them to discuss, comment on, and recommend changes in the job descriptions for positions. This makes development of job descriptions a cooperative venture, leading to consensus, effective management, and effective performance appraisal. Language used in the job descriptions should be simple and understandable. Job descriptions are guides, and rigid application can result in negative behavior. Job descriptions should define minimum standards for effective job performance and employment and should not be too detailed. "Performs other duties as directed" is evasive and should not be put into a job description.

A format is needed for quality and thoroughness of job descriptions. Kennedy recommends the following elements.[28]

1. Header: job title, name and location of incumbent, immediate superiors.
2. Principal purpose or summary; overall contribution of incumbent.
3. Principal responsibilities, including percentage of time spent on each.
4. Job skills: knowledge, skills, and education.
5. Dimension or scope: quantifies such areas as the budget, size of reporting organizations, impact on bottom line.
6. Organization chart.
7. Problem-solving examples.
8. Environment.
9. Key contacts.
10. References guiding incumbent's actions.
11. Supervision given and received.

Exhibit 27–4 presents a job description for a bedside nurse in a U.S. hospital in 1887. Exhibit 27–5 is a current job description for a generalized clinical nurse.

Performance Appraisal and Job Descriptions.   Tom Peters has a low opinion of job descriptions. "Performance appraisal should be ongoing, based upon a simple, written 'contract' between the person being appraised and his or her boss. Limit objectives to no more than three per period (quarter, year). Eliminate job descriptions."[29] Performance appraisal, the setting of objectives, and job descriptions are control devices. As such they are increasingly bureaucratic, run by "experts," and out of touch with the world of human relations, since they promote stability at the expense of flexibility. Most job descriptions are not read or adhered to by successful workers. The alternative is coaching and teaching values.

Exhibit 27–4   1887 Job Description

In its publication, *Bright Corridor,* Cleveland's Lutheran Hospital published this job description for a bedside nurse in a U.S. hospital in 1887.

In addition to caring for your fifty patients, each bedside nurse will follow these regulations:

1. Daily sweep and mop the floors of your ward; dust the patient's furniture and window sills.
2. Maintain an even temperature in your ward by bringing in a scuttle of coal for the day's business.
3. Light is important to observe the patient's condition. Therefore, each day fill kerosene lamps, clean chimneys, and trim wicks. Wash the windows once a week.
4. The nurse's notes are important in aiding the physician's work. Make your pens carefully; you may whittle nibs to your individual tastes.
5. Each nurse on day duty will report every day at 7:00 A.M. and leave at 8:00 P.M., except on the Sabbath, on which day you will be off from 12:00 noon to 2:00 P.M.

6. Graduate nurses in good standing with the director of nursing will be given an evening off each week for courting purposes, or two a week if you go regularly to church.
7. Each nurse should lay aside from each payday a goodly sum of [her] earnings for her benefits during her declining years, so that she will not become a burden. For example, if you earn $30 a month you should set aside $15.
8. Any nurse who smokes, uses liquor in any form, gets her hair done at a beauty shop, or frequents dance halls will give the director of nurses good reason to suspect her worth, intentions, and integrity.
9. The nurse who performs her labors, serves her patients and doctors faithfully and without fault for a period of five years will be given an increase by the hospital administration of $.05 a day, providing there are no hospital debts that are outstanding.

Job Evaluation

Job evaluation is a process used to measure exact amounts of base elements found in a job. Laws require men and women to be paid equally for equal work requiring equal skill, knowledge, effort, and responsibility under similar working conditions. This is an important factor in the fight to achieve pay equity for women and hence for nurses.[30]

The Hay system attempts to measure exact amounts of base elements found in all jobs, including (1) know-how, (2) problem solving, and (3) accountability. Know-how includes practical procedures, specialized techniques, scientific disciplines, managerial know-how, and human relations skills. Problem solving includes the thinking challenge created by the environment. Accountability includes freedom to act, input of the job on the corporation, and the magnitude of the job.[31]

Work Classification

Helton reports a system for work classification to improve white-collar work. The system includes four categories: specialist, professional, support, and clerical. Professional and specialist jobs involve a significant amount of cognitive effort, are not routine, and are challenging. Criteria used to classify white-collar work are (1) work range, (2) work structure, (3) control, and (4) cognitive effort. Applied to nursing, the MSN nurse would be a specialist, the BSN nurse

Exhibit 27–5   Position Description

Title: Generalized Clinical Nurse (GCN)

General Description. The GCN is a professional nurse with academic preparation at the BSN level or above who provides expert nursing care based upon scientific principles; delivers direct patient care and serves as a consultant or technical advisor in the area of health professions; and serves as a role model in the leadership, management, and delivery of quality nursing care by integrating the role components of clinician, administrator, teacher, consultant, and researcher.

QUALIFICATIONS

A. **Educational**
   1. Graduation from an accredited school of nursing.
   2. Bachelor of Science in Nursing degree required.

B. **Personal and professional**
   1. Current state professional nursing license.
   2. Knowledge of and experience in preventive care (screening and teaching).
   3. Demonstrated knowledge and competence in nursing, communication, and leadership skills.
   4. Ability to analyze situations, recognize problems, search for pertinent facts, and make appropriate decisions.
   5. Ability to coordinate orientation and continuing education of clinic staff utilizing appropriate teaching strategies.
   6. Ability to apply principles of change, organizational theory, and decision making.
   7. Membership and participation in professional organizations desirable.
   8. Recognition of civic responsibilities of nursing.
   9. Ability to communicate effectively both in writing and verbally.
   10. Evidence of professional manner and conduct.
   11. Optimum physical and emotional health.

Organizational Relationships. The GCN is administratively responsible and accountable to the nurse administrator. He or she is responsible for assessing, teaching, coordinating, providing appropriate care, and making referrals when necessary.

ACTIVITIES

A. **Clinician**
   1. Give direct patient care in selected patient situations and serve as a behavioral model for excellence in practice.
   2. Assist the nursing personnel in assessing individual patient needs and formulation of a plan of nursing care; write nursing orders, when appropriate, for implementation of nursing plan; assist the nursing personnel in documenting the effectiveness of the individualized care.
   3. Set, evaluate, and reevaluate standards of nursing practice; communicate these standards to the nursing personnel; change standards as necessary.
   4. Evaluate nursing care given to patients within the clinical area (assessing and teaching); when appropriate, make recommendations for improvement of that care.
   5. Function as a change agent; identify the barriers to more comprehensive health-care delivery, modify behavior, and introduce new approaches to patient care.
   6. Collaborate with other health-care providers and make appropriate referrals when necessary.

B. **Teacher**
   1. Provide an atmosphere conducive to learning.
   2. Teach appropriate prevention measures to clients.
   3. Direct the orientation of new staff and student nurses to ease their role transition and improve their skills, attitudes, and practices.
   4. Consider the needs of the adult learners (nursing personnel) as well as the clinicians' knowledge and expertise when planning continuing education to the clinical practice.
   5. Initiate or assist with the planning, presenting, and evaluating of continuing education programs for clinic staff.
   6. Guide and assist staff and nursing students as they assume the responsibility of patient teaching.

Exhibit 27–5   Position Description *(Continued)*

C. Administrator

1. Function as a change agent and appraise leadership, communication, and change processes in the organization and assist with direct strategies for change as necessary.
2. Work collaboratively with hospital personnel and other health-care providers in planning care and making referrals.
3. Make recommendations relative to improving patient care and staff and student requirements to the appropriate administrative personnel.
4. Support and interpret the clinical policies and procedures.

D. Self-Development

1. Assume responsibility for identifying own educational needs and upgrade deficit areas through independent study, seminar attendance, or requesting staff development programs.
2. Evaluate own nursing practice and instruction of others and the effect these have on the quality of patient care.

E. Consultant

1. Conduct informal conferences with nursing personnel concerning patient care of specific health problems, the problem patient, or other pertinent problems related to nursing as suggested by the staff.
2. Assist personnel to develop awareness of community agencies/resources available in planning patient care.
3. Serve as a resource person to patients and their families.

F. Researcher

1. Determine research problems related to preventive care, nursing clinics, etc.
2. Conduct research studies to upgrade independent nursing practice.
3. Demonstrate knowledge of the current research applicable to the clinical area and apply this knowledge in nursing care when appropriate.
4. Research clinical nursing problems through the development and testing of relevant theories, evaluation, and implementation of research findings for nursing practice.
5. Promote interest in reading and reviewing of current publications dealing with the delivery of preventive care to ambulatory patients.

---

a professional, the AD/Diploma/LPN nurse a support person, and aides and clerks equivalent to clerical workers.[32]

Job redesign uses job enlargement and job enrichment. Job enlargement uses horizontal loading to add tasks of equal difficulty and responsibility to jobs. Job enrichment uses vertical loading to add tasks that increase difficulty and responsibility of jobs. Both have beneficial results, including increased productivity. In thirty-two experiments involving job redesign, thirty indicated impact; the median increase in productivity was 6.4 percent. Employee satisfaction increased in twenty cases and was tied to more pay for increased work plus less supervision and more worker autonomy.

To make job redesign effective, nurse managers need to make accurate diagnosis and real job changes. They need to address technological and personnel system constraints; support autonomy; have a bureaucratic climate; have union cooperation and top management and supervising management support; have individuals ready to fill the jobs; and have contextual satisfaction with pay, supervision, promotion opportunities, and co-workers.[33] While some persons indicate that autonomy and bureaucracy are incompatible, bureaucratic activities that support professional nurses' autonomy are desirable.

TRAINING

Nurse managers should be educated to do effective performance appraisal that will maintain employees' productivity. Training will entail coverage of such subjects as motivational environment, appropriate job assignment, proper supervision, establishing job expectancies, appropriate job training, interpersonal relationships, providing feedback, coaching, counseling, interviewing, and performance appraisal methods.

Training raters makes performance appraisal work. The goal of such training is improved productivity. A training program can give nurses a conceptual understanding of performance appraisal as a management system for transmitting, reinforcing, and rewarding the behaviors desired by the organization. Raters need to know how performance appraisals will be used. Research indicates that raters have been found to vary ratings depending upon their use. Refresher training is recommended after one year. Performance appraisal training can be conducted with other management development programs.[34]

Feedback

Feedback was discussed in chapter 20. An analysis of 69 articles reporting 126 experiments in which feedback was applied indicated that feedback with goal setting and/or behavioral consequences was much more consistently effective than feedback alone. Daily and weekly feedback produced more consistent effects than monthly feedback. Also, feedback accompanied by money or fringe benefits of food and gasoline produced improvements in behavior more often than praise. Graphs were the feedback mechanism producing the highest proportion of consistent effects. The conclusion is that feedback graphically presented at least weekly along with tangible rewards yields effective work performance.[35]

Training will include providing specific feedback to raters on timeliness, completeness, rating errors, and quality and consistency of ratings. Training methods include case studies, role playing, behavioral modeling, discussion, and writing exercises that evaluate actual appraisals by relating them to job descriptions.[36]

Coaching

The appraisal rater is a leader and a coach. Coaching for job performance is similar to coaching for athletic performance. As a coach, the rater does continuous reinforcement of tasks done well and helps with other tasks. In addition, the rater uses knowledge of adult education to train the employees to accomplish assigned work, does two-way communication, and has the necessary resources to do the job.

Coaching can include observing and listening for examples of work, good or bad. The rater coach praises the good and helps improve the bad with a joint action plan. Coaching makes performance evaluation useful.[37]

Coaching is year-long evaluation and discussion of performance. It eliminates surprises. Progress discussions can be brief, regular, frank, open, and factual and can include the employee's viewpoint. In the latter instance, the rater does not try to achieve truth but tries to discuss perceptions. The coach also removes obstacles to satisfactory performance. If the consequences are not working to improve unsatisfactory performance, the coach changes them. The ultimate resort is to transfer or terminate the employee.[38]

Progressive discipline combined with performance evaluation results in compliant employees. Effective leaders are coaches who gain commitment from employees. Today's employees will put forth effort if stimulated, challenged, and recognized for their efforts. They do not want to be managed, so managers must manage, lead, and coach.

Coaching prevents discipline. The nurse manager as coach is available to observe behavior, provide feedback, and encourage employees to do their best. Coaching is done on a regular basis and is nonjudgmental. The employee believes the coach manager is supporting him or her to do better, to be successful, to excel.

The following are some characteristics of an effective manager/coach:[39]

- Listens.
- Views employee as a person.
- Cares about employee and helps with personal problems.
- Sets a good example.
- Stretches employee.
- Encourages employee.
- Helps get the work done.
- Keeps employee informed.
- Praises a job well-done, criticizes a poor job in a forthright manner.

An employee who can do the job as if his or her life depended on it, but does not, needs coaching. Coaching is personal. It is a process that involves time, interviews, observation, feedback, and help to make employees successful. The process may be repeated as necessary.

Exercise 27–1   Determine the extent to which a nurse manager exhibits coaching behavior. Apply it to yourself or have a group of peers apply it to themselves and use the results for discussion.

Counseling

Counseling can be the most productive function of supervision. Counseling interviews are for the purpose of advising and assisting an individual to grow and develop self-direction, self-discipline, and individual responsibility. The counseling interview is a helping relationship involving direct interaction between the counselor (rater) and the counselee (ratee). In a counseling interview, a personal face-to-face relationship takes place. One person helps another recognize, accept, examine, and solve a certain problem.

Nurses can use the counseling interview to offer support and to

- Help workers develop realistic pictures of themselves, their abilities, their potential, and their deficiencies.
- Explore courses of action.
- Explore sources of assistance.
- Accept incontestable limitations and learn to live with them, whether physical, emotional, or intellectual.
- Make choices and improve capabilities.

Unless they have had special training, most nurses are not qualified for in-depth, extensive counseling in areas involving personality structure or analysis of psychological or emotional conditions. Nurse managers must beware of tampering with the psyche of the worker. They should in such cases know and be able to recommend sources of help.

Although counseling interviews are conducted to promote desirable behavior, the term *counseling* should not be used synonymously with the term *reprimand*. Reprimands belong more properly in the progress and informational type of interview. One often hears a supervisor say, "I have counseled him on what will happen if he does not improve." This is *not* counseling; this is informing a worker of the consequences of certain types of behavior or performance.

Performance counseling results from observation and evaluation of performance based on job standards. Anecdotal records may be kept and will yield facts to support written ratings or reports.

When counseling employees on performance problems, the rater uses a problem-solving approach. Such an approach includes reaching agreement that a problem exists, discussing alternative solutions, agreeing on a solution, and following up on progress.[40]

Interviewing

Interviewing is covered in chapter 8. For appraisal interviews, the problem-solving approach is more effective than tell-and-see or tell-and-listen. High ratee participation produces greater rater satisfaction. The problem-solving rater has a helpful and constructive attitude, does mutual goal setting with the ratee, focuses on solutions of problems, and acts with the knowledge that high criticism does not improve behaviors.[41]

PEER RATINGS

Research has shown that an individual's peers—the people the individual works with from day to day—are a more reliable source for identifying the capacity for leadership than are the person's superiors. The armed services have found that peer nominations for leadership are significant predictors of future performance. Democratic procedures, having peers select the person to be promoted, would probably be threatening to many nurses. It has been found that peer selection differs little from selections by superiors. Occasionally, peers see a member of their group as a leader when superiors do not. Peer rating is valid if the members of the group have sufficient interaction and are reasonably stable over time. It is also valid if the position is important within the organization. Where several individuals are equally qualified for a position, peer ratings may single out the one with the highest informal leadership status.[42]

Peer rating is the professional model of appraisal used by physicians and is gaining in interest and use among professional nurses. It is advocated as part of a system to make performance appraisals more objective, the theory being that multiple ratings will give a more objective appraisal. Ratings can be obtained from multiple managers, project leaders, peers, and even patients.[43]

Peer review is a performance appraisal process among persons with similar competencies who are in active practice. These people critically review others' practice using established standards of performance.[44] Peer review is self-regulation and supports the principle of autonomy.[45] It consists of colleagues examining the goal-directed care of colleagues with standards that are specific, critical indicators of care written by the colleagues.[46]

The purposes of peer review are to measure accountability, evaluate and improve delivery of care, identify workers' strengths and weaknesses, develop new or altered policies, identify a worker's need for more knowledge (competence), increase workers' self-awareness from feedback (critical reflection), and increase professionalism.[47]

Implementation of a peer review rating or evaluation system would include the following:

1. Planning by management and clinical nurses. It may be done by a steering committee representing these categories of nurses plus those from the domains of research and education.
2. Having a shared-governance type of environment.
3. Defining the peer review process and who is a peer.
4. Setting of goals.
5. Outlining the process through consultation with management, human resource personnel, and a labor attorney. A decision is made as to who gathers the data. It can be the employee, with a clinical nurse specialist as coordinator. Decisions are also made as to when and how often the interview will be done and how the outcome will be handled.
6. Developing a tool using the job description.
7. Obtaining multiple inputs—peer reports, self-reports, and coach reports. The manager acts as coach and counselor.

The process may be developed using three distinct phases of establishing a peer review program: familiarization, utilization, and internalization.[48] These phases are outlined in Exhibit 27–6.

Exhibit 27–6   Three Phases of Peer Review

Phase I: Familiarization
Characterized by the development of trust, the talking through of the process and its related problems, and the realization that performance, not human worth, is being evaluated.

Phase II: Utilization
Marked by trial-and-error responses. Objectives are refined. Colleagues become more open with each other. The peer review process takes a sharper focus.

Phase III: Internalization
Occurs with complete actualization of the entire peer review process. Staff no longer feel threatened. Objectives are well-defined. On-site, hands-on evaluations are conducted, charts audited, and results discussed in peer review conferences. If indicated, findings are acted upon.

Source: M. E. Jacobs and J. D. Vail, "Quality Assurance: A Unit-Based Plan," *Journal of the Association of Nurse Anesthetists,* June 1986, 265–271. Reprinted with permission.

SELF-RATING

Self-rating is another method of performance appraisal that is little used. In the Fortune 1300 study, 96 percent of appraisals were done by immediate supervisors.[49] Problems with self-rating are the same as with supervisor rating, indicating the need for training of the self-rater as well as the supervisor rater.[50]

Somers and Birnbaum studied a sample of 198 staff nurses from a large urban hospital. They found "no evidence of leniency error or restriction of range in self-appraisal job performance."[51] Convergence between self and supervisory ratings was also evident and was interpreted as an effect of "halo error," a tendency to rate all employees as outstanding. Self-rating requires employees be trained in its use and a focus on core job skills to make it work.

A format for self-evaluation and peer evaluation is depicted in Appendix 27–1. The objective of the emergency medical services (EMS) unit using this format was to determine competence. Qualification for peer evaluation included the amount of time peers worked together. Results indicated the following:[52]

- Peer rated partners higher than partners rated selves in intubation, EKG recognition, ACLS, EMT-P skills, and EMT-A skills.
- Self-ratings were higher than peer ratings in communication, scene management, trauma, patient assessment, and report-rating skills, which are more subjective areas.
- Both peer evaluation and self-ratings indicated that patients who were system abusers received the lowest quality of care and that the higher the socioeconomic group, the better the care received.

Peer and supervisor ratings have been found to be relatively highly correlated; self-supervisor and self-peer ratings, only moderately correlated. In an assessment center study, peer evaluations were better predictors of subsequent job advancement than were other ratings, including self-ratings. Peer and self-ratings predicted management potential. Behavioral information was important to peer rating and self-evaluation.[53]

OTHER RATING METHODOLOGIES

Other rating methodologies are less common than supervisor ratings, peer ratings, and self-ratings. They include team evaluation consensus (TEC), behavior-anchored rating scales (BARS), and task-oriented performance evaluation system (TOPES). These methodologies measure job-related behaviors.[54]

PERFORMANCE EVALUATION PROBLEM AREAS

It is largely assumed that merit-rating systems of performance evaluation help to develop subordinates and attest to their readiness for pay increases, promotions, selected assignments, or penalties. When such systems have been scrutinized, three main problem areas have been found:[55]

1. Subordinates have not been motivated to want to change.
2. Even when people recognize a need for a change, they are unable to change.
3. Subordinates become resentful and anxious when the merit system is conscientiously implemented.

Effective Performance Appraisal

Contrast two situations in which the same job standards are applied. In the first situation, the subordinate is handed a completed rating form and is told to read it and sign it. She does so but immediately appeals to the next highest level of supervision, saying that the rating is the lowest she has received in fifteen years of work and that she has never been counseled about the fact that the quality of her performance has been slipping. Even though the situation is resolved in favor of the subordinate, this employee is no longer satisfied to work for the supervisor and has to be transferred.

In the other situation, the job standards are discussed with the subordinate before they are used. The subordinate is asked to identify those performance factors and responsibilities that are really important to the success of the unit. She is asked also to write out the goals of her job as she sees them. The goals are fully discussed between supervisor and subordinate. Progress is discussed at the request of the subordinate and at stated intervals. As a result, the subordinate is assisted in planning educational activities that she will accomplish in preparation for the career she desires.

Which of the two situations meets the criteria of an effective performance appraisal?

Weaknesses of Performance Appraisal

What are some of the weaknesses of performance appraisal? The rater is influenced by the most recent period of performance, an influence that may be positive or negative. Without objective measurements and records, raters tend to focus on the few outstanding activities that are vivid in their minds. Personal feelings can influence raters, causing positive "halo" or negative "horns" effects. In many instances, the performance is appraised without clear job definitions, job descriptions, and job standards. The employee seldom knows the yardsticks by which performance is being measured. Raters are either lenient or tough, making a great variance in value judgments. Attitudes about whether the employee deserves a pay increase influence the rater. Some managers believe that all employees are average, and they project their beliefs by rating everyone the same.[56]

Other rating errors include the following:

- *Leniency/stringency error.* The rater tends to assign extreme ratings of either poor or excellent.
- *Similar-to-me-error.* The rater rates according to how he/she views him/herself.
- *Central tendency error.* All ratings are at the middle of the scale.
- *First-impression error.* The rater views early behavior that may be good or bad and rates all subsequent behaviors similarly.

Other problems of performance appraisal include racial bias, focus on longevity, and complacency of managers. In their usual form, performance appraisals are intrinsically confrontational, emotional, judgmental, and complex. A survey of 360 managers in 190 corporations indicated that 69 percent viewed objectives as unclear; 40 percent saw some payoff, but 29 percent saw minimal benefits; 45 percent were only partially involved in setting objectives for their own performance; 81 percent indicated that regular progress reviews were not conducted; 52 percent said that guidelines for collecting performance data were haphazard or nonexistent; a scant 19 percent viewed performance appraisal as properly planned; only 37 percent viewed meetings as highly productive; and 30 percent saw no worthwhile results.[57]

The Future of Performance Appraisals

Deming advocated the abolition of performance appraisals. Performance appraisal is the deadliest of Deming's deadly diseases that stand in the way of total quality management. Performance appraisals embody a win-lose philosophy that destroys people psychologically and poisons healthy relationships. A win-win philosophy emphasizes cooperation, participation, and leadership, directed at continuous improvement of quality.[58]

Deming's system provides for three ratings for performance appraisal using process data. Using the statistic of variation, ratings will fall within the system, outside the system on the high side, or outside the system on the low side. If the rating is within the system, pay should be according to seniority. If outside the system on the high side, pay should be based on merit. If outside the system on the low side, the employee should be coached or replaced.[59]

EFFECTIVE MANAGEMENT OF PERFORMANCE APPRAISAL

How do we overcome these pitfalls or deficiencies? First, we must be aware of them. Second, we can learn the management by objectives approach and treat people as people. As a result, employees will know by what yardsticks they will be measured. The appraisal will be a joint project. It will be a helpful situation for rater and ratee. Usually, if the situation is working right, ratees will push themselves.

A complex and lengthy evaluation form has not proved effective in rating personnel. Many managers have reduced their rating system to a limited checklist and a write-up that asks for employee strengths and weaknesses, with specific examples to justify each. Many nurses will agree to the following principles for a rating system:[60]

1. The system should be simple and effective, efficient and administratively feasible.
2. The procedures and uses of the system should be understood and agreed upon by line management and the employees being rated.
3. Factors to be rated should be measurable and agreed upon by managers and subordinates.
4. Raters should understand the purpose and nature of the performance review. They should be taught to use the system; observe; write notes, including a critical incident file; organize notes and write evaluations that include examples of evidence; edit their reports; and conduct effective review interviews.
5. Raters should understand the meanings of the dimensions rated, including the dimensions' relative weights. Managers are reported to be able to distinguish among only three levels of performance: poor, satisfactory, and outstanding.
6. Criticism should promote warmth and the building of self-esteem with both the rater and the ratee.
7. The process should be organized and used to manage people on a daily basis according to their need to be coached.
8. Praise or suggestions for improvement should be done at the time of the event.
9. Standards of performance should be set and modified at the time of the event.
10. Performance standards should be valid, reliable, and fair.
11. Managers should be rewarded for good performance evaluation skills.
12. Professionally accepted procedures should be used for job analysis, developing job-related observable performance criteria, and job classifications. Fairness is ensured when processes are applied systematically and uniformly throughout the organization.
13. A fair employment posture committed to equal opportunity should be used. A conscientious and equitable appraisal system reduces lawsuits and assures fairness and confidence. Such a system should be congruent with administrative and legal guidelines.

14. Work output, not habits and traits such as loyalty, should be measured *unless* the latter are described by observed behavior examples.

15. Quality, constant innovation, and functional barrier distraction should be emphasized.

16. Appraisal should be less time-consuming through time management: daily feedback, preparation time for annual or semiannual evaluation, spread-out execution time, and group time for consultation and coordination of appraisal criteria with peers. The last provides for fairness and equity throughout the organization.

17. The number of performance categories should be small, and no forced ranking should be used. Raters should keep it simple: 10 percent to 20 percent of the total, superior (bonus × 2); 70 percent to 85 percent, satisfactory (bonus); and 5 percent to 10 percent, questionable/unsatisfactory (no bonus).

18. The form and process should be kept simple: a one- to two-page written contract drafted with subordinate and containing one to two specific annual or semiannual objectives, one to two personal/group/team growth or career-enhancement objectives, one to two objectives to improve skills, and one objective related to the team's strategic theme (such as QI). The manager should use an open-ended prose as format, do formal reviews bimonthly or more often, and be able to recall the content of every contract.

19. Performance goals should be straightforward, emphasizing the manager's desired results and considering what is important to the continuing success of the business.

20. Pay decisions should be made public. No one will be embarrassed if there is no inequity.

21. Formal appraisal should be made a small part of overall recognition that includes listening, celebrating, pay, and involvement.

22. Multiple ratings, including those of ratees' subordinates, should be used.

Exercise 27–2   With a group of peers where you work, discuss whether the performance appraisal system your employer uses is too complicated. If it is, discuss how it can be simplified and still meet accreditation and legal requirements. Are these requirements keeping the system too complicated? If so, how?

Exercise 27–3   With a group of peers where you work, discuss how the job descriptions can be modified consistent with the vision of the organization. The goal is to make job descriptions objective and usable.

WEB ACTIVITIES

- Visit www.jbpub.com/swansburg, this text's companion website on the Internet, for further information on Appraising Performance.
- What sites would you recommend for learning more about appraisal performance methods?
- Explore the Internet to locate various discussion areas on the practice of performance appraisals.

SUMMARY

Performance appraisal is a major component of the evaluating or controlling function of nursing management. It is disliked by both raters and ratees. If used appropriately and conscientiously, the performance appraisal process will govern employee behavior to produce goods and services in high volume and of high quality.

Purposes or uses of performance evaluation are multiple. In nursing, performance evaluation is used to motivate employees to produce high-quality patient care. The results of performance appraisal are often used for promotion, selection, and termination and to improve performance.

Performance appraisal is a part of the science of behavioral technology and should be viewed as part of that body of knowledge that relates to the management of human behavior. Nurse managers need this knowledge to manage the clinical nurse effectively and efficiently as a human resource.

Performance appraisal should be done as a system with

1. Clearly defined performance standards developed by rater and ratee.
2. Objective application of the performance standards—with both rater and ratee measuring the latter's performance against the standards.
3. Planned interval feedback with agreed-upon improvements when indicated.
4. A continuous cycle. (Raters and ratees should trust each other.)

Job analysis and job description are essential instruments of behavior technology used in performance appraisal. They provide objectivity and discriminate among jobs.

Coaching, counseling, and interviewing are skills of an effective performance appraisal system. Performance appraisal can include supervisor ratings, peer ratings, and self-ratings, among others.

Problems with performance appraisal systems include poor preparation of raters and ratees, problems of recency, halo and horns effects, lack of use of standards, leniency/stringency errors, similar-to-me errors, central tendency errors, and first-impression errors.

A simple, well-planned performance appraisal system can be devised. It will be successful when understood by employees and will require considerable supervisory effort using nursing management theory.

NOTES

1. S. Krantz, "Five Steps to Making Performance Appraisal Writing . . .," *Supervisory Management,* December 1983, 7–10.
2. R. Zemke, "Is Performance Appraisal a Paper Tiger?" *Training,* December 1985, 24–32.
3. S. Krantz, op. cit.
4. C. J. Fombrun and R. L. Land, "Strategic Issues in Performance Appraisal: Theory and Practice," *Personnel,* November–December 1983, 23–31.
5. B. P. Moroney and M. R. Buckley, "Does Research in Performance Appraisal Influence the Practice of Performance Appraisal?: Regretfully Not!" *Public Personnel Management,* summer 1992, 185–195.
6. R. D. Bretz, G. T. Milkovich, and W. Read, "The Current State of Performance Appraisal Research and Practice: Concerns, Directions and Implications," *Journal of Management,* June 1992, 321–352.
7. C. J. Fombrun and R. L. Land, op. cit.
8. C. E. Schneier, A. Geis, and J. A. Wert, "Performance Appraisals: No Appointment Needed," *Personnel Journal,* November 1987, 80–87.
9. R. Zemke, op. cit.; R. D. Moen, "The Performance Appraisal System: Deming's Deadly Disease," *Quality Progress,* November 1989, 62–66.
10. A. Levenstein, "Feedback Improves Performance," *Nursing Management,* February 1984, 65–66.
11. R. Zemke, op. cit.
12. D. L. Kirkpatrick, "Performance Appraisal: When Two Jobs Are Too Many," *Training,* March 1986, 65, 67–69.
13. Ibid.
14. R. E. Kopelman, "Linking Pay to Performance Is a Proven Management Tool," *Personnel Administrator,* October 1983, 60–68.
15. Ibid.
16. Ibid.
17. N. R. Deets and D. T. Tyler, "How Xerox Improved Its Performance Appraisals," *Personnel Journal,* April 1986, 50–52.
18. D. C. Mosley, P. H. Pietri, and L. C. Megginson, *Management: Leadership in Action* (New York: HarperCollins, 1996), 497–500.
19. B. Blai, "An Appraisal System That Yields Results," *Supervisory Management,* November 1983, 39–42.
20. M. G. Friedman, "10 Steps to Objective Appraisals," *Personnel Journal,* June 1986, 66–71.
21. M. R. Edwards and J. R. Sproull, "Safeguarding Your Employee Rating System," *Business,* April–June 1985, 17–27.
22. S. Price and J. Graber, "Employee-Made Appraisals," *Management World,* February 1986, 34–36.
23. D. Ignatavicius and J. Griffith, "Job Analysis: The Basis for Effective Appraisal," *Journal of Nursing Administration,* July–August 1982, 37–41.

24. J. Dienemann and C. Shaffer, "Faculty Performance Appraisal Systems: Procedures and Criteria," *Journal of Professional Nursing,* May–June 1992, 148–154.

25. D. K. Denton, "Redesigning a Job by Simplifying Every Task and Responsibility," *Industrial Engineering,* August 1992, 46–48.

26. C. Berenson and H. O. Ruhnke, "Job Descriptions: Guidelines for Personnel Management," *Personnel Journal,* January 1966, 14–19.

27. P. R. Webb and R. J. Cantone, "Performance Evaluation: Triumph or Torture?" *Journal of Home Health Care Practice,* February 1993, 14–19.

28. W. R. Kennedy, "Train Managers to Write Winning Job Descriptions," *Training and Development Journal,* April 1987, 62–64.

29. T. Peters, *Thriving on Chaos* (New York: Harper & Row, 1987), 596–597.

30. A. Waintroob, "Comparable Worth Issue: The Employer's Side," *The Hospital Manager,* July–August 1985, 6–7.

31. TNA's Professional Services Committee, "Nurses and the Comparable Worth Concept," *Texas Nursing,* April 1985, 12–16; "How to Establish the Comparable Worth of a Job—Or One Way to Compare Apples and Oranges," *California Nurse,* March/April 1982, 10–11.

32. B. R. Helton, "Will the Real Knowledge Worker Please Stand Up?" *Industrial Management,* January–February 1987, 26–29.

33. R. G. Kopelman, "Job Redesign and Productivity: A Review of the Evidence," *National Productivity Review,* summer 1985, 237–255.

34. D. C. Martin and K. M. Bardol, "Training the Raters: A Key to Effective Performance Appraisal," *Public Personnel Management,* summer 1986, 101–109.

35. F. Balcazar, B. L. Hopkin, and Y. Suarez, "A Critical, Objective Review of Performance Feedback," *Journal of Organizational Behavior Management,* fall 1985/winter 1985–86, 65–89.

36. D. C. Martin and K. M. Bardol, op. cit.; M. G. Friedman, op. cit.

37. C. E. Schneier, A. Geis, and J. A. Wert, op. cit.

38. V. D. Lachman, "Increasing Productivity Through Performance Evaluation," *Journal of Nursing Administration,* December 1984, 7–14.

39. L. P. Frankel and K. L. Ofuzo, "Employee Coaching: The Way to Gain Compliance," *Employment Relations Today,* autumn 1992, 311–320.

40. V. D. Lachman, op. cit.

41. D. C. Martin and C. M. Bardol, op. cit.

42. G. S. Booker and R. W. Miller, "A Closer Look at Peer Ratings," *Personnel,* January–February 1966, 42–47.

43. M. G. Friedman, op. cit.

44. J. Jambunathan, "Planning a Peer Review Program," *Journal of Nursing Staff Development,* September/October 1992, 235–239.

45. J. B. Jurf, L. Ecoff, W. Haley, P. L. Keegan, and P. A. Williams, "First Steps Toward Peer Review," *Journal of Nursing Staff Development,* July/August 1992, 184–186.

46. M. E. Jacobs and J. D. Vail, "Quality Assurance: A Unit-Based Plan," *Journal of the Association of Nurse Anesthetists,* June 1986, 265–271.

47. Ibid; J. Jambunathan, op. cit.

48. M. E. Jacobs and J. D. Vail, op. cit; J. B. Jurf, L. Ecoff, W. Haley, P. L. Keegan, and P. A. Williams, op. cit.; J. Jambunathan, op. cit.

49. C. J. Fombrun and R. L. Land, op. cit.

50. R. Zemke, op. cit.

51. M. J. Somers and D. Birnbaum, "Assessing Self-Appraisal of Job Performance as an Evaluation Device: Are the Poor Results a Function of Method or Methodology?" *Human Relations,* October 1991, 1081–1091.

52. J. Ballinger and J. Ferko III, "Peer Evaluations," *Emergency,* April 1989, 28–31.

53. I. H. Shore, L. H. Shole, and G. C. Thornton III, "Construct Validity of Self-and Peer Evaluation of Performance Dimensions in an Assessment Center," *Journal of Applied Psychology,* February 1992, 42–54.

54. M. R. Edwards and J. R. Sproull, op. cit.; R. Zemke, op. cit.; S. C. Bushardt and A. R. Fowler, Jr., "Performance Evaluation Alternatives," *Journal of Nursing Administration,* October 1988, 40–44.

55. W. M. Fox, "Evaluating and Developing Subordinates," *Notes and Quotes,* April 1969, 4.

56. J. C. Coyant, "The Performance Appraisal: A Critique and an Alternative," *Business Horizons,* June 1973, 73–78.

57. R. E. Lofton, "Performance Appraisal: Why They Go Wrong and How to Do Them Right," *National Productivity Review,* winter 1985, 54–63.

58. R. D. Moen, op. cit.

59. L. E. Mainstone and A. S. Levi, "Fundamentals of Statistical Process Control," *Journal of Organizational Behavior Management* 9, no. 1 (1987): 5–21.

60. S. Krantz, op. cit; D. C. Martin and K. M. Bardol, op. cit.; C. Logan, "Praise: The Powerhouse of Self-Esteem," *Nursing Management,* June 1985, 36, 38; M. G. Friedman, op. cit.; C. E. Schneier, J. A. Geis, and J. A. Wert, op. cit.; M. R. Edwards and J. R. Sproull, op. cit.; E. Y. Breeze, "The Performance Review," *Manage,* May 1968, 6–11; J. Dienemann and C. Shaffer, op. cit.; T. Peters, op. cit.

Confidential (Nondepartmental) Self-Evaluation

Name _____ Age _____ Sex _____

Time of EMT-P Certification: _____ years _____ months

A B C D F	Knowledge		A B C D F
□ □ □ □ □	EMT-A Knowledge	ACLS Knowledge	□ □ □ □ □
□ □ □ □ □	EMT-P Knowledge	Trauma Knowledge	□ □ □ □ □

A B C D F	Skill Competency		A B C D F
□ □ □ □ □	EMT-A Skill Competency	EKG Recognition	□ □ □ □ □
□ □ □ □ □	EMT-P Skill Competency	Intubation Competency	□ □ □ □ □
□ □ □ □ □	ACLS Skill Competency	Trauma Skill Competency	□ □ □ □ □
□ □ □ □ □	Report Writing	Scene Management Skills	□ □ □ □ □
□ □ □ □ □	Patient Assessment Skills	Communication Skills	□ □ □ □ □

A B C D F	Quality of Care When Encountering . . .		A B C D F
□ □ □ □ □	Lower Socioeconomic Groups	Intoxicated Patients	□ □ □ □ □
□ □ □ □ □	Higher Socioeconomic Groups	System Abusers	□ □ □ □ □
□ □ □ □ □	Patients of Different Race	Homosexual Patients	□ □ □ □ □
□ □ □ □ □	Drug Abusers		

A B C D F	Other		A B C D F
□ □ □ □ □	Fair Treatment of Partner	Motivation Level	□ □ □ □ □
□ □ □ □ □	Ability to Relate to Patients	Compassion for Patients	□ □ □ □ □
□ □ □ □ □	Decision-Making Under Overwhelming Conditions		
□ □ □ □ □	Stress Management Skills/Emotional Stability		
□ □ □ □ □	Overall Quality of Patient Care		

Confidential (Nondepartmental) Evaluation of Colleague

Colleague Evaluated: _____ His/Her Sex _____ Age _____

Approximate Time of Colleague's EMT-P Certification: _____ years _____ months

Number of Shifts Worked With Colleague (last six months): _____

Time of Your EMT-P Certification: _____years _____ months   Your Sex _____ Age _____

A B C D F	Knowledge		A B C D F
□ □ □ □ □	EMT-A Knowledge	ACLS Knowledge	□ □ □ □ □
□ □ □ □ □	EMT-P Knowledge	Trauma Knowledge	□ □ □ □ □

A B C D F	Skill Competency		A B C D F
□ □ □ □ □	EMT-A Skill Competency	EKG Recognition	□ □ □ □ □
□ □ □ □ □	EMT-P Skill Competency	Intubation Competency	□ □ □ □ □
□ □ □ □ □	ACLS Skill Competency	Trauma Skill Competency	□ □ □ □ □
□ □ □ □ □	Report Writing	Scene Management Skills	□ □ □ □ □
□ □ □ □ □	Patient Assessment Skills	Communication Skills	□ □ □ □ □

A B C D F	Quality of Care When Encountering . . .		A B C D F
□ □ □ □ □	Lower Socioeconomic Groups	Intoxicated Patients	□ □ □ □ □
□ □ □ □ □	Higher Socioeconomic Groups	System Abusers	□ □ □ □ □
□ □ □ □ □	Patients of Different Race	Homosexual Patients	□ □ □ □ □
□ □ □ □ □	Drug Abusers		

A B C D F	Other		A B C D F
□ □ □ □ □	Fair Treatment of Partner	Motivation Level	□ □ □ □ □
□ □ □ □ □	Ability to Relate to Patients	Compassion for Patients	□ □ □ □ □
□ □ □ □ □	Decision-Making Under Overwhelming Conditions		
□ □ □ □ □	Stress Management Skills/Emotional Stability		
□ □ □ □ □	Overall Quality of Patient Care		

Source: J. Ballinger and J. Ferko, III, "Peer Evaluation," *Emergency,* April 1989, 31. Reprinted with permission of *Emergency.* To become a regular subscriber to *Emergency,* phone 1-800-854-6449.

PAY FOR PERFORMANCE

"If you want more, then work more."

John A. Parnell[1]

OBJECTIVES

- Distinguish among the major types of pay for performance.
- Identify the criteria being used in a pay-for-performance plan.
- Discuss the design of a pay-for-performance plan.

KEY CONCEPTS

Pay for performance
Individual plan
Group plan
Merit pay

Manager behavior: Directs how a pay-for-performance program will be administered.

Leader behavior: Solicits input from employee representatives before directing how pay-for-performance programs will be administered.

Pay for performance is based upon equity theory, expectancy theory, the law of effect, and psychological fulfillment. Equity theory indicates that people want to be treated equally and fairly by employers. Expectancy theory says that people believe they can achieve certain levels of performance and, if they do, they expect to be rewarded. The law of effect states that behavior will be rewarded when repeated. Equity theory, expectancy theory, and the law of effect, individually or combined, apply when the employee says, "I believe that when I increase my efforts or inputs to produce sustained greater outputs, my employer will increase my rewards." Increased pay that is linked as a reward to increased employee inputs and outputs is termed *pay for performance.* If used effectively, the compensation system should reward superior, excellent, and satisfactory performance. People perceive an imbalance in this theory when they put forth greater effort than others but receive the same rewards. They perceive compensation to be inequitable, and pay becomes a dissatisfier.[2] Pay for performance is an incentive program that links pay to employee or corporate performance.[3]

Performance, not longevity, is fast becoming the basis for pay increases in institutions of all sizes. This may apply only to the managerial staff, or it can apply down to the lowest-paid employees in an organization.[4]

Since the recession of 1982, pay for performance has become the mode for pay increases in business and industry. Of 1,080 Canadian companies surveyed in 1990, 64 percent indicated they would use a merit-only pay increase in 1991. Thirty-two percent would use a general-plus-merit system for pay increases.[5] A 1990 survey of 250 manufacturers indicated 76 percent had incentive-based programs.[6] A 1993 survey of 2,000 U.S. companies indicated 68 percent of this sample did pay for performance.[7]

EXPECTED OUTCOMES

Expectancy theory postulates that individuals will choose among alternatives in a rational manner to maximize expected rewards. A study designed to test subjects' choice of a pay plan from among piece rate, fixed rate, and bonus concluded the following:[8]

- Pay choice has a strong impact on subjects' behavior.
- High-ability individuals choose a piece-rate plan or a bonus plan over a fixed-rate plan.
- Individuals tend to choose a pay plan that maximizes their expected rewards.
- Pay choice results in higher pay satisfaction.

Studies of managers and administrators show a positive relationship between pay-for-performance perception and pay satisfaction. Also, pay higher than the outside market gives greater employee satisfaction. Pay system fairness is a function of factors that pertain to organizational justice, such as participation in pay system development, perceived fairness of allocation procedures, and greater understanding of the pay system.[9]

A company's ability to compete and its employee relations are improved by creatively managed compensation systems. Performance-based pay affects profitability, with profits increasing when high or good performance is rewarded with pay incentives. Variable pay affects profitability more than base pay.[10]

There may be a limit to the ratio of pay for performance. A study of seventy-five college students that related performance to 0 percent, 10 percent, 30 percent, 60 percent, or 100 percent of base pay as incentives indicated that while 0 percent produced no significant incentive, the productivity of subjects in the 10, 30, 60, and 100 percent incentive groups did not differ. They all produced significant incentive.[11]

Compensation is a part of business strategy. A direct link exists between compensation and achievement of established goals. Increased compensation is an incentive for employees to do well. An employee will work to achieve predetermined goals if there are predetermined rewards.[12]

The following are some reasons for basing pay on performance:[13]

1. Performance-based pay increases job satisfaction. Subordinates who are involved in developing a work plan feel ownership of the process, and as a result they will work harder to make their plan successful.
2. Performance-based pay reduces absenteeism.
3. Performance-based pay increases productivity. Workers will perform clearly identified behaviors that are rewarded. (Mediocrity should not be rewarded.)

4. Performance-based pay decreases voluntary turnover, which says, "I believe I am worth more. Other employers will pay me more."

5. Performance-based pay improves the quality of the employee mix. It attracts and keeps higher-level performers.

A study of 984 engineering employees of two large U.S. high-technology companies offering pay incentive awards confirmed that "extremely high and moderately low performers are likely to remain in firms offering [pay incentive] contracts while moderately high and extremely low performers are likely to depart."[14] The contracts with these companies aggressively rewarded extreme performance and largely ignored moderate performance limits. To correct this, the employer can design a system to retain above-average performers and reduce turnover to only the extremely low performers.

Pay for performance rewards what is valued by the employer. This may be time-in-grade and longevity, but in a competitive business environment, employers are more apt to value new job skills and new knowledge by paying more for performance that demonstrates their use than for longevity.[15]

Exhibit 28–1   Major Types of Pay for Performance (Compensation) Programs

Type	Characteristics
Merit pay	Probably most common. Usually a percentage of base pay. Sometimes part of a pay raise—a percentage for merit and a percentage for longevity. Pay raises are established for each job or group of jobs. Progression at fixed intervals based on observation of performance. Standards of employees' success are not established a priori. When given as merit pay, a bonus is not added to base pay. An individual incentive plan.
Gain sharing	A profit-sharing plan, usually a group incentive plan. A specific share of the organization's profits is distributed to a group of employees based on production measures, financial performance, and quality of service. (See also chapter 16, "Decentralization and Participatory Management.")
Cash or lump-sum bonuses	Usually a share of the profits. Also a group incentive. May be a uniform bonus paid to all or most employees organizationwide.
Pay for knowledge	Pay is linked to learning new skills and being able to work at a higher level or at more than one specialty.
Employee stock ownership plans (ESOPs)	Profit-sharing plan. Some pay cash from interest and dividends. Most are deferred plans. See Chapter 15, "Decentralization and Participatory Management." Risky link between pay and performance for these plans. The direct pay contingency is typically quite small and linked to company performance.
Individual incentive	Compensation is paid for individual performance.
Small group incentive	Each member of a group is compensated for achieving predetermined objectives.
Instant incentive	Individual compensation for noteworthy achievements.
Recognition programs	Performance awards to individuals or groups. May be money, education programs, vacation/travel, certificates, or other symbolic award.

TYPES OF COMPENSATION PROGRAMS

Exhibit 28–1 lists the major types of compensation programs.[16]

PAY-FOR-PERFORMANCE PROCESS

The following are elements of a pay-for-performance process:[17]

1. Compensation should be part of the strategic planning process. When done with employees or their representatives as part of a task force, the compensation plan is more apt to be perceived as fair and to elicit their trust. Company mission, philosophy, objectives, vision, values, and business plans can be a guide to developing a compensation plan. Decisions are made on how to link compensation to employee and/or company performance, and hence to individuals versus groups. It is best to use more than one kind of incentive. The plan should be customized to the organizational culture and to the core values of a pay system. An obvious link exists between effort and performance, and reward. The organization should consider the need for change and the level(s) of organizational participation. It should assess the current compensation system for gaps, holes, and overfunding and then assign potential plan types to close the gaps.

2. Goals should be carefully set. They should be achievable to avoid system errors. When goals are set with employees, employees assume ownership of the goals. Organizational performance goals may relate to improving employee motivation, engendering a culture of employees who genuinely care about organizational effectiveness, and tying labor costs to the organization's ability to pay specific amounts. Goals should be made job-specific. Exhibits 28–2 and 28–3 give examples of criteria for establishing a pay-for-performance plan and policy.

3. Standards for measurement should be precise, since they are the benchmarks against which performance is met. The standards should be able to be influenced by participants. They may include the following:

   ■ Quality standards related to TQM or CQI for eliminating defects or errors.
   ■ Safety standards related to all customers, internal and external.
   ■ Attendance standards such as pay for unused sick time or paid days off.
   ■ Productivity standards related to volume of inputs versus outputs.
   ■ A pay-for performance matrix (see Exhibit 28–4).
   ■ Job descriptions that include specific objectives of each position and measure the accomplishments of those objectives. Job descriptions can be developed with input from incumbents. When job descriptions are related to pay for knowledge, new technology may require help from experts and outside vendors. End results of these job descriptions include such items as "trained and motivated crew" and "safety." Each end result has one to three or four measures of

Exhibit 28–2   Criteria Established for the Pay-for-Performance Plan

- The plan must create or better establish a link between pay and plant and division performance (performance should be a factor in considering appropriate wage adjustments).
- The plan must provide a fair and equitable method of compensation or rewards to attract, retain, and motivate good employees.
- The plan should be based on criteria that allow employees to contribute to and have an impact on the organization's objectives.
- Costs of the plan must be consistent with the financial state of the business.
- The plan should be consistent with plant and division objectives.

- The plan must fit the culture of the organization.
- The plan should provide a stable level of compensation to foster commitment among participants.
- The plan should involve a high level of communication and employee participation.

Source: Reprinted by permission of publisher from J. P. Guthrie and E. P. Cunningham, "Pay for Performance for Hourly Workers: The Quaker Oats Alternative," *Compensation & Benefits Review,* March/April © 1992, 20, American Management Association, New York. All rights reserved.

Exhibit 28–3   The Pay-for-Performance Policy

- If wages are more than 5 percent greater than the market average, then the annual hourly wage adjustment will be a lump sum determined by the performance matrix (0–6.5 percent cash bonus of last 12 months' wages).
- If wages are less than 5 percent greater than the market average, then an across-the-board annual adjustment, determined by the performance matrix,

will be given. It is, however, our policy to keep wages at 5 percent above the market average.

Source: Reprinted by permission of publisher from J. P. Guthrie and E. P. Cunningham, "Pay for Performance for Hourly Workers: The Quaker Oats Alternative," *Compensation & Benefits Review,* March/April © 1992, 20, American Management Association, New York. All rights reserved.

accomplishment, such as "responsiveness to customer's needs" and "number of machine breakdowns." Preparation to meet pay for knowledge includes massive training efforts that may be done in cooperation with vendors, consultants, and educational institutions. An extensive set of training modules can be developed so that training is directly related to the job descriptions.

- Organizational performance—profitability, financial performance.
- Management by objectives.
- Critical incidents: innovation, new products and services, market penetration, and targets.
- Economic value added (EVA). Some companies are awarding bonuses and stock options to managers on the basis of economic value added. EVA, which is a way of increasing a company's real profitability, equals the operating profits minus taxes minus the total annual cost of capital. The cost of capital includes interest paid on

Exhibit 28–4   Summary of Pay-for-Performance Matrix

1. Financial (0–2% possible payout)
   a. Raw materials
      Meet (lower) target rate = .5% payout
      Meet (higher) target rate = 1% payout
   b. Conversion
      Meet (lower) target rate = .5% payout
      Meet (higher) target rate = 1% payout
2. Safety (0–1% possible payout)
   Safety goals:
   a. OSHA incidence rate (target rate)
   b. Days away severity rate (target rate)
   c. Lost workdays case incidence rate (target rate)
      Achieve two of three safety rates = .5% payout
      Achieve all three safety rates = 1% payout
3. Quality (0–1% possible payout)
   a. Comply with target specifications = .5% payout
   b. Meet reduction target in plant controllable complaints = .5% payout

4. Sanitation (0–1% possible payout)
   a. Make an excellent rating on corporate audits = .5% payout
   b. Quality assurance audits meet absolute/variance standards = .5% payout
5. Focus (0–1% possible payout)
   a. This will change from year to year to reflect an area of special emphasis during the upcoming pay-for-performance cycle
6. Division performance (0–5% possible payout)
   a. Division meets operating income goal = .5% payout

Source: Reprinted by permission of publisher from J. P. Guthrie and E. P. Cunningham, "Pay for Performance for Hourly Workers: The Quaker Oats Alternative," *Compensation & Benefits Review,* March/April © 1992, 22, American Management Association, New York. All rights reserved.

borrowed capital (less deductible tax) plus equity capital, the money provided by the shareholders. Equity includes investment in human capital. A positive EVA means wealth is being created, while a negative EVA means that capital is being destroyed. EVA can be used for service businesses. It can be raised by using less capital and giving shareholders higher dividends. Stock prices go up!

- Cooperation among individuals or groups.
- Specific competencies, such as ability to communicate, customer focus, dealing with change, interpersonal skills, team relationships, leadership.
- Cultural diversity.

4. An objective performance appraisal system needs to be established that measures the achievement of the standards as employee outputs. The following are some examples:
   - Completion of specific education and training programs.
   - Absence or reduction (including prevention) of accidents, injuries, and illnesses and measurable reduced pollution.
   - Specific problems solved.
   - Reduced supply inventories and supply use.
   - Reduced patient stays.
   - Increased responsibility.
   - Reduced costs.
   - Demonstrated mastery of knowledge, skills, and abilities.

   Supervisors should be trained to use the performance appraisal system effectively. The system must be objective. Some companies separate performance appraisals from salary reviews. They focus on career development—improvement, job skills, career growth—during performance appraisals. During the salary review, the focus is on worth—objectives, potential to learn new skills.

Performance standards should not be confused with results or accomplishments. If cultural diversity is a standard and it is measured and rewarded, it will be accomplished.

5. A plan needs to be decided upon (refer to Exhibit 28–1). The structure of the plan should be tailored to the performance dimensions of the job.
6. Needed policies and procedures for implementing the plan must be written and communicated to the participants. All employees need to understand the system, what it is, and how it works. Exhibit 28–5 suggests guidelines for performance-based salary increases.
7. The plan is then implemented and monitored.
8. The effectiveness of the plan is evaluated.

Exhibit 28–6 summarizes the process for designing a pay-for-performance plan.

GROUP VERSUS INDIVIDUAL INCENTIVE PLANS

Group Plans

Group incentive plans include small groups or work units where rewards are allocated for group performance exceeding predefined standards, productivity improvement plans, and profit-sharing plans. These plans are designed to encourage teamwork and cooperation with shared profits, information, responsibility, accountability, and participation in decision making.

Group variable pay is used for meeting goals based on collaborative performance and teamwork. It encourages communication. Quality can become a team sport and a win-win affair. Group variable pay is flexible and can respond to multiple goals and measures and to change. Group variable pay should be funded independently of other pay plans.[18]

Exhibit 28–5   Guidelines for Performance-Based Salary Increases

Appraisal Factor	Weight	Salary Increase
Unsatisfactory	0–20 points	0%
Satisfactory	21–41 points	3%
Excellent	42–62 points	5%
Superior	63+ points	7%

Source: J. T. Browdy, "Performance Appraisal and Pay for Performance Start at the Top," *Health Care Supervisor,* April 1989, 31–41. Reprinted with permission.

Exhibit 28–6   Designing a Pay-for-Performance Plan

The following principles, objectives, and design standards provide a framework; each organization can tailor the specific pay-for-performance programs that are compatible with its environment.

Overall Principles
Pay-for-performance programs should

- Be designed to ensure that each unit's programs meet overall corporate policies, thereby supporting the overall philosophy and intentions of the firm.
- Offer decentralized units within the firm the operational flexibility to strengthen pay for performance in ways that take into account their unique circumstances while simultaneously adhering to corporate personnel policies and strategy.

All pay-for-performance programs must

- Adhere to the philosophy of a meritocracy.
- Ensure fair employee/labor relations.
- Improve the firm's quality of services and operations.

- Support corporate personnel strategies and philosophy.
- Be consistent with and supported by the appropriate corporate compensation system.
- Be cost effective/affordable.
- Maintain/enhance the reputation and legitimacy of the firm.

Specific Program Objectives
Each unit's pay-for-performance program must be designed to

- Help improve the unit's quality of services and performance.
- Sharpen employees' focus on unit purposes and results.
- Contain costs/enhance affordability.
- Support fair labor/employee relations.
- Take advantage of the unit's unique features.
- Adhere to and be consistent with corporate personnel policies.

Program Design Standards
To ensure a technically sound design, companies should follow these design standards:

Objective(s)	Make objectives specific yet flexible.
Measures	Specify appraisals, measures, and results to measure objectives.
Eligibility	Specify which employees are eligible, which are not, rationales, etc.
Funding	Examine how the plan will be funded and its effects on labor costs.
Data sources	Detail information systems that exist or need to be developed to support measurements.
Labor/Employee relations	Specify how employees and/or their units will participate in the plan.
Payouts	Specify the nature of payouts, timing, etc.
Simulation of scenarios	Give a detailed analysis of payouts/nonpayouts and anticipated effects under various conditions.
Modifications/Termination	Consider how the program will or can be adapted and/or terminated as conditions change.
Dispute-resolution procedures	Specify how issues will be handled.
Communications/Expectations management	Consider how employees and managers will understand and react to the plan; anticipate effects on employee satisfaction. Communicate how participants can influence achievement.
Administration	Consider ease of administration and administrative roles and responsibilities.
Fit with total compensation	Keep in mind that pay-for-performance programs are part of a total compensation approach. Ensure that these programs are not conceived in isolation from rest of the firm's pay system.
Evaluation of effects	Detail how the effects of plan on the unit's mission will be evaluated.
Measurements	Ensure that these are known and understood by participants. Make them as simple as possible. Ensure that documentation enables examination or audit.

Source: Reprinted by permission of publisher from G. Milkovich and C. Milkovich, "Strengthening the Pay-For-Performance Relationship: The Research," *Compensation & Benefits Review,* November/December © 1992, 61, American Management Association, New York. All rights reserved.

Increasingly, teams, not individuals, are being rewarded for good work, resulting in innovation, better cost control, and better morale. Team leaders or managers set up worthwhile goals that are easy to measure. Everyone—from plant manager on down—gets the same annual raise for achieving or exceeding goals. The percentage of pay is set by goals that may be divided between those of the unit and organizational goals. Employees are involved in designing team-based incentive programs. A trusting work relationship is needed. Some companies have teams of twenty-five to fifty employees who supervise themselves and have no time clock and no foreperson. After a three-month probation, teams take over evaluation. If performance is below standards, the team recommends improvement programs, probation, or termination. The team helps hire new employees. Team members identify free-riders, or lay-abouts.[19]

Individual Plans

Individual merit pay can create internal competition for pay raises and the withholding of information from each other by competing employees. It encourages individuals to try to improve the system on their own, a difficult task to accomplish. Individual merit pay also uses individual quality outcome measures, which are difficult to develop meaningfully. It encourages a microfocus, decreases flexibility, and becomes an anxiety producer.[20]

Stars are best rewarded individually with career development, promotional tracking, and distinguished service awards. Be sure their performance is not distractive if they achieve at the expense of others.[21]

Competency Model

Individual accomplishments are temporary and variable, whereas competencies and salaries are additive over time. Competency reflects individual performance; accomplishments can result from both individual and group efforts. A value-added pay system combines base salary to employee competency and rewards individual or team accomplishment with one-time lump-sum awards. Employees are paid and rewarded for actual accomplishments, and fixed payroll costs are reduced. As employees move through competency levels, the salaries are planned to reflect this. Thus, employees are paid what they are worth to the organization. Those who exceed goals accomplish beyond expectation and add value to the position they fill. The value-added compensation approach is motivational while it controls costs.[22]

Benner's research, using the Dreyfuss Model of Skills Acquisition, could be used as the competency model for a pay-for-performance system. Base pay would mirror the five levels of proficiency: novice, advanced beginner, competent, proficient, and expert. A nurse who bettered the time line for achieving a higher level of proficiency could be paid a lump-sum bonus for the accomplishment.[23] Exhibit 28–7 is a simplified pay-for-competency plan.

Exhibit 28–7   Simplified Pay-for-Competency Plan

	Performance Criteria*					
	Common Skills	Primary Craft Skills	Blended Craft Skills	Process Equipment Skills	Leadership & Team Skills	Wages
Skill block III	[1]	[1]	40%	100%	100%	$ _____
Skill block II	[1]	100%	20%	66%	66%	$ _____
Skill block I	100%	50%	0	33%	33%	$ _____
Entry level	Specific skills, experiences, and/or aptitudes and abilities required to enter					

Notes
* Participant must demonstrate the required skills (performance criteria) in each category of the skill block prior to moving into the next skill block.
[1] Continued proficiency in previously demonstrated skills.
% Percent of total skills listed in the category.

Source: R. M. Williamson, "Reward What You Value and Reach New Maintenance Levels." Reprinted from *Plant Engineering,* 12 August 1992, 118, with permission of Reed Publishing USA, © 1992.

Peer Review

The subjectivity of pay for performance can be partially eliminated by peer review. At one Motorola plant, employees are working on peer review for pay. In the early stages, peer review represented 20 percent of annual pay, with a goal of 50 percent. Employees vote on one another's performance. This puts enormous pressure on fellow workers to perform better. Under the Motorola pay system, all factory workers reach a maximum base pay after thirty-nine weeks on the job. The rest of their pay is based on the individual's performance.[24]

PAY DESIGNS

Many employees are willing to risk fat bonuses for superb results. The risk is that bonuses go down with recession. Bonuses hold down fixed costs, while merit raises increase them, driving up retirement benefits.[25]

A study by Schwab and Olson produced the following findings:

Conventional merit systems achieve a considerably better link between pay and performance than does a bonus system with periodic adjustments in base wages. A bonus system without periodic adjustments in base wages also performs less well than conventional merit systems, because merit systems benefit from the consistency of true performance over time. One surprising finding is that even very substantial error in the measurement of performance has only a modest effect on the pay performance correlation.[26]

Rewards should be consistent, fair, and timely and should relate to work. They should also be ample.[27] In a pay-for-performance system, the outcomes include increased productivity from "overpaid" performers and rewards for underpaid performers.[28]

Money to fund some programs has come from senior managers who gave up their bonuses. Other companies use money from attrition.[29]

The Quaker Oats pet-food plant at Lawrence, Kansas, paid employees 5 percent to 10 percent above market to attract and retain above-average employees and remain nonunion.[30] (Exhibit 28–8 illustrates the Quaker Oats pay-for-performance policy.) To achieve maximum effect on employees, base pay must be kept at a level at or above the industry average. Also, labor costs must be reduced and controlled by using incentives not added into base pay (see Exhibit 28–9.

Exhibit 28–8   The Pay-for-Performance Policy: An Illustration

Employee: Ed Norton
Hourly wage: $12.00
Annual salary: Ed worked 1,900 hours at regular pay and 100 hours of overtime.
$(1{,}900 \times \$12.00) + (100 \times \$18.00) = \$24{,}600$

Scenario 1 (A):
- Performance matrix determines payout of 5.5 percent
- Lawrence plant is 6.25 percent above the "market."
- Since plant wages are greater than 5 percent above market, payout takes form of lump sum, based on Ed's total earnings for the previous year.
- Ed's lump sum payment = $1,353 ($24,600 × .055).

Scenario 1 (B):
- Performance matrix determines payout of 5.5 percent.
- Lawrence plant is 4.5 percent above the "market."
- Since plant wages are less than 5 percent above market, payout takes the form of a base wage increase.
- Ed's adjusted hourly wage = $12.66 ($12.00 × 1.055).

Source: Reprinted by permission of publisher from J. P. Guthrie and E. P. Cunningham, "Pay for Performance for Hourly Workers: The Quaker Oats Alternative," *Compensation Benefits Review,* March/April © 1992, 21, American Management Association, New York. All rights reserved.

Exhibit 28–9   Does Performance-Based Pay Matter?

	Level of Performance Measurement	
	Individual	Group
Added Into base	Merit	
Not added in	Awards	Gain sharing
	Piece rates	Profit sharing
	Commissions	Stock options
	Bonuses	

Source: Reprinted by permission of publisher from G. Milkovich and C. Milkovich, "Strengthening the Pay-for-Performance Relationship: The Research," *Compensation & Benefits Review,* November/December © 1992, 56, American Management Association, New York. All rights reserved.

Exhibit 28–10   Standards for Evaluation of Pay-for-Performance Programs

1. There are pay-for-performance programs.
2. They were developed with input from employees.
3. They are based on company philosophy, goals, objectives, and vision.
4. They have policies and procedures.
5. The goals are job-specific.
6. There are standards for measurement.
7. The standards are linked to an objective performance appraisal system.
8. Rewards are linked to effort and performance.
9. Employees are informed about the programs.
10. Employees trust the programs.
11. Managers are well-trained and skilled in administering the programs.
12. The programs are funded or budgeted.
13. An evaluation program is in place to monitor the programs.
14. Productivity and performance outcomes are being measured.
15. The plans are accomplishing the stated objectives.

Exercise 28–1   Use Exhibit 28–10 above to evaluate the pay-for-performance programs in the health-care organization for which you work. These programs may be merit increases, individual rewards, individual piece rates, individual commissions, and group rewards such as gain sharing, profit sharing, stock options, or bonuses. How can the programs be improved? Make a management plan for improving them and present it to your supervisor and the director of human resources.

Exercise 28–2   If no pay-for-performance programs exist in your organization, prepare a proposal for one. Present it to your supervisor and the director of human resources. You may want to do this as a group exercise.

WEB ACTIVITIES

- Visit www.jbpub.com/swansburg, this text's companion website on the Internet, for further information on Pay for Performance.
- What organizations or journals could you search for information on pay for performance?
- Are there separate sources for the different types of pay for performance?

SUMMARY

Incentive programs are very common in organizations. The trend is to link pay to the employee or corporate performance, as the linkage motivates employees to increase productivity, especially when tied to such operational measures as attendance, quality, and safety. The most common individual performance-based pay plans are merit, awards, piece rates, and commissions. Gain sharing, profit sharing, and stock options are the most common performance-based group awards. Bonuses are common as both individual and group awards. In many instances, merit pay is added to base pay, while other awards are given on a one-time basis and are less expensive over time.

A pay-for-performance plan should be communicated well, have measures that can be influenced by participants, be consistent and fair, provide ample and timely rewards linking them to work, and be trusted.

Participants in a pay-for-performance plan often risk the choice of earning less now for the chance to earn more later through higher retirement benefits. Pay for performance starts with reduced wages and salaries, although the base should equal or slightly exceed the industry standard.

Equity theory, expectancy theory, and the law of effect are the basis for pay for performance. People expect equal pay for equal work; increased rewards for increased output.

Teams are effective in implementing pay-for-performance plans.

NOTES

1. J. A. Parnell, "Five Reasons Why Pay Must Be Based on Performance," *Supervision,* February 1991, 6–8.
2. S. H. Appelbaum and B. T. Shapiro, "Pay for Performance: Implementation of Individual and Group Plans," *Management Decision: Quarterly Review of Management Technology,* November 1992, 86–91.
3. J. Grossmann, "Pay, Performance and Productivity," *Small Business Reports,* October 1992, 50–59.
4. J. D. Browdy, "Performance Appraisal and Pay for Performance Start at the Top," *Health Care Supervisor,* April 1989, 31–41.
5. S. H. Appelbaum and B. T. Shapiro, op. cit.
6. J. Grossmann, op. cit.
7. S. Tully, "Your Paycheck Gets Exciting," *Fortune,* 1 November 1993, 83–84, 88, 95, 98.
8. Jiing-Lih Farh, R. W. Griffith, and D. B. Balkin, "Effects of Choice of Pay Plans on Satisfaction, Goal Setting, and Performance," *Journal of Organizational Behavior* 12 (1991): 55–62.
9. M. P. Miceli, I. Jung, J. P. Near, and D. B. Greenberger, "Predictions and Outcomes of Reactions to Pay-for-Performance Plans," *Journal of Applied Psychology,* April 1991, 508–521.
10. G. Milkovich and C. Milkovich, "Strengthening the Pay-Performance Relationship: The Research," *Compensation and Benefits Review,* November–December 1992, 53–62.
11. C. J. Frisch and M. A. Dickinson, "Work Productivity as a Function of the Percentage of Monetary Incentives to Base Pay," *Journal of Organizational Behavior Management* 11, no. 1 (1990): 13–33.

12. S. Berger and J. Moyer, "Launching a Performance-Based Pay Plan," *Modern Health-care,* 19 August 1991, 64.

13. J. A. Parnell, op. cit.

14. T. R. Zenger, "Why Do Employers Only Reward Extreme Performance? Examining the Relationships Among Performance, Pay, and Turnover," *Administrative Science Quarterly,* June 1992, 198–219.

15. R. M. Williamson, "Reward What You Value and Reach New Maintenance Performance Levels," *Plant Engineering,* 13 August 1992, 113–114.

16. S. H. Appelbaum and B. T. Shapiro, op. cit.; J. Grossman, op. cit.; M. A. Conte and D. Kruse, "ESOPs and Profit-Sharing Plans: Do They Link Employee Pay to Company Performance?" *Financial Management,* winter 1991, 91–100; D. P. Schwab and C. A. Olson, "Merit-Pay Practice Implications for Pay-Performance Relationships," *Industrial and Labor Relations Review,* February 1990, 237S–255S; D. W. Jones and M. C. Hanser, "Putting Teeth into Pay-for-Performance Programs," *Healthcare Financial Management,* September 1991, 32, 34–35, 40, 42.

17. J. Grossmann, op. cit.; S. H. Appelbaum and S. H. Shapiro, op. cit.; J. P. Guthrie and E. P. Cunningham, "Pay for Performance for Hourly Workers: The Quaker Oats Alternative," *Compensation and Benefits Review,* March–April 1992, 18–23; G. J. Meng, "Using Job Descriptions, Performance and Pay Innovations to Support Quality: A Paper Company's Experience," *National Productivity Review,* spring 1992, 247–255; "Performance Reviews Key in Pay for Performance and Pay," *The Wall Street Journal,* 10 May 1993, B1; G. Milkovich and C. Milkovich, op. cit.; S. Berger and J. Moyer, op. cit.; S. Tully, "The Real Key to Creating Wealth," *Fortune,* 20 September 1993, 38–39, 44–45, 48, 50; B. P. MacLean, "Value-Added Pay Beats Traditional Merit Programs," *Personnel Journal,* September 1990, 46, 48–50, 52; J. Greenwald, "Workers: Risks and Rewards," *Time,* 15 April 1991, 42–43; L. Thornburg, "Pay for Performance: What You Should Know," *HR Magazine,* June 1992, 58–61; L. Thornburg, "How Do You Cut the Cake?" *HR Magazine,* October 1992, 66–68, 70, 72; K. A. McNally, "Compensation as a Strategic Tool," *HR Magazine,* December 1992, 38–40; J. D. Browdy, op. cit.

18. P. K. Zingheim and J. R. Schuster, "Linking Quality and Pay," *HR Magazine,* December 1992, 55–59.

19. L. M. Sixel, "Team Incentives Gain Popularity as Reward Method," *San Antonio Express-News,* 24 July 1994, 8H.

20. P. K. Zingheim and J. R. Schuster, op. cit.

21. L. Thornburg, "Pay for Performance: What You Should Know," op. cit.

22. B. P. MacLean, "Value-Added Pay Beats Traditional Merit Programs," *Personnel Journal,* September 1990, 46–52.

23. P. Benner, *From Novice to Expert* (Menlo Park, Calif.: Addison-Wesley, 1984).

24. F. Swoboda, "Motorola Tests Peer Review of Performance for Pay," *San Antonio Express-News,* 24 July 1994, 8H.

25. S. Tully, "Your Paycheck Gets Exciting," op. cit.

26. D. P. Schwab and C. A. Olson, op. cit.

27. L. Thornburg, "How Do You Cut the Cake?" op. cit.

28. S. H. Appelbaum and B. T. Shapiro, op. cit.

29. L. Goff, "Working Harder to Get the Same Raise," *Computerworld,* 2 March 1992, 76.

30. J. P. Guthrie and E. P. Cunningham, op. cit.

REFERENCES

"A Master Class in Radical Change." 1993. *Fortune* (13 December): 82–96.

Abruzzese, R. S. 1989. "Management Development of the Head Nurse: The Program and Evaluation of the Program." *Journal of Continuing Education in Nursing* 20, no. 4: 186–187.

Ackerman, L. 1970. "Let's Put Motivation Where It Belongs—Within the Individual." *Personnel Journal* (July): 559–562.

Ackoff, R. L. 1986. "Our Changing Concept of Planning." *Journal of Nursing Administration* (October): 35–40.

Adams, R., and P. Duchene. 1985. "Computerization of Patient Acuity and Nursing Care Planning." *The Journal of Nursing Administration* (April): 11–17.

Adamski, M. G., and B. R. Hagen. 1990. "Using Technology to Create a Professional Environment for Recruitment and Retention." *Nursing Administration Quarterly* (Summer): 32–37.

"Advance Directives . . . Is the Law Clear?" 1991. *Healthcare Alabama* (January/February): 3, 5–7, 21.

Afo, G. V., J. A. Thomason, and S. E. Karel. 1991. "Better Management for Better Health Services." *World Health Forum* 12, pp. 161–167.

"Agencies Tout CM as Value Added for Prenatal Clients." 1994. *Case Management Advisor*™ (May): 64–66.

Al-Shehri, A. 1992. "The Market and Educational Principle in Continuing Medical Education for General Practice," *Medical Education* 26, pp. 384–387.

Allen, D. 1990. "Decentralization: Problems and Approaches." *Aspen's Advisor for Nurse Executives* (November): 1, 3–5.

Alt-White, A. C., M. Charns, and R. Strayer. 1983. "Personal Organizational and Managerial Factors Related to Nurse-Physician Collaboration." *Nursing Administration Quarterly* (Fall): 8–18.

American Academy of Nursing, 1977. *Primary Care by Nurses: Sphere of Responsibility and Accountability*, Kansas City, Mo.: The Academy.

American Hospital Association. 1980. *Managerial Cost Accounting for Hospitals*. Chicago: American Hospital Publishing.

American Nurses Association. 1991. *Standards of Clinical Nursing Practice*. Washington, D.C.: American Nurses Publishing.

———. 1994. *Nursing: A Social Policy Statement*. Washington, D.C.: American Nurses Association.

———. 1995. *Scope and Standards for Nurse Administrators*. Kansas City, Mo.: American Nurses Association.

Andrusyszyn, M. A. 1990. "Faculty Evaluation: A Closer Look at Peer Review." *Nurse Education Today* (December): 410–414.

Anthony, C. E., and D. delBueno. 1993. "A Performance-Based Development System." *Nursing Management* (June): 32–34.

Applegeet, C. J. 1989. "AORN's Budget—Planning and Forecasting Uncover Future Needs." *AORN Journal* (August): 212, 214.

Aranjo, M. D., and S. M. Carballo. 1993. "Creating the Future." *Health Progress* (June): 22–24, 58.

Argyris, C. 1967. "How Tomorrow's Executives Will Make Decisions." Reprint from *THINK Magazine*, IBM.

———. 1982. *Reasoning, Learning and Action.* San Francisco: Jossey-Bass.

Arikian, V. L. 1991. "Total Quality Management: Applications to Nursing Service." *Journal of Nursing Administration* (June): 46–50.

Arndt, M. J., and B. Underwood. 1990. "Learning Style Theory and Patient Education." *Journal of Continuing Education in Nursing* 21, 1: 28–31.

Artinian, B. M., F. D. O'Connor, and R. Brock. 1984. "Comparing Past and Present Nursing Productivity." *Nursing Management* (October): 50–53.

Ash, S. 1992. "A Big Job: How to Psych Yourself Up." *Supervisory Management* (April): 9.

Auger, B. Y. 1967. "How to Run an Effective Meeting." *Commerce* (October).

Auger, J. A., and V. Dee. 1983. "A Patient Classification System Based on the Behavioral System Model of Nursing: Part I." *Journal of Nursing Administration* (April): 38–43.

Ayers, A. F. 1988–89. "Defined Objectives Helping Management to Reach for Stars." *Presidential Issue,* pp. 70–72, 74.

Baker, H. K., and P. Morgan. 1986. "Building a Professional Image: Using 'Feeling-Level' Communication." *Supervisory Management* (January): 20–25.

Baker, K. G. 1980. "Application of a Group Theory in Nursing Practice." *Supervisor Nurse* (March): 22–24.

Baldwin, S. R., and M. McConnell. 1988. "Strategic Planning: Process and Plan Go Hand in Hand." *Management Solutions* (June): 29–36.

Ballengee, N. B. 1990. "Developing a Performance Appraisal System." *Management Accounting* (September): 52–54.

Barber, A. E., R. B. Dunham, and R. A. Formisano. 1992. "The Impact of Flexible Benefits on Employee Satisfaction: A Field Study." *Personal Psychology* (Spring): 55–75.

Barnett, J., and G. Anderson. 1987. "Performance Appraisal Revived." *Senior Nurse* (December): 20–22.

Barnum, B. S., and K. M. Kerfoot. 1995. *The Nurse as Executive.* 4th ed. Gaithersburg, MD: 296–308.

Basford, P., and C. Downie. 1990. "How to . . . Organize Brainstorming." *Nursing Times* (4 April): 63.

Bauerhaus, P. I. 1996. "Creating a New Place in the Competitive Market." *Nursing Policy Forum* (March/April): 18–20.

Beeber, L. S., and M. H. Schmitt. 1986. "Cohesiveness in Groups: A Concept in Search of a Definition." *Advances in Nursing Science* (January): 1–11.

Beeler, J. R., P. A. Young, and S. M. Dull. 1990. "Professional Development Framework." *Journal of Nursing Staff Development.* (November/December): 296–301.

Beissner, K. L. 1992. "Use of Concept Mapping to Improve Problem Solving." *Journal of Physical Therapy Education* (Spring): 22–27.

Bengtsson, J. 1991. "Education, Training and Labor Market Development." *Futures* (December): 1085–1106.

Bermas, N. F., and A. Van Slyck. 1984. "Patient Classification Systems and the Nursing Department." *Hospitals* (November): 99–100.

Bertinasco, L. G. 1990. "Strategies for Resolving Conflict." *Health Care Supervisor* (July): 35–37.

Beyers, M. 1984. "Getting on Top of Organizational Change: Part 2. Trends in Nursing Service." *Journal of Nursing Administration* (November): 31–37.

Bice, M. 1990. "Behavior Is the Most Effective Communicator." *Hospitals* (20 October): 78.

"Biomedical Ethics and the Bill of Rights." (1989). *National Forum* (Fall).

Bircher, A. U. 1975. "One Development and Classification of Diagnoses." *Nursing Forum* (January): 11–29.

Blake, L. 1992. "Reduce Employees' Resistance to Change." *Personnel Journal* (September): 72–76.

Blanchard, K., and N. V. Peale. 1988. *The Power of Ethical Management.* New York: Fawcett Crest.

Blanchard, K., and S. Johnson. 1982. *The One Minute Manager.* New York: William Morrow.

Blanchard, K. H., and A. B. Sargent. 1986. "The One Minute Manager Is an Androgynous Manager." *Nursing Management* (May): 43–45.

Boissoneau, R., and B. Schwada. 1989. "Participatory Management: Its Evaluation, Current Usage." *AORN Journal* (November): 1079–1086.

Bolman, L. G., and T. E. Deal. 1991. *Reframing Organizations: Artistry, Choice, and Leadership.* San Francisco: Jossey-Bass.

Bolster, C. J. 1991. "Work Redesign: More Than Rearranging Furniture on the Titanic." *Aspen's Advisor for Nurse Executives* (August): 4–7.

Bolton, L. B., C. Aydin, G. Popolow, and J. Ramseyer. 1992. "Ten Steps for Managing Organizational Change." *Journal of Nursing Administration* (June): 14–20.

Bower, K. 1992. *Case Management by Nurses,* 2d ed. Washington, D.C.: American Nurses Publishing.

Bower, K. A., and J. G. Somerville. 1988. "Managed Care and Case Management Outcome-Based Practice: Creating the Environment." Program at Sheraton Grand Hotel, Tampa, Florida, February 15–16.

Boyd, M., L. Collins, J. Pepitone, E. Balk, and P. Kapustay. 1990. "Theory Z as a Framework for the Application of a Professional Practice Model in Increasing Nursing Staff Retention on Oncology Units." *Journal of Advanced Nursing* 15, pp. 1226–1229.

Brider, P. 1992. "The Move to Patient-Focused Care." *American Journal of Nursing* (September): 26–33.

Brothers, J. 1994. "Some Techniques That Can Help You . . . Turn a Drawback into a Strength." *Parade Magazine* (10 April): 4–6.

Brown, D. S. 1966. "Shaping the Organization to Fit People." *Management of Personnel Quarterly* (Summer).

Bryan, E. L., and R. E. Welton. 1986. "Let Your Business Plan Be a Road Map to Credit." *Business* (July–September): 44–47.

Buerhaus, P. I. 1996. "Creating a New Place in the Competitive Market." *Nursing Policy Forum* (March/April): 13–20.

Buhler, P. 1993. "Managing in the 90s." *Supervision* (March): 17–19.

Bunch, D. 1995. "The Next Frontier in Managed Care." *AARC Times* (December): 48–49.

Burcham, M. R. 1994. "Strategic Planning for Managed Care." *Rehab Management* (April/May): 93, 95–96, 99.

Burda, D. 1988. "Provider Looks to Industry for Quality Models." *Modern Healthcare* (July 15): 24–26, 28, 30, 32.

Butler, K. 1996. "Managed Care: Emerging Issues in Clinical Ethics." *ASHA* (Summer): 7.

Butterfield, P. G. 1988. "Nominal Group Process as an Instructional Method with Novice Community Health Nursing Students." *Public Health Nursing* (March): 12–15.

Cain, C., and V. Laschinger. 1978. "Management by Objectives: Applications to Nursing." *Journal of Nursing Administration* (January): 35–38.

Call, A. 1992. "Building Bridges." *Nursing Times* (2 December): 44–45.

Campbell, J. M., and E. S. Kinion. 1993. "Teaching Leadership/Followership to RN-to-MSN Students." *Journal of Nursing Education* (March): 138–140.

Caplan, A. 1991. "Bush Must Avert Medical Disaster." *San Antonio Light* (17 November): F4.

Caramanica, L. 1984. "What? Another Committee?" *Nursing Management* (September): 12–14.

Carse, J. 1994. "Diversity in the World's Religions." *National Forum* (Winter): 26–27.

Carson, K. P., R. L. Cardy, and G. H. Dobbins. 1992. "Upgrade the Employee Evaluation Process." *HR Magazine* (November): 88–92.

Castaldi, T. M. 1989. "Adult Learning: Transferring Skills from the Workplace to the Classroom." *Lifelong Learning: An Omnibus of Practice and Research* 12, no. 6: 17–19.

Cavanagh, S. J. 1990. "Educational Aspects of Cardiopulmonary Resuscitation (CPR) Training." *Intensive Care Nursing* 6, pp. 38–44.

Cericola, S. A. 1995. "Facing Challenges of Managed Care." *Plastic Surgical Nursing* (Winter): 219.

Chase, M. 1992. "Cancer Doctors Aim to Improve Chemotherapy." *The Wall Street Journal* (21 May): 88.

Chinn, P. L., and M. K. Jacobs. 1987. *Theory and Nursing: A Systematic Approach.* St. Louis, Mo.: C. V. Mosby.

Chu, N. L., and J. A. Schmele. 1990. "Using the ANA Standards as a Basis for Performance Evaluation in the Home Health Care Setting." *Journal of Nursing Quality Assurance* (May): 25–33.

Ciske, K. I. 1978. Response to Zander's "Primary Nursing Won't Work . . . Unless the Head Nurse Lets It." *Journal of Nursing Administration* (January): 26, 43, 50.

Clark, C. M., A. Steinbinder, and R. Anderson. 1994. "Implementing Clinical Paths in a Managed Care Environment." *Nursing Economics* (July–August): 230–234.

Clark, L. H. Jr. 1992. "Service Center Faces Task of Cutting Costs Without Trimming Quality of Its Product." *The Wall Street Journal* (2 April): B9A.

Clegg, C. W., and Wall, T. D. 1984. "The Lateral Dimension to Employee Participation." *Journal of Management Studies* (October): 429–442.

Clifford, M. 1992. "Can Do, Make Do." *Far Eastern Economic Review* (5 March): 53–54.

Coaly, P. R., and P. R. Sackett. 1987. "Effects of Using High- Versus Low-Performing Job Incumbents as Sources of Job Analysis Information." *Journal of Applied Psychology* (August): 434–437.

Cochran, Sr. Jeanette. 1979. "Refining a Patient-Acuity System Over Four Years." *Hospital Progress* (February): 56–60.

Coeling, H.V.E., and J. R. Wilcox. 1990. "Using Organizational Culture to Facilitate the Change Process." *ANNA Journal* (June): 231–236.

Cohen, L. 1988. "Quality Function Deployment: An Application Perspective from Digital Equipment Corporation." *National Productivity Review* (Summer): 197–208.

Cohen, M. H., and M. E. Ross. 1982. "Team Building: A Strategy for Unit Cohesiveness." *Journal of Nursing Administration* (January): 29–34.

Cohen, S. S. 1995. "National Committee for Quality Assurance." *Rehab Management* (October/November): 13, 109.

Coile, R. C., Jr. 1995. "Integration, Capitation, and Managed Care: Transformation of Nursing for 21st Century Health Care." *Advanced Practice Nursing Quarterly* (Fall): 77–84.

Colavecchio, R. 1982. "Direct Patient Care: A Viable Career Choice." *Journal of Nursing Administration* (July–August): 17–22.

Cole, R. 1988. "What Was Deming's Real Influence?" *Mechanical Engineering* (January): 49–51.

Collins, J. 1996. "The Classics: The Complete Guide to the Best Business and Management Books Ever Written." *Inc.* (December): 53–56, 60, 62.

"Comprehensive CM in Integrated Care Presents Exciting New Career Opportunity." 1994. *Case Management Advisor*™ (August): 105–106, 108.

Connors, K. 1996. "Managed Care and Case Management." *Australian Nursing Journal* (May): 32–34.

Conway-Rutkowski, B. 1984. "Labor Relations: How Do You Rate?" *Nursing Management* (February): 13–16.

Conway-Welch, C. 1996. "Trends in Health Care Impact on Nursing Education." *NSNA Imprint* (April–May): 37–38.

Corder, K. T., J. Phoon, and M. Barter. 1996. "Managed Care: Employers' Influence on the Health Care System." *Nursing Economic$* (July–August): 213–217.

Corley, M. C., and B. E. Satterwhite. 1993. "Forecasting Ambulatory Clinic Workload to Facilitate Budgeting." *Nursing Economic$* (March–April): 77–81, 114.

Cortes, C. E. 1994. "Limits to Pluribus, Limits to Unum." *National Forum* (Winter): 6–8.

Covin, T. J., and R. H. Kilmann. 1990. "Participant Perceptions of Positive and Negative Influences on Large-Scale Change." *Group & Organizational Studies* (June): 233–248.

Cox, C. L. 1980. "Decentralization: Uniting Authority and Responsibility." *Supervisor Nurse* (March): 28, 32.

Crosby, P. B. 1984. *Quality Without Tears: The Art of Hassle-Free Management.* New York: McGraw-Hill.

Cummings, C., and R. McCaskey. 1992. "A Model Combining Centralized and Decentralized Staff Development." *Journal of Nursing Staff Development* (January/February): 22–25.

Cunningham, J. B., and T. Eberle. 1990. "A Guide to Job Enrichment and Redesign." *Personnel* (February): 56–61.

Curtin, L. L. 1990. "Creating a Culture of Competence." *Nursing Management* (September): 7–8.

D'Andrea, G. 1996. "Introduction to Managed Care." *Journal of AHIMA* (January): 42–46.

Davenport, J. III. 1987. "Is There Any Way Out of the Andragogy Morass?" *Lifelong Learning: An Omnibus of Practice and Research* vol. 11, no. 3: 17–20.

Davidson, J. R., and T. Davidson. 1996. "Confidentiality and Managed Care: Ethical and Legal Concerns." *Health and Social Work* (August): 208–215.

Davis, B., and D. Milbank. 1992. "If the U.S. Work Ethic Is Fading, 'Laziness' May Not Be the Reason." *The Wall Street Journal* (7 February): 1, A5.

Davis, C. K., D. Oakley, and J. A. Sochalsk. 1982. "Leadership for Expanding Nursing Influence on Health Policy." *Journal of Nursing Administration* (January): 15–21.

Davis, D. L. 1984. "Assessing and Improving Productivity in the Operating Room." *AORN Journal* (October): 630, 632, 634.

Davis, D. S., A. E. Greig, J. Burkholder, and T. Keating. 1984. "Evaluating Advance Practice Nurses." *Nursing Management* (March): 44–47.

Davis, G. S. 1996. "Learning the Ropes of Contracting." *Provider* (July): 32–34.

Dawkins, C., D. Oakley, J. Davis, and N. Erwin. 1991. "Collaboration as an Organizational Process." *Journal of Nursing Education* (April): 189–191.

Dearhammer, W. G. 1991. "Con: Promotion Calls for Proper Preparation." *Business Credit* (April): 27–28.

Dee, V., and J. A. Auger. 1983. "A Patient Classification System Based on the Behavioral System Model of Nursing: Part II." *Journal of Nursing Administration* (May): 18–23.

Dennis, K. E. 1983. "Nursing's Power in the Organization: What Research Has Shown." *Nursing Administration Quarterly* (Fall): 47–60.

Denton, D. K. 1986. "Problem Solving by Keeping in Touch." *Business* (July–September): 40–42.

DeSilets, L. 1986. "Self-Directed Learning in Voluntary and Mandatory Continuing Education Programs." *Journal of Continuing Education in Nursing* (May/June): 81–83.

Deutsch, B. J. 1991. "A Conversation with Philip Crosby." *Bank Marketing* (April): 22–27.

"Development of an Organizational Strategic Planning Process for a Hospital Department." 1990. *Health Care Supervisor* (September): 1–20.

DeWeese, S., and D. Satecki. 1986. "Combining Management Education with an Assessment Center." *Nursing Management* (August): 80–81.

Dickoff, J., P. James, and E. Wiedenbach. 1968. "Theory in a Practice Discipline, Part I. Practice Oriented Theory." *Nursing Research* (September–October): 415–435.

———. 1968. "Theory in a Practice Discipline, Part II. Practice Oriented Research." *Nursing Research* (November–December): 545–554.

Dienemann, J., and T. Glazner. 1992. "Restructuring Nursing Care Delivery Systems." *Nursing Economic$* (July–August): 253–258, 310.

Dixon, I. L. 1993. "Continuous Quality Improvement in Shared Leadership." *Nursing Management* (January): 40–41, 44–45.

Dixon, N. 1984. "Participative Management: It's Not as Simple as It Seems." *Supervisory Management* (December): 2–8.

Dobyns, L., and C. Crawford-Mason. 1991. *Quality or Else: The Revolution in World Business* (New York: Houghton Mifflin).

Doering, L. 1990. "Recruitment and Retention: Successful Strategies in Critical Care." *Heart and Lung* (May): 220–224.

Donadio, P. J. 1992. "Capturing the Principles of Motivation." *Business Credit* (March): 40.

Donaldson, T. 1992. "Individual Rights and Multinational Corporate Responsibilities." *National Forum* (Winter): 7–9.

Dowless, R. 1992. "Motivating Salespeople: One Order of Empowerment, Hold the Carrots." *Training* (February): 16, 73–74.

Dowling, G. F. 1991. "Case Management Nursing: Indications for Material Management." *Hospital Material Management Quarterly* (February): 26–32.

Drucker, P. F. 1990. "The Emerging Theory of Manufacturing." *Harvard Business Review* (May–June): 94–100.

Dumaine, B. 1993. "Payoff from the New Management." *Fortune* (13 December): 103–104, 108, 110.

Duncan, R. P., E. C. Fleming, and T. G. Gallati. 1991. "Implementing a Continuous Quality Improvement Program in a Community Hospital." *Quality Review Bulletin* (April): 106–112.

Eason, F. R. 1988. "Quality Circles—A Summation for Inservice Educators: Using Circles to Increase Staff Nurse Participation in Problem Solving." *Journal of Nursing Staff Development* 4, 3: 131–132.

Eason, F. R., and R. W. Corbett. 1992. "Effective Teacher Characteristics Identified by Adult Learners in Nursing." *Journal of Continuing Education in Nursing* (January): 21–23.

Eddy, D. M., and J. Billings. 1988. "The Quality of Medical Evidence: Implications for Quality of Care." *Health Affairs* (Spring): 19–32.

Editorial. 1993. "Executive Pay: It Doesn't Add Up." *Business Week* (26 April): 122.

Emblen, J. D., and G. T. Gray. 1990. "Comparison of Nurses' Self-Directed Learning Activities." *Journal of Continuing Education in Nursing* 21, 2: 56–61.

Erdman, A. 1992. "What's Wrong with Workers." *Fortune* (10 August): 18.

Ernst, C. J. 1984. "A Relational Expert System for Nursing Management Control." *Human Systems Management* (Fall): 286–293.

Ertl, N. 1984. "Choosing Successful Managers: Participative Selection Can Help." *Journal of Nursing Administration* (April): 27–33.

Esmond, T. H. Jr. 1982. *Budgeting Procedures for Hospitals 1982 Edition.* Chicago: American Hospital Publishing.

Esterhuysen, P. 1993. "Budgeting—A Serious Matter." *Nursing News* (May): 8.

Ethridge, J. R. 1990. "Criteria for Evaluating Performance: An Empirical Study for Nonprofit Hospitals." *Health Care Supervisor* (September): 49–56.

Etzioni, A. 1992. "Too Many Rights Too Few Responsibilities." *National Forum* (Winter): 4–6.

Eubanks, P. 1992. "The CEO Experience: TQM/CQI." *Hospitals* (5 June): 24–36.

"Evaluation." 1992. *Advisor* (January): 4.

Fadden, T. C., and G. K. Seiser. 1984. "Nursing Diagnosis: A Matter of Form." *American Journal of Nursing* (April): 470–472.

Farley, M. J. 1991. "Teamwork in Perioperative Nursing: Understanding Team Development, Effectiveness, Evaluation." *AORN Journal* (March): 730–738.

Farnham, A. 1993. "State Your Values, Hold the Hot Air." *Fortune* (19 April): 117–124.

Fay, M. S., and A. K. Morrill. 1985. "The Grievance-Arbitration Process: the Experience of One Nursing Administration." *Journal of Nursing Administration* (June): 11–16.

Felton, G. 1975. "Increasing the Quality of Nursing Care by Introducing the Concept of Primary Nursing: A Model Project." *Nursing Research* (January–February): 27–32.

Ferketish, B. J., and J. W. Hayden. 1992. "HRD & Quality: The Chicken or the Egg?" *Training & Development Journal* (January): 39–42.

Filmer, D. 1985. "Improving Communications in Large Organizations." *Work and People* (February): 12–14.

Finkler, S. A. 1991. "Variance Analysis Part II, Use of Computers." *Journal of Nursing Administration* (September): 9–15.

———. 1992. *Budgeting Concepts for Nurse Managers,* 2d ed. Philadelphia: W. B. Saunders.

Finsher, S. 1985. "Rework, Revise, Rewrite." *Business* (July–September): 54–55.

Fisher, D. W., and E. Thomas. 1975. "A 'Premium Day' Approach to Weekend Nurse Staffing." *Staffing: A Journal of Nursing Administration Reader.* Wakefield, Mass.: Contemporary Publishing.

Fong, C. M. 1993. "A Longitudinal Study of the Relationship Between Overload, Social Support and Burnout Among Nursing Educators." *Journal of Nursing Education* (January): 24–29.

Fouracre, S., and A. Wright. 1986. "New Factors in Job Evaluation." *Personnel Management* (May): 40–43.

Francisco, P. D. 1989. "Flexible Budgeting and Variance Analysis." *Nursing Management* (November): 40–43.

French, P., and D. Cross. 1992. "An Interpersonal-Epistemological Curriculum Model for Nurse Education." *Journal of Advanced Nursing* 17, pp. 83–89.

Friedman, M. D., M. H. Bailit, and J. O. Michel. 1995. "Vendor Management: A Model for Collaboration and Quality Improvement." *Journal of Quality Improvement* (November): 635–645.

Froebe, D. 1975. "Scheduling: By Team or Individually." *Staffing: A Journal of Nursing Administration Reader.* Wakefield, Mass.: Contemporary Publishing.

Fulmer, R. M., and S. G. Franklin. 1982. *Supervision: Principles of Professional Management,* 2d ed. New York: Macmillan.

Galbraith, J. K. 1967. *The New Industrial State.* Boston: Houghton Mifflin.

Ganong, W. L., and J. M. Ganong. 1972. "Reducing Organizational Conflict Through Working Committees." *Journal of Nursing Administration* (January–February): 12–19.

Gardner, D. L. 1991. "Assessing Career Commitment: The Role of Staff Development." (November/December): 263–266.

Garre, P. P. 1990. "A Computerized Recruitment Program." *Journal of Nursing Administration* (January): 24–27.

Gebhardt, A. N. 1982. "Computers and Staff Allocation Made Easy." *Nursing Times* (September): 1471–1473.

Gelfand, L. I. 1970. "Communicate Through Your Supervisors." *Harvard Business Review* (November–December): 101–104.

Genasci, L. 1994. "Downsizing Not Always Effective, Experts Say." *San Antonio Express-News* (24 July): 3H.

Gentile, G. 1989. "Fun Becoming Part of Corporate Culture." *Augusta Chronicle* (30 July): 7.

Gevedon, S. 1992. "Leadership Behaviors of Deans of Top-Ranked Schools of Nursing." *Nursing Education* (May): 221–224.

Gibson, J. L., J. W. Ivancevich, and J. H. Donnelly, Jr. 1993. *Organizations: Behavior, Structure, Processes,* 8th ed. Burr Ridge, Ill.: Richard D. Irwin.

Gillies, D. A., M. Franklin, and D. A. Child. 1990. "Relationship Between Organizational Climate and Job Satisfaction of Nursing Personnel." *Nursing Administration Quarterly* (Summer): 15–22.

Ginnodo, W. L. 1985–86. "Consultative Management: A Fresh Look at Employee Motivation." *National Productivity Review* (Winter): 78–80.

Ginsburg, L., and N. Miller. 1992. "Value-Driven Management." *Business Horizons* (May–June): 23–27.

Gitlow, H. S., S. J. Gitlow, A. Oppenheim, and R. Oppenheim. 1990. "Telling the Quality Story." *Quality Progress* (September): 41–46.

Glazner, L. 1992. "Understanding Corporate Cultures: Use of Systems Theory and Situational Analysis." *AAOHN Journal* (August): 383–387.

Glover, D. 1993. "Everett Hospitals to Unify Management." *Seattle Post-Intelligencer* (21 July): B2.

Goetz, J. F., and H. L. Smith. 1980. "Zero Base Budgeting for Nursing Services: An Opportunity for Cost Containment." *Nursing Forum* (February): 122–137.

Goldberg, D. 1978. "What Makes a Leader?" *Mississippi Press* (23 November): 6D.

Golde, R. A. 1972. "Are Your Meetings Like This One?" *Harvard Business Review* (January–February): 68–77.

Goldstein, M., D. Scholthaver, and B. B. Kleiner. 1985. "Management on the Right Side of the Brain." *Personnel Journal* (November): 40–45.

Golembienski, R. T., and B. Sun. 1991. "Public-Sector Innovation and Predisposing Situational Features: Testing Covariants of Successful QWC Applications." *PAQ* (Spring): 106–131.

———. 1989. "Positive-Findings Bias in Quality of Work Life Research: Public-Private Comparisons." *Public Productivity & Management Review* (Winter): 145–154.

Goodale, J. G. 1992. "Improving Performance Appraisal." *Business Quarterly* (Autumn): 65–70.

Goodpaster, K. E., and G. Atkinson. 1992. "Stakeholders, Individual Rights, and the Common Good." *National Forum* (Winter): 14–17.

Goodroe, J. H., and D. A. Murphy. 1994. "The Algebra of Managed Care." *Hospital Topics* (Fall): 14–18.

Goodson, J. R., and G. W. McGee. 1991. "Enhancing Individual Perceptions of Objectivity in Performance Appraisal." *Journal of Business Research* (June): 293–303.

Grandori, A. 1984. "Prescriptive Contingency View of Organizational Decision Making." *Administrative Science Quarterly* (June): 192–209.

Gray, B. 1995. "Managed Health Care Plans Pose Employment Risk for NPs." *NP News* 3, no. 3: 1, 8.

Gray, D. H. 1986. "Uses and Misuses of Strategic Planning." *Harvard Business Review* (January–February): 89–97.

Grazman, T. E. 1983. "Managing Unit Human Resources: A Microcomputer Model." *Nursing Management* (July): 18–22.

Greiner, L. E., D. P. Leitch, and D. P. Barnes. 1970. "Putting Judgment Back Into Decisions." *Harvard Business Review* (March–April): 59–67.

Grimaldi, P. L. 1985. "HMOs and Medicare." *Nursing Management* (April): 16, 18, 20.

Gunden, E., and S. Crissman. 1992. Leadership Skills for Empowerment." *Nursing Administration Quarterly* (Spring): 6–10.

Gupta, A. K., and A. Singhal. 1993. "Managing Human Resources for Innovation and Creativity." *Resource Technology Management* (May–June): 41–48.

Guy, M. E. 1986. "Interdisciplinary Conflict and Organizational Complexity." *Hospital & Health Services Administration* (January/February): 111–121.

Hagglund, K., and R. G. Frank. 1996. "Rehabilitation Psychology Practice, Ethics, and a Changing Health Care Environment." *Rehabilitation Psychology* 41, 1: 19–32.

Haislett, J., R. B. Hughes, G. Atkinson, and C. L. Williams. 1993. "Success in Baccalaureate Nursing Programs: A Matter of Accommodation?" *Journal of Nursing Education* (February): 64–70.

Hall, R. H. 1963. "The Concept of Bureaucracy: An Empirical Assessment." *American Journal of Sociology* (July): 32–40.

Hallows, D. A. 1982. "Budget Processes and Budgeting in the New Authorities." *Nursing Times* (4 August): 1309–1311.

Han, P. E. 1983. "The Informal Organization You've Got to Live With." *Supervisory Management* (October): 25–28.

Hancock, C. 1982. "The Nursing Budget." *Nursing Mirror* (20 October): 47–48.

Hanks, J. H. 1992. "Empowerment in Nursing Education: Concept Analysis and Application to Philosophy, Learning and Instruction." *Journal of Advanced Nursing* 17, pp. 607–618.

Hanson, C., C. R. Menkiena, and E. Meterko. 1990. "Successful Implementation of an Automated Nurse-Information System, Staff Development's Role." *Journal of Nursing Staff Development* (September/October): 229–232.

Harris, C. 1992. "Work Redesign Calls for New Pay and Performance." *Hospitals* (5 October): 56, 58, 60.

Hatcher, L. L., and T. L. Ross. 1985. "Organizational Development Through Productivity Gainsharing." *Personnel* (October): 42, 44–50.

Hayes, E. 1993. "Managing Job Satisfaction for the Long Run." *Nursing Management* (January): 65–67.

Heilriegel, D., and J. W. Slocum. 1972. "Organizational Climate: Measures Research and Contingencies." *Academy of Management Journal* (June): 255–280.

Helmer, F. T., and S. Gunatilake. 1988. "Quality Control Circles: A Supervisor's Tool for Solving Operational Problems in Nursing." *Health Care Supervisor* (July): 63–71.

Helms, L. 1988. "Tides of Change at Seafirst." *ABA Banking Journal* (November): 69–70, 74.

Hendricks, D. E. 1982. "Avoiding Cultural Myopia: What The Japanese Can Teach Nurses About Management." *Nursing Leadership* (June): 11–15.

Hendrickson, M. F. 1993. "The Nurse Engineer: A Way to Better Nursing Information Systems." *Computers in Nursing* (March/April): 67–71.

Henney, C. R., and R. N. Bosworth. 1980. "A Computer-Based System for the Automatic Production of Nursing Workload Data." *Nursing Times* (10 July): 1212–1217.

Henry, B., C. Arndt, M. DiVincenti, and A. Mariner-Tomey, eds. 1989. *Dimensions of Nursing Administration: Theory, Research, Education, Practice.* Boston: Blackwell.

Herbert, G. R., and D. Doverspike. 1990. "Performance Appraisals in the Training Needs Analysis Process: A Review and Critique." *Public Personnel Management* (Fall): 253–270.

Hern-Underwood, M. J., and L. L. Workman. 1993. "Group Climate: A Significant Retention Factor for Pediatric Nurse Managers." *Journal of Professional Nursing* (July–August): 233–238.

Hicks, L. 1993. "The Rise in Temps." *San Antonio Express-News* (12 December): 1–H, 6–H.

Hicks, L. L., and K. E. Boles. 1984. "Why Health Economics?" *Nursing Economic$* (May–June): 175–180.

Hillebrand, P. L. 1992. "12 Commandments to Communication in a Decentralized System." *Nursing Management* (August): 56–57.

Hirsch, J. 1987. "Organizational Structure and Philosophy." *Nursing Administration Quarterly* (Summer): 47–51.

"HMOs Win Physician Support but Quality Questions Remain." 1985. *Medical Staff News* (July): 3.

Hobson, C. J., M. E. Meade, and D. Soverly. 1985. "CE: Out-Dated Notions Can't Update Nurses." *Nursing Management* (May): 35–36, 38.

Hodgetts, R. M., and Howe, R. L. 1975. *Workbook to Accompany Management, Theory, Process, and Practice.* Philadelphia: W. B. Saunders.

Hoffman, W. M., and E. S. Petry, Jr. 1992. "Abusing Business Ethics." *National Forum* (Winter): 10–13.

Holland, H. K. 1968. "Decision-Making and Personality." *Personnel Administration* (May–June): 24–29.

Hotter, A. N. 1992. "The Clinical Nurse Specialist and Empowerment: Say Good-bye to the Fairy Godmother." *Nursing Administration Quarterly* (Spring): 11–15.

Howle, C. O. 1972. *The Design of Education.* San Francisco: Jossey-Bass.

Huber, D. 1996. *Leadership and Nursing Care Management.* Philadelphia: W. B. Saunders.

Huey, J. 1994. "The New Post-Heroic Leadership." *Fortune* (21 February): 42–44, 48, 50.

Hughes, J. M. 1992. "Total Quality Management in a 300-Bed Community Hospital: The Quality Improvement Process Translated to Health Care." *Quality Review Bulletin* (September): 311–318.

Hutchins, B. 1996. "Managing Cost and Quality." *REHAB Management* (April/May): 25–26.

Hutton, J., and D. Moss. 1982. "Budgetary Control—The Role of the Director of Nursing Services and Treasurers." *Nursing Times* (11 August): 1364–1365.

Hyett, K. 1987. "A Meeting of Minds." *Nursing Times* (18 February): 53–54.

Idaszak, J. R., and F. Drasgow. 1987. "A Revision of the Job Diagnostic Survey: Elimination of a Measurement Artifact." *Journal of Applied Psychology* (February): 69–74.

"Integrated Care Reduces Costs, Gives CM a Boost." 1994. *Case Management Advisor*™ (December): 166–168.

"Is Anybody Listening?" 1950. *Fortune* (September): 77+.

Jablin, F. M. 1982. "Formal Structural Characteristics of Organizations and Superior-Subordinate Communication." *Human Communication Research* (Summer): 338–347.

Jacobsen-Webb, M. 1985. "Team Building: Key to Executive Success." *Journal of Nursing Administration* (February): 16–20.

Jacobson, B., and B. L. Kaye. 1986. "Career Development and Performance Appraisal: It Takes Two To Tango." *Personnel* (January): 26–32.

Jecmen, C., and Stuerke, N. M. 1983. "Computerization Helps Solve Staff Scheduling Problems." *Nursing Economic$* (November–December): 209–211.

Jelinek, R. C., T. K. Zinn, and J. R. Brya. 1973. "Tell the Computer How Sick the Patients Are and It Will Tell How Many Nurses They Need." *Modern Hospital* (December): 81–85.

Jennings, E. E. 1962. "The Anatomy of Leadership." *Notes & Quotes* No. 274 (March): 1, 4.

Joblin, F. M. 1982. "Formal Structural Characteristics of Organizations and Superior-Subordinate Communication." *Human Communication Research* (Summer): 338–347.

Johnson, K. P. 1982. "Revenue Budgeting/Rate Setting." Pp. 279–311 in *Handbook of Health Care Accounting and Finance,* ed. W. O. Cleverly. Rockville, Md.: Aspen.

Johnson, L. M., J. R. Happel, J. Edelman, and S. J. Brown. 1983. "A Model of Participatory Management with Decentralized Authority." *Nursing Administration Quarterly* (Fall): 30–36.

Jones, G. R. 1983. "Forms of Control and Leader Behavior." *Journal of Management* (Fall): 159–172.

Jones L. 1991. "Integrating Research Activities, Practice Changes, and Monitoring and Evaluation: A Model for Academic Health." *Quality Review Bulletin* (July): 229–239.

Jones, L. C., T. D. Gubereski, and K. L. Soeken. 1990. "Nurse Practitioners: Leadership Behaviors and Organizational Climate." *Journal of Professional Nursing* (November–December): 327–333.

Joyce, W. F., and J. Slocum. 1982. "Climate Discrepancy: Refining the Concepts of Psychological and Organizational Climate." *Human Relations* 11, pp. 951–972.

Juran, J. M. 1989. "Universal Approach to Managing for Quality." *Executive Excellence* (May): 15–17.

Kabb, M. 1989. "Participatory Management in Nursing as an Alternative to Traditional Management." *Health Matrix* (April): 39–44.

Kaestle, P. 1990. "A New Rationale for Organizational Structure." *Planning Review* (July/August): 20–22, 27.

Kaluzny, A. D., C. P. McLaughlin, and K. Simpson. 1992. "Applying Total Quality Management Concepts to Public Health Organizations." *Public Health Reports* (May–June): 257–263.

Kaprowski, E. J. 1968. "Toward Innovative Leadership." *Notes & Quotes* No. 351 (August): 2.

Keenan, M. J., P. S. Hoover, and R. Hoover. 1985. "Leadership Theory Lets Clinical Instructors Guide Students Toward Autonomy." *Nursing and Health Care* (February): 83–86.

Keller, J. M. 1983. "Motivational Design of Instruction." *Instructional Design Theories and Models: An Overview of Their Current Status,* ed. C. M. Riegeluth. Hillsdale, N.J.: Erlbaum.

Kelly, K. J. 1990. "Administrator's Forum." *Journal of Nursing Staff Development* (September–October): 225–257.

———. 1992. "Administrators' Forum." *Journal of Nursing Staff Development* (March/April): 90–91.

Kersey, J. H. Jr. 1985. "Responsibility Accounting: Making Decisions Efficiently." *Nursing Management* (May): 14, 16–17.

Kin, C. S. 1995. "Managed Care: Is It Moral?" *Advanced Practice Nursing Quarterly* (Winter): 7–11.

King, G. B. 1990. "Performance Appraisal on the Automated Environment." *Journal of Library Administration* (Midwinter): 195–204.

Kintgen-Andrews, J. 1991. "Critical Thinking and Nursing Education: Perplexities and Insights." *Journal of Nursing Education* (April): 152–157.

Kipnis, D. 1987. "Psychology and Behavioral Technology." *American Psychologist* (January): 30–36.

Kirby, P. 1992. "An Aberration: Supervisors Who Like Performance Appraisal?" *Supervision* (October): 14–17.

Klann, S. 1989. "Mastering the OR Budgeting Process Is Key to Success." *OR Manager* (October): 10–11.

Klimaski, R., and L. Inks. 1990. "Accountability Forces in Performance Appraisal." *Organizational Behavior and Human Decision Processes* (April): 194–208.

Knowles, M. 1980. *The Modern Practice of Adult Education: From Pedagogy to Andragogy*, 2d ed. Chicago: Follet.

Koleszar, A. J. 1990. "The Great Debate." *CWRU* (February): 16–20.

Konstam, P. 1992. "'Quality' Should Begin at Home." *San Antonio Light* (1 March): D1.

Koontz, H. 1965. "Challenges for Intellectual Leadership or Management." *Notes & Quotes* No. 315 (August): 1, 4.

Koziol-McLain, J., and M. K. Maeve. 1993. "Nursing Theory in Perspective." *Nursing Outlook* (March/April): 79–81.

Krampitz, S. D., and M. Williams. 1983. "Organizational Climates: A Measure of Faculty and Nurse Administrator Perception." *Journal of Nursing Education* (May): 200–206.

Kreitlow, B. W., ed. 1981. *Examining Controversies in Adult Education*. San Francisco: Jossey-Bass.

La Violette, S. 1979. "Classification Systems Remedy Billing Inequity." *Modern Healthcare* (September): 32–33.

Lachman, V. D. 1986. "Nine Ways to Make Better Decisions." *Nursing 86* (June): 73–74.

Lammers, T. 1992. "The Improved Organization Chart." *Inc.* (October): 147–149.

Lancaster, J. 1985. "Creating a Climate for Excellence." *Journal of Nursing Administration* (January): 16–19.

Lane, A. J. 1992. "Using Havelock's Model to Plan Unit-Based Change." *Nursing Management* (September): 58–60.

Lant, T. W., and D. Gregory. 1984. "The Impact of 12-Hour Shift: An Analysis." *Nursing Management* (October): 38A–38B, 38D–38 F, 38 H.

Laschinger, H. K. S. 1992. "Impact of Nursing Learning Environments on Adaptive Competency Development in Baccalaureate Nursing Students." *Journal of Professional Nursing* (March–April): 105–114.

Lawler, F. E. III. 1986. "What's Wrong with Point Factor Job Evaluation?" *Management Review* (November): 44–48.

Lee, M. A. 1987. "How to Use Job Analysis Technique." *Restaurant Management* (April): 84–85.

Leebov, W. 1984. "Problems, Plans, and Sharing: A Format for Productive Meetings." *Supervisory Management* (June): 35–37.

Leininger, M. 1988. "Leininger's Theory of Nursing: Culture Care Diversity and Universality." *Nursing Science Quarterly* 1, 4: 152–160.

———. 1993. "Culture Care Theory: The Comparative Global Theory to Advance Human Care Theory and Practice." Pp. 3–18 in *A Global Agenda for Caring,* ed. D. A. Gaut. New York: National League for Nursing.

———. 1994. "Quality of Life from a Transcultural Nursing Perspective." *Nursing Science Quarterly* 7, 1: 22–28.

———. 1995. *Transcultural Nursing: Concepts, Theories, Research & Practices,* 2d ed. New York: McGraw-Hill.

Leo, M. 1984. "Avoiding the Pitfalls of ManagemenThink." *Business Horizons* (May–June): 44–47.

Levenstein, A. 1984. "Negotiation vs. Confrontation." *Nursing Management* (January): 52–53.

———. 1984. "Where Nurses Differ." *Nursing Management* (March): 64–65.

———. 1984. "Leadership Under the Microscope." *Nursing Management* (November): 68–69.

Levin, T., and R. Long. 1981. *Effective Instruction* (Alexandria, Va.: Association for Supervision and Curriculum Development.

Levinson, R. E. 1985. "Why Decentralize?" *Management Review* (October): 50–53.

Lindberg, G. E. 1995. "The Any Willing Provider Controversy." *Rehab Economics* 3, no. 6: 79–81.

Little, D. E., and D. L. Carnevali. 1976. *Nursing Care Planning,* 2d ed. Philadelphia: Lippincott.

Llewelyn, S., and G. Fielding. 1982. "Forming, Storming, Norming and Performing." *Nursing Mirror* (21 July): 14–16.

———. 1982. "Under the Influence." *Nursing Mirror* (28 July): 37–39.

Locke, E. A., D. M. Schweiger, and G. P. Latham. 1986. "Participation in Decision Making: When Should It Be Used?" *Organizational Dynamics* (Winter): 65–79.

Logan, C. 1985. "Praise: The Powerhouse of Self-Esteem." *Nursing Management* (June): 36, 38.

Longnecker, C. O., and S. J. Goff. 1992. "Performance Appraisal Effectiveness: A Matter of Perspective." *SAM Advanced Management Journal* (Spring): 17–23.

Lorentzon, M. 1992. "Authority, Leadership, and Management in Nursing." *Journal of Advanced Nursing* (April): 525–527.

Love, A. A. 1998. "National Health Care Spending Tops $1 Trillion." *San Antonio Express-News* (January 13): 1F, 3F.

Lovell, R. B. 1980. *Adult Learning.* New York: Wiley.

Lovrich, M. P. 1985. "The Dangers of Participative Management: A Test of Unexamined Assumptions Concerning Employee Involvement." *Review of Public Personnel Administration* (Summer): 9–25.

Lublin, J. S. 1992. "Trying to Increase Worker Productivity, More Employers Alter Management Style." *The Wall Street Journal* (13 February): B1, B7.

Luconi, F. L., T. W. Malone, and M. S. Scott Morton. 1986. "Expert Systems: The Next Challenge for Managers." *Sloan Management Review* (Summer): 3–14.

Ludeman, K. 1992. "Using Employee Surveys to Revitalize TQM." *Training* (December): 51–57.

Lynch, E. M. 1966. "So You're Going to Run a Meeting." *Personnel Journal* (January): 22+.

Lyne, M. 1983. "Grasping the Challenge." *Nursing Times* (23 November): 11–12.

Lynn, M. R. 1989. "Poster Sessions: A Good Way to Communicate Research." *Journal of Pediatric Nursing* (June): 211–213.

MacDicken, R. A. 1991. "Managing the Plateaued Employee." *Association Management* (July): 37–39, 57.

Maciorowski, T. J., E. Larson, and A. Keane. 1985. "Quality Assurance: Evaluate Thyself." *Journal of Nursing Administration* (June): 38–42.

Mackelprang, R., and P. B. Johnson. 1995. "Managed Care: Balancing Costs, Quality and Access." *SCI Psychosocial Process* (November): 175–178.

Mackenzie, A. E. 1992. "Learning from Experience in the Community: An Ethnographic Study of District Student Nurses." *Journal of Advanced Nursing* 17, pp. 682–691.

Mackie, R., R. Peddie, and R. Pendleton. 1984. "Perioperative Care Plan Guides." *AORN Journal* (August): 192–201.

Mailhot, C. B. 1985. "Setting OR's Course Toward Greater Productivity." *Nursing Management* (October): 42I, J, L, M, P.

Mann, L. M., C. F. Burton, M. T. Presti, and J. E. Hirsch. 1990. "Peer Review in Performance Appraisal." *Nursing Administration Quarterly* (Summer): 9–14.

Manthey, M. 1991. "Empowering Staff Nurse: Decision on the Action Level." *Nursing Management* (February): 16–17.

Manthey, M. 1992. "Leadership: A Shifting Paradigm." *Nurse Educator* (September/October): 5–14.

Manz, C. 1990. "Preparing for an Organizational Change: The Managerial Transition." *Organizational Dynamics* 19, pp. 15–26.

Margotta, M. H. Jr. 1991. "Pro: Continuing Education Leads to Promotion." *Business Credit* (April): 26–28.

Markowitz, J. 1987. "Managing the Job Analysis Process." *Training and Development Journal* (August): 64–66.

Marriner, A. 1979. "Development of Management Thought." *Journal of Nursing Administration* (September): 21–31.

———. 1980. "Budgetary Management." *Journal of Continuing Education in Nursing* (November/December): 11–14.

Marszaleck-Goucher, E., and V. D. Eelsenhans. 1988. "Intrapreneurship: Tapping Employee Creativity." *Journal of Nursing Administration* (December): 20–22.

Martin, D. C., and K. M. Bectal. 1991. "The Legal Ramifications of Performance Appraisal: An Update." *Employee Relations Law Journal* (Autumn): 257–286.

Maslow, A. H. 1964. *Religion, Values and Peak Experiences.* Columbus: Ohio State University Press.

———. 1968. *Toward a Psychology of Being,* 2d ed. New York: Van Nostrand Reinhold.

Masys, D. R. 1996. "The Informatics of Health Care Reform." *Bulletin of The Medical Library Association* (January): 11–16.

Mathes, K. 1992. "Will Your Performance Appraisal System Stand Up in Court?" *HR Forum* (August): 5.

Mathews, J., and P. Katel. 1992. "The Cost of Quality." *Newsweek* (7 September): 48–49.

Matteson, P., and J. W. Hawkins. 1990. "Concept Analysis of Decision Making." *Nursing Forum* 25, 4–10.

Maturen, V., and L. Van Dyck. 1996. "Using Outcome-Based Critical Paths to Improve Documentation." *Home Health Care Management & Practice* (February): 48–58.

McAllister, M. 1990. "A Nursing Integration Framework Based on Standards of Practice." *Nursing Management* (April): 28–31.

McCabe, W. J. 1992. "Total Quality Management in a Hospital." *Quality Review Bulletin* (April): 134–140.

McCarthy, J. P. 1991. "A New Focus on Achievement." *Personnel Journal* (February): 74–76.

McCarty, P. 1979. "Nursing Administrators Control Millions." *The American Nurse* (20 September): 1, 8, 19.

McCloskey, J. C., and B. McCain. 1988. "Nurse Performance: Strengths and Weaknesses." *Nursing Research* (September/October): 308–313.

McCormick, V. E. 1991. "Software Helps with Hard Decisions." *Training* (August): 23–24.

McDaniel, C., and G. A. Wolf. 1992. "Transformational Leadership in Nursing Service." *Journal of Nursing Administration* (February): 60–65.

McGee, K. G. 1992. "Making Performance Appraisal a Positive Experience." *Nursing Management* (August): 36–37.

McGuire, J. B., and J. R. Liro. 1986. "Flexible Work Schedules, Work Attitudes, and Perceptions of Productivity." *Public Personnel Management* (Spring): 65–73.

McKenzie, M. E. 1985. "Decisions: How You Reach Them Makes a Difference." *Nursing Management* (June): 48–49.

McLaughlin, C. 1994. "Thinking About Diversity." *National Forum* (Winter): 16–18.

McLaughlin, C. P., and A. D. Kaluzny. 1990. "Total Quality Management in Health: Making It Work." *Health Care Management Review* 15, 3: 7–14.

Meisenheimer, C. 1991. "The Customer: Silent or Intimate Player in the Quality Revolution." *Holistic Nurse Practitioner* (April): 39–50.

Mendlen, J., S. Goss, and K. Heist. 1996. "Managing Data for Managed Care." *Provider* (July): 66–68.

Merchant, J. 1991. "Task Allocation: A Case of Resistance to Change?" *Nursing Practice* 4, 2: 16–18.

Mercy Health Services Nurses' Council. 1991. "Mercy Health Services: Systemwide Redesign of Patient Care Services." *Nursing Administration Quarterly* (Fall): 38–45.

Messmer, M. 1992. "Strategic Staffing." *Management Accounting* (June): 28–30.

Metcalf, M. L. 1982. "The 12-Hour Weekend Plan—Does the Nursing Staff Really Like It? *Journal of Nursing Administration* (October): 16–19.

Meyer, A. L. 1984. "A Framework for Assessing Performance Problems." *Journal of Nursing Administration* (May): 40–43.

Meyers, M. E. 1992. "Motivating High-Tech Workers." *Best's Review—Life-Health Insurance Edition* (June): 86–88.

Miller, J. O., and S. J. Carey. 1993. "Work Role Inventory: A Guide to Job Satisfaction." *Nursing Management* (January): 54–62.

Miller, M. 1984. "Putting More Power into Management Decisions." *Management Review* (September): 12–16.

Mills, P. K., and B. Z. Posner. 1982. "The Relationships Among Self-Supervision, Structure, and Technology in Professional Service Organizations." *Academy of Management Journal* (June): 437–443.

Moffic, H. S., and J. D. Kinzie. 1996. "The History of Cross Cultural Psychiatric Services." Community Mental Health Journal (December): 581–582.

Moore, J. 1992. "Senator Says Mental Hospital Abuses Not Limited to Texas." *San Antonio Light* (29 April): D6.

Moore, K. F. 1996. "Cost or Quality When Selecting a Health Plan?" *National Policy Forum* (March/April): 24.

Morstain, B. R., and J. C. Smart. 1977. "A Motivational Typology of Adult Education." *Journal of Higher Education* (November–December): 665–679.

Mosley, D. C., P. H. Pietri, and L. C. Megginson. 1996. *Management: Leadership in Action.* 5th ed. New York: HarperCollins.

Mossholder, K. W., W. F. Giles, and M. A. Weslowski. 1991. "Information Privacy and Performance Appraisal: An Examination of Employee Perceptions and Reactions." *Journal of Business Ethics* (February): 151–156.

Muczyk, J. P., and B. C. Reimanu. 1987. "Has Participative Management Been Oversold?" *Personnel* (May): 52–56.

Mullaby, C. M. 1995. "What Next for Case Management? *TCM* (Convention): 82–84, 86–88, 90.

Murphy, K. R. 1991. "Criterion Issues in Performance Appraisal Research Behavioral Accuracy Versus Classification Accuracy." *Organizational Behavior and Human Decision Processes* 50, pp. 45–50.

Murphy, K. R., B. A. Gannett, B. M. Herr, J. A. Chen. 1986. "Effects of Subsequent Performance on Evaluation of Previous Performance." *Journal of Applied Psychology* (August): 427–431.

Nagelkerk, J. M., and B. M. Henry. 1990. "Strategic Decision Making." *Journal of Nursing Administration* (July/August): 18–23.

Nalley, E. A., and J. E. Braithwaite, Jr. 1992. "Communication: Key to a Vital future." *Phi Kappa Phi Newsletter* (June): 1–3.

Narayanasamy, A. 1990. "Evaluation of the Budgeting Process in Nurse Education." *Nurse Education Today* (August): 245–252.

Nathan, B. R., A. M. Mohrman, Jr., and J. Milliman. 1991. "Interpersonal Relations as a Context for the Effects of Appraisal Interviews on Performance and Satisfaction: A Longitudinal Study," *Academy of Management Journal* (June): 352–369.

"Negotiating Managed Care Contracts." *Laboratory Medicine* (September 1996): 587–596.

Nelson, M. F., and R. H. Christenson. 1995. "The Focused Review Process: A Utilization Management Firm's Experience with Length of Stay Guidelines." *Journal of Quality Improvement* (September): 477–487.

Netzel, L. 1995. "A Primer On Capitation: Another Step in Managed Care." *The Surgical Technologist* (November): 16–18.

Newcomb, D. P., and R. C. Swansburg. 1953, 1971. *The Team Plan* New York: Putnam.

Newman, M. A. 1984. "Nursing Diagnosis: Looking at the Whole." *American Journal of Nursing* (December): 1496–1499.

Nielsen, B. B. 1992. "Applying Andragogy in Nursing Continuing Education." *Journal of Continuing Education in Nursing* (July/August): 148–151.

Nightingale, Florence. 1959. *Notes on Nursing*. Philadelphia: J. B. Lippincott.

Nikolajski, P. Y. 1992. "Investigating the Effectiveness of Self-Learning Packages in Staff Development." *Journal of Nursing Staff Development* (July/August): 179–182.

Norman-Culp, S. 1993. "No Mercy for Dying Man, Wife Says." *San Antonio Express-News* (23 May): 3F.

Norris, J. E. S. 1992. "Eight Steps to Strategic Planning." *Nursing Management* (March): 78–79.

O'Neal, C. R. 1991. "It's What's Up Front That Counts." *Marketing News* (4 March): 9, 28.

O'Reilly, B. 1994. "Reengineering the MBA." *Fortune* (24 January): 38–40, 42, 44, 46–47.

O'Toole, J. 1985. "Employee Practices at the Best Managed Companies." *California Management Review* (Fall): 35–65.

Odiorne, G. S. 1984. *Strategic Management of Human Resources*. San Francisco: Jossey-Bass.

Ondrack, D. A., and M. G. Evans. 1986. "Job Enrichment and Job Satisfaction in Quality of Working Life and Nonquality of Working Life Work Sites." *Human Relations* (September): 871–889.

Osley, M. 1995. "Legislative Update." *Journal of Legal Nurse Consulting"* (October): 12–13.

Padberg, R. M., and L. F. Padberg. 1990. "Strengthening the Effectiveness of Patient Education: Applying Principles of Adult Education." *Oncology Nursing Forum* 17, 1: 65–69.

Palesy, S. R. 1980. "Motivating Line Management Using the Planning Process." *Planning Review* (March): 3–8, 44–48.

Parfitt, B. A. 1989. "A Practical Approach to Creative Thinking: An Experiment." *Journal of Advanced Nursing* 14, pp. 665–677.

Parker, R. S. 1990. "Measuring Nurses' Moral Judgments." *Image* (Winter): 213–218.

Parlish, C. 1987. "A Model for Clinical Performance Evaluation." *Journal of Nursing Education* (October): 338–339.

Pattan, J. E. 1991. "Nurse Recruitment: From Selling to Marketing" (September): 16–20.

Patterson, B. H. 1986. "Creativity and Andragogy: A Boon for Adult Learners." *Journal of Creative Behavior* 20, 2: 99–110.

Paul, N. 1992. "For the Record: Information on Individuals." *National Forum* (Winter): 34–38.

Paul, R. N., and J. W. Taylor. 1986. "The State of Strategic Planning." *Business* (January–March): 37–43.

Pearce, W. H. 1986. "I Thought I Knew What Good Management Was." *Harvard Business Review* (March–April): 59–65.

Pell, A. R. 1992. "Motivation: Praise." *Manager's Magazine* 67, 8: 30–31.

Pelle, D., and L. Greenhalgh. 1987. "Developing the Performance Appraisal System." *Nursing Management* (December): 37–40, 42, 44.

Pender, N. J. 1992. "The NIH Strategic Plan. How Will It Affect the Future of Nursing Science and Practice?" *Nursing Outlook* (March/April): 55–56.

Pesut, D. J. 1992. "Self-Regulation, Self-Management and Self-Care." *South Carolina Nurse* (Summer): 22–23.

Peters, T. 1991. "Family Gives 'Teams' Plenty of Experience." *San Antonio Light* (12 November): E3.

———. "Ingersoll-Rand Retools the Way It Makes Tools." *San Antonio Light* (12 February): D1.

———. "Letting Go of Controls." *Across the Board* (June): 14–15, 18.

———. 1992. "Listening to What's Wrong and Right." *San Antonio Light* (20 October): D2.

———. 1992. "McKenzie Exemplifies Structureless Corporation of Future." *San Antonio Light* (12 November): B1, B8.

———. 1992. "'Must Do' Ideas Help Keep Business Afloat." *San Antonio Light* (11 February): B8.

———. 1992. "'Gee Whiz' 'Wow' Factors Significant." *San Antonio Light* (21 July): B3.

Petersen, B. A. 1996. "Nurse-Midwifery in a Managed Care Environment." *Journal of Nurse Midwifery* (July/August): 267–268.

Philp, T. 1992. "Getting Down to Some Serious Work on Staff Appraisal." *CA Magazine* (June): 26, 28.

Phoon, J., K. Corder, and M. Barter. 1996. "Managed Care and Total Quality Management: A Necessary Integration." *Journal of Nursing Care Quality* (January): 25–32.

Pike, O. 1987. "Rutan, Yeager Showed What Leadership Is About." *Mobile Press Register* (January): 4A.

Pilette, P. C., and K. K. Kirby. 1991. "Expectations and Responsibilities of the Nursing Director Role." *Nursing Management* (March): 77–80.

Podeschi, R. L. 1987. "Andragogy: Proofs or Premises?" *Lifelong Learning: An Omnibus of Practice and Research* vol. 11, no. 3: 14–16, 20.

Podsakoff, P. M., W. D. Todor, and R. S. Schuler. 1983. "Leader Expertise as a Moderator of the Effects of Instrumental and Supportive Leader Behaviors." *Journal of Management* (Fall): 173–185.

Pope, T. 1995. "Case Managers Help Define Managed Care." *TCM* (April/May/June): 109–111.

Potter, P. A. 1998. *Pocket Guide to Health Assessment,* 4th ed. St. Louis: Mosby.

Port, O. 1987 "How to Make It Right the First Time." *Business Week* (8 June): 142–143.

Powell, J. T. 1986. "Stress Listening: Coping with Angry Confrontations." *Personnel Journal* (May): 27–29.

Price, S., and J. Graber. 1986. "Employee-Made Appraisals." *Management World* (February): 34–36.

Prien, E. P., I. L. Goldstein, W. H. Macey. 1987. "Multidomain Job Analysis: Procedures and Applications." *Training and Development Journal* (August): 68–72.

Pritchard, R. D., and B. W. Karasick. 1973. "The Effects of Organizational Climate on Managerial Job Performance and Job Satisfaction." *"Organizational Behavior and Human Performance* 9, pp. 126–143.

Probst, M. R., and J. M. Noga. 1980. "A Decentralized Nursing Care Delivery System." *Supervisor Nurse* (January): 57–60.

Purcell, J. 1989. "How to Manage Decentralized Bargaining." *Personnel Management* (May): 53–55.

Rachal, J. R., W. L. Pierce, R. Leonard, and V. DeCoux. 1992. "Nurses and Adult Educational Philosophy: A Comparison of Nurses and Non-Nurses in a Graduate Adult Education Program." *Journal of Continuing Education in Nursing* (November/December): 253–258.

Ratcliffe, T. A., and D. J. Logsdon. 1980. "The Business Planning Process—A Behavioral Perspective." *Managerial Planning* (March/April): 32–38.

Rauer, R. 1990. "Practicing Participative Management." *Nursing Management* (June): 48A–48B, 48F, 48H.

"Recruitment & Retention: A Positive Approach." 1984. *Nursing Management* (April): 15–17.

Redman, L. N. 1983. "The Planning Process." *Managerial Planning* (May/June): 24–30, 40.

Rempusheski, V. F. 1991. "Incorporating Research Role and Practice Role." *Applied Nursing Research* (February): 46–48.

Richard, S. B. 1995. "Financial Considerations for Managed Care." *Journal of Home Health Care Practice* (August): 24–30.

Richmond, B. 1992. "Teachers Must Stand Up to School Board Group." *San Antonio Light* (12 December): F5.

Rigdon, J. E. 1992. "Using Lateral Moves to Spur Employees." *The Wall Street Journal* (26 May): B1, B5.

Rigg, M. 1992. "Reasons for Removing Employee Evaluations from Management Control." *Industrial Engineering* (August): 17.

Riverin-Simard, D. 1988. "Phases of Working Life and Adult Education." *Lifelong Learning: An Omnibus of Practice and Research* vol. 12, no. 2: 24–26.

Roberts, V. 1985. "The Head Nurse Meeting: Who, What, When and Where." *Nursing Management* (August): 10, 12.

Rogers, M. 1970. *An Introduction to the Theoretical Basis of Nursing.* Philadelphia: F. A. Davis.

Rogers, M., J. Riordan, and D. Swindle. 1991. "Community-Based Nursing Care Management Pays Off." *Nursing Management* (March): 30–34.

Rondeau, K. V. 1992. "Morale Boosters for Off-Shift Staff." *Medical Laboratory Observer* (August): 40–41.

Rosen, C. 1989. "Value of Ownership." *Executive Excellence* (February): 14–15.

Ross, H. T., and M. M. Oumsby. 1990. "Teamwork Breeds Quality at Hearing Technology." *National Productivity Review* (Summer): 321–327.

Rothrock, J. C. 1984. "Nursing Diagnosis in the Days of Florence Nightingale." *AORN Journal* (August): 189–190.

Rowsell, G. 1981. "Economics of Health Care." *AARN Newsletter* 37 no. 7 (July/August): 6–8.

Roy, S. C. 1976. *Introduction to Nursing: An Adaptation Model.* Englewood Cliffs, N.J.: Prentice-Hall.

Rubin, I. M., R. E. Fry, and M. S. Plovnick. 1978. *Managing Human Resources in Health Care Organizations.* Reston, Va.: Reston Publishing.

Rulon, V. 1996. "Measurement Systems Beyond HEDIS: The Evolution of Healthcare Data Analysis in Managed Care." *Journal of AHIMA* (February): 48, 50–52.

Ruskowski, U. 1980. "A Budget Orientation Tool for Nurse Managers." *Dimensions in Health Service* (December): 30–31.

Sanderson, D. R. 1989. Mid-Career Support: An Approach to Lifelong Learning in an Organization." *Lifelong Learning: An Omnibus of Practice and Research* vol. 12, no. 7: 7–10.

Sarvela, P. D., D. R. Holcomb, and J. A. Odulana. 1992. "Designing a Safety Program for a College Health Service." *Journal of College Health* (March): 231–233.

Sashkin, M. 1986. "Participative Management Remains an Ethical Imperative." *Organizational Dynamics* (Spring): 62–75.

Sayers, W. K. 1990. "ESOPs Are No Fable." *Small Business Reports* (June): 57–60.

Schaffner, R. J., and C. C. Bowman. 1992. "Increasing the Impact of the Clinical Nurse Specialist Through Activity in a Shared Governance Organization." *Clinical Nurse Specialist* 6, 4: 211–216.

Schauffler, H. H., and J. Wolin. 1996. "Community Health Clinics Under Managed Competition: Navigating Uncharted Waters." *Journal of Health Politics, Policy and Law* (Fall): 461–488.

Schmele, J. A., M. E. Allen, S. Butler, and D. Gresham. 1991. "Quality Circles in the Public Health Sector: Implementation and Effect." Public Health Nursing (September): 190–195.

Schmeling, W. H., J. R. Futch, D. Moore, and J. W. MacDonald. 1991. "The Interactive Planning/Management Model." *Nursing Administration Quarterly* (Fall): 14, 31.

Schnake, M. G., and M. P. Dumler. 1985. "Affective Response Bias in the Measurement of Perceived Task Characteristics." *Journal of Occupational Psychology* (June): 159–166.

Schneider, B., and D. T. Hall. 1972. "Toward Specifying the Concept of Work Climate: A Study of Roman Catholic Diocesan Priests." *Journal of Applied Psychology* (June): 447–455.

Schrader, S. F. 1993. "Labor Budgeting." *AORN Journal* (April): 925–927.

Schuster, M. H., and C. S. Miller. 1985. "Employee Involvement: Making Supervisors Believers." *Personnel* (February): 24–28.

Seawell, V. L. 1994. *Chart of Accounts for Hospitals: An Accounting and Reporting Reference Guide.* Burr Ridge, Ill.: Probus.

Servais, S. H. 1991. "Nursing Resource Applications Through Outcome Based Nursing Practice." *Nursing Economic$* (May–June): 171–174, 179.

Sherman, J. L. Jr., and S. K. Fields. 1978. *Guide to Patient Evaluation,* 3d ed. Garden City, N.Y.: Medical Examination Publishing.

Sherman, S. 1994. "Leaders Learn to Heed the Voice Within." *Fortune* (22 August): 92–94, 96, 98, 100.

Shindul-Rothschild, J. 1995. "The Economics of Managed Care." *The Massachusetts Nurse* (October/November): 4, 6.

Shukla, R. K. 1981. "Structure vs. People in Primary Nursing: An Inquiry." *Nursing Research* (July–August): 236–241.

Shultz, J. N. 1992. "Group Dynamics Can Change Attitudes." *Nursing Management* (November): 95–97.

Simpson, R. D., and W. W. Anderson. 1992. "Science Education and the Common Good." *National Forum* (Winter): 30–33.

Smeltzer, C. H. 1992. "Brainstorming: A Process for Cost Reduction." *Nursing Economic$*. (January–February): 74–75.

Smith, H. L. 1992. "Genetic Technologies: Can We Do Responsibly Everything We Can Do Technically?" *National Forum* (Winter): 26–29.

Smith, H. L., F. D. Reinow, and R. A. Reid. 1984. "Japanese Management: Implications for Nursing Administration." *Journal of Nursing Administration* (September): 33–39.

Smith, J. L., M. K. V. Mackey, and J. Markham. 1985. "Productivity Monitoring: A Recovery Room System for Economizing Operations." *Nursing Management* (May): 34A–D, K–M.

Smith, L. 1994. "Burned-Out Bosses." *Fortune* (25 July): 44–46, 50, 52.

Solomon, J. 1993. "The Fall of the Dinosaurs." *Newsweek* (8 February): 42–44.

Sonberg, V., and K. E. Vestal. 1983. "Nursing as a Business." *Nursing Clinics of North America* 18, no. 3 (September): 491–498.

Sorrentino, E. A. "Overcoming Barriers to Automation." *Nursing Forum* (Mar. 1991): 21–23.

Southern Council on Collegiate Education for Nursing. 1985. *Preparing Nurses for Decision Making in Clinical Practice: A White Paper.* Atlanta: SCCEN.

Sovie, M. D. 1993. "Hospital Culture—Why Create One?" *Nursing Economic$* (March–April): 69–75.

Sparer, M. S. 1996. "Medicaid Managed Care and the Health Reform Debate: Lessons from New York and California." *Journal of Health Politics, Policy and Law* (Fall): 433–460.

Spicer, J. G., M. J. Craft, and K. C. Ross. 1988. "A Systems Approach to Customer Satisfaction." *Nursing Administration Quarterly* (Spring): 79–83.

Spitzer-Lehman. R. 1995. "Managed Care: What's Ahead." *Surgical Services Management* (January): 18–21.

———. 1990. "Recruitment and Retention of Our Greatest Asset." *Nursing Administration Quarterly* (Summer): 66–69.

Spitzer-Lehman, R., and K. J. Yahn. 1992. "Patient Needs Drive an Integrated Approach to Care." *Nursing Management* (August): 30–32.

Stengrevics, S. S., K. K. Kirby, and E. R. Ollis. 1991. "Nurse Manager Job Satisfaction: The Massachusetts Perspective." *Nursing Management* (April): 60–64.

Stewart, T. A. 1993. "Welcome to the Revolution." *Fortune* (13 December): 66–80.

———. 1994. "Rate Your Readiness to Change." *Fortune* (27 February): 106–107, 110.

Strong, A. G. 1992. "Case Management and the CNS." *Clinical Nurse Specialist* (Summer): 64.

Strong, A. G., and N. V. Sneed. 1991. "Clinical Evaluation of a Critical Path for Coronary Artery Bypass Surgery Patients." *Progress in Cardiovascular Nursing* (January–March): 29–37.

Stuerke, N. 1984. "Computers *Can* Advance Nursing Practice." *Nursing Management* (July): 27–28.

Styles, M., S. Allen, S. Armstrong, M. Matsurra, D. Stannard, and J. S. Ordway. 1991. "Entry: A New Approach." *Nursing Outlook* (September/October): 200–203.

Suding, M. J. 1984. "Decision Making Controlling the Computer Input." *Nursing Management* (July): 44, 46, 48–52.

Suver, J. D. 1982. "Zero Base Budgeting." Pp. 353–376 in *Handbook of Health Care Accounting and Finance,* ed. W. O. Cleverly. Gaithersburg, Md.: Aspen.

Swansburg, R. C. 1977. *The Organizing Function of Nursing Service Administration.* Hattiesburg: University of Southern Mississippi School of Nursing.

———. 1968. *Team Nursing: A Programmed Learning Experience,* 4 Volumes. New York: Putnam.

———. 1978. *Nurses & Patients: An Introduction to Nursing Management.* Hattiesburg, Miss.: Impact III.

Swansburg, R. C., and P. W. Swansburg. 1988. *The Nurse Manager's Guide to Financial Management.* Rockville, Md.: Aspen.

Taft, S., and J. Stearns. 1991. "Organizational Change with a Nursing Agenda: Lessons from the Strengthening Hospital Nursing Program." *Journal of Nursing Administration* 21, no. 2: 12–21.

Taft, S. H., P. K. Jones, and E. L. Minch. 1992. "Strengthening Hospital Nursing, Part 2: Characteristics of Effective Planning Processes." *Journal of Nursing Administration* (June): 36–46.

Taguchi, G., and D. Clausing. 1990. "Robust Quality." *Harvard Business Review* (January–February): 65–75.

Talone, P. 1996. "Ethics and Managed Care: Beyond Helplessness" *MEDSURG Nursing* (June): 212–214.

Taylor, B. A., and A. deSimone. 1983. "Taking the First Steps to Become a Nurse Manager." *Nursing Administration Quarterly* (Winter): 17–22.

Theile, J. R. 1983. "The Anatomy of an Organization." *Nursing Administration Quarterly* (Winter): 42–45.

Thomas, B. 1983. "Using Nominal Group Technique to Identify Researchable Problems." *Journal of Nursing Education* (October): 335–337.

Thomas, J. 1992. "Package Deals." *Nursing Times* (15 July): 48–49.

Thomas, L. H. 1992. "Qualified Nurse and Nursing Auxiliary Perceptions of Their Work Environment in Primary, Team, and Functional Nursing Wards." *Journal of Advanced Nursing* (March): 373–382.

Thomas, N. M., and G. G. Newsome. 1992. "Factors Affecting the Use of Nursing Diagnosis." *Nursing Outlook* (July/August): 182–186.

Thurgood, J. 1993. "Definitions and Explanations of the New Financial Vocabulary." *British Journal of Nursing* (March): 295–296.

Thurston, N. E., S. C. Tenove, and J. M. Church. 1990. "Hospital Nursing Research Is Alive and Flourishing." *Nursing Management* (May): 50–53.

Tichy, N. M. 1993. "Revolutionize Your Company." *Fortune* (13 December): 114–118.

Tingey, S. 1967. "Six Requirements for a Successful Company Publication." *Personnel Journal* (November): 638–642.

Towers, J. 1996. "What Do You Know About NCQA?" *Nursing Policy Forum* (May/June): 30.

Trofino, J. 1984. "Managing the Budget Crunch." *Nursing Management* (October): 42–47.

Tumulty, G. 1992. "Head Nurse Role Redesign." *Journal of Nursing Administration* (February): 41–48.

Tushman, M., and D. Nadler. 1986. "Organizing for Innovation." *California Management Review* (Spring): 74–92.

Tuttle, D. M. 1992. "A Transfer Fair Approach to Staffing." *Nursing Management* (December): 72–74.

Ubell, E. 1997. "You Can Get Quality Care in an HMO World." *Parade Magazine* (14 September): 10–11.

Ulrich, D. 1992. "Strategic and Human Resource Planning: Linking Customers to Employees." *Strategic and Human Resources Planning* 15, no. 2: 47–62.

Van Gorder, B. 1990. "Moving Back to Centralization." *Credit Magazine* (May/June): 12–13, 15–16.

Vasilash, G. S. 1981. "Crosby Says Get Fit For Quality." *Production* (January): 51–52, 54.

Vian, J. J. 1990. "Theory Z: "Magic Potion" for Decentralized Management." *Nursing Management* (December): 34–36.

Vic, A. G., and R. C. McKay. 1982. "How Does the 12-Hour Shift Affect Patient Care?" *Journal of Nursing Administration* (January): 12.

Vlcek, D. J. Jr. 1987. "Decentralization: What Works and What Doesn't." *Journal of Business Strategy* (Fall): 71–74.

Vracin, R. A. 1982. "Capital Budgeting." Pp. 323–351 in *Handbook of Health Care Accounting and Finance*. ed. W. O. Cleverly. Gaithersburg, Md.: Aspen.

Wagel, W. H. 1987. "Working" (and Managing) Without Supervisors." *Personnel* (September): 8–11.

Wagner, L., B. Henry, G. Giovinco, and C. Blanks. 1988. "Suggestions for Graduate Education in Nursing Administration." *Journal of Nursing Education* (May): 210–218.

Waldman, D. A., and R. S. Kenett. 1990. "Improve Performance by Appraisal." *HR Magazine* (July): 66–69.

Walton, M. 1987. "Deming's Parable of the Red Beads." *Across the Board* (February): 43–48.

Ward, D. L. 1993. "Operational Finance and Budgeting." Pp. 281–298 in *The Managed Care Handbook,* 2d ed. ed. P. R. Kongstvedt. Gaithersberg, Md.: Aspen.

Waterstradt, C. R., and T. L. Phillips. 1990. "A Productivity System for a Hospital Education Department." *Journal of Nursing Staff Development* (May/June): 139–144.

Webber, J. B., and M. A. Dula. 1974. "Effective Planning Committees for Hospitals." *Harvard Business Review* (May–June): 133–142.

Weingard, M. 1984. "Establishing Comparable Worth Through Job Evaluation." *Nursing Outlook* (March/April): 110–113.

Werning, S. C. 1993. "A Primer on Managed Care." *Healthcare Trends and Transition* (October): 10–13, 26–28, 46–47.

White, J. A. 1992. "When Employees Own Big Stake, It's a Buy Signal for Investors." *The Wall Street Journal* (13 February): C1.

Wilbers, S. 1993. "Performance Reviews Can Be Easier." *San Antonio Express-News* (23 May): 3G.

Williams, B. 1992. "Ten Commandments for Group Leaders." *Supervisory Management* (September): 1–2.

Williams, R. 1991. "Putting Deming's Principles to Work." *The Wall Street Journal* (4 November): A18.

———. 1992. "Nurse Case Management: Working with the Community." *Nursing Management* (December): 33–34.

Williams, S. L., and M. L. Hummert. 1990. "Evaluating Performance Appraisal Instruments Dimensions Using Construct Analysis." *Journal of Business Communication* (Spring): 117–133.

Wilson, H. S., and S. A. Hutchison. 1986. *Applying Research in Nursing: A Resource Book* (Menlo Park, Calif.: Addison-Wesley.

Wlodkowski, R. 1972. *Enhancing Adult Motivation to Learn.* San Francisco: Jossey-Bass.

Wolff, G. M. 1986. "Systems Management: Evaluating Nursing Departments as a Whole." *Nursing Management* (February): 40–43.

Woods, M. D. 1989. "New Manufacturing Practices—New Accounting Practices." *Production and Inventory Management Journal* (Fourth Quarter): 8–12.

"Workplace Trends: Who Gets the Promotion?" 1992. *Small Business Reports* 17, no. 10: 28.

Wrapp, H. E. 1967. "Good Managers Don't Make Policy Decisions." *Harvard Business Review* (September/October): 91–99.

Yanker, M. 1986. "Flexible Leadership Styles: One Supervisor's Story." *Supervisory Management* (January): 2–6.

Yoder Wise, P. S. 1995. *Leading and Managing in Nursing.* St. Louis: C. V. Mosby.

Yoder, M. E. 1984. "Nursing Diagnosis: Application During Perioperative Practice." *AORN Journal* (August): 183–188.

Zachry, B. R., and R. L. Gilbert. 1992. "Director of Nursing Planning and Finance: A New Role." *Nursing Management* (February).

Zander, K. S. 1977. "Primary Nursing Won't Work . . . Unless the Head Nurse Lets It." *Journal of Nursing Administration* (October): 19–23.

Zawackie, R. A., and C. A. Norman. 1991. "Breaking Appraisal Tradition." *Computerworld* (1 April): 78.

Zebelman, E., K. Davis, and E. Larsen. 1983. "Helping Staff Nurses Use Learning Modules." *Nursing and Health Care* (April): 198–199.

Zeira, Y., and J. Aredisian. 1989. "Organizational Planned Change: Assessing the Chances for Success." *Organizational Dynamics* (Spring): 31–45.

Zelman, W. N., and D. L. Parham. 1990. "Strategic, Operational, and Marketing Concerns of Product-Line Management in Health Care." *Health Care Management Review* (Winter): 29–35.

Ziegler, J. C., and N. K. Van Ellen. 1992. "Implementation of a National Nursing Standards Program." *Journal of Nursing Administration* (November): 40–46.

Zyoman, R. S. 1996. "Building Customer-Supplier Relationships for Performance Management and Quality Improvement: Hospital and Health Plan Partnerships." *Journal of AHIMA* (May): 57–60.

INDEX